National Key Book Publishing Planning Project of the 13th Five-Year Plan

"十三五"国家重点图书出版规划项目

International Clinical Medicine Series Based on the Belt and Road Initiative

"一带一路"背景下国际化临床医学丛书

U0337381

Surgery

外科学（上）

Chief Editors　Ma Qingyong　Liang Guiyou　Bai Yuting　Qiu Xinguang　Wang Wenjun　Wu Xuedong

主编　马清涌　梁贵友　白育庭　邱新光　王文军　吴学东

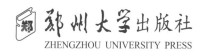

郑州大学出版社

ZHENGZHOU UNIVERSITY PRESS

图书在版编目(CIP)数据

外科学 = Surgery：英文 / 马清涌等主编. — 郑州：郑州大学出版社，2020.12
("一带一路"背景下国际化临床医学丛书)
ISBN 978-7-5645-7692-9

Ⅰ. ①外… Ⅱ. ①马… Ⅲ. ①外科学 - 英文 Ⅳ. ①R6

中国版本图书馆 CIP 数据核字(2020)第 272606 号

外科学 = Surgery：英文

项目负责人	孙保营　杨秦予	策划编辑	李龙传
责任编辑	陈文静	装帧设计	苏永生
责任校对	张彦勤	责任监制	凌　青　李瑞卿

出版发行	郑州大学出版社有限公司	地　址	郑州市大学路 40 号(450052)
出版人	孙保营	网　址	http://www.zzup.cn
经　销	全国新华书店	发行电话	0371-66966070
印　刷	河南文华印务有限公司		
开　本	850 mm×1 168 mm　1 / 16		
总印张	77.25	总字数	2 976 千字
版　次	2020 年 12 月第 1 版	印　次	2020 年 12 月第 1 次印刷
书　号	ISBN 978-7-5645-7692-9	总定价	389.00 元(上、下)

本书如有印装质量问题,请与本社联系调换。

Staff of Expert Steering Committee

Chairmen

Zhong Shizhen   Li Sijin   Lü Chuanzhu

Vice Chairmen

Bai Yuting   Chen Xu   Cui Wen   Huang Gang   Huang Yuanhua

Jiang Zhisheng   Li Yumin   Liu Zhangsuo   Luo Baojun   Lü Yi

Tang Shiying

Committee Member

An Dongping   Bai Xiaochun   Cao Shanying   Chen Jun   Chen Yijiu

Chen Zhesheng   Chen Zhihong   Chen Zhiqiao   Ding Yueming   Du Hua

Duan Zhongping   Guan Chengnong   Huang Xufeng   Jian Jie   Jiang Yaochuan

Jiao Xiaomin   Li Cairui   Li Guoxin   Li Guoming   Li Jiabin

Li Ling   Li Zhijie   Liu Hongmin   Liu Huifan   Liu Kangdong

Song Weiqun   Tang Chunzhi   Wang Huamin   Wang Huixin   Wang Jiahong

Wang Jiangang   Wang Wenjun   Wang Yuan   Wei Jia   Wen Xiaojun

Wu Jun   Wu Weidong   Wu Xuedong   Xie Xieju   Xue Qing

Yan Wenhai   Yan Xinming   Yang Donghua   Yu Feng   Yu Xiyong

Zhang Lirong   Zhang Mao   Zhang Ming   Zhang Yu'an   Zhang Junjian

Zhao Song   Zhao Yumin   Zheng Weiyang   Zhu Lin

Staff of Editor Steering Committee

Chairmen

Cao Xuetao   Liang Guiyou   Wu Jiliang

Vice Chairmen

Chen Pingyan   Chen Yuguo   Huang Wenhua   Li Yaming   Wang Heng

Xu Zuojun   Yao Ke   Yao Libo   Yu Xuezhong   Zhao Xiaodong

Committee Member

Cao Hong	Chen Guangjie	Chen Kuisheng	Chen Xiaolan	Dong Hongmei
Du Jian	Du Ying	Fei Xiaowen	Gao Jianbo	Gao Yu
Guan Ying	Guo Xiuhua	Han Liping	Han Xingmin	He Fanggang
He Wei	Huang Yan	Huang Yong	Jiang Haishan	Jin Chengyun
Jin Qing	Jin Runming	Li Lin	Li Ling	Li Mincai
Li Naichang	Li Qiuming	Li Wei	Li Xiaodan	Li Youhui
Liang Li	Lin Jun	Liu Fen	Liu Hong	Liu Hui
Lu Jing	Lü Bin	Lü Quanjun	Ma Qingyong	Ma Wang
Mei Wuxuan	Nie Dongfeng	Peng Biwen	Peng Hongjuan	Qiu Xinguang
Song Chuanjun	Tan Dongfeng	Tu Jiancheng	Wang Lin	Wang Huijun
Wang Peng	Wang Rongfu	Wang Shusen	Wang Chongjian	Xia Chaoming
Xiao Zheman	Xie Xiaodong	Xu Falin	Xu Xia	Xu Jitian
Xue Fuzhong	Yang Aimin	Yang Xuesong	Yi Lan	Yin Kai
Yu Zujiang	Yu Hong	Yue Baohong	Zeng Qingbing	Zhang Hui
Zhang Lin	Zhang Lu	Zhang Yanru	Zhao Dong	Zhao Hongshan
Zhao Wen	Zheng Yanfang	Zhou Huaiyu	Zhu Changju	Zhu Lifang

Gao Hui	Hubei University of Science and Technology
Gao Jie	The First Affiliated Hospital of Xi'an Jiaotong University
Geng Zhimin	The First Affiliated Hospital of Xi'an Jiaotong University
Huang Jun	The Second Xiangya Hospital of Central South University
Huo Xiongwei	The First Affiliated Hospital of Xi'an Jiaotong University
Ke Xixian	The Affiliated Hospital of Zunyi Medical University
Li Jian	The Affiliated Hospital of Guizhou Medical University
Li Junhui	The Second Affiliated Hospital of Xi'an Jiaotong University
Li Ruichun	The First Affiliated Hospital of Xi'an Jiaotong University
Li Shaobo	The First Affiliated Hospital of Dali University
Liu Daxing	The Affiliated Hospital of Zunyi Medical University
Liu Qing	The Third Xiangya Hospital of Central South University
Liu Senyuan	The First Affiliated Hospital of Zhengzhou University
Liu Yang	The Second Affiliated Hospital of Xi'an Jiaotong University
Lu Le	The Second Affiliated Hospital of Xi'an Jiaotong University
Ma Xing	The First Affiliated Hospital of Xi'an Jiaotong University
Mao Ping	The First Affiliated Hospital of Xi'an Jiaotong University
Mao Xinzhan	The Second Xiangya Hospital of Central South University
Ouyang Zhihua	The First Affiliated Hospital of University of South China
Qi Lei	The First Affiliated Hospital of Xi'an Jiaotong University
Qiu Guanglin	The First Affiliated Hospital of Xi'an Jiaotong University
Qu Kai	The First Affiliated Hospital of Xi'an Jiaotong University
Shan Tao	The Second Affiliated Hospital of Xi'an Jiaotong University
Shen Xin	The First Affiliated Hospital of Xi'an Jiaotong University
Song Yongchun	The First Affiliated Hospital of Xi'an Jiaotong University
Wang Ning	The First Affiliated Hospital of Dali University
Wang Suoliang	The First Affiliated Hospital of Xi'an Jiaotong University
Wang Wei	The First Affiliated Hospital of Xi'an Jiaotong University
Wu Tao	The Second Affiliated Hospital of Xi'an Jiaotong University
Xu Gang	The Affiliated Hospital of Zunyi Medical University
Xu Kedong	The First Affiliated Hospital of Xi'an Jiaotong University
Xue Wujun	The First Affiliated Hospital of Xi'an Jiaotong University
Yan Yiguo	The First Affiliated Hospital of University of South China
Yao Nüzhao	The First Affiliated Hospital of University of South China
Yi Guoliang	The First Affiliated Hospital of University of South China
Yin Ke	The First Affiliated Hospital of University of South China
Zha Wenliang	Hubei University of Science and Technology
Zhang Dong	The First Affiliated Hospital of Xi'an Jiaotong University
Zhang Hanchong	Shenzhen People's Hospital
Zhang Yangchun	The First Affiliated Hospital of University of South China
Zheng Jianbao	The First Affiliated Hospital of Xi'an Jiaotong University
Zheng Xin	The First Affiliated Hospital of Xi'an Jiaotong University

Zhu Guodong   The First Affiliated Hospital of Xi'an Jiaotong University
Zhu Yulin   The First Affiliated Hospital of Xi'an Jiaotong University

Editor

Sun Wenjuan   The First Affiliated Hospital of Xi'an Jiaotong University

作者名单

名誉主编

李玉民　兰州大学

主　编

马清涌　西安交通大学第一附属医院

梁贵友　贵州医科大学

白育庭　湖北科技学院

邱新光　郑州大学第一附属医院

王文军　南华大学附属第一医院

吴学东　大理大学第一附属医院

副主编

马振华　西安交通大学第一附属医院

王曙逢　西安交通大学第一附属医院

范晋海　西安交通大学第一附属医院

曹　罡　西安交通大学第二附属医院

王　拓　西安交通大学第一附属医院

王　铮　西安交通大学第一附属医院

王　程　南华大学附属第一医院

编　委（以姓氏汉语拼音排序）

柏宏亮　西安交通大学第一附属医院

蔡庆勇　遵义医科大学附属医院

陈　晨　西安交通大学第一附属医院

陈　魏　南华大学附属第一医院

陈志伟　南华大学附属第一医院

崔飞博　西安交通大学第一附属医院

崔俊成　南华大学附属第一医院

戴　祝　南华大学附属第一医院

邓幼文　中南大学湘雅三医院

丁晨光　西安交通大学第一附属医院

丁小明　西安交通大学第一附属医院

樊　林　西安交通大学第一附属医院

范伟杰　南华大学附属第一医院

亢 丹	湖北科技学院
高 洁	西安交通大学第一附属医院
耿智敏	西安交通大学第一附属医院
黄 俊	中南大学湘雅二医院
霍雄伟	西安交通大学第一附属医院
柯希贤	遵义医科大学附属医院
李 剑	贵州医科大学附属医院
李军辉	西安交通大学第二附属医院
李瑞春	西安交通大学第一附属医院
李绍波	大理大学第一附属医院
刘达兴	遵义医科大学附属医院
刘 擎	中南大学湘雅三医院
刘森源	郑州大学第一附属医院
刘 阳	西安交通大学第二附属医院
卢 乐	西安交通大学第二附属医院
马 兴	西安交通大学第一附属医院
冒 平	西安交通大学第一附属医院
毛新展	中南大学湘雅二医院
欧阳智华	南华大学附属第一医院
祁 磊	西安交通大学第一附属医院
仇广林	西安交通大学第一附属医院
曲 凯	西安交通大学第一附属医院
单 涛	西安交通大学第二附属医院
申 新	西安交通大学第一附属医院
宋永春	西安交通大学第一附属医院
王 宁	大理大学第一附属医院
王锁良	西安交通大学第一附属医院
王 炜	西安交通大学第一附属医院
吴 涛	西安交通大学第二附属医院
徐 刚	遵义医科大学附属医院
许克东	西安交通大学第一附属医院
薛武军	西安交通大学第一附属医院
晏怡果	南华大学附属第一医院
姚女兆	南华大学附属第一医院
易国良	南华大学附属第一医院
尹 科	南华大学附属第一医院
查文良	湖北科技学院
张 东	西安交通大学第一附属医院
张晗翀	深圳市人民医院
张阳春	南华大学附属第一医院
郑见宝	西安交通大学第一附属医院
郑 鑫	西安交通大学第一附属医院

朱国栋　　西安交通大学第一附属医院
朱宇麟　　西安交通大学第一附属医院
编　辑
孙文娟　　西安交通大学第一附属医院

Preface

At the Second Belt and Road Summit Forum on International Cooperation in 2019 and the Seventy-third World Health Assembly in 2020, General Secretary Xi Jinping stated the importance for promoting the construction of the "Belt and Road" and jointly build a community for human health. Countries and regions along the "Belt and Road" have a large number of overseas Chinese communities, and shared close geographic proximity, similarities in culture, disease profiles and medical habits. They also shared a profound mass base with ample space for cooperation and exchange in Clinical Medicine. The publication of the International Clinical Medicine series for clinical researchers, medical teachers and students in countries along the "Belt and Road" is a concrete measure to promote the exchange of Chinese and foreign medical science and technology with mutual appreciation and reciprocity.

Zhengzhou University Press coordinated more than 600 medical experts from over 160 renowned medical research institutes, medical schools and clinical hospitals across China. It produced this set of medical tools in English to serve the needs for the construction of the "Belt and Road". It comprehensively coversaspects in the theoretical framework and clinical practicesin Clinical Medicine, including basic science, multiple clinical specialities and social medicine. It reflects the latest academic and technological developments, and the international frontiers of academic advancements in Clinical Medicine. It shared with the world China's latest diagnosis and therapeutic approaches, clinical techniques, and experiences in prescription and medication. It has an important role in disseminating contemporary Chinese medical science and technology innovations, demonstrating the achievements of modern China's economic and social development, and promoting the unique charm of Chinese culture to the world.

The series is the first set of medical tools written in English by Chinese medical experts to serve the needs of the "Belt and Road" construction. It systematically and comprehensively reflects the Chinese characteristics in Clinical Medicine. Also, it presents a landmark achievement in the implementation of the "Belt and Road" initiative in promoting exchanges in medical science and technology. This series is theoretical in nature, with each volume built on the mainlines in traditional disciplines but at the same time introducing contemporary theories that guide clinical practices, diagnosis and treatment methods, echoing the latest research findings in Clinical Medicine.

As the disciplines in Clinical Medicine rapidly advances, different views on knowledge, inclusiveness, and medical ethics may arise. We hope this work will facilitate the exchange of ideas, build common ground while allowing differences, and contribute to the building of a community for human health in a broad spectrum of disciplines and research focuses.

Nick Lemoine

Foreign Academician of the Chinese Academy of Engineering

Dean, Academy of Medical Sciences of Zhengzhou University

Director, Barts Cancer Institute, London, UK

6th August, 2020

Foreword

With the development of medical international communication and education in China, there is an urgent need for an English version of surgery textbooks to meet the domestic demand for clinical medical English teaching in the current Chinese education system. In view of this, we compiled this textbook, together with 9 medical colleges and universities in China. In the process of compiling, we use the syllabus of undergraduates in clinical medicine as the basis, draw on the contents of the Chinese version of the textbook of surgery, and refer to the presentation, typesetting and professional vocabulary of textbooks in overseas medical schools. On the basis of following the principles of surgical treatment, this book highlights the characteristics of disease spectrum, diagnosis and treatment in China. We wish this book could be used as a bridge and link between domestic and foreign surgeon training methods, and could be widely used in medical schools in China.

The content of the book is mainly for international students and undergraduates, while it can also be used for the continuing education of domestic undergraduates and graduate students. We believe this book can bring you professional improvement. At the same time, we hope everyone can improve their English level. Regarding the shortcomings in the book, we really appreciate if you can give us valuable advices.

Authors

Contents

Part 1

Introduction

The management of surgical disorders requires not only the application of technical skills and training in the basic sciences to the problems of diagnosis and treatment but also genuine sympathy and indeed love for the patient. The surgeon must be a doctor in the old fashioned sense, an applied scientist, an engineer, an artist, and a minister of his or her fellow human beings. Because life or death often depends upon the validity of surgical decisions, the surgeon's judgment must be matched by courage in action and by a high degree of technical proficiency.

Chapter 1

Origin of Surgical Diseases

All somatic diseases, regardless of what specialties treat them, have their origins in following six basic pathological processes: congenital defects, inflammations, neoplasms, trauma, metabolic defects and degeneration, and collagen defects.

Four phenomena that result from these fundamental pathological processes are responsible for almost all surgical diseases and for many nonsurgical diseases as well. These phenomena areobstruction, perforation, erosion, and tumors or masses.

1.1 Obstruction

Cerebrovascular disease (strokes) and coronary heart disease (coronaries) are two of the leading causes of death in the United States. Both result from obstruction of vital arteries carrying blood to the brain or to the heart muscle, respectively. Glaucoma, one of the two leading causes of blindness in the United States also results from obstruction, in this case obstruction to the outflow of fluid from the anterior chamber of the eye.

Free flow of blood, urine, cerebrospinal fluid (CSF), lymph, and other fluids, as well as air, is essential for health. Table 1-1-1 shows a wide variety of diseases that result from obstruction.

Table 1-1-1 Diseases resulting from obstruction

System	Disease	Nature of obstruction
CNS	Hydrocephalus	Congenital obstruction of cerebrospinal fluid
ENT	Middle ear infection	Eustachian tube obstruction
Eye	Glaucoma	Obstruction of aqueous humor
Lung	Atelectasis	Mucus plug in bronchus
Biliary tract	Cholecystitis	Cystic duct stone
GI	Appendicitis	Fecalith in appendix
GU	Prostatism	Prostatic hypertrophy
Extremity	Intermittent claudication	Arteriosclerosis

CNS: Central nervous system; ENT: ear nose throat Branch; GI: Gastrointestinal; GU: gonococcal urethritis.

1.2 Perforation

Perforation, similarly, is the direct cause of many surgical diseases. Perforation is often such an intensely dramatic event that few medical students will forget the boardlike abdomen of the patient with a ruptured peptic ulcer or the shock that overwhelms the patient with a ruptured aortic aneurysm. Examples are given in Table 1-1-2.

Table 1-1-2 Examples of perforation

System	Disease	Nature of perforation
CNS	Cerebral hemorrhage	Rupture of CNS artery
ENT	Perforation of tympanic membrane	Infection with pressure
Lung	Spontaneous pneumothorax	Rupture of bleb
Biliary tract	Rupture of gallbladder	Obstruction, distension, necrosis
GI	Duodenal ulcer	Perforation of ulcer
GU	Ruptured bladder	Obstruction and distension
Vascular	Aortic aneurysm	Rupture of aneurysm

1.3 Erosion

Erosion is a "partial perforation", a slower process of ulceration (i. e. , a break in the continuity of a tissue surface). Examples of erosion are given in Table 1-1-3.

Table 1-1-3 Examples of erosion

System	Disease	Nature of erosion
CNS	Meningitis	Erosion of abscess wall; mastoiditis
ENT	Pharyngeal carcinoma	Bleeding; erosion into blood vessels
Lung	Tuberculosis	Bleeding; granulomatous erosion into blood vessels
GI	Duodenal ulcer	Bleeding; ulcer erosion into blood vessels
GU	Bladder stone	Bleeding; erosion into bladder wall
Extrimity	Reynaud's phenomenon	Digital ulceration; ischemic erosion of skin

1.4   Tumors

The most subtle of these phenomena is a tumor or mass. This explains in large measure why cancer is so often detected only after it induces one of the three processes. Because no vital flow is obstructed and perforation or erosion of the skin occurs very late symptoms, and consequently diagnosis, are delayed, often tragically.

Chapter 2

Approach to the Surgical Patient

2.1 History

At their first contact, the surgeon must gain the patient's confidence and convey the assurance that help is available and will be provided. The surgeon must demonstrate concern for the patient as a person who needs help and not just as a case to be processed through the surgical ward. This is not always easy to do, and there are no rules of conduct except to be gentle and considerate. Most patients are eager to like and trust their doctors and respond gratefully to a sympathetic and understanding person. Some surgeons are able to establish a confidental relationship with the first few words of greeting; others can only do so by means of a stylized and carefully acquired bedside manner. It does not matter how it is done, so long as an atmosphere of sympathy, personal interest, and understanding is created. Even under emergency circumstances, this subtle message of sympathetic concern must get across.

Eventually, all histories must be formally structured, but much can be learned by letting the patient ramble a little. Discrepancies and omissions in the history are often due as much to over structuring and leading questions as to the unreliability of the patient, The enthusiastic novice asks leading questions; the cooperative patient gives the answer that seems to be wanted; and the interview concludes on a note of mutual satisfaction with the wrong answer thus developed.

2.1.1 Building up the history

History taking is detective work. Preconceived ideas, snap judgments, and hasty conclusions have no place in this process. The diagnosis must be established by inductive reasoning. The interviewer must first determine the facts and then search for essential clues, realizing that the patient may conceal the most important symptom, e. g., the passage of blood by rectum in the hope (born of fear) that if it is not specifically inquired about or if nothing is found to account for it in the physical examination, it can not be very serious.

Common symptoms of surgical conditions that require special emphasis in history taking are discussed in the following paragraphs.

(1) Pain

Pain is a distressing feeling often caused by intense or damaging stimuli. Pain motivates the individual to withdraw from damaging situations, to protect a damaged body part while it heals, and to avoid similar experiences in the future. Pain is the most common reason for physician consultation in most developed countries. It is a major symptom in many medical conditions, and can interfere with a person's quality of life and general functioning. A careful analysis of the nature of pain is one of the most important features of surgical history. The examiner must first ascertain how the pain began. Was it explosive in onset, rapid or gradual? What is the precise character of the pain? Is it so severe that it can not be relieved by medication? Is it constant or intermittent? Are there classic associations, such as the rhythmic pattern of small bowel obstruction or the onset of pain preceding the limp of intermittent claudication?

One of the most important aspects of pain is the patient's reaction to it. The overreactor's description of pain is often obviously inappropriate, and so is a description of excruciating pain offered in a casual or jovial manner. A patient who shrieks and thrashes about is either grossly overreacting or suffering from renal or biliary colic. Very severe pain due to infection, inflammation, or vascular disease usually forces the patient to restrict all movement as much as possible.

Moderate pain is made agonizing by fear and anxiety. The reassurance of a sort calculated to restore the patient's confidence in the care being given is often a more effective analgesic than an injection of morphine.

(2) Vomiting

Vomiting, also known as emesis and throwing up, among other terms, is the involuntary, forceful expulsion of the contents of one's stomach through the mouth and sometimes the nose. Vomiting can be caused by a wide variety of conditions; it may present as a specific response to ailments like gastritis or poisoning, or as a non-specific sequela of disorders ranging from brain tumors and elevated intracranial pressure to overexposure to ionizing radiation. The feeling that one is about to vomit is called nausea, which often precedes, but does not always lead to vomiting.

Before the diagnosis wo must make sure what did the patient vomit? How much? How often? What did the vomitus look like? Was vomiting projectile? It is especially helpful for the examiner to see the vomitus.

(3) Change in bowel habits

A change in bowel habits is a common complaint that is often of no significance. However, when a person who has always had regular evacuations notices a distinct change, particularly toward intermittent alternations of constipation and diarrhea, colon cancer must be suspected. Too much emphasis is placed upon the size and shape of the stool, many patients who normally have well-formed stools may complain of irregular small stools when their routine is disturbed by travel or a change in diet.

(4) Hematemesis or hematochezia

Bleeding from any orifice demands the most critical analysis and can never be dismissed as due to some immediately obvious cause, The most common error is to assume that bleeding from the rectum is attributable to hemorrhoids. The character of the blood can be of great significance. Does it clot? Is it bright or dark red? Is it changed in any, as in the coffee ground vomitus of slow gastric bleeding or the dark, tarry stool of upper gastrointestinal bleeding? The full details and variations can not be included here but will be emphasized under separate headings elsewhere.

(5) Trauma

Trauma occurs so commonly that it is often difficult to establish a relationship between the chief complaint and an episode of trauma. Children in particular are subject to all kinds of minor trauma. And the family may attribute the onset of an illness to a specific recent injury. On the other hand, children may be subjected to sever trauma though their parents are unaware of it. The possibility of trauma having been inflicted by a parent must not be overlooked.

When there is a history of trauma, the details must be established as precisely as possible. What was the patient's position when the accident occurred? Was consciousness lost? Retrograde amnesia (inability to remember events just preceding the accident) always indicates some degree of cerebral damage. If a patient can remember every detail of an accident, has not consciousness, and has no evidence of external injury to the head, brain damage can be excluded.

In the case of gunshot wounds and stab wounds, knowing the nature of the weapon, its size and shape, the probable trajectory. And the position of the patient when hit may be very helpful in evaluating the nature of the resultant injury.

The possibility that an accident might have been caused by preexisting disease such as epilepsy, diabetes, coronary artery disease, or hypoglycemia must be explored.

When all of the facts and essential clues have been gathered, the examiner is in a position to complete the study of the present illness. By this time, it may be possible to rule out (by inductive reasoning) all but a few possible diagnoses. A novice diagnostician asked to evaluate the causes of shoulder pain in a given patient might include ruptured ectopicpregnancy in the list of possibilities. The experienced physician will automatically exclude that possibility on the basis of sex or age.

2.1.2　Family history

The family history is of great significance in a number of surgical conditions. Polyposis of the colon is a classic example, but diabetes, Peutz Jeghers syndrome (a familial disorder characterized by diffuse gastrointestinal polyposis and mucocutaneous pigmentation), chronic pancreatitis, multiglandular syndromes, other endocrine abnormalities, and cancer are often better understood and better evaluated in the light of careful family history.

2.1.3　Past history

The details of the past history may illuminate obscure areas of the present illness, It has been said that people who are well are almost never sick. And people who are sick are almost never well. It is true that a patient with a long and complicated history of diseases and injuries is likely to be a much poorer risk than even a very old patient experiencing a major surgical illness for the first time.

In order to makesure that important details of the past history will not be overlooked, the system review must be formalized and thorough. It's better to review the past history in the same way, the experienced examiner never omits significant details. Many skilled examiners find it's easy to review the past history by inquiring about each system as they perform the physical examination on that part of the body.

In reviewing the past history, it is important to consider the nutritional background of the patient. There is an increasing awareness throughout the world that the underprivileged malnourished patient responds poorly to disease, injury, and operation. Indeed, there is some evidence that various lesions such as carcinoma may be more fulminating in malnourished patients. Malnourishment may not be obvious on physical examination and must be elicited by questioning.

Acute nutritional deficiencies, particularly fluid and electrolyte losses, can be understood only in the light of the total (including nutritional) history. For example, a low serum sodium may be due to the use of diuretics or a sodium restricted diet rather than to acute loss. In this connection, the use of any medication must be carefully recorded and interpreted.

A detailed history of acute losses by vomiting and diarrhea and the nature of the losses is helpful in estimating the probable trends in serum electrolytes. Thus, the patient who has been vomiting persistently with evidence of bile in the vomitus is likely to have acute pyloric stenosis associated with benign ulcer, and hypochloremic alkalosis must be anticipated. Chronic vomiting without bile and particularly with evidence of changed and previously digested food is suggestive of chronic obstruction, and the possibility of carcinoma should be considered.

It is essential for the surgeon to think in terms of nutritional balance. It is often possible to begin therapy before the results of laboratory tests have been obtained, because the specific nature and probable extent of fluid and electrolyte losses can often be estimated on the basis of the history and the physician's clinical experience. Laboratory data should be obtained as soon as possible, but a knowledge of the probable fluids will provide sufficient grounds for the institution of appropriate immediate therapy.

2.1.4   The patient's emotional background

Psychiatric consultation is seldom required in the management of surgical patients, but there are times when it is of great help. Emotionally and mentally disturbed patients require surgical operations as often as others. And full cooperation between psychiatrist and surgeon is essential. Furthermore either before or after an operation, a patient may develop a major psychotic disturbance that is beyond the ability of the surgeon to appraise or manage. Prognosis, drug therapy, and overall management require the participation of a psychiatrist.

On the other hand, there many situations in which the surgeon can and should deal with the emotional aspects of the patient's illness rather than resorting to psychiatric assistance. Most psychiatrists prefer not to be brought in to deal with minor anxiety states. As long as the surgeon accepts the responsibility for the care of the whole patient, such services are superfluous.

This is particularly true in the care of patients with the malignant disease or those who must undergo mutilating operations such as amputation of an extremity, ileostomy, or colostomy. In these situations, the patient can be supported more effectively by the surgeon and the surgical team than by a consulting psychiatrist.

Surgeons are becoming increasingly more aware of the importance of psychosocial factors in surgical convalescence. Recovery from a major operation is greatly enhanced if the patient is not worn down with worry about emotional, social, and economic problems that have nothing to do with the illness itself. Incorporation of these factors into the record contributes tothe better total care of the surgical patient.

2.2   The Physical Examination

The complete examination of the surgical patient includes the physical examination, certain special procedures such as gastroscopy and esophagoscopy, laboratory tests, X-ray examination, and follow up examination. In some cases, all of these may be necessary; in others, special examinations and laboratory tests can be kept to a minimum. It is just as poor practice to insist on unnecessary thoroughness as it is to overlook procedures that may contribute to the diagnosis. Painful, inconvenient, and costly procedures should not be ordered unless there is a reasonable chance that the information gained will be useful in making clinical decisions.

2.2.1   The elective physical examination

The elective physical examination should be done in an orderly and detailed fashion. One should acquire the habit of performing a complete examination in exactly the same sequence so that no step is omitted. When the routine must be modified, as in an emergency, the examiner recalls without conscious effort what must be done to complete the examination later. The regular performance of complete examinations has the added advantage of familiarizing the beginner with what is normal so that what is abnormal can be more readily recognized.

All patients are sensitive and somewhat embarrassed at being examined. It is both courteous and clinically useful to put the patient at ease. The examining room and table should be comfortable, and drapes should be used if the patient is required to strip for the examination. Most patients will relax if they are allowed to talk a bit during the examination, which is another reason for taking the past history while the examination is being done.

A useful rule is to first observe the patient's habitus and then to carefully inspect the hands. Many systemic diseases show themselves in the hands (cirrhosis of the liver, hyperthyroidism, Reynaud's disease, pulmonary insufficiency, heart disease and nutritional disorders).

Inspection, palpation, and auscultation are the time-honored essential steps in appraising both the normal and the abnormal. Comparison of the two sides of the body often suggests a specific abnormality. The slight droop of one eyelid characteristic of Horner syndrome can only be recognized by careful comparison with the opposite side. Inspection of the female breasts, particularly as the patient raises and lowers her arms, will often reveal slight dimpling indicative of an infiltrating carcinoma barely detectable on palpation.

Successful palpation requires skill and gentleness. Spasm, tension, and anxiety caused by painful examination procedures may make an adequate examination almost impossible particularly in children. Another important feature of palpation is the laying on of hands that has been called part of the ministry of medicine. A disappointed and critical patient often will say of a doctor, "He hardly touched me." Careful, precise, and gentle palpation not only gives the physician the information being sought but also inspires confidence and trust. When examining for areas of tenderness, it may be necessary to use only one finger in order to precisely localize the extent of the tenderness. This is of particular importance in examination of the acute abdomen.

Auscultation, once thought to be the exclusive province of the physician, is now more important in surgery than it is in medicine. Radiologic examinations, including cardiac catheterization, have relegated auscultation of the heart and lungs to the status of preliminary scanning procedures in medicine. In surgery, however, auscultation of the abdomen and peripheral vessels has become absolutely essential. The nature of ileus and the presence of a variety of vascular lesions are revealed by auscultation. Bizarre abdominal pain in a young woman can be ascribed to hysteria or anxiety on the basis of a negative physical examination and X-rays of the gastrointestinal tract. Auscultation of the epigastrium, however, may reveal a murmur due to obstruction of the celiac artery.

2.2.2   Examination of the body orifices

A complete examination of the ears, mouth, rectum, and pelvis is accepted as part of a complete examination. The palpation of the mouth and tongue is as essential as inspection. Inspection of the rectum with a sigmoidoscope is now regarded as part of a complete physical examination; every surgeon should acquire familiarity with the use of the ophthalmoscope and sigmoidoscope and should use them regularly in doing complete physical examinations.

2.2.3　The emergency physical examination

In an emergency, the routine of the physical examination must be altered to fit the circumstances. The history may be limited to a single sentence, or there may be no history the patient is unconscious and there are no other informants. Although the details of an accident or injury may be very useful in the total appraisal of the patient, they must be left for later consideration. The primary considerations are the following: Is the patient breathing? Is the airway open? Is there a palpable pulse? Is the heart beating? Is massive bleeding occurring?

If the patient is not breathing, airway obstruction must ruled out by thrusting the fingers into the mouth and pulling the tongue forward. If the patient is unconscious, the respiratory tract should be intubated and mouth to mouth respiration started. If there is no pulse or heartbeat, start cardiac resuscitation.

Every victim of major blunt trauma should be suspected of capable of causing damage to the spinal cord unless rough handling is avoided.

Some injuries are so life threatening that action must be taken before even a limited physical examination is done. Penetrating wounds of the heart, large open sucking wounds of the chest, massive crush injures with flail chest, and massive external bleeding, all require emergency treatment before any further examination can be done.

In most emergencies, however, after it has been established that the airway is open, the heart is beating, and there is no massive external hemorrhage and after anti-shock measures have been instituted, if necessary a rapid survey examination must be done. Failure to perform such an examination can lead to serious mistakes in the care of the patient. It takes no more than 2 or 3 minutes to carefully examine the head, thorax, abdomen, extremities, genitalia (particularly in females) , and back, if cervical cord damage has been rule out, it is essential to turn the injured patient and carefully inspect the back, buttocks, and perineum.

Tension pneumothorax and cardiac tamponade may easily be overlooked if there are multiple injuries.

Upon completion of the survey examination, control of pain, splinting of fractured limbs, suturing of lacerations, and other types of emergency treatment can be started.

Chapter 3

Laboratory and Diagnostic Examinations

3.1 Laboratory Examination

Laboratory examinations in surgical patients have the following objectives: ①screening for asymptomatic disease that may affect the surgical result (e. g. , unsuspected anemia or diabetes). ②appraisal of diseases that may contraindicate elective surgery or require treatment before surgery (e. g. , diabetes, heart failure). ③diagnosis of disorders that require surgery (e. g. , hyperparathyroidism, pheochromocytoma). ④evaluation of the nature and extent of metabolic or septic complications.

Patients undergoing major surgery, even though they seem to be in excellent health except for their surgical disease, should have a complete blood and urine examination. A history of renal, hepatic, or heart disease requires detailed studies. Latent, asymptomatic renal insufficiency may be missed, since many patients with chronic renal disease have varying degrees of nitrogen retention without proteinuria. A fixed urine specific gravity is easily overlooked, and preoperative determination of the blood urea nitrogen and creatinine is frequently required. Patients who have had hepatitis may have no jaundice but may have severe hepatic insufficiency that can be precipitated into acute failure by blood loss or shock.

Medical consultation is frequently required in the total preoperative appraisal of the surgical patient, and there is no more rewarding experience than the thorough evaluation of a patient with heart disease or gastrointestinal disease by a physician and a surgeon working together. It is essential, however, that the surgeon could not become totally dependent upon the medical consultant for the preoperative evaluation and management of the patient. The total management must be the surgeon's responsibility and is not to be delegated. Moreover, the surgeon is the only one with the experience and background to interpret the meaning of laboratory tests in the light of other features of the case particularly the history and physical findings.

3.2 Imaging Examination

Modern patient care calls for a variety of critical radiologic examinations. The closest cooperation between the radiologist and the surgeon is essential if serious mistakes are to be avoided. This means that the surgeon must not refer the patient to the radiologist, requesting a particular examination, without providing an adequate account of the history and physical findings. Particularly in emergency situations, review of the films and consultation are needed.

When the radiologic diagnosis is not definitive, the examinations must be repeated in the light of the history and physical examination. Despite the great accuracy of X-ray diagnosis, a negative gastrointestinal study still does not exclude either ulcer or a neoplasm; particularly in the right colon, small lesions are easily overlooked. At times, the history and physical findings are so clearly diagnostic that operation is justifiable despite negative imaging studies.

3.3   Special Examinations

Special examinations such as cystoscopy, gastroscopy, esophagoscopy, colonoscopy, angiography, and bronchoscopy are often required in the diagnostic appraisal of surgical disorders. The surgeon must be familiar with the indications and limitations of these procedures and be prepared to consult with colleagues in medicine and the surgical specialties as required.

Part 2

Asepsis

Asepsis is a basic practice in clinical medicine. For surgery, it is particularly important. Various microorganisms are ubiquitous in the human and the surrounding environment. In the process of surgery, puncture, intubation, injection and dressing change, a series of strict measures must be taken to prevent microorganisms from entering the wound or tissue through contact, air or droplets, otherwise it may infect. Aseptic technique is a series of preventive measures against microorganisms and infection pathways.

In theory, sterilization means killing all living microorganisms, including spores. Disinfection refers to the killing of pathogenic microorganisms and other harmful microorganisms but does not require the removal or killing of all microorganisms. From a clinical point of view, all pathogenic microorganisms must be killed, whether sterilized or disinfected, to meet the requirements of clinical aseptic technique. The items that are usually used for the surgical area or wound are treated according to sterilization requirements—all the microorganisms on the related items are completely destroyed by physical methods (high temperature, etc.) or chemical methods (such as glutaraldehyde) beforehand; some special operations, the instruments, the surgeon's arm, the patient's skin, and the air in the operating room are treated according to the disinfection standard to remove harmful microorganisms.

The content of the aseptic technique involves not only a variety of sterilization and disinfection methods, but also the relevant operating rules and management systems that are very important. In the process of medical care operations, medical personnel must follow a set of operating procedures to keep sterile articles, sterile areas from being contaminated, and to prevent pathogenic microorganisms from invading the human body. All medical personnel must consciously abide by and strictly implement these rules and regulations to ensure the implementation of aseptic technique.

With the development of society and economy, many hospitals in China have updated their instruments and equipment in the past few years, which has greatly improved the appearance of aseptic technique. The establishment of laminar flow rooms, the widespread use of ethylene oxide and plasma gas sterilization, and the preparation of disposable medical materials have significantly improved the effectiveness of sterilization and disinfection, and have played a role in the clinical work of the surgery.

Chapter 1

Sterilization and Disinfection of Surgical Instruments and Articles

1.1 Sterilization of High-pressure Steam

The application of the sterilization method with the high pressure steam method is the most common and the effect is also very reliable. High-pressure steam sterilizers can be divided into two types: lower exhaust type and pre-vacuum type. The exhaust vent sterilizer has many styles, such as portable, horizontal and vertical, but its basic structure and function are the same. It consists of a high-pressure boiler with two walls. The steam enters the sterilizing room, accumulates to increase the pressure, and the temperature in the room also increases. When the vapor pressure reaches a certain temperature and time, it can kill all the microorganisms including the bacterial spores with indomitable resistance.

Many hospitals have now adopted a more advanced pre-vacuum steam sterilizer. Its characteristic is that the air in the sterilizer is firstly pumped to a vacuum state, and then the vapor is directly input into the sterilization chamber by the central gas supply system. This ensures that the vapor distribution in the sterilization chamber is even. The entire sterilization process takes time and the damage to the item is also slighter (Table 2-1-1).

Table 2-1-1　Sterilization parameters of pressure steam sterilizer

Equipment	Goods	Temperature	Shortest time	Pressure
lower exhaust	dressing	121 ℃	30 min	102.9 kPa
		121 ℃	20 min	102.9 kPa
pre-vacuum	instrument dressing	132-134 ℃	4 min	205.8 kPa

The high-pressure steam method is applicable to large logarithmic medical articles, including surgical instruments, disinfecting cloths, and cloth dressings. In order to ensure the effect of autoclaving, there are strict rules in the process. ①The various packages to be sterilized should not be too large, the upper volume limit is: length 40 cm, width 30 cm, height 30 cm. Packing should not be too tight. ②The package inside the sterilizer should not be too dense, the capacity of the bottom row steam sterilizer is 10% –80% of the volume of the cabinet, and the load of the pre-vacuum type steam sterilizer is 5% –90%, so as not to interfere with the penetration of steam and affect the sterilization effect. ③Preset special package and package external sterilization instruction tape, when the pressure and temperature reach the sterilization requirement, the special package internal card (also called the crawler card) changes from colorless to black, and the external package indicates that Black streaks appear. ④Sterile items should be marked with a valid date, usually two weeks.

1.2　Chemical Gas Sterilization Method

This type of method is applicable to the sterilization of medical materials that are not resistant to high temperatures and heat, such as electronic instruments, optical instruments, endoscopes and special instruments, cardiac catheters, catheters, and other rubber products. At present, ethylene oxide gas sterilization, hydrogen peroxide plasma cryogenic sterilization and formaldehyde vapor sterilization are mainly used.

1.2.1　Ethylene oxide gas sterilization method

The effective gas concentration is 450 – 1200 mg/L. The temperature in the sterilization chamber is 37–63 ℃. It takes 1–6 hours to reach the sterilization requirements. The article is sealed in a special paper bag and placed in a sterilization chamber. The sterilization period is limited to 6 months.

1.2.2　Hydrogen peroxide plasma cryogenic sterilization

The principle of this method is to stimulate the glow discharge in the sterilization equipment and use hydrogen peroxide as a medium to form a low-temperature plasma that plays a role in sterilization. The concentration of hydrogen peroxide is >6 mg/L, the temperature is 45–65 ℃, and the time is 28–75 minutes. The article should be fully dried before sterilization.

1.2.3　Low-temperature formaldehyde vapor sterilization

The effective gas concentration is 3–11 mg/L, the sterilization temperature is 50–80 ℃, and the sterilization time is 30–60 minutes.

After the ethylene oxide and formaldehyde steam sterilization treatment, residual gas emissions can not be naturally volatilized, but dedicated exhaust system emissions should be set.

1.3　Boiling Method

This method applies to metal equipment, glass products and rubber and other items. Boil in water to 100 ℃ for 15–20 minutes. Normal bacteria can be killed, but bacteria with spores need to be boiled for at least 1 hour to be killed. This method is simple and easy to use and has a positive effect. It is used in some primary medical units or emergency services. In order to save time and ensure the quality of sterilization, high pressure cookers can be used for boiling sterilization in plateau areas. Pressure steam pressure cooker is generally 127.5 kPa, the maximum temperature in the pot up to about 124 ℃, sterilization can be 10 minutes.

1.4   Chemical Liquid Soaking

Sharp surgical instruments, endoscopes, etc. , can also be soaked with chemical liquids for disinfection purposes. At present, most of the clinical use of 2% neutral glutaraldehyde as soaking solution, 30 minutes to achieve disinfection effect, sterilization time is 10 hours. Other soaking liquids used for disinfection include 10% formaldehyde, 70% ethanol, 1 : 1000 benzalkonium bromide, and 1 : 1000 chlorhexidine.

1.5   Dry Heat Sterilization

This is suitable for the sterilization of heat, moisture, steam or gas that can not penetrate the product, such as glass, powder, oil and other items sterilized. The dry heat temperature reached 160 ℃ , the shortest sterilization time was 2 hours, 170 ℃ was 1 hour, and 180 ℃ was 30 minutes.

1.6   Ionizing Radiation Method

The method belongs to the industrialized sterilization method and is mainly applied to aseptic medical consumables (disposable syringes and silk threads) and certain drugs. The commonly used ^{60}Co releases γ−rays or electron rays generated by an accelerator for sterilization.

Chapter 2

Preparation of Surgical Staff and Patient Surgical Region

2.1 Preoperative Preparation for the Surgeon

2.1.1 General preparation

After the surgeon enters the operating room, he must first wear clean shoes and underwear prepared in the operating room and wears a hat and a mask. The hat should cover all hair and the mask should cover the nostrils. Cut your nails and remove the deposits under the edges. When the hand or arm skin is damaged or purulent infection occurs, surgery cannot be performed.

2.1.2 Arm disinfection

There are microbial communities on the surface of human skin. Some of them are found in deep skin wrinkles and pores. They are often colonized, and include coagulase-negative staphylococci, coryneform bacteria, propionic acid bacteria, and acinetobacter, and are not easily rubbed. The other part of the skin surface of temporary bacteria, mostly from the environment, loosely attached to the skin surface. The arm disinfection can remove almost all temporary bacteria and a few resident bacteria on the skin surface. During surgery, these deep-seated bacteria can gradually move to the surface of the skin. Therefore, after disinfecting the arm, wear sterile rubber gloves and sterile surgical gowns to prevent these bacteria from contaminating the surgical wound.

Disinfection of the arm includes cleaning and disinfecting in two steps: firstly, using soap or hand sanitizer, wash the arm thoroughly with a "seven-step handwashing method" to remove various stains on the surface; secondly, use a disinfectant for skin disinfection. Currently used skin disinfectants are ethanol, isopropanol, chlorhexidine, iodophor and so on. Limit methods include brushing, rinsing, and flushing. Surgical hand disinfection is the most commonly used brushing technique. It can wash the arm in a certain sequence for 3 minutes to reach the surgical hand disinfection standard.

Traditional arm disinfection methods include soapy water washing and ethanol soaking, which take 15 minutes to complete. And it is now rarely used. The emergence of new-type hand sanitizers has made the sterilization process simpler, and the use requirements of various disinfectants have been slightly different, but all emphasize the skin cleansing steps before disinfection.

2.2   Preparation of the Patient's Operating Area

Temporary bacteria and resident bacteria are also present on the surface of the patient's skin. These bacteria enter the cut tissue and may cause infection. The purpose of the patient's surgical field preparation is to eliminate temporary bacteria on the skin at and around the surgical incision and to inhibit the movement of resident bacteria. Minimize surgical site−related infections.

Skin near the surgical area should be removed before surgery if it is thick and may affect exposure and handling. The day before the operation, the patient is allowed to bathe in his/her health condition. If the skin has more oil or adhesive plaster residue, you can wipe off with gasoline or turpentine.

In addition to local anesthesia, skin disinfection prior to surgery should be performed after anesthesia, the traditional skin disinfection method is to use 2.5%−3% iodine rubbed the operating area, wait until it is dry after being rubbed twice with 70% ethanol to remove iodine. Because of the exact effect of iodine disinfection, this method is thrown into use. In recent years, special skin disinfectants containing active iodine or active chlorine have been successively introduced and widely used in clinics. The new disinfectants have little skin irritation and can stay on the skin surface for a long time, and have a long−lasting antiseptic and antibacterial effect.

Note: ①When rubbing the above−mentioned liquid medicine, should rub around from the central part of the operation area. If it is an infected wound or an anal area operation, it should be applied to the infected wound or the perineum and anus from the periphery of the surgical field. The liquid gauze that has been in contact with the contaminated site should not be returned to the clean room. ②The range of skin disinfection in the surgical site should include a 15 cm area around the surgical incision. If the surgery has the possibility of prolonging the incision, the scope of skin disinfection should be expanded accordingly.

Disinfect the surgical area and lay sterile cloths. The purpose is to cover the non−surgical area beyond the minimal skin area necessary to reveal the surgical incision, minimize the contamination during surgery, and provide an adequate sterile surface for the surgical procedure. In addition to the incision site, the surgical incision must be covered with four or more sterile towels. The principle of drape is to lay the relatively unclean area (abdomen, perineum) first, and then lay the side close to the operator, and use a cloth towel clamp to clamp the corners to prevent movement. After the sterile towel is laid, it can not be moved freely. If the position is not accurate, it can only be moved out of the operating area and can not be moved from the outside to the inside. Then, according to the specific situation of the surgical site, then spread the single or large single. The head of the large cloth should be covered by the anesthesia shelf, and the sides and foot ends should hang down more than 30 cm from the side of the operating table. Upper and lower extremity surgery should be performed after the skin is sterilized. Limb proximal surgery commonly used double sterile towel will be hand (foot) department of the package. The hand (foot) surgery needs to be wrapped around the proximal end of the limb with a sterile towel. For some major surgeries, a sterile plastic film can be applied to the skin in the surgical incision area after the procedure is completed, which can further reduce the displacement of the common resident bacteria in the deep skin adjacent to the surgery and contaminate the surgical field.

Chapter 3

Aseptic Principles in Operation

At the beginning of the surgery, the surgical instruments and articles were sterilized. The surgeons completed arm disinfection, wearing sterile surgical gowns and gloves, and the patient's surgical area was sterilized and covered with a sterile cloth sheet. All this has provided a sterile operating environment for surgery. However, in the course of surgery, if there is no certain regulation to maintain this sterile environment, the sterilized and disinfected items or the surgical area may still be contaminated, resulting in wounds and even deep infections. This may cause the surgery to fail and even affect the patient's life. Therefore, all personnel who participate in the surgery must carefully implement the rules for aseptic operation:

(1) After the surgeon wears a sterile surgical gown and sterile gloves, the personal sterile space is below the shoulders, in front of the waist, in front of the body, and on both arms. After laying a sterile sheet on the operating table and instrument cart, the table top area is also a sterile area. All surgical personnel must always maintain a clear awareness of the need to strictly protect sterile areas during the operation. Hands should not touch the back, below the waist, or above the shoulders. These areas are considered to be commensurate with the zone; likewise, do not touch the rags under the edge of the operating table. If accidental contamination occurs, it needs to be replaced or re-sterilized immediately.

(2) Do not send surgical instruments and supplies behind the surgeon. Articles of equipment falling outside of sterile towels or operating tables are treated as contaminants.

(3) If the glove breaks or comes into contact with the bacteria in the operation, the sterile gloves should be replaced. If the forearm or elbow touch the bacteria place, should replace thesterile surgical gown or add sterile sleeve. Such as sterile towels, cloth and other items have been soaked, their sterile isolation is no longer complete, should be covered with dry sterile cloth.

(4) Before the operation begins, check the equipment and dressings. At the end of the operation, check the body cavity such as the chest and abdomen. After checking the number of devices and dressings correctly, close the incision so as to avoid foreign matter being left in the cavity and causing serious consequences.

(5) Before making a skin incision and suturing the skin, disinfect the skin with 70% ethanol.

(6) The incision margin should be covered with a sterile gauze pad or surgical towel. For example, after abdominal operation, the sterile towel is sutured to the peritoneum to protect the abdominal wall incision. Now incision protection devices are available. After the abdomen is opened, the incision protector is placed in the abdominal cavity. After the eversion of the sterile film, the entire incision can be covered and the incision has a good protection.

(7) Before cutting the hollow organ, use a gauze pad to protect the surrounding tissue to prevent or reduce contamination.

(8) During the operation, if the same side surgeon needs to change the position, one person should step back one step at a time and turn back to another position to prevent touching the unclean area on the other side.

(9) The person who visits the operation must not be too close to the operation personnel or stand too high, nor can he walk around often to reduce the chance of contamination.

(10) Ventilation or fans should not be used to open the window during operation, nor can the air outlet of the room air conditioner be blown to the operating table so as to avoid dust and contaminate the air inside the operating room.

(11) All participating surgical personnel must strictly abide by the aseptic system. Everyone should maintain a high sense of responsibility in responding to the principle of asepsis. For suspected contaminated items, they should be treated as contaminants.

Chapter 4

Management of Operating Room

The operating room needs a strict management system to ensure its clean environment. Related pork belly includes disinfection, hygiene system, preservation and monitoring of sterilized items, and treatment of equipment items used in special infection patients. The relevant rules and regulations are summarized as follows:

(1) The layout of the operating room should follow the principle of prevention and control of hospital infections, so that the layout is reasonable, the zoning is clear, the marks are clear, and the basic principles of reasonable function flow and separation of the contaminated areas are met. The operating room should be provided with access for staff, access to patients, and the logistics should be separated and the flow should be reasonable.

(2) The staff members who enter the operating room strictly abide by the various operating room systems, such as the changing of the shoes, the visit system, the patient safety management system, the check-up system, and the use of equipment and equipment.

(3) The modern laminar flow operating room adopts air purification technology to treat microorganisms with different degrees of treatment, not only providing clean air, but also controlling the flow direction of the air flow, forming a positive pressure environment in the operating room, and making the air flow from a clean operation. The area flows into areas of low cleanliness and forms a closed clean environment. When the door is closed, the air pressure in the room is greater than the outdoor air pressure, so that the clean air in the operating room is only discharged outwards, and the outdoor air does not enter the room. Open the door to reduce the positive pressure inside the room, there will be a small amount of air outside the door into the room, affecting the cleanliness of indoor air. During the operation, the number of open operations in the operation room should be minimized, and it is forbidden to open the door for operation.

(4) There are multiple surgeries within the same operation room during the day, and arrangements must be made to follow the principle of doing contaminated or infected surgery after performing a sterile operation. Patients with special infectious diseases such as hepatitis B, syphilis, and AIDS should be placed after surgery without infectious diseases.

(5) The operating area of the operating room should be cleaned and disinfected once every 24 hours. After the surgery is completed, the surgery room should be cleaned and disinfected in a timely manner. Thoroughly clean the operating room once a week, including floors, walls, ceilings, instrument surfaces, etc. Monthly bacterial culture of the fingers after washing hands, air culture of the operating room bacteria, and

bacterial culture of disinfected articles.

(6) Disinfection of special infections Gas gangrene and Pseudomonas aeroginosa infections are fumigated with 40% formaldehyde + potassium permanganate (40% formaldehyde 200 mL + 100 g potassium permanganate per 100 m^3). For hepatitis, Pseudomonas aeruginosa infection, and open tuberculosis patients, all surgical instruments were first immersed in 2000 mg/L available chlorine solution for 60 minutes, then washed, autoclaved, and drained in 2000 mg/L available chlorine solution. After immersed for 60 minutes, it is poured into a fixed sewer, and the hospital uniformly processes the used dressing and sends it to the laundry room for treatment.

In recent years, a hybrid operating room with CT, MRI, or digital subtraction imaging equipment and surgical facilities has a complex internal structure, a large space, and a large number of equipments, which imposes higher requirements on aseptic management.

Part 3

Fluid, Electrolyte and Acid-base Disorders

Fluid status, electrolyte homeostasis, and acid-base balance are clinical parameters of critical significance in surgical patients. Understanding normal physiology and pathophysiology related to these parameters is crucial. Surgical patients are at high risk for derangements of body water distribution, electrolyte homeostasis, and acid-base physiology. These disturbances may be secondary to trauma, preexisting medical conditions which alter normal physiology, or the nature of the surgery. This chapter describes the etiology, pathophysiology, compensation mechanism, clinical manifestations, diagnosis and treatment measures of fluid, electrolyte and acid-base imbalance in surgical diseases.

Chapter 1

Summary

Total body mass is 45% –60% water. The percentage in any individual is influenced by age and lean body mass, therefore the percentage is higher in men compared to women, in children compared to adults, and in people of normal body habits compared to the obese. Body fluid includes intracellular and extracellular fluid. 2/3 of total body water, 30% –40% of body mass, is intracellular; 1/3, 15% –20% of total body mass, is extracellular. The extracellular fluid is divided into two compartments, with 80% (12% –16% of total body mass) in the interstitial compartment, and 20% (3% –4%) in the intravascular compartment. 1/5 of intravascular fluid is proximal to the arterioles, the remaining 4/5 is distal to the arterioles.

The intracellular, interstitial, and intravascular compartments each hold fluid characterized by markedly different electrolyte profiles. The main intracellular cation is the potassium ion (K^+), while the main extracellular cation is the sodium ion (Na^+). Not only the electrolyte profile, but also the protein composition of the fluids differs: intracellular cations are electrically balanced mainly by the polyatomic ion phosphate (PO_4^{3-}) and negatively charged proteins, while extracellular cations are balanced mainly by the chloride ion (Cl^-). The intravascular fluid has a relatively higher concentration of protein and lower concentration of organic acids than the interstitial fluid. This higher concentration of protein, chiefly albumin, is the main cause of the high colloid osmotic pressure of serum, which in turn is the chief regulator of the fluid distribution between the two extracellular compartments. The relationship between colloidosmotic pressure and hydrostatic pressure governs the movement of water across the capillary membrane, and is modeled by the Starling equation.

The body's volume status and electrolyte composition are determined largely by the kidneys. The kidneys maintain a constant volume and osmolality by modulating how much free water and Na^+ is reabsorbed from the renal filtrate. Antidiuretic hormone (ADH), also known as arginine vasopressin, is the chief regulator of osmolality. The peptide hormone is released from the posterior pituitary in response to increased serum osmolality. ADH induces translocation of aquaporin channels to the collecting duct epithelium, increasing permeability to water and causing reabsorption of free water from the renal filtrate. Thus water is retained, and the urine concentrated. In the absence of ADH, the collecting duct is impermeable to water, leading to water loss and production of dilute urine. At high physiologic levels ADH has a direct vasoconstrictive effect on arterioles.

The main determinant of Na^+ reabsorption is the Na^+ load in the renal filtrate. Most filtered Na^+ (60% – 70%) is reabsorbed in the proximal tubule. A further 20% –30% of filtered Na^+ is reabsorbed in the thick ascending limb of the loop of Henle; reabsorption here is determined by the Na^+ load delivered to the loop and a variety of hormones. The remaining distal tubule reabsorbs 5% –10% of filtered Na^+; again, the exact percentage is determined by the Na^+ load and a variety of hormonal factors, particularly aldosterone. The collecting duct reabsorbs a small percentage of filtered Na^+ under the influence of aldosterone and natriuretic hormone. Under normal circumstances the kidneys will adjust excreted water and Na^+ to match a wide spectrum of dietary intake.

Although the movement of ions and proteins between the different fluid compartments is normally restricted, water itself is freely diffusible between them. Consequently the osmolality of the different fluid compartments is identical, normally approximately 290 mOsm/kg. Control of osmolality occurs through regulation of water intake through diet and excretion through urine and insensible loses.

Chapter 2

Maladjustment of Body Fluid

There are three forms of imbalance in body fluid: volume disorder, concentration disorder and component disorder. Volume disorder which is isotonic dehydration only changes amount of extracellular fluid and does not impact amount of intracellular fluid. Concentration disorder that is change of water in extracellular fluid further impact osmotic pressure. Owing to 90% osmotic pressure is provided by Na^+ in extracellular fluid, the concentration imbalance occurs at this time majorly is hyponatremia and hypernatremia. Other ion concentration disorder such as hypokalemia and hyperkalemiain in extracellular fluid does not obviously impact osmotic pressure owing to small amount.

2.1 Isotonic Dehydration

Isotonic dehydration is also called acute lack of water or mixed type of water shortage. Hypovolemia commonly occur in surgical patients, both following elective surgery and in the setting of trauma and acute care surgery. Volume disturbances run the gamut from being clinically insignificant to being immediately life threatening. The underlying cause of any volume disorder must be sought and addressed while the volume disorder itself is managed.

Etiology: It is typically caused by loss of isotonic fluids in the setting of hemorrhage, gastrointestinal losses (e. g. , gastric suctioning, emesis, and diarrhea), sequestration of fluids in the gut lumen (e. g. , bowel obstruction, ileus, and enteric fistulas), burns, and excessive diuretic therapy. In resource poor settings sweat is often an additional important fluid loss, for example, in a non-air-conditioned operating room. In all of these cases, loss of isotonic fluid results in loss of Na^+ and water without significantly affecting the osmolality of the extracellular fluid compartment, thus there is very little shift of water into or out of the intracellular compartment. Hypovolemia stimulates aldosterone secretion from the zona glomerulosa of the adrenal cortex, leading to increased reabsorption of Na^+ and water from the renal filtrate and excretion of low volumes (oliguria) of hypertonic urine with a low Na^+ concentration.

Clinical manifestation: Nausea, anorexia, weak, oliguria is major clinical symptoms. Sign include tongue dry, eyehole sunken, skin dry, skin slack, etc. , except thirsty. Once lossof fluid accounts for 5% of body weight (25% extracellular fluid) at short period, the patients performance symptom includes pulse tachycardia, acromelic wet, blood pressure instability, etc. When fluid volume further loss to 6% -7% of body weight

(30%-35% extracellular fluid), the patients will be subjected to shock.

Diagnosis: Hypovolemia is suggested by a patient's history, physical examination, and laboratory data. Diagnosis by physical examination alone in the immediate postoperative setting is difficult, especially when volume loss is mild to moderate, and especially in very old and very young patients. Laboratory evidence includes blood concentration include elevated red blood cell count, Hb, and hematocrit. Serum Na^+, Cl^- concentration does not reduce. No single highly sensitive test to diagnose hypovolemia exists, thus the diagnosis must be made by examining all available data with a high index of suspicion.

Treatment: It is very important to treatment the primary disease. Hypovolemia is corrected with intravenous administration of an isotonic fluid such as balance salt solution. To the patients with pulse tachycardia, or blood pressure instability (also mean loss of fluid accounts for 5% of body weight), we should rapidly apply intravenous infusion with 3000 mL balance salt solution. Coexistent electrolyte abnormalities should be addressed simultaneously. Care must be taken in patients in renal or heart failure not to exacerbate these conditions. If hypovolemia is allowed to worsen unimpeded it will eventually lead to circulatory collapse and shock, which is covered elsewhere. Additionally, we must monitor cardiac function such as heart rate, central venous pressure, or pulmonary artery wedge pressure when rapidly intravenous infusion balance salt solution. To the patient with insufficient blood volume is not assured, we may apply intravenous infusion with half above solution (1500-2000 mL). Additionally, it should also be supplemented with 2000 mL water/daily and 4.5 g NaCl/ daily.

2.2　Hypotonic Dehydration

Hypotonic dehydration is also called chronic lack of water or secondary type of water shortage. Hypotonic dehydration often occur in surgical patients with water and sodium simultaneously loss, the loss amount of sodium is more than water, total body Na^+ may be decreased. The compensatory mechanism of the body is antidiuretic hormone secretion decrease, so that osmotic pressure in extracellular fluid is increase owing to decease reabsorb water in collecting duct. But this could be make extracellular fluid become more less, it force intercellular fluid inflow blood circulation to supplement blood volume. Once to the certain extent, the body will not take into account the maintenance of osmotic pressure. The following renin-aldosterone system is excited, increase in the secretion of antidiuretic hormone, reabsorb water is added and oliguria emergence. If blood volume further worsen, the patients will be subjected to shock.

Etiology: Hyponatremia is common in surgical patients postoperatively, as ADH is secreted in response to pain, nausea and vomiting, opiate administration, and positive-pressure ventilation. Typically, this hyponatremia is mild and inconsequential; however, it may be exacerbated by rapid parenteral administration of hypotonic fluids. Hyponatremia may result from severe hyperglycemia, or any other condition in which an osmotically active solute draws water from the intracellular space to the extracellular space. In the setting of hyperglycemia,

Clinical manifestation: It is different from sodium loss status. The signs of hyponatremiaare nausea, vomit, dizzy, visual vagueness, weak and feeble, but not thirsty. Hypotonic dehydration can be divided into three degrees according to the degree of sodium deficiency. Mild $Na^+ < 135$ mmol/L, the signs of patients are tired, dizzy, deadlimb, sodium reduction in urine. Moderate $Na^+ < 130$ mmol/L, the signs of patients are tired, dizzy, deadlimb, nausea, vomit, pulse tachycardia, blood pressure instability, stand fainting, no NaCl in the urine. Severe $Na^+ < 120$ mmol/L, the signs of patients are delirious, muscle spasmodic pain, diminished or disappearing of tendon reflex,stupor,coma and shock.

Diagnosis:Hyponatremia is suggested by a patient's history,physical examination. Further laboratory examine:①urine examination,urine specific gravity<1. 010, Na^+, Cl^- obvious reduction in urine. ②serum Na^+ examination, Na^+<135 mmol/L,the disease is worse when the blood sodium is lower. ③elevated red blood cell count,Hb,hematocrit,and urea nitrogen.

Treatment:Hypertonic saline should not be used to correct hyponatremia. Unless serum Na^+ falls very rapidly,it should be corrected slowly,as too-rapid correction has the devastating complication of osmotic demyelination. No consensus exists on the appropriate rate of correction. Sodium levels should not be corrected beyond what is needed to alleviate central nervous system(CNS) disturbances. Correction of Na^+ does not replace pharmacologic intervention in a seizing patient.

One formula used to calculate the expected change in Na^+ from intravenous administration of 1 L of any fluid is as below:

$$Na^+_{supplement}(mmol/L) = [Na^+_{normal}(mmol/L) - Na^+_{measured}(mmol/L)] \times body\ mass(kg) \times 0.6(0.5\ for\ female)$$

Total body water is estimated as a fraction of body mass. Hyponatremia causing CNS disturbances should prompt admission to an intensive care unit given the close monitoring needed in such patients,the need for rapid intervention,and the potentially devastating consequences of delays in management.

2.3 Hypertonic Dehytration

Hypertonic dehydration is also called primary lack of water. Hypertonic dehydration often occur in surgical patients with water and sodium simultaneously loss,the loss amount of water is more than sodium,total body Na^+ may be increased and osmotic pressure in extracellular fluid sequently increased. It will result in intracellular and extracellular fluid decreasion when intracellular fluid move out to extracellular at severe water shortage. The compensatory mechanism of the body is firstly the patient's thirst center in the hypothalamus be stimulated and drink water to reduce osmotic pressure. Secondly,antidiuretic hormone secretion increase and osmotic pressure in extracellular fluid is decrease owing to incease reabsorb water in collecting duct.

Etiology:Loss of free water alone occurs when patients do not have access to water (e. g. ,preverbal, bed-bound or otherwise incapacitated patients) ,in diabetes insipidus,in the setting of high fevers,and in patients in whom enteral feeds do not contain adequate water.

Clinical manifestation:It is different from water loss status. Hypertonic dehydration can be divided into three degrees according to the degree of water deficiency. Mild water loss is equal to 2% -4% body mass, the signs of patients are majorly thirsty. Moderate water loss is equal to 4% -6% body mass,the signs of patients are thirsty,tired,dizzy,deadlimb,pulse tachycardia,blood pressure instability,stand fainting,oliguria and urine specific gravity increasion. Severe water loss is equal to >6% body mass,the signs of patients are delirious,muscle spasmodic pain,diminished or disappearing of tendon reflex,stupor,coma and shock.

Diagnosis:Hypernatremia is suggested by a patient's history,physical examination. Further laboratory examine including the following:①urine examination,urine specific gravity>1. 010. ②serum Na^+ examination, Na^+>150 mmol/L. ③elevated red blood cell count,Hb,hematocrit.

Treatment:It is very important to treatment the primary disease. To the patient that can't be taken orally,we should provide parenteral administration of free water,typically as 5% dextrose in water and 0. 45%

NaCl solution. If the patient's hypernatremia developed over a period of hours it may safely be corrected at a rate of 1 mmol/(L · h). In patients whose hypernatremia developed more slowly, a rate of 0.5 mmol/(L · h) is safe. At the same time monitoring the concentration of blood sodium is important and normal requirements 2000 mL water/daily should be supplement. In addition, Sodium should be supplemented as appropriate to prevent hyponatremia.

2.4 Water Intoxication

Water intoxication is also called diluent hypernatremia. Water intoxication seldom occur in surgical patients with water excessive intake and plasma osmotic pressure decreasion.

Etiology: ①A variety of causes leading to the increase in the antidiuretic hormone secretion. ②Renal insufficiency. ③Excessive intake of water in the body.

Clinical manifestation: Acute water intoxication firstly causes brain cell edema and increase intracranial pressure, finally cause a series of mental symptoms. The signs are headache, sleepiness, dysphoria, abnormal orienteering, delirium, and coma. Once the occurrence of cerebral hernia, the corresponding neuropositioning sign is appear. The signs of chronic water intoxication is often covered by primary diseases including nausea, vomit, dizzy, visual vagueness, weak and feeble. Further laboratory examine including decreased red blood cell count, Hb, hematocrit, and osmotic pressure.

Treatment: It should be stop ingest water once water intoxication is diagnosed. To the mild patients, the signs of water intoxication soon relieve when water is discharged, To the severe patients, we should use diuretic to relieve the signs of water intoxication.

Chapter 3

Maladjustment of Potassium

Potassium is the major intracellular cation. Plasma potassium ion (K^+) concentration is determined primarily by two factors. The first is acid−base homeostasis. Hydrogen ion (H^+) and K^+ are exchanged between the intracellular and extracellular spaces, thus disturbances of acid−base balance (below) tend to cause disturbances in serum K^+. The second is the size of the total body K^+ pool. Intracellular stores of K^+ are large, but may be exhausted, especially in the setting of prolonged ketoacidosis.

3.1 Hypokalemia

Etiology: Hypokalemia is common in surgical patients postoperatively ($K^+ < 3.5$ mmol/L). In the surgical setting, total body K^+ is typically decreased by gastrointestinal losses, excessive diuretic administration, and prolonged malnutrition, particularly in alcoholic patients. Prolonged alkalosis that also results in hypokalemia (e. g., due to gastric losses of hydrochloric acid and K^+) results in a so−called "paradoxical aciduria" as the nephron conserves K^+ at the expense of H^+, which maintains the alkalosis instead of correcting it an attempt to prevent life−threatening hypokalemia.

Clinical manifestation: The earliest clinical manifestation is myasthenia, from the numbness of the limbs to the trunk and respiratory muscle. It can lead to dyspnea, asphyxia. Additionally, the patients could appear anorexia, nausea and vomiting, abdominal distention, diminished intestinal peristalsis. The hallmark signs of hypokalemia are decreased muscle contractility eventually leading to diaphragmatic paralysis, electrocardiogram(EKG) changes including a flattened or inverted T wave and a prominent U wave, and cardiac arrhythmias, which may present an immediate threat to life.

Diagnosis: Hypokalemia is suggested by a patient's history, physical examination. Further electrocardiogram examine can be used as an auxiliary diagnosis. $K^+ < 3.5$ mmol/L is very important.

Treatment: When hypokalemia develops acutely it should be corrected with parenteral supplementation. Parenteral administration of K^+ must be done carefully so as not to cause iatrogenic hyperkalemia. In cases of chronic hypokalemia in which neuromuscular and cardiac manifestations are absent, oral supplementation (either through dietary changes or oral potassium chloride administration) should suffice.

3.2 Hyperkalemia

Etiology：In the surgical setting，hyperkalemia is often caused by crush injuries，burns and other catabolism-inducing events，renal insufficiency，adrenal insufficiency，and excessive K^+ administration. Acidosis may cause hyperkalemia as the intracellular space buffers acidemia by exchanging H^+ from the extracellular space for K^+ from within cells.

Clinical manifestation：The clinical manifestation is not specificity. It can lead to consciousness，abnormal sensation，weak and feeble. Hyperkalemia has few outward signs and symptoms until potentially lethal cardiac arrhythmias manifest. Initial ECG changes include flattened P waves and peaked T waves. Widening of the QRS complex is a later finding and demands immediate intervention，as it portends the imminent onset of ventricular fibrillation.

Diagnosis：Hyperkalemia is suggested by a patient's history，physical examination. Further electrocardiogram examine can be used as an auxiliary diagnosis. $K^+>5.5$ mmol/L is very important.

Treatment：A serum K^+ of 6.5 mmol/L or greater is a medical emergency and must prompt immediate intervention. The patient must be placed on continuous ECG monitoring. Initial treatment should consist of intravenous administration of 50% dextrose in water，10 units of regular insulin，and calcium gluconate，as well as inhaled β-adrenergic agonists like albuterol. Insulin，glucose，and β-agonists drive K^+ from the extracellular space into the intracellular space，while calcium gluconate increases the excitability threshold of the myocardium，protecting against arrhythmias. If these measures are unsuccessful，hemodialysis may be required. Slowly developing hyperkalemia not severe enough to warrant intravenous interventions may be treated with oral sodium polystyrene sulfonate，which causes a slow enteral K^+ wasting.

Chapter 4

Maladjustment of Magnesium

Magnesium: The magnesium ion (Mg^{2+}) is an essential cofactor in many of the most important biochemical reactions in the body. Adenosine triphosphate (ATP) must be bound to Mg^{2+} to be biologically active. Mg^{2+} is required for every step of DNA transcription and translation, nerve conduction, ion transport and Ca^{2+} channel activity. 50%–60% of total body magnesium is found in the bones. The large majority of the rest is intracellular, and approximately 1% is extracellular. A constant proportion of dietary Mg^{2+} is absorbed by the gut. If gut absorption exceeds Mg^{2+} needs, the excess is excreted by the kidneys. If dietary intake is insufficient the kidney retains Mg^{2+}, with urinary levels dropping to nearly zero.

4.1 Hypomagnesemia

Etiology: Hypomagnesemia occurs in the setting of malnutrition (especially malnutrition associated with alcoholism), gastrointestinal losses (especially prolonged diarrheal loses), diuretic or aminoglycoside use, hyper–or hypocalcemia, and hypophosphatemia.

Presentation: In the surgical setting, hypomagnesemia most commonly presents as hypokalemia refractory to parenteral K^+ administration. Hypomagnesemia may cause sedation, muscle paralysis, tetany, seizures, and coma.

Treatment: Parenteral administration of Mg^{2+} is generally preferred to oral supplementation, as orally–administered magnesium is a cathartic agent.

4.2 Hypermagnesemia

Etiology: Hypermagnesemia is rare in the surgical setting, but may develop in acute renal failure.

Presentation: At high concentrations, Mg^{2+} acts as a Ca^{2+} antagonist. Thus although hypermagnesemia may cause lethargy, weakness and diminished deep tendon reflexes, it most often presents as cardiac arrhythmias. Peaked T waves and widening of the QRS complex occur, which may progress to complete heart block, arrhythmias, and eventually asystole.

Treatment: If hypermagnesemia is mild and caused by supplementation, withdrawal of supplementation, and close monitoring should be sufficient treatment. If hypermagnesemia is significant and causing ECG changes, calcium gluconate should be administered intravenously so as to overwhelm the Ca^{2+}-antagonizing effect of Mg^{2+} in neuromuscular function. Diuretic therapy may be required. In severe cases and in cases caused by renal failure, hemodialysis may be required.

Chapter 5

Maladjustment of Calcium

Calcium (Ca^{2+}) is involved in a wide variety of physiologic processes, from maintenance of bone strength to neuromuscular function. Half of serum Ca^{2+} is protein-bound, chiefly to albumin. The unbound fraction is physiologically active, while the bound fraction is not; this unbound (or "ionized") fraction is normally held constant across a wide range of plasma Ca^{2+}. Ca^{2+} homeostasis is influenced by vitamin D, parathyroid hormone, calcitonin, acid-base balance, and PO_4^{3-} homeostasis. Standard laboratory tests measure total serum Ca^{2+}, including the fraction bound to albumin. Thus, a low Ca^{2+} value on a serum chemistry may reflect hypoalbuminemia rather than true hypocalcemia.

5.1 Hypocalcemia

Etiology: In the surgical setting is often caused by hypothyroidism and hypoparathyroidism (either organic or iatrogenic after thyroid or parathyroid surgery), pancreatitis, renal insufficiency, crush injuries, severe soft tissue infections, and necrotizing infections like necrotizing fasciitis.

Presentation: Hypocalcemia manifests as neuromuscular dysfunction, causing hyperactive deep tendon reflexes, Chvostek sign, muscle cramps, abdominal pain, and in severe cases tetany and cardiac arrhythmias.

Treatment: In persistent hypocalcemia, whole blood pH must be determined, and any alkalosis corrected. Calcium supplementation, enterally if possible and parenterally if necessary, may be required. Chronic hypoparathyroidism and hypothyroidism require chronic vitamin D and Ca^{2+} supplementation, and may require aluminum hydroxide to decrease PO_4^{3-} absorption from the gut.

5.2 Hypercalcemia

Etiology: Hypercalcemia in the surgical setting is often caused by primary or tertiary hyperparathyroidism, hyperthyroidism, bony cancer metastases, paraneoplastic syndromes in which parathyroid hormone-related peptide is elaborated, and as a complication of thiazide diuretic use.

Presentation: Signs and symptoms of acute hypercalcemia include anorexia, nausea and vomiting, polydipsia, polyuria, depression, confusion, memory loss, stupor, coma, psychosis, and cardiac arrhythmias. Dyspepsia, constipation, acute pancreatitis, nephrolithiasis, osteoporosis, osteomalacia, and osteitis fibrosa cystica are indicative of chronic hypercalcemia. Untreated longstanding hypercalcemia, especially in conjunction with untreated hyperphosphatemia and especially in patients with chronic renal failure, may lead to calciphylaxis and high morbidity and mortality.

Treatment: In a patient with healthy kidneys, administration of large volumes of normal saline over 1 – 3 days will often correct even a profound hypercalcemia. Treatment may be followed by targeting a urine output of 2–3 mL/(kg · h) and monitoring serum Ca^{2+} levels closely. Loop diuretics (e. g. , furosemide) inhibit Ca^{2+} reabsorption in the nephron, and will aid in calciuresis, but should not be used until the patient is clinically euvolemic. Calcitonin increases osteoblastic activity and inhibits osteoclastic activity, locking Ca^{2+} into the skeleton. In severe hypercalcemia or hypercalcemia secondary to renal failure, hemodialysis may be required. In patients whose hypercalcemia is caused by malignancy, bisphosphonates may provide a means of controlling Ca^{2+} levels in the medium and long term. In hypercalcemia caused by hyperparathyroidism, parathyroidectomy is potentially curative, but is reserved for the elective setting unless the patient is in hypercalcemic crisis which is refractory to optimal medical management.

Chapter 6

Maladjustment of Phosphate

Phosphate: Like Ca^{2+} and Mg^{2+}, the majority of PO_4^{3-} is found in the skeleton. The large majority of the remainder is found intracellularly, where it functions as a constituent of ATP. Like Mg^{2+}, it is essential to energy metabolism.

6.1 Hypophosphatemia

Etiology: Chronic hypophosphatemia is typically found in malnourished patients, especially alcoholic patients. It may also occur in patients who consume large amounts of antacids, and following liver resection. An important and often overlooked cause of hypophosphatemia is refeeding syndrome. This syndrome occurs after a patient who has been without significant caloric intake for at least 5 days begins to eat again. Severe hypophosphatemia may occur as phosphofructokinase binds PO_4^{3-} to glucose to begin glycolysis, and as PO_4^{3-} is consumed in production of large amounts of ATP. The syndrome usually manifests within 4 days of starting refeeding.

Presentation: Hypophosphatemia results in muscular and neurologic dysfunction. Muscle weakness, diplopia, depressed cardiac output, respiratory depression due to diaphragmatic weakness, confusion, delirium, coma, and death may all develop. An uncommon presentation is with rhabdomyolysis. Hypophosphatemia may leave a patient ventilator-dependent as they are unable to replenish ATP stores for proper functioning of the muscles of respiration.

Treatment: Severe hypophosphatemia is a medical emergency, requiring parenteral administration of Na_3PO_4 or K_3PO_4, depending on the patient's electrolyte profile. If hypophosphatemia is not severe it may be treated with oral supplementation, either with sodium phosphate/potassium phosphate or with high-phosphate foods like milk.

6.2 Hyperphosphatemia

Etiology: Hyperphosphatemia is unusual in the surgical setting, typically developing in the setting of severe renal disease or after severe trauma.

Presentation: Hyperphosphatemia is usually asymptomatic, but it may cause hypocalcemia as calcium phosphate precipitates and is deposited in tissues.

Treatment: Hyperphosphatemia is treated by diuresis, administration of phosphate-binders like aluminum hydroxide, or hemodialysis in the setting of renal failure.

Chapter 7

Acid–base Disorders

The body's handling of hydrogen ion (H^+) is a particularly complex example of electrolyte management, as it involves not only dietary intake and renal clearance but also extracellular and intracellular buffer systems and respiratory as well as renal excretion.

7.1 Normal Physiology

An acid is a chemical that donates a H^+ in solution, for example, HCl or H_2CO_3. A base is a chemical that accepts H^+ in solution, for example, Cl^- or HCO_3^-. The concentration of H^+ in a solution determines the acidity of the solution. Acidity of a solution is measured by pH, which is the negative logarithm of H^+ concentration expressed in mol/L. The strength of an acid is determined by its degree of dissociation into H^+ and the corresponding base, as expressed in the Henderson–Hasselbalch (H–H) equation:

$$pH = pK \times \log [A^-]/[HA]$$

where K = dissociation constant, $[A^-]$ = concentration of acid, $[HA]$ = concentration of base. Stronger acids have a higher K than weaker acids. The main buffer system in human blood is a carbonic acid/bicarbonate (H_2CO_3/HCO_3^-) system. Using the H–H equation, the pH of this buffer system is calculated as below:

$$pH = pK \times \log [HCO_3^-]/[H_2CO_3]$$

H_2CO_3 in the blood exists mostly as CO_2 (the so-called "volatile acid"); conversion of one to the other is catalyzed by the enzyme carbonic anhydrase. The dissociation constant of CO_2 is 0. 03. Making these substitutions into the equation:

$$pH = pK \times \log [HCO_3^-]/[PCO_2 \times 0.03]$$

where PCO_2 is the partial pressure of CO_2. The pK for this buffer system is 6. 1. In arterial blood, HCO_3^- normally ranges from 21 to 37 mmol/L, while PCO_2 ranges from 36 to 44 mmHg. Thus, arterial pH normally ranges from 7. 36 to 7. 44. Venous blood is easier to sample than arterial blood. Venous blood gas sampling varies significantly between institutions, and between central, mixed, and different peripheral sites of sampling, and thus must be interpreted with caution.

7.2 Acid-base Disorders

The fundamental acid-base disorders are as follows:

Acidemia: pH below the normal range.

Alkalemia: pH above the normal range.

Acidosis: a process that lowers the pH of the extracellular fluid.

Alkalosis: a process that raises the pH of the extracellular fluid.

There are four primary or simple (as opposed to mixed) acid-base disorders:

Metabolic acidosis: a disorder in which decreased HCO_3^- causes decreased pH.

Metabolic alkalosis: a disorder in which increased HCO_3^- causes increased pH.

Respiratory acidosis: a disorder in which increased PCO_2 causes decreased pH.

Respiratory alkalosis: a disorder in which decreased PCO_2 increased pH are found.

Acid-base disorders are classified as simple or mixed. In a simple acid-base disorder, only one primary acid-base disorder is present, and the compensatory response is appropriate. In a mixed acid-base disorder, more than one primary acid-base disorder is present. Mixed acid-base disorders are suspected from a patient's history, from a lesser or greater than expected compensatory response, and from analysis of the serum electrolytes and anion gap (AG).

The use of a systematic approach to identifying and diagnosing acid-base disorders is essential. One must first determine alkalemia or academia based on pH. One must then determine whether a metabolic derangement with respiratory compensation or a respiratory derangement with metabolic compensation exists, based on the HCO_3^- and PCO_2 values(Table 3-7-1).

Table 3-7-1 Changes in HCO_3^- and PCO_2 in primary acid-base disorders

Disorder	pH	HCO_3^-	PCO_2
Metabolic acidosis	↓	↓	↓ (compensatory)
Metabolic alkalosis	↑	↑	↑ (compensatory)
Respiratory acidosis	↓	↑ (compensatory)	↑
Respiratory alkalosis	↑	↓ (compensatory)	↓

Whether the disturbance is primarily respiratory or metabolic, some degree of compensatory change occurs in an attempt to maintain normal pH. Changes in PCO_2 (respiratory disorders) are compensated for by changes in HCO_3^- (metabolic/renal compensation), and vice versa.

Acute respiratory disorders may develop in matter of moments. Such circumstances may not allow sufficient time for renal compensation, resulting in severe pH changes without significant compensatory changes. By contrast, chronic respiratory disturbances allow the full range of renal compensatory mechanisms to function. In these circumstances, pH may remain normal or nearly normal despite wide variations in PCO_2. By contrast, respiratory compensation for metabolic disorders occurs quickly. Thus there is little difference in respiratory compensation for acute and chronic metabolic disorders.

7.2.1 Metabolic acidosis

Metabolic acidosis is caused by increased production of H^+ or by excessive loss of HCO_3^-. In the surgical setting,metabolic acidosis is commonly encountered in trauma,critically ill,and postoperative patients,and especially in patients in shock. The body's response to metabolic acidosis is respiratory hyperventilation,"blowing off" H_2CO_3 as CO_2 and correcting the acidosis. This response is rapid,beginning within 30 minutes of the onset of acidosis and reaching full compensation within 24 hours. The adequacy of the respiratory response to metabolic acidosis is evaluated using Winter's formula:

$$PCO_2 = (1.5 \times HCO_3^- \text{ in mmol/L}) + (8 \pm 2)$$

If compensation is inadequate or excessive—that is,if PCO_2 is not within the range predicted by Winter's formula—one must evaluate for a mixed acid-base disorder.

Etiology:①Excessive basic substance loss:diarrhea,intestinal fistula,biliary fistula,pancreatic fistula leads to HCO_3^- loss. ②Excessive acid production:shock leads to circulation failure and tissue ischemic anoxia,it finally lead to lactic acidosis. Diabetes or long term inability to eat lead to overadipose decomposition and ketoacidosis. ③Renal insufficiency:endogenetic H^+ can not expulate in vitro and HCO_3^- reabsorption reduction lead to acidosis.

Clinical manifestation:Mild metabolic acidosis has no special symptoms,the symptoms of severe patients are vertigo,abnormal sensation,weak and feeble,dullness and irritability. The most obvious change is that the breathing becomes deeper and faster. Breathing can reach 40 times/min.

Exhaled gas with ketone taste. The signs of patients are cheek flush,tachycardia,low blood pressure.

Diagnosis:Metabolic acidosis is suggested by a patient's diarrhea,intestinal fistula,shock history,deeper and faster breathing sign. Further blood gas analysis examine can be used as an auxiliary diagnosis including $H^+ \downarrow$, $HCO_3^- \downarrow$. Compensable pH can be in the normal range,but HCO_3^- ,BE,PCO_2 appear a certain degree of reduction.

Treatment:Treatment of metabolic acidosis involves identifying the underlying cause of the acidosis and correcting it. Usually,this is sufficient. If this is not sufficient,correction may require administration of exogenous alkali in the form of $NaHCO_3^-$ to correct the derangement in pH. The degree of restoration is estimated by subtracting the plasma HCO_3^- from the normal value (24 mmol/L at our institution)and multiplying the resulting number by half TBW. This is a useful empiric formula,as in practice it is unwise (and unnecessary)to administer enough $NaHCO_3^-$ to completely correct pH. Doing so will likely cause fluid overload from the large Na^+ load delivered,and will likely over correct the acidosis. In patients with a chronic metabolic acidosis,often seen in chronic renal failure,alkali may be administered chronically as oral $NaHCO_3^-$. Efforts to minimize the magnitude of HCO_3^- loss in these patients must be undertaken as well.

7.2.2　Metabolic alkalosis

Etiology:Metabolic alkalosis is often encountered in surgical patients. The pathogenesis is complex,but often involves the following:①Loss of H^+,usually via gastric losses of HCl. ②Hypovolemia. ③Total body K^+ depletion. All three are commonly encountered with vomiting or gastric suctioning,diuretic use,and renal failure. HCl is secreted by chief cells in the gastric mucosa;simultaneously,HCO_3^- is absorbed in the blood. $NaHCO_3$ is then secreted by the pancreas into the lumen of the duodenum,neutralizing the gastric acid,after which the neutralized acid and base are reabsorbed by the small intestine. Thus,under normal circumstances there is no net alteration of acid-base balance in the function of the gastrointestinal tract. However,when H^+ is lost from the gastric lumen,for example,through emesis,gastric suctioning or gastric drainage—the result is loss of H^+ from the gastric lumen and a corresponding gain of HCO_3^- in the blood,leading to metabolic alkalosis. Normally,the kidneys excrete excess HCO_3^-;however,if volume depletion accompanies HCO_3^- excess,the kidneys attempt to maintain normovolemia by increasing tubular reabsorption of Na^+,which is reabsorbed in an electrically neutral fashion by increasing reabsorption of Cl^- and HCO_3^-. This impairs HCO_3^- excretion, perpetuating the metabolic alkalosis. Severe K^+ depletion further exacerbates metabolic alkalosis. To preserve K^+, Na^+ is exchanged for H^+ in the kidney, through the Na^+-K^+ and Na^+-H^+ ATPases in the distal renal tubule. This explains why severe metabolic alkalosis with hypokalemia results in paradoxical aciduria. In such cases, urine Na^+, K^+, and Cl^- concentrations are low, and the urine is acidic. In simple volume depletion, urine Cl^- alone is low and the urine is alkaline. Severe metabolic alkalosis may lead to tetany and seizures, as seen in hypokalemia and hypocalcemia. Adequate respiratory compensation for metabolic alkalosis should raise PCO_2 by 0.7 mmHg for every 1 mmol/L elevation in HCO_3^-. Generally, respiratory compensation will not raise PCO_2 beyond 55 mmHg. Thus a PCO_2 greater than 60 mmHg in the setting of metabolic alkalosis suggests a mixed metabolic alkalosis and respiratory acidosis.

Clinical manifestation: Mild metabolic acidosis often has no special symptoms, the symptoms of severe patients are vertigo, abnormal sensation, weak and feeble, sleepiness and delirium. The most obvious change is that the breathing becomes shallow and slowly.

Diagnosis: Metabolic acidosis is suggested by a patient's history, shallow and slowly breathing sign. Further blood gas analysis examine can be used as an auxiliary diagnosis including BE $\uparrow$, HCO_3^- $\uparrow$. Compensable pH can be in the normal range, but at the decompensation status pH and HCO_3^- is increased.

Treatment of metabolic alkalosis includes fluid administration, usually normal saline. With adequate fluid repletion, tubular reabsorption of Na^+ is diminished, and the kidneys will excrete excess HCO_3^-. K^+ must be repleted, both to allow for correction of the alkalosis and to prevent life-threatening hypokalemia. Repletion of volume with normal saline and of potassium with KCl also provides the nephron with needed Cl^-, allowing for reabsorption of K^+ and Na^+ with Cl^- instead of HCO_3^-. Acetazolamide, a carbonic anhydrase inhibitor diuretic, may also be used to treat metabolic alkalosis as long as the patient is euvolemic. Administration of exogenous acid in the form of HCl may be employed in the case of profound alkalosis.

7.2.3 Respiratory acidosis

Acute respiratory acidosis occurs when ventilation suddenly becomes inadequate. CO_2 accumulates in the blood, and as carbonic anhydrase coverts it to H_2CO_3, acidosis develops.

Etiology: Acute respiratory acidosis is most common in conditions where gas exchange is physically impaired, resulting in decreased ventilation. These conditions typically involve decreased oxygenation as well. They include respiratory arrest, acute airway obstruction, pulmonary edema, pneumonia, saddle pulmonary embolus, aspiration of intraoral contents, and acute respiratory distress syndrome. Hypoventilation may occur in patients postoperatively who are oversedated (e. g. , from narcotics, benzodiazepines, or as they recover from general anesthesia). Pain, especially from large abdominal incisions or from rib fractures, leads to respiratory splinting and hypoventilation. Excess ethanol ingestion decreases respiratory drive, thereby impairing ventilation. Head trauma, either by direct damage to central nervous system respiratory centers or by global brain damage and brainstem herniation, may impair ventilation. Patients with obesity hypoventilation syndrome and obstructive sleep apnea may develop a periodically recurring acute respiratory acidosis, leading eventually to some renal compensation. True chronic respiratory acidosis arises from chronic respiratory failure in which impaired ventilation leads to persistently elevated PCO_2, for example, as seen in chronic obstructive pulmonary disease. Chronic respiratory acidosis is usually well tolerated with adequate renal compensation, thus pH may be normal or near normal. Over 80% of increased acid produced in respiratory acidosis is buffered by the body's tissues and intracellular hemoglobin. The remaining minority is buffered by HCO_3^- in the blood, which the kidney reclaims and reabsorbs. Thus, metabolic (renal) compensation for respiratory disorders is a much slower process than respiratory compensation for metabolic disorders. Furthermore, in acute respiratory acidosis renal mechanisms may not have had time to function at all, and HCO_3^- may be within normal limits. Adequate renal compensation for respiratory acidosis involves an increase in HCO_3^- of 1 mmol/L for every 10 mmHg increase in PCO_2.

Clinical manifestation: the symptoms of patients are chest tightness, dyspnea, restlessness, headache and cyanosis. Along with acidosis aggravation, the patients could appear blood pressure instability and coma.

Diagnosis: Respiratory acidosis is suggested by a patient's history, symptom and sign. Further blood gas analysis examine can be used as an auxiliary diagnosis including pH ↓, PCO_2 ↑, HCO_3^- can be in the normal range, but at the chronic respiratory acidosis status pH ↓ and PCO_2, HCO_3^- is increased.

Treatment of respiratory acidosis involves restoration of adequate ventilation by treating the underlying cause. Aggressive chest physical therapy and pulmonary toilet should beinstituted on all postsurgical patients. Patients with pulmonary edema should receive appropriate diuretic therapy, and patients with pneumonia should receive appropriate antibiosis. Naloxone or flumazenil should be used as needed in the setting of narcotic or benzodiazepine overdose, respectively. If necessary, endotracheal intubation and mechanical ventilation should be employed in order to correct PCO_2. Acute respiratory acidosis should be corrected rapidly. However, too rapid correction of chronic respiratory acidosis risks causing posthypercapnic metabolic alkalosis syndrome, characterized by muscle spasms and by potentially lethal cardiac arrhythmias.

7.2.4   Respiratory alkalosis

Hyperventilation decreases PCO_2, leading to a respiratory alkalosis.

Etiology: In the surgical setting, anxiety, agitation, and pain are common causes of respiratory alkalosis. Hyperventilation and respiratory alkalosis may be an early sign of sepsis and of moderate pulmonary embolism. Chronic respiratory alkalosis occurs in chronic pulmonary and liver disease.

Treatment: Acute respiratory alkalosis is treated by addressing the underlying cause. Patients may require pain control, sedation/anxiolytics, and even paralyzation and mechanical ventilation if necessary. Well-compensated chronic respiratory alkalosis does not require treatment. In these cases, rapid correction of PCO_2 leads to so-called posthypocapnic hyperchloremic metabolic acidosis, which is often severe. The renal response to respiratory alkalosis is decreased reabsorption of filtered HCO_3^- and increased urinary HCO_3^- excretion. HCO_3^- decreases as Cl^- increases, since Na^+ is reabsorbed with Cl^- instead of with HCO_3^-. This same pattern is seen in hyperchloremic metabolic acidosis; the two are distinguished only by pH measurements. Adequate renal compensation for respiratory alkalosis involves a decrease in HCO_3^- of 2 mmol/L for every 10 mmHg decrease in PCO_2.

7.2.5   Mixed acid-base disorders

Many common pathophysiologic processes cause mixed acid-base disorders. In these situations, pH may be normal or near normal, but compensatory changes are either inadequate or exaggerated. One way of determining the presence of a simple versus mixed disorder is to plot the patient's acid-base disorder on a nomogram. If the set of data falls outside one of the confidence bands, then by definition the patient has a mixed disorder. If the acid-base data falls within one of the confidence bands, the patient more likely has a simple acid-base disorder.

Acid-base nomogram for use in evaluation of clinical acid-base disorders. Hydrogen ion concentration (top) or blood pH (bottom) is plotted against plasma HCO_3^- concentration; curved lines are isopleths of CO_2

tension ($PaCO_2$, mmHg). Knowing any two of these variables permits estimation of the third. The circle in the center represents the range of normal values; the shaded bands represent the 95% confidence limits of four common acid-base disturbances: I, acute respiratory acidosis; II, acute respiratory alkalosis; III, chronic respiratory acidosis; IV, sustained metabolic acidosis. Points lying outside these shaded areas are mixed disturbances and indicate two primary acid-base disorders. As with simple acid-base disorders, a systematic approach to mixed acid-base disorders is essential. First, determine the primary acid-base disorder. Next, determine whether or not adequate compensation has occurred, using the equations and rules given above. If compensation is "inadequate," meaning too little or too much, the patient has a mixed acid-base disorder.

- Expected compensation in primary acid-base disorders.
- Metabolic acidosis Winter's formula: $PCO_2 = 1.5 \times HCO_3^- + (8 \pm 2)$.
- Metabolic alkalosis ⇑ PCO_2 0.7 mm Hg for every 1 mmol/L increase in HCO_3^-.
- Respiratory acidosis ⇑ HCO_3^- 1 mmol/L for every 10 mm Hg increase in PCO_2.
- Respiratory alkalosis ⇓ HCO_3^- 2 mmol/L for every 10 mm Hg decrease in PCO_2.

An additional step is needed in the case of metabolic acidosis. Axer AG has been calculated, the "delta-delta" or "delta ratio" or "gap-gap" (three names for the same parameter) should be calculated: $\Delta\Delta = \Delta AG/\Delta HCO_3^-$ where $\Delta\Delta$ = delta-delta, ΔAG = AG-maximum normal AG, ΔHCO_3^- = normal HCO_3^- - HCO_3^-.

At our institution, maximum normal AG is 12 mmol/L and normal HCO_3^- concentration is 24 mmol/L, thus $\Delta\Delta = (AG-12)/(24-HCO_3^-)$. $\Delta\Delta < 1$ indicates the coexistence of an AG and a non-AG metabolic acidosis, that is, a metabolic acidosis caused by increased production of acid and by renal loss of HCO_3^-. This may occur in the setting of diabetic ketoacidosis. $\Delta\Delta > 1$ indicates the coexistence of an AG metabolic acidosis and a metabolic alkalosis. This can occur in the intensive care unit in patients who have an underlying AG metabolic acidosis and are also undergoing diuresis or gastric suctioning, leading to the concurrent metabolic alkalosis. The most common mixed acid-base disorder in surgical patients is a metabolic acidosis superimposed on a respiratory alkalosis. This occurs in patients with septic shock and hepatorenal syndrome, and also in the case of salicylate poisoning. Since the two acid-base disorders disrupt H^+ homeostasis in opposite directions, the patient's pH may be normal or near normal. Mixed respiratory acidosis and metabolic alkalosis is less common, occurring in the setting of cardiorespiratory arrest, which is a medical emergency.

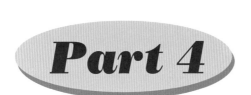

Part 4

Shock

Chapter 1

Introduction of Shock

Shock may be defined as acute circulatory failure with inadequate or inappropriate perfusion resulting in generalized cellular hypoxia. Inadequate tissue perfusion for whatever reason causes cellular hypoxia, thereby precipitating a number of intracellular reactions and a cytokine cascade, culminating in a metabolic acidosis. The latter, by altering vascular permeability, creates a vicious circle: there are increasing plasma losses from the circulation with reducing cardiac output (CO) and further acidosis, so that the state of shock becomes irreversible.

1.1　Classification of Shock

There are many classifications of shock, but there is no consensus. This chapter divides shock into five categories: hypovolemic, infective, cardiogenic, neurogenic and anaphylactic shock. The shock caused by trauma and hemorrhagic stroke is classified as hypovolemic shock, but hypovolemic and septic shock are most common in surgery.

1.2　Pathophysiology

The reduction of effective circulating blood volume and insufficient tissue perfusion and the production of inflammatory mediators are the common pathophysiological basis of all kinds of shock.

1.2.1　Changes in microcirculation

In the process of shock caused by insufficient effective circulation, the microcirculation, which accounts for 20% of the total circulating capacity, correspondingly changes at different stages.

(1) Microcirculation systole period

In the early stage of shock, due to the significant decrease in effective circulating blood volume, the capacity of circulation decreased and arterial blood pressure decreased. At this point, the body adjusts and corrections the pathological changes through a series of compensatory mechanisms. Including aortic arch and carotid sinus baroreceptor cause vasomotor reflex, the sympathetic adrenal axis excitation leads to a large number of catecholamine release and the increase of renin-angiotensin secretion, which can cause a faster heart rate, increased cardiac output to maintain the relative stability of the circulation, and through selective contraction. The small vessels of the peripheral (skin, skeletal muscle) and viscera (such as liver, spleen and gastrointestinal tract) redistribute the circulating blood volume and ensure effective perfusion of vital organs such as heart and brain. The effects of visceral small movement, vascular smooth muscle and the anterior sphincter of capillaries were strongly affected by catecholamine and other hormones such as catecholamine and other hormones. The short circuit was open and the peripheral vascular resistance and the blood circulation increased. The contraction of the sphincter and the sphincter of the capillaries were helpful to the reabsorption and blood of the tissue. The capacity is partially compensated. However, the microcirculation is caused by the contraction of the anterior contracted muscles, resulting in "no blood coming out," and the blood volume is reduced, and the tissue is still in low perfusion and anoxia. If we can remove the cause and recover at this time, shock is often easier to be corrected.

(2) Microcirculation expansion period

If the shock continues to progress, the microcirculation will be further open to the arteriovenous short circuit and the direct passage, which makes the original inadequacy of the tissue perfusion more serious, and the cells are in the anaerobic metabolism due to severe hypoxia, and the release of energy deficiency, the accumulation of lactic acid products and the mediators of the vasodilator, such as histamine and bradykinin, will be released. These substances can directly cause the relaxation of the sphincter of the anterior sphincter, and the sphincter is still in a state of contraction due to its low sensitivity. Results the blood stagnation, the increase of blood pressure in the capillary network, the increase of blood pressure in the capillary network, the increase of the permeability of blood plasma, the concentration of blood and the increase of blood viscosity in the capillary network, thus further reducing the blood circulation, the decrease of the cardiac output, the insufficient perfusion of the heart and brain, and the aggravation of shock. At this time, the characteristics of microcirculation are extensive expansion. Clinically, patients are manifested as progressive decline in blood pressure, confusion in consciousness, cyanosis and acidosis.

(3) Microcirculation failure period

If the disease continues to develop, it will enter irreversible shock. The sticky blood in the microcirculation is high in the acid environment. Red blood cells and platelets tend to accumulate and form microthrombus in the blood vessels, and even cause diffuse intravascular coagulation. At this time, because of the lack of blood perfusion in the tissue, the cells are in the condition of severe anoxia and lack of energy. The lysosome membrane in the cell is broken and various acidic hydrolysate in the enzyme is spillover, causing autolysis and damaging the other cells around it. It eventually causes damage to large tissues, organs and even multiple organs.

1.2.2　Metabolic change

(1) Metabolic acidosis caused by anaerobic metabolism

Anaerobic release of glycolysis occurs when oxygen release does not meet the oxygen demand of cells. Pyruvate changes into lactic acid in the cytoplasm, thus, as the oxygen supply decreases, the production of lactic acid increases and the concentration of pyruvate decreases, that is, the increase of blood lactate concentration and the increase of lactic acid/pyruvic acid (L/P) ratio. Lactate content and L/P ratio can reflect the condition of hypoxia in patients without lactic acidosis. When pH<7.2 was developed to severe acidosis, the responsiveness of cardiovascular to catecholamine decreased, which showed slow heartbeat, dilatation of blood vessels and the decrease of cardiac output, and the dissociation curve of oxygenated hemoglobin moved right.

(2) Energy metabolism disorder

Trauma and infection make the body stress state, sympathetic adrenal medullary system and hypothalamus pituitary adrenocortical Zhou Xingfen, which make the body catecholamine and adrenocortical hormone rise significantly, thus inhibiting protein synthesis and promoting protein decomposition in order to provide energy and synthesis of acute phase protein materials for the body. The above changes in hormone levels can also promote gluconeogenesis and inhibit carbohydrate degradation, leading to elevated blood glucose levels.

In stress state, protein is consumed as a substrate. When proteins with special functions are consumed, the complex physiological process can not be completed, which leads to multiple organ dysfunction syndrome. The metabolism of fat is obviously enhanced when stress is stressed, and it is the main source of energy for critical patients.

(3) Release of inflammatory mediators and ischemia-reperfusion injury

Severe trauma, infection and shock can stimulate the body to release excessive inflammatory mediators to form "waterfall like" chain amplification reactions. Inflammatory mediators include interleukin, tumor necrosis factor, colony-stimulating factor, interferon and vasodilator nitric oxide (NO). Reactive oxygen species can cause lipid peroxidation and cell membrane disruption.

Metabolic acidosis and energy deficiency also affect the barrier function of various cell membranes. After the damage of cell membrane, besides the increase of permeability, there are dysfunction of ion pump on cell membrane, such as Na^+-K^+ pump and calcium pump. The abnormal distribution of ion and body fluid, such as sodium and calcium ion, can not be discharged into the human cell and the potassium ion can not enter the cell outside the cell, which causes the decrease of sodium and the increase of blood potassium, and the extracellular fluid enters the cell with sodium ion, causing the decrease of extracellular fluid and the cell swelling and death, while a large number of calcium ions are added into the cell. In addition to activation of lysosomes, human cells also increase calcium in mitochondria and destroy mitochondria in many ways. After the rupture of the lysosome membrane, many toxic factors such as MDF and bradykinin can also be produced in addition to the release of many hydrolases that cause cell autolysis and tissue damage. After the mitochondrial membrane damage, the membrane lipid degradation produces the toxic products such as thromboxane and leukotrienes, which show the swelling of mitochondria, the disappearance of mitochondrial crista, and the oxidative phosphorylation of cells to influence the generation of energy.

1.2.3　Secondary damage of visceral organs

(1) Lung

Hypoxia can damage the capillary endothelial cells and alveolar epithelium in the lungs and reduce the surfactant. In the process of resuscitation, if a large amount of blood is used in the process of recovery, a large number of micropolymers can cause pulmonary microcirculation embolism, and some alveoli are collapsing, inflexible and edema, some of the pulmonary blood tubes are incarcerated or inadequately perfused, causing pulmonary shunt and the pulmonary shunt. Dead space ventilation increased, leading to acute respiratory distress syndrome (ARDS). The risk of ARDS is higher in elderly patients. The mortality of elderly patients over 65 years old is correspondingly increased. The mortality of ARDS patients with systemic infection is also increased significantly. ARDS often occurs in shock stage or within 48-72 hours after stabilization.

(2) Kidney

Because of the decrease of blood pressure and catecholamine secretion, the renal vascular involvement and effective circulation capacity decreased, and the renal filtration rate decreased significantly, resulting in oliguria. During shock, the blood flow in the kidney redistributes and turns to the medulla, so it can not only reduce the amount of urine, but also lead to the renal tubular ischemic necrosis in the cortical area, and the acute renal failure can occur.

(3) Brain

Cerebral perfusion pressure and descent of blood flow will lead to cerebral anoxia. Ischemia, CO_2 retention and acidosis can cause swelling of brain cells and increase of vascular permeability, resulting in brain edema and intracranial pressure increase. Patients may develop mental disorders. Severe cases can cause hernia and coma.

(4) Heart

Coronary artery blood flow decreases, leading to ischemia and acidosis, thereby damaging the myocardium. When the myocardial microcirculation is thrombosis, it can cause focal necrosis of the myocardium. The myocardium is rich in xanthine oxidase and is vulnerable to ischemia-reperfusion injury. Abnormal electrolyte will affect the contractile function of the myocardium.

(5) Gastrointestinal tract

Because the density of angiotensin II receptor in the mesenteric vessels is higher than that of other parts, it is highly sensitive to vasopressin, and the blood flow of the superior mesenteric artery can be reduced by 70% in shock. Intestinal mucosa suffers from hypoxic injury due to insufficient perfusion. In addition, intestinal mucosal cells are also rich in xanthine oxidase system and produce ischemia-reperfusion injury, which can cause gastric stress ulcers and enteric infection. As the barrier function of normal mucosal epithelial cells is damaged, the bacteria in the intestinal tract or its toxin translocation through the lymph or portal vein, called bacterial translocation and endotoxin translocation, and form enteric infection, which is an important cause of the development of shock and the formation of multiple organ dysfunction syndrome.

(6) Liver

Shock can cause liver ischemia and hypoxic injury, which can destroy the function of liver synthesis and metabolism. In addition, harmful substances from the gastrointestinal tract can activate liver Kupffer cells and release inflammatory mediators. Histologically, central lobe bleeding and necrosis of liver cells were observed. Biochemical examination showed abnormal metabolism of ALT and blood ammonia. The detoxification and metabolic capacity of the damaged liver decreased, which could lead to endotoxemia and aggravate the existing metabolic disorders and acidosis.

1.3　Clinical Manifestation

According to the pathogenesis of shock, it can be divided into shock compensation stage and shock inhibition stage, or early shock stage or shock stage.

1.3.1　Shock compensatory period

As the body has the corresponding compensatory ability in the early period of the effective circulation of blood, the patient's central nervous system is excitable and the sympathetic adrenal axis is excited. It is manifested as mental tension, excitement or irritability, pale skin, cold limbs, heart rate, pulse pressure, breathing and urine volume. At this point, if handled promptly and properly, shock can be corrected quickly. Otherwise, the disease will continue to develop and enter the stage of shock suppression.

1.3.2　Shock inhibition period

The manifestation: the patient is indifferent, the reaction is slow, even can appear the consciousness blurred or the coma; the cold sweat, the lip acrocyanosis, the pulse speed, the blood pressure drop. In severe cases, the skin and mucous membranes of the whole body are markedly cyanotic, with cold extremities, unclear pulse, blood pressure not detected, and even less urine. If the skin and mucous membrane appear ecchymosis or gastrointestinal bleeding, it indicates that the disease has developed to the stage of disseminated intravascular coagulation. Acute respiratory distress syndrome should be considered if progressive dyspnea, pulse speed, irritability, cyanosis, and general oxygen intake do not improve breathing status. Table 4-1-1 lists the main points of the clinical manifestation of shock.

1.4　Diagnosis

The key is to find shock early in time. The main point is that any serious injury, massive bleeding, severe infection, and allergic patients and people with a history of heart disease should think of the possibility of concurrence with shock; in clinical observation, shock should be suspected for those with symptoms of sweating, excitement, heart rate acceleration, low pulse pressure, or less urine. If the patient has indifference, slow reaction, pale skin, shallow breathing, and systolic pressure below 90 mmHg and less urine, the patient has entered a period of shock inhibition.

1.5　Shock monitoring

Through monitoring, we can not only understand the patient's condition and treatment response, but also provide an objective basis for adjusting the treatment plan.

1.5.1　General monitoring

1.5.1.1　Mental state

It is a reflection of hemoperfusion and circulatory system of brain tissue. For example, the patient's mind is clear, the external stimulus can be reacted normally, indicating that the patient's circulating blood volume is basically sufficient; on the contrary, if the patient's expression is indifferent, uneasy, taunting or drowsiness and coma, it reflects the disorder of the brain due to poor circulation of blood.

1.5.1.2　Skin temperature, color and lustre

It is a sign of the condition of the body surface perfusion. If the patient's extremities are warm, the skin is dry, and the nail or lip is lightly pressed, the temporary ischemia is pale, and the color and lustre quickly turns to normal, indicating the recovery of the end circulation and the improvement of shock; on the contrary, the condition of shock still exists.

Table 4-1-1   The clinical manifestation and degree of shock

Stages	Degree	Spirits	Drgee of thirst	Skin and mucous membrane		Pulse	Blood pressure	Body surface vessel	Urine volume	Estimated blood loss
				Color and lustre	temperature					
Shockcom-pensatory period	Light	With a clear mind, a painful expression, a mental tension	thirsty	Begin to be pale	Normal or cool	Under 100 times/min, there is still strength	Systolicblood pressure is normal or slightly elevated, diastolic blood pressure is increased, pulse pressure is reduced	normal	normal	20% below (below 800 mL)
Shock inhibition period	moderate	The expression is clear, the expression is indifferent	Very thirsty	pale	cold	100-200 times/min	The systolic pressure is 70-90 mmHg, and the pulse pressure is small	Superficial vein collapse, capillary filling is slow	Less urine	20% - 40% (800 - 1600 mL)
	severe	A vague sense of consciousness, even a coma	Very thirsty, there may be no main complaint	Purplish of extremities	Cold(the end of the limb is more obvious)	Fast, weak, or obscure	The systolic pressure is below 70mmHg or can not be measured	Superficial vein collapses, capillary filling is very slow.	Less urine or no urine	More than 40% (above 1600 mL)

1.5.1.3   Blood pressure

Maintaining stable blood pressure is very important in shock treatment. However, blood pressure is not the most sensitive indicator of shock. It is generally considered that systolic blood pressure (<90 mmHg) and pulse pressure (<20 mmHg) are the manifestations of shock. The rise of blood pressure and pulse pressure are signs of shock improvement.

1.5.1.4   Pulse rate

The changes in the pulse rate appear before the change of blood pressure. When the blood pressure is still low, but the pulse rate has been restored and the limbs are warm, the shock tends to improve. Common pulse rate/systolic blood pressure (mmHg) was used to calculate the shock index. The index is <0.5, which indicates no shock. The index >1.0-1.5 indicates shock; The index >2.0 is severe shock.

1.5.1.5   Urine volume

It is a useful index to reflect the condition of renal blood perfusion. Oliguria is usually an incomplete manifestation of early shock and shock resuscitation. The urine volume of <25 mL/h and the increase of specific gravity indicate that there are still renal vasoconstriction and insufficient blood supply, and those with normal blood pressure but low urine volume and low specific gravity suggest that acute renal failure is possible. When urine volume is above 30 mL/h, shock is corrected. In addition, the patients who use hypertonic solution in the resuscitation of the trauma patients may have obvious diuresis, and the brain injury involved in the posterior pituitary may appear in the diabetes insipidus, and the urinary tract injury leads to the oliguria and no urine.

1.5.2　Special monitoring

Including the following multiple hemodynamic monitoring projects:

(1) Central venous pressure

Central venous pressure(CVP) represents the change of pressure in the right atrium or in the thoracic cavity, reflecting the relationship between systemic blood volume and right ventricular function. The normal value of CVP is 0.49-0.98 kPa (5-10 cmH_2O). When CVP<0.49 kPa, the blood volume is insufficient; higher than 1.47 kPa (15 cmH_2O), not heart failure, vein bed overcontraction, or pulmonary circulation resistance increased; if 1.96 kPa (20 cmH_2O), the presence of congestive heart failure. In clinical practice, continuous measurement is usually carried out to dynamically observe the change trend to accurately reflect the preload of the right heart.

(2) Pulmonary capillary wedge pressure

Pulmonary artery pressure (PAP) and pulmonary capillary wedge pressure (PCWP) can be measured by Swan-Ganz floating catheter, reflecting the function of pulmonary vein, left atrium and left ventricle. The normal value of PAP is 1.3-2.9 kPa (10-22 mmHg); the normal value of PCWP is 0.8-2 kPa (6-15 mmHg), which is close to the left atrial pressure. PCWP is below normal and reflects insufficient blood volume (CVP sensitivity). Increased PCWP can reflect increased left atrial pressure, such as acute pulmonary edema. Therefore, when PCWP is found to be elevated clinically, even if CVP is still normal, the amount of fluid infusion should be limited to avoid or aggravate pulmonary edema. In addition, blood samples can be obtained at PCWP for mixed venous blood gas analysis to understand the changes of pulmonary arteriovenous shunt or pulmonary ventilation/perfusion ratio in the lungs. However, it must be pointed out that the pulmonary artery catheter technique is a invasive examination, with the possibility of serious complications (3%-5%), so the indications should be strictly mastered.

(3) Cardiac output and heart index

Cardiac output(CO) is the product of heart rate and stroke volume, which can be measured by Swan-Ganz catheter thermal dilution method. The normal value of adult CO is 4-6 L/min; the cardiac output of unit body surface area is called cardiac index (CI), and the normal value is 2.5-3.5 L/ (min · m^2).

(4) Arterial blood gas analysis

The normal value of arterial oxygen partial pressure (PO_2) was 10.7-13 kPa(80-100 mmHg); the normal value of arterial carbon dioxide partial pressure ($PaCO_2$) was 4.8-5.8 kPa (36-44 mmHg). Shock can be caused by insufficient ventilation in the lungs, and the accumulation of carbon dioxide in the body increases significantly in $PaCO_2$. On the contrary, if the patient has no lung disease, excessive ventilation can lead to lower $PaCO_2$; if $PaCO_2$ exceeds 5.9-6.6 kPa (45-50 mmHg), the pulmonary alveolar ventilation dysfunction is often suggested; PaO_2 is lower than 8.0 kPa (60 mmHg), and the inhalation of pure oxygen is still not improved. A person may be a precursor of ARDS. The arterial blood pH is normal from 7.35-7.45. By monitoring the dynamic changes of pH, buffer excess(BE), buffer base (BB) and standard bicarbonate (SB), we can understand the acid-base balance in shock. base deficit (BD) can reflect systemic acidosis, severity of reaction and recovery.

(5) Determination of arterial blood lactate

Insufficient tissue perfusion in shock patients can cause anaerobic metabolism and high lactic acidemia. Monitoring helps to estimate the trend of shock and resuscitation. The normal value is 1–1.5 mmol/L, and the critically ill patients are allowed to 2 mmol/L. In addition, the condition can be judged by other parameters, such as the increase of lactate/pyruvate(L/P)ratio in anaerobic metabolism, the normal ratio is 10 : 1, and the increase of the L/P ratio in hyperlactic acid.

(6)Detection of disseminated intravascular coagulation

For patients suspected of having disseminated intravascular coagulation(DIC), the number and quality of platelets, the consumption of coagulation factors, and the multiple indicators of fibrinolytic activity should be determined. When the following five examinations showed more than three abnormalities combined with the symptoms of thromboembolism and bleeding, the DIC could be diagnosed: ①the platelet count was lower than 80×10^9 L; ②the prothrombin time was longer than the control group for more than 3 seconds; ③plasma fibrinogen was lower than 1.5 g/L or progressive reduction; ④plasma positive for protamine secondary coagulation; ⑤red blood cells in blood smears exceeded 2%.

1.6　Treatment

For shock, which is caused by different causes, but with common clinical manifestations, the following corresponding treatment should be taken in response to the causes of shock and the important physiological disorders in different stages of shock. The key to treatment shock is to restore perfusion and provide sufficient oxygen for tissue. In recent years, the concept of resuscitation that emphasizes the excess oxygen supply and oxygen consumption should reach the following criteria: $DO_2 > 600$ mL/(min $\cdot$ m^2), $VO_2 > 170$ mL/(min $\cdot$ m^2), and cardiac index CI>4.5 L/(min $\cdot$ m^2); the ultimate aim is to prevent multiple organ dysfunction syndrome (MODS).

1.6.1　General emergency treatment

It includes active treatment of primary injuries and diseases that cause shock. Such as trauma, bleeding, and respiratory tract patency. The head and trunk were raised 20–30 degrees and the lower limbs were raised 15–20 degrees to increase the amount of blood. Establish venous access early and medication (see later) to maintain blood pressure. Early nasal tube or mask oxygen inhalation. Pay attention to heat preservation.

1.6.2　Supplemental blood volume

It is the key to correct hypoxic and hypoxia induced by shock. On the basis of continuous monitoring of arterial blood pressure, urine volume and CVP, combined with the patient's skin temperature, peripheral circulation, pulse amplitude and capillary filling time and other microcirculation, the effect of supplemental blood volume should be judged. First, crystal fluid and artificial colloid fluid were resuscitated, and component blood transfusion was necessary. 3%–7.5% hypertonic saline solution is also used for shock resuscitation.

1.6.3　Actively dealing with primary disease

Most of the shock caused by surgical diseases, such as the control of large visceral hemorrhage, the resection of necrotic intestinal loop, the repair of the digestive tract perforation, and the drainage of the pus. It is necessary to recover the effective blood circulation as soon as possible and treat the primary lesions in time so as to effectively treat shock. In some cases, the operation should be carried out at the same time of active anti shock, so as not to delay the rescue time.

1.6.4 Correcting the maladjustment of acid-base balance

Acidic internal environment has inhibitory effects on myocardium, vascular smooth muscle and renal function. In the early stage of shock, hyperventilation may also result in hypocapnia and respiratory alkalosis. According to the law of hemoglobin oxygenation and dissociation curve, alkalosis makes the hemoglobin oxygen dissociation curve move left, oxygen is not easy to release from hemoglobin, and can make the tissue anoxia aggravate. Therefore, we do not advocate the early use of basic drugs. The acidic environment is conducive to the dissociation of oxygen from hemoglobin, thereby increasing tissue oxygen supply. The fundamental measure is to improve tissue perfusion and provide basic drugs in a timely and appropriate manner. At present, the treatment of acid-base balance claims to be acid rather than alkaline. Acidic environment can increase the dissociation of oxygen and hemoglobin, thereby increasing oxygen release to tissues, which is beneficial to recovery. In addition, the use of basic drugs must first ensure that the respiratory function is intact, otherwise it will lead to CO_2 retention and secondary respiratory acidosis.

1.6.5 The application of vasoactive drugs

Vasoactive drugs are needed to maintain organ perfusion under the premise of adequate capacity resuscitation. With the in-depth study of the pathogenesis and pathophysiology of shock, the application and efficacy of vasoactive drugs are constantly reappraise. Vasoactive drugs can improve circulation and elevated blood pressure rapidly, especially in patients with septic shock, and increasing blood pressure is the primary goal for the application of vasoactive drugs. Ideal vasoactive agents should rapidly increase blood pressure, improve heart and cerebral blood flow, and improve blood perfusion in organs such as kidneys and intestines.

1.6.6 Vasoconstrictor

There are dopamine, norepinephrine and hydroxylamine.

Dopamine is the most commonly used vasoactive agent. It has the function of stimulating alpha, beta 1 and dopamine receptors. Its pharmacological action is related to dose. Small dose of <10 μg/ (min · kg), mainly beta 1 and dopamine receptors, can enhance myocardial contractility and increase CO, and expand the visceral organs such as kidney and gastrointestinal tract; large doses of >15 μg/ (min · kg) act as alpha receptor and increase peripheral vascular resistance. The main effect of anti shock is to strengthen the heart and expand the blood vessels of the viscera. In order to raise blood pressure, low dose dopamine can be combined with other vasoconstrictor drugs without increasing dopamine dose.

The positive inotropic effect of dobutamine on myocardium is stronger than dopamine, which can increase CO, decrease PCWP and improve cardiac pumping function. The common dose is 2.5-10 μg/ (kg · min), and the small dose has a slight vasoconstriction effect. The combination of norepinephrine and dobutamine is the best vasoactive agent in the treatment of septic shock. Dobutamine can increase systemic oxygen transport and improve mesenteric blood perfusion. Stimulation of beta receptors increases cardiac output and oxygen delivery, improves intestinal perfusion, and significantly decreases arterial lactate levels.

Norepinephrine is a vasoconstrictor, which excites the alpha receptor and excites the beta receptor slightly. It can stimulate the myocardium, constrict the blood vessels, raise the hypertension and increase the blood flow of the coronary artery, and the time of action is short. The usual dosage was 0.5-2 mg and 5%

glucose solution was injected intravenously into 100 mL.

Methylephrine (Alam) indirectly excite alpha and beta receptors, acting on the heart and blood vessels with norepinephrine, but the effect is weak, and the maintenance time is about 30 minutes. Commonly used amount 2–10 mg intramuscular injection or 2–5 mg intravenous injection, also can 10–20 mg add 5% glucose solution 100 mL intravenous drip.

Isopropyl adrenaline is a beta agonist which can enhance myocardial contraction and increase heart rate. The dosage is 0.1–0.2 mg and is dissolved in 100 mL infusion. It can not be used for cardiogenic shock because of its strong contractile effect on myocardium and arrhythmia.

1.6.7   Vasodilator

It is divided into two types: alpha receptor blocker and anticholinergic drug. The former includes phentolamine, phenacetin and so on, which can relieve small vessel contraction and microcirculation stasis caused by norepinephrine and enhance left ventricular contractility. Among them, phentolamine has a quick effect and a short duration. The dosage is 0.1–0.5 mg/kg plus 100 mL intravenous infusion. Phenacetin is an alpha blocker, and it has the role of indirect reflex excitatory beta receptor. It can slightly increase cardiac contractility, cardiac output and heart rate, and increase coronary blood flow, reduce peripheral circulation resistance and blood pressure. The effect can be maintained for 3–4 days. Dosage is 0.5–1.0 mg/kg, add 5% glucose solution or 0.9% sodium chloride solution 200–400 mL, 1–2 hour dripping.

Anticholinergic agents include atropine, anisodamine and scopolamine. The most clinically used shock treatment is anisodamine (artificial synthetic 654–2), which can counteract the vasodilatation of the smooth muscle spasms caused by acetylcholine and improve the microcirculation. It can also protect the cells by inhibiting the metabolism of peanut four acid and reducing the release of leukotriene and prostaglandins. It is a good cell membrane stabilizer. Especially in peripheral vasospasm, it is more effective in improving blood pressure, improving microcirculation and stabilizing the disease. Usage is 10 mg every time, once every 15 minutes, intravenous injection, or 40–80 mg/h continue to pump until the clinical symptoms improve.

1.6.8   Cardio drug

Drugs such as dopamine and dobutamine, as well as dopamine and dobutamine, such as dopamine and dobutamine, and other strong glycosides such as carotene (seroside), can enhance cardiac contractility and slow down heart rate. When the central venous pressure is monitored, the infusion volume is full but the arterial pressure is still low and its central venous pressure is up to 1.47 kPa (15 cmH$_2$O), the intravenous injection of 0.8 mg/d can be injected intravenously for the first time, and the initial dose of 0.4 mg is slow intravenous injection, and the maintenance amount can be given again when it is effective.

The choice of vasoactive drugs in shock should be associated with the main condition of the time, such as the main disease in the early stage of the shock and the microvascular spasm of the capillaries; later, it was related to the microvenous and small venous spasms. Therefore, vasodilators should be used in combination with dilatation therapy. When the expansion is not completed, if necessary, vasoconstrictor can be used in moderation, but the dosage should not be too large and the time should not be too long.

In order to take into account the perfusion levels of important organs, vasoconstrictor and dilator are often combined. For example, the combined intravenous drip of norepinephrine 0.1–0.5 μg/ (kg · min) sodium nitroprusside 1.0–10 μg/ (kg · min) can increase the heart index by 30%, reduce the peripheral resistance by 45%, increase the blood pressure to above 80 mmHg, and maintain the urine volume above 40 mL/h.

1.6.9   Treatment of DIC and improving microcirculation

For diagnostic DIC, heparin can be used for anticoagulation, general 1. 0 mg/kg, 6 hours, and adults can be 10 000 U for the first time (LMG is equivalent to 125 U). Aspirin, Pan Shengding and small molecule dextran are also used to resist platelet adhesion and aggregation, such as aminoacid and aminohexanoic acid.

1.6.10   The application of corticosteroids and other drugs

Corticosteroids can be used for septic shock and other severe shock. The main function is to block the excitatory effect of alpha receptor, dilate blood vessels, reduce peripheral vascular resistance, and improve microcirculation. Protect the lysosomes in cells and prevent lysosome rupture; strengthen myocardial contractility and increase cardiac output; increase the function of mitochondria and prevent leukocyte agglutination. It is reduced to glucose and alleviated acidosis. It is generally advocated to apply large doses, intravenous drip, and once dripping. To prevent side effects after corticosteroid use, it is usually 1−2 times.

We should strengthen nutrition metabolism support and immunomodulation therapy, and proper enteral and parenteral nutrition can reduce the catabolism of the tissue. In combination with growth hormone, glutamine has synergistic effect. Glutamine is the main energy source of intestinal mucosal cells and the synthetic material of nucleic acid.

Other drugs include the following: ①calcium channel blockers such as Vera Pammy, nifedipine and diltiazem, which can prevent calcium ion inflow and protect cell structure and function; ②morphine antagonist naloxone can improve tissue hemoperfusion and prevent cell dysfunction; ③oxygen free radical scavenger, such as superoxide dismutation, can be used. Enzyme(SOD) can reduce the destruction of oxygen free radicals to tissue in ischemia−reperfusion injury; ④regulate the body prostaglandin (PGS), such as the infusion of prostacyclin (PGI_2) to improve microcirculation; ⑤the use of adenosine triphosphate−magnesium chloride (ATP−$MgCl_2$) therapy has the effect of increasing intracellular energy, restoring the membrane sodium potassium pump, and prevention and treatment the effect of cell swelling and recovery of cell function.

Chapter 2

Hypovolemic Shock

Hypovolemic shock is usually caused by massive bleeding or fluid loss or fluid volume in the third space, resulting in a reduction in effective circulating volume. Hemorrhagic shock caused by rupture of large vessels or visceral hemorrhage; traumatic shock with loss of blood and loss of plasma at the same time after a variety of injuries or major operations.

The main manifestations of hypovolemic shock are the decrease of CVP, the decrease of the blood circulation, the decrease of CO, the peripheral vasoconstriction caused by the neuroendocrine mechanism, the increase of vascular resistance and the rate of heart rate, and the various tissue and organ dysfunction and pathological changes caused by the microcirculation disorder. Timely replenishment of blood volume, treatment of its etiology and prevention of continued blood loss and fluid loss are the key to the treatment of this type of shock.

2.1 Hemorrhagic Shock

Hemorrhagic shock is very common in surgical shock. It is often seen in the rupture of the large vessels, the rupture of the spleen, the blood of the stomach and the duodenum, the blood of the duodenum, and the rupture of the veins of the esophagus and the fundus of the stomach. Shock usually occurs when rapid blood loss exceeds 20% of the total blood volume of the body. Severe body fluid loss can cause a large number of extracellular fluid and plasma loss, resulting in reduced effective blood circulation and shock.

Treatment

It mainly includes two aspects: blood volume supplement, active treatment of primary disease and prevention of bleeding. Attention should be paid to two aspects at the same time, so as to avoid further development of the disease and cause organ damage.

(1) Supplemental blood volume

Blood loss can be estimated according to the change of blood pressure and pulse rate, as shown in Table 4-2-1. Although hemorrhagic shock is mainly caused by blood loss, it is not necessary to replenish blood when supplementing blood volume. Instead, we should seize the opportunity to increase venous return in time. First, a rapid infusion of a balanced salt solution and a colloidal solution can be used quickly, in which the rapid input of the colloid fluid is easier to restore the intravascular volume and maintain the stability of the hemodynamics, and the colloid osmotic pressure can be maintained at the same time, and the duration of the colloid is longer. It is generally believed that the maintenance of hemoglobin concentration at 100 g/L and HCT at 30% is good. If the concentration of hemoglobin is greater than 100 g/L, blood transfusion is not necessary; lower than 70 g/L can be used to concentrate red blood cells; at 70 – 100 g/L, the transfusion of red blood cells can be determined according to the patient's compensatory ability, general condition and other organ functions, and 30% of the acute blood loss exceeds the total amount of the whole blood. Theamount of the input liquid should be evaluated according to the cause, the amount of urine and the hemodynamics, and the blood pressure combined with the central venous pressure is often used to guide the fluid.

Table 4-2-1 The relationship between central venous pressure and fluid infusion

Central venous pressure	Blood pressure	Reason	Handling principles
Low	Low	Severe insufficiency of blood volume	Full rehydration
Low	Normal	Insufficiency of blood volume	Appropriate rehydration
High	Low	Insufficiency of heart function or relative excessive volume of blood	Cardio drugs, Correct acidosis, vasodilation
High	Normal	Excessive vasoconstriction	Vasodilation
Normal	Low	Cardiac insufficiency or insufficiency of blood volume	Rehydration test

Rehydration test: Isotonic saline 250 mL was injected into the vein within 5 – 10 minutes. If the blood pressure is elevated, the central venous pressure does not change. This indicates that the blood volume is insufficient. If the blood pressure is constant, the central venous pressure rises 0. 29 – 0. 49 kPa (3 – 5 cmH$_2$O), suggesting cardiac insufficiency.

With the recovery of blood volume and venous return, the lactic acid accumulated in the tissue can enter the circulation. Sodium bicarbonate should be given to correct acidosis. Hypertonic saline can also be used to dilate small vessels, improve microcirculation, increase myocardial contractility and increase CO. The mechanism is related to the increase of sodium ion and the recovery of extracellular fluid volume. However, high blood sodium also has the risk of lowering blood pressure, secondary hypokalemia, phlebitis and platelet aggregation.

(2) Hemostasis

In addition to blood volume, if there is still bleeding, it is difficult to maintain stable blood volume, and shock is not easy to correct. For patients with acute active upper gastrointestinal bleeding, we should actively prepare for operation while maintaining blood volume, and stop bleeding early.

2.2 Traumatic Shock

Traumatic shock is seen in severe trauma, such as rupture of large blood vessels, complex fractures, compression injuries, or major operations, causing loss of blood or plasma, inflammatory swelling and exudation of the body fluid, which can lead to low blood volume. Histamine, protease and other vasoactive substances can be found in the damaged body, causing microvascular dilatation and increased permeability, resulting in a further reduction in effective circulating blood volume. On the other hand, trauma can stimulate the nervous system, cause pain and neuroendocrine system reaction, affect the cardiovascular function; some trauma, such as chest injury can directly affect the heart and lung, paraplegia can reduce the amount of blood back temporarily, craniocerebral injury can sometimes reduce blood pressure and so on. So the condition of traumatic shock is often complicated.

Treatment: Because traumatic shock is also a hypovolemic shock, it is necessary to expand blood volume in first aid, which is basically the same as hemorrhagic shock. However, due to the presence of blood clot, plasma and inflammatory fluid infiltration in the body cavity and deep tissue, detailed examination is necessary to accurately estimate the amount of loss. Patients with severe pain and pain should be properly treated with analgesic sedatives; proper temporary fixation (braking) of the injured part; and emergency treatment for life-threatening trauma such as open or tension pneumothorax and flail chest. Surgery and other complex treatments should generally be performed after stable blood pressure or after a preliminary recovery. Antibiotics should also be used to prevent secondary infection after trauma or major surgery.

Chapter 3

Septic Shock

Septic shock is more common in surgery and is rather difficult to treat, with a mortality rate of over 50%. It is common in acute peritonitis, biliary tract infection, strangulated intestinal obstruction and urinary tract infection. The main pathogenic bacteria are G-bacillus, and the released endotoxin is the main cause of shock, so it can also be called endotoxic shock. After binding to complement, antibody or other components in the body, endotoxin stimulates sympathetic vasospasm and damages vascular endothelial cells. At the same time, endotoxin can promote the release of inflammatory mediators such as histamine, kinin, prostaglandin and lysosomal enzyme, causing systemic inflammatory reaction, and eventually lead to microcirculation disorder, metabolic disorder and organ dysfunction. A lot of progress has been made in the study of related cytokines of severe surgical infection, and the concept of systemic inflammatory response syndrome (SIRS) has been widely recognized. Further development of SIRS can lead to shock and multiple organ failure (MOF).

The hemodynamic changes in patients with septic shock are more complicated, and they are involved in three aspects: cardiac output, blood volume and peripheral vascular resistance. In the early stage of shock, the cardiac output increased significantly (increased by several times) and decreased significantly in the later stage. A small number of severe cases had a significant reduction in cardiac output at an early stage. Due to abnormal distribution of body fluid, the effective circulating blood volume of patients with septic shock has been reduced, but to a certain extent. The difference in the resistance of peripheral vessels is greater. Some patients have significantly increased resistance, characterized by cold skin on the extremities, and warm skin on the contrary. In the past, the theory of "warm shock" and "cold shock" is nothing but a reflection of the state of peripheral vascular resistance. It is difficult to diagnose the cause of this disease. Because of sepsis caused by G+ and G- bacteria, it may be warm in the early stage of shock due to fever and dilatation of the surrounding blood vessels; and it is wet cold in the late shock. Moreover, the hemodynamic state of patients will change with the development process of their disease (improvement or deterioration). Therefore, the clinician should master the patient's immediate hemodynamic state (including cardiac function, blood volume and peripheral vascular resistance) and formulate anti shock measures to achieve better therapeutic effect.

Treatment: The pathophysiological changes of septic shock are relatively complex, and treatment is difficult. The treatment principle is to rectify shock and control infection equally. In the presence of shock, it is obvious that the anti shock measures should be taken first and the infection should be considered. After shock correction, infection control becomes the focus.

3.1 Supplemental Blood Volume

It is advisable to infuse the balanced salt solution with the appropriate infusion of colloid solution (artificial colloid, blood or whole blood, etc.) to restore enough circulating blood volume. Central venous pressure (CVP) should be monitored as a routine. In order to ensure normal heart filling pressure, arterial oxygen content and ideal blood viscosity, the hemoglobin concentration is adjusted to 70–80 g/L, and the ratio of blood cells to 25% –30% is the best state. Patients with septic shock often suffer from impaired heart and kidney function. We should be vigilant against the adverse consequences resulting from excessive transfusion.

3.2 Control of Infection

If the patient's pathogen has not yet been determined, the most probable pathogenic bacteria can be deduced according to the clinical rules and experience, and sensitive antibiotics should be selected accordingly. Or, a powerful broad-spectrum antibiotic can be selected. For example, most of the intraperitoneal infection is caused by a variety of pathogenic bacteria in the intestine. Third or fourth generation cephalosporins, such as cefoperazone sodium, ceftazidin or ceftazidine, or metronidazole or tinidazole, can be considered, and penicillin or broad-spectrum penicillin can also be added. When sensitive pathogens are known, antibiotics with a narrow sensitivity should be chosen. Most surgical patients with septic shock have a clear primary infection, such as diffuse peritonitis, liver abscess, obstructive suppurative cholangitis and so on. It should be treated as early as possible, including the necessary surgery (such as abscess or drainage of the bile duct). Timely surgical management may be a turning point in correcting shock.

3.3 Correction of Acid–base Imbalance

Septic shock is often accompanied by severe acidosis, which occurs earlier and must be corrected in time. 5% sodium bicarbonate 200 mL can be injected from another vein while supplementing blood volume. After 1 hours, the arterial blood gas analysis was reviewed, and the additional dosage was determined according to the results.

3.4 Application of Cardiovascular Drugs

When blood volume is increased and acidosis is corrected, vasodilator drugs should be added if shock does not improve. Sometimes it can be combined with a–receptor excitation, with a mild excitatory beta receptor vasoconstrictor and a a–receptor blocker with a beta receptor action to counteract vasoconstriction, maintain, enhance beta receptor excitation, and not increase the rate of heart rate, such as anisodamine and dopamine. Or norepinephrine combined with dopamine (or dobutamine).

Recently, it is reported that adding a small dose of pituitrin (vasopressin) can improve the average arterial pressure in patients with septic shock when the two drugs are still ineffective.

Cardiac function is often impaired in septic shock. Cardiac function can be improved by cardiac glycoside.

3.5   Corticosteroid Therapy

Glucocorticoids are important natural inhibitors of proinflammatory cytokines that regulate host defense responses at all levels. It can inhibit the release of various inflammatory mediators and stabilize lysosomal membrane and alleviate SIRS. Glucocorticoids should be used as early as possible in the course of disease. The dosage should be large, up to 10−20 times as much as the normal dosage. It is generally advocated for short term use, not more than 48 hours. However, some people think that prolonging the time of medication can improve the therapeutic effect.

3.6   Other Treatment

It includes nutrition support, treatment of important organ dysfunction.

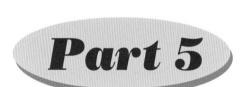

Part 5

Multiple Organ Dysfunction Syndrome

Chapter 1

Introduction

1.1 Definition

Multiple organ dysfunction syndrome (MODS), also known as multiple organ failure (MOF), total organ failure (TOF) or multisystem organ failure (MSOF), is defined as "the presence of altered organ function in an acutely ill patient requiring medical intervention to achieve homeostasis". The exact incidence of MODS in people is difficult to estimate because there is no true consensus for the definition of dysfunction in each individual organ system; but it has been estimated that 15% of all people admitted to the intensive care unit (ICU) will develop MODS. Mortality rates for surgical and medical ICU patients with MODS range from 44% to 76%.

1.2 Cause

The condition of MODS usually results from sepsis, major trauma, burns, pancreatitis, aspiration syndromes extracorporeal circulation (e. g. , cardiac bypass), multiple blood transfusion, ischaemia−reperfusion injury, autoimmune disease, heat−induced illness, eclampsia and poisoning/toxicity.

The primary cause triggers an uncontrolled inflammatory response. Sepsis is the most common cause of MODS and may result in septic shock. Multiple organ dysfunction syndrome is well established as the final stage of a continuum: SIRS + infection, sepsis, severe sepsis, multiple organ dysfunction syndrome.

1.3 Pathophysiology

The pathophysiology of MODS is complex, multi−factorial, and poorly understood. First, a dysregulated immune response to critical illness plays a central role in the pathogenesis of MODS. Second, following resuscitation from severe trauma or circulatory shock, an inflammatory response in gut evolves that promotes dysfunction in distant organs. Third, nosocomial or iatrogenic insults ("hits") that occur in the post resuscitation period promote an exaggerated immune response that leads to organ dysfunction and MODS. Fourth, patients can recover completely from MODS, which is consistent with a functional rather than structural etiology. Finally, the mechanism(s) by which critical illness induces dysfunction of individual organs is not uniform.

Nevertheless, recognition of several key concepts can facilitate our understanding of the syndrome. Respiratory failure is common in the first 72 hours. Subsequently, one might see liver failure (5-7 days), gastrointestinal bleeding (10-15 days) and kidney failure (11-17 days).

1.4 Symptoms

The following six organ systems characterize MODS and they include respiratory, renal, cardiovascular, neurologic, hepatic, hematologic.

The signs and symptoms of end-organ dysfunction in the above organ systems consist of the following:

Lung or respiratory system-will show a dysfunction of normal exchange of gas, revealed mainly in "arterial hypoxemia" which is insufficient oxygen getting into the blood system. Many pathologic features add to this impaired gas exchange.

Kidney or renal system-is revealed in the impairment of the normal selective excretory function first in oliguria or low output of urine despite adequate intravascular volume, but later in a rising creatinine level and electrolyte and fluid problems of sufficient magnitude that in some cases dialysis may be required.

Heart and cardiovascular system-dysfunction of this system consist of abnormalities predisposed to impaired delivery of oxygen and therefore contribute to the injury of other organ systems.

Hepatic system-dysfunction of the hepatic system is reflected in excess bilirubin circulating in the blood as well as lack of bile flowing from the liver.

Neurologic system-there is an altered level of consciousness, which is reflected in the reduction in the Glasgow coma score which is the scale of consciousness of a individual due to multiple causes

Hematologic system-the most widely cited manifestation of dysfunction of the blood system consist of thrombocytopenia which in critical illness is cause by a multiple of factors.

1.5 Clinical Phases

The European Society of Intensive Care organized a consensus meeting in 1994 to create the "Sepsis-Related Organ Failure Assessment (SOFA)" score to describe and quantitate the degree of organ dysfunction in six organ systems. Using similar physiologic variables the multiple organ dysfunction score was developed.

Four clinical phases have been suggested:

Stage 1: the patient has increased volume requirements and mild respiratory alkalosis which is accompanied by oliguria, hyperglycemia and increased insulin requirements.

Stage 2: the patient is tachypneic, hypocapnic and hypoxemic; develops moderate liver dysfunction and possible hematologic abnormalities.

Stage 3: the patient develops shock with azotemia and acid-base disturbances; has significant coagulation abnormalities.

Stage 4: the patient is vasopressor dependent and oliguric or anuric; subsequently develops ischemic colitis and lactic acidosis.

1.6   Treatment

Presently there is no medical agent that reverses organ failure. Therapy is limited therefore to only supportive care, such as safeguarding hemodynamics and respiration. The principal aim is to maintain adequate tissue oxygenation. Beginning enteral nutrition within 36 hours of the admission to an intensive care unit has been shown to reduce complications caused by infections.

1.7   Prognosis

The mortality rate varies from 30% –100% with the chance of surviving diminishing as the number of organs involved increases. Since approximately the 1980s this mortality rate has not changed.

Chapter 2

Acute Renal Failure

2.1 Definition

Acute renal failure (ARF), also known as acute kidney injury, means decreased kidney function (reduced glomerular filtration rate) over a relatively short period of time. This can occur in the setting of previously normal kidney function or as an acute-on-chronic phenomenon.

2.2 Etiology

ARF will occur when parts of this system are disrupted.

(1) Pre-renal conditions

Poor flow of blood to the glomeruli. Usually related to volume depletion and relative hypotension. Possible etiologies include hemorrhage, volume loss from stool or urine, heart failure, shock.

(2) Renal conditions

Injury to the kidney itself that interrupts glomerular and/or tubular function, including glomerular disease (e. g. ,acute glomerulonephritis), tubulointerstitial disease (e. g. , interstitial nephritis, acute tubular necrosis), vascular disease (e. g. , vasculitis).

(3) Post-renal conditions

Obstruction of the drainage system distal to the renal tubules. This could be at any point along the urinary tract but is frequently seen at the bladder outlet. ARF usually requires bilateral obstruction, or obstruction of the one functioning kidney. Causes include kidney stones, congenital obstructions (UPJ obstruction, posterior urethral valves), tumor and strictures.

There are two main forms of ARF associated with MODS. One form involves a more traditional definition of kidney failure which is characterized by renal epithelial necrosis; renal hypoperfusion and ischemia often are cited in the pathogenesis. This form is the least common. The 2nd form of ARF is specific to MODS and is apoptosis caused by inflammatory cytokines (e. g. ,TNF-α) and endotoxin appears to be a predominant mechanism of this form of sepsis-induced ARF. Apoptosis is difficult to appreciate on routine histopathology, which may explain the lack of histopathologic damage in ARF. Instead of global hypoperfusion during sepsis, renal blood flow is adequate or increased which may explain the lack of acute tubular necrosis. It has been proposed that during sepsis-induced ARF, the efferent arteriole dilates to a greater degree than the afferent arteriole resulting in increased renal blood flow, decreased glomerular capillary pressure, and decreased glomerular filtration rate.

ARF is an important form of organ dysfunction in people because it markedly increases mortality. A multinational, multicenter study in humans found that ARF had a prevalence of 5%-6% and only 40% of these people survived to discharge. Septic shock was the most common cause of ARF in this study.

2.3 Diagnosis

The diagnosis of ARF is traditionally based on a rise in serum creatinine and/or fall in urine output. The definition has evolved from the risk, injury, failure, loss, end-stage (RIFLE) criteria in 2004 to the AKI Network (AKIN) classification in 2007.

(1) Thorough history and physical examination. Pay attention to time course, systemic complaints, drugs or exposures, family history, urinary symptoms, blood pressure, fluid balance.

(2) Check and follow the serum creatinine. Consider the appropriate level for the size/age of the patient. A rising creatinine suggests ARF.

(3) Check the urine. Look for evidence of blood, protein and casts in the urine. A bland urine with little or no findings might be seen in interstitial nephritis. Urinary indices (e. g. , fractional excretion of sodium (FENa)) can sometimes be useful.

(4) Evaluate the volume/perfusion status. Determine if the patient is volume overloaded or volume deplete. Assess the perfusion of vital organs.

(5) Consider imaging studies. Renal ultrasound is often a good test to look for hydronephrosis (suggestive of obstruction) or intrinsic renal structural abnormalities.

(6) Consider additional tests. Blood tests can point to some causes of ARF (HUS, acute glomerulonephritis, vasculitis). Sometimes a kidney biopsy is needed.

2.4 Management

Management of ARF depends on the etiology and severity of the ARF. For any patient with persistent ARF, it is important to maintain fluid and electrolyte balance.

(1) Pre-renal ARF: Improve renal blood flow by replacing lost volume and/or optimizing perfusion. Bevery careful about using potassium in this setting.

(2) Post-renal ARF: Relieve the identified obstruction. This may require placement of a Foley catheter or a percutaneous nephrostomy, removal of a stone, etc. Following relief of obstruction, there may be a very brisk post-obstructive diuresis with very high urine output and electrolyte loss, putting your patient at risk for pre-renal ARF. Be prepared.

(3) Renal causes of ARF: Specific therapy depends on the diagnosis.

Chapter 3

Acute Respiratory Distress Syndrome

3.1 Definition

Acute respiratory distress syndrome(ARDS)refers to acute diffuse lung injury caused by various intra-lung and extrapulmonary pathogenic factors and then acute respiratory failure. The main pathological features are the damage of pulmonary microvascular endothelium and alveolar epithelium caused by the inflammatory response, increased pulmonary microvascular permeability, alveolar leakage of protein-rich fluid, leading to pulmonary edema and the formation of transparent membranes. The main pathophysiological changes were lung volume reduction, lung compliance reduction and severe ventilation/blood flow imbalance.

3.2 Etiology

There are many causes or risk factors for ARDS, which can be divided into intrapulmonary factors (direct factors) and extrapulmonary factors (brief factors) (Table 5-3-1). However, these direct and indirect factors, as well as their inflammatory reactions, influence changes and pathophysiological responses, often overlap with each other.

Table 5-3-1　Common risk factors for acute respiratory distress syndrome

pneumonia	severe burn
non-pulmonary infection-poisoning	non-cardiogenic shock
stomach contents inhaled	drug overdose
massive trauma	transfusion related acute lung injury
lung contusion	pulmonary vasculitis
pancreatitis	drowning
aspiration lung injury	

The pathogenesis of ARDS has not been fully clarified. Although some pathogenic factors can cause direct damage to the alveolar membrane, ARDS is essentially a variety of inflammatory cells (macrophages, neutrophils, vascular endothelial cells, platelets) and their released inflammatory mediators and cytokines indirectly mediate the pulmonary inflammatory response. ARDS is a systemic inflammatory response (systemic inflammatory response syndrome, SIRS) of the lung. SIRS refers to the inflammatory cascade reaction of self-continuous amplification and self-destruction of the body. The body with SIRS and launched a series of endogenous anti-inflammatory reaction called compensatory anti-inflammatory response syndrome (compensatory anti-inflammatory response syndrome, CARS). Multiple organ dysfunction syndrome (MODS) can be caused if SIRS and CARS have imbalance in the course of disease development. ARDS is the earliest involvement or most common manifestation of organ dysfunction in the occurrence of MODS, and is the injury response mode of lung tissue to a variety of acute and severe intrapulmonary and extrapulmonary injuries.

Inflammatory cells and inflammatory mediators are two main factors that initiate early inflammatory response and maintain inflammatory response, which play a key role in the occurrence and development of ARDS. Inflammatory cells to produce a variety of inflammatory mediators and cytokines, the most important thing is that the tumor necrosis factor alpha (TNF-α) and interleukin-1 (IL-1), resulting in a large number of neutrophils in the lungs, activation, and through the outbreak of "breathing" release oxygen free radicals, protease and inflammatory medium, cause damage to the target cells, characterized by pulmonary capillary endothelial cells and alveolar epithelial cell damage, increased pulmonary microvascular permeability and stomach thrombosis, a large number of high in protein and fiber protein liquid seeps to the pulmonary interstitial and alveolar, forming non cardiac pulmonary edema and transparent membrane. If the damage repair process is normal and orderly, pulmonary reepithelialization and structural function recovery can be completed. If the damage repair process is abnormal and disordered, the post-ARDS pulmonary fibrosis will evolve into an abnormal remodeling process and eventually form an irreversible fibrosis lesion.

3.3　Diagnosis

According to the definition of ARDS Berlin, the following four conditions are satisfied before diagnosing ARDS.

Identify acute or progressive dyspnea that occurs within 1 week of cause.

Chest X-ray plain film/chest CT showed bilateral lung infiltration, which could not be fully explained by pleural effusion, pulmonary lobe/atelectasis and nodules.

Respiratory failure can not be fully explained by cardiac failure and fluid overload. If there are no clinical risk factors, cardiogenic pulmonary edema should be assessed using objective examination (e. g. , Echocardiography).

Hypoxemia confirmed the diagnosis of ARDS according to PaO_2/FiO_2, and its severity was divided into mild, moderate and severe. It should be noted that the PaO_2 monitoring in the above oxygenation index is measured under the condition that the mechanical ventilation parameter PEEP/CPAP is not lower than 5 cmH_2O. When the local altitude exceeds 1 000 m, the PaO_2/FiO_2 should be corrected, and the corrected $PaO_2/FiO_2 = (PaO_2/FiO_2) \times (\text{the local atmospheric pressure value} /760)$.

Mild: 200 mmHg<$PaO_2/FiO_2 \leqslant$300 mmHg.

Moderate: 100 mmHg<$PaO_2/FiO_2 \leqslant$200 mmHg.

Severe: $PaO_2/FiO_2 \leqslant$100 mmHg.

3.4   Treatment

The treatment principle is the same as that of general acute respiratory failure. The main treatment measures include active treatment of primary disease, oxygen therapy, mechanical ventilation and ventilation and regulation of fluid balance.

(1) Treatment of primary disease

As the first principle and basis of treating ARDS, the primary disease should be actively looked for and treated thoroughly. Infection is a common cause of ARDS, which is also the first risk factor for ARDS, and ARDS is prone to co-infection. Therefore, the possibility of infection should be suspected in all patients, unless there are other specific reasons for ARDS. Broad-spectrum antibiotics should be selected for treatment.

(2) Correct hypoxia

Take effective measures to improve PaO_2 as soon as possible. Generally, high concentration of oxygen is required to make PaO_2 greater than 60 mmHg or SaO_2 greater than 90%. For mild cases, oxygen can be given by mask, but most patients need mechanical ventilation.

(3) Mechanical ventilation

Although there is no uniform standard for the indications of ARDS mechanical ventilation, most scholars believe that mechanical ventilation should be carried out as soon as possible once being diagnosed as ARDS. Patients with mild ARDS can try non-invasive positive pressure ventilation (NIPPV). The purpose of mechanical ventilation is to maintain adequate ventilation and oxygenation to support organ function.

(4) Liquid management

To reduce pulmonary edema, the fluid intake should be reasonably limited to allow a lower circulation capacity to maintain effective circulation and keep the lungs in a relatively "dry" state.

(5) Nutrition support and monitoring

ARDS are in a high metabolic state of the body and should be supplemented with sufficient nutrition.

Part 6

Anesthesiology

Chapter 1

Introduction

Anesthesiology is clinical medicine specialized in the study of theory, technology and anesthetic drugs as an independent discipline. The term of anesthesia is derived from the Greek language. Early meaning refers to the loss of perception or sensation, especially the loss of pain to the patient in order to better perform surgical therapy or medical treatment.

In ancient times, opium, ethanol or even bloodletting were used to make the patients feel painless. There were also ways to achieve local painlessness by pressing nerve trunk or freezing. As early as Dong Han Dynasty, the Chinese famous doctor Hua Tuo had used Mafeisan for surgical treatment. However, the modern anesthesiology started in the middle of 19th Century. In October 16, 1846, Morton publicly demonstrated the ether anesthesia in Massachusetts General Hospital, and was considered to be a milestone in the development of anesthesiology. Its significance not only found a safe and effective drug and a method for clinical practice, but also promoted the study of anesthetic methods, anesthetic pharmacology and anesthetic physiology. But the impact of surgery on the body is not only pain, but also changes such as nerve reflex, organ function, endocrine and metabolism. Anesthesia should not only solve the problem of pain, but also how to maintain and regulate the physiological function of the patient during the operation and anesthesia, and the difficulty and depth and breadth of the required knowledge are more difficult and complex than the simple elimination of the operation pain. Correct understanding and rational application of anesthetic drugs and improving the anesthesia level and anesthesia management are important links to improve the quality and safety of anesthesia.

In the modern anaesthesia, eliminating the pain of the operation is not the whole content of the anaesthesia. It has also accumulated rich experience in emergency resuscitation, critical medicine, acute and chronic pain diagnosis and treatment, and has carried out extensive scientific research, and gradually formed a more complete theoretical system. The combination of practice and theory constitutes anesthesiology.

The theory and technology of anesthesiology is not only used for surgical treatment, but also plays an active role in the medical work outside the operation room. But clinical anesthesia is still one of the main contents of anesthesiology. The purpose of anesthesia is to eliminate operative pain, ensure patient safety and create favorable conditions for surgery. The production of anesthetic effects mainly involves the use of anesthetic drugs or anesthetic techniques to induce temporary and completely reversible inhibition of the central nervous system or certain parts of the nervous system.

Chapter 2

Pre-anesthesia Preparation and Pre-anesthesia Medication

The purpose of preparation before anaesthesia is to ensure the safety of patients during anesthesia and operation, enhance the patient's tolerance to anesthesia and operation, and avoid or reduce the complications during perioperative period. The contents of pre-anesthesia preparation include evaluating the adaptability of patients to anesthesia and operation and possible physiological or pathological changes. According to the needs of the operation, we choose the appropriate anesthesia and intraoperative treatment; for surgical patients with internal medical or other systemic diseases, pre-anesthesia preparation should make the patient's internal medicine or other diseases to be treated in the best state, so as to better adapt to anesthesia and surgery.

2.1 Preoperative Assessment

2.1.1 Reasons

Perioperative risk factors — operation (stress response), anesthetic agents and anesthetic manipulation, concomitant disease.

2.1.2 Contents

Preoperative visit.

Purposes: ①Establish rapport with the patients. ②Obtain a history and perform a physical examination. ③Order special investigation. ④Assess the risk of anesthesia and surgery and if necessary postpone or cancel the surgery. ⑤Institute preoperative management. ⑥Prescribe premedication and plan the anesthetic management.

2.1.3　ASA grading system

The ASA grading system is shown in Table 6-2-1.

Table 6-2-1　ASA grading system and perioperative mortality rate

ASA rating[*]	Physical status scale	Mortality rate
I	A normally healthy individual	0.06-0.08
II	A patient with mild systemic disease	0.27-0.40
III	A patient with severe systemic diaease that is not incapacitating	1.82-4.30
IV	A patient with incapacitating systemic disease that is a constant threat to life	7.80-23.0
V	A moribund patient who is not expected to survive 24 h or without operation	9.40-50.7

Note: ※Add "E" as a suffix for emergency operation.

2.2　Preparation Before Anesthesia

2.2.1　Mental preparation

Mental preparation for patients focuses on eliminating patients' scruples and anxieties. Because emotional agitation, anxiety insomnia can cause the central nerve or sympathetic nerve hyperactivity, reduce the patient's tolerance to anesthesia and operation. Therefore, when visiting patients, we should dispel their mental anxieties and anxieties with care and encouragement. we should patiently listen and answer questions raised by patients, and get patient's understanding, trust and cooperation. For those who are too nervous to control themselves, they can treated with drugs. Those with mental disorders should be treated by the Psychiatrist.

2.2.2　Physical preparation

Before operation, we should improve the patient's malnutrition as much as possible, correct the disorder of water, electrolyte and acid-base imbalance. Surgical patients were often accompanied internal medical diseases. Anesthesiologists should fully understand their pathophysiological changes, make a correct evaluation of their severity, and ask medical experts to assist in diagnosis and treatment when necessary. Patients with complex condition often received some drugs before operation. The interaction between these drugs should be considered before anesthesia, so as to prevent adverse reactions during anesthesia. Patients with hypertension are controlled by internal medicine to maintain blood pressure stable. When choosing antihypertensive drugs, central hypotensive drugs should be avoided to avoid intractable hypotension and bradycardia during anaesthesia. Other antihypotensive drugs can be continued to the day of operation to avoid dramatic fluctuations in blood pressure due to withdrawal. Pulmonary function and arterial blood gas should be checked before operation for patients with respiratory diseases; stop smoking for at least 2 weeks, and perform respiratory function exercise. Aerosol inhalation and chest physical therapy can promote sputum excretion.

2.2.3 Gastrointestinal preparation

Patients undergoing elective surgery should take regular fasting before operation, avoid perioperative gastric reflux, aspiration and asphyxia and aspiration pneumonia. Adult elective surgery should be fasted for 8–12 hours, and be fasted water for 4 hours before anesthesia, so as to ensure gastric emptying. Those who are full stomach and must have general anesthesia can consider tracheal intubation under conscious state, which is beneficial to avoid or reduce the risk of vomiting and aspiration. In emergency patients, there is a risk of vomiting and aspiration even if regional block or intraspinal anesthesia is applied.

2.2.4 Preparation of equipment, apparatus and drugs

In order to ensure the safety and stability of anesthesia and operation, and to prevent the occurrence of accidents, the preparation and examination of anesthesia and monitoring equipment, anesthesia equipment and drugs must be carried out before anesthesia. No matter what kind of anesthesia is applied, anesthetic machines, first-aid equipment and medicines must be prepared. During anesthesia, the patient's vital signs must be monitored, such as blood pressure, respiration, ECG, pulse and end expiratory carbon dioxide pressure ($ETCO_2$), invasive arterial pressure, central venous pressure (CVP), and so on. Before the implementation of anesthesia, we should recheck the prepared equipment, appliances and drugs. The drugs used in operation must be checked before being used.

2.2.5 Informed consent

Before anesthesia, the patients and (or) family members should be given a description of the anaesthesia, unexpected accidents and complications that may occur during the perioperative period, and the perioperative notes, and an informed consent form should be signed.

2.3 Premedication

2.3.1 Purpose

①It can eliminate the patient's tension and anxiety, so that patients can be stable and cooperative before anesthesia and operation. At the same time, it also enhances the effect of general anesthetics, and reduces the dosage and side effects of general anesthetics. It has a forgetting effect on some adverse stimuli. ②It can elevate the pain threshold, relieve the pain caused by primary disease or invasive manipulation before anesthesia. ③It can inhibit secretion function of respiratory glands and reduce saliva secretion, so as to prevent aspiration. ④It can eliminate adverse reflex caused by surgery or anesthesia, such as vagus reflex. Inhibition of sympathetic excitation caused by excitation or pain can maintain hemodynamic stability.

2.3.2 Drug selection

Appropriate drugs, dosage and route of administration should be chosen according to anesthesia method and condition before anaesthesia. Generally speaking, the patients with general anesthesia are mainly used sedative and anticholinergic. The use of narcotic analgesics in patients with severe pain can not only relieve pain, but also enhance the effect of general anesthetics. Patients who are very nervous or unable to cooperate with spinal canal anesthesia can be given sedatives properly. The dose of sedative drugs in patients with coronary heart disease and hypertension can be appropriately increased, while those with heart valvular disease, poor heart function and serious condition should be reduced in doses of sedative and analgesic drugs, and the anticholinergic drugs are suitable for scopolamine. Patients who are generally ill, old, weak, cachexia and hypothyroidism are very sensitive to sedatives and analgesics, and the dosage should be reduced. And in young and strong patients or hyperthyroidism, the dosage should be increased. Premedication is usually administered intramuscularly injection within 30-60 minutes before anesthesia. For those with mental stress, oral sedative drugs should be taken the night before operation, so as to eliminate patients' nervousness.

2.3.3   Drugs in common use

(1) Benzodiazepine sedatives: They have sedative, hypnotic, anxiolytic and anticonvulsant effects, and can prevent the toxic reaction of local anesthetics. The commonly used drugs are diazepam, midazolam, etc.

(2) Barbiturates: It mainly inhibits the cerebral cortex, which has sedative, hypnotic and anticonvulsant effects. It also has some preventive effects on the toxicity of local anesthetics. The commonly used drugs are phenobarbital, etc.

(3) Analgesics: It can eliminate or relieve pain and change the emotional reaction to pain. The commonly used drugs are pethidine, morphine, etc. Intramuscular injection is generally used half an hour before anesthesia.

(4) Anticholinergics: The cholinergic receptor on the cholinergic innervated effector of the postganglionic nerve can be blocked to inhibit the secretion of glands, so as to keep the respiratory tract unobstructed and relax the smooth muscle of the gastrointestinal tract. The commonly used drugs are atropine and scopolamine. Atropine can inhibit vagal reflex and increase heart rate.

(5) H_2 receptor blocker: Antihistamine effect of cimetidine, ranitidine, can make the stomach acid pH increased significantly, while acid capacity decreased.

Chapter 3

General Anesthesia

3.1　General Anesthetics

3.1.1　Inhalation anesthetics

Inhalation anesthetics is the drug that produce general anesthesia through inhalation by respiratory tract. It is generally used for general anesthesia maintenance, and sometimes for anesthesia induction.

3.1.1.1　Physicochemical properties and pharmacological properties

Commonly used inhalation anesthetics are mostly halogens, inhaled into the alveolus through the respiratory tract, spread to the blood, and eventually enter the central nervous system, resulting in general anesthesia. The oil/gas partition coefficient (liposolubility) and blood/gas partition coefficient of inhaled anesthetics have a significant effect on their anesthetic performance. The intensity of inhalation anesthetics is related to the oil/gas partition coefficient. The minimum alveolar concentration (MAC) is used to measure the inhalation anesthetics. MAC refers to the minimum alveolar concentration when inhaling anesthetics to relieve pain in 50% patients at a single atmospheric pressure. From Table 6-3-1, we can see that the intensity of inhalation anesthetics is positively correlated with the oil/gas partition coefficient. The higher the oil/gas partition coefficient, the greater the anesthetic intensity, and the smaller the MAC value. The controllability of inhaled anesthetics are related to their blood/gas partition coefficients. The lower the blood/gas distribution coefficient is, the easier the partial pressure in alveoli, blood and brain tissues to reach equilibrium state, thus the easier to control in the central nervous system. As shown in Table 6-3-1, the blood/gas partition coefficient of desflurane and sevoflurane are relatively low, so the induction and recovery rate are faster.

3.1.1.2　Factors affecting the concentration of alveolar drugs

Alveolar concentration (FA) is the concentration of inhaled anesthetics in alveoli. Inspired concentration (FI) refers to the concentration of drugs entering the respiratory tract from the loop. In clinic, FA/FI is often used to compare the rising speed of alveolar concentration of different drugs. The rising speed of FA and FA/FI depends on the speed of the transportation of anesthetics and the uptake of pulmonary circulation. The influencing factors include the following:

(1) Ventilatory effect

Alveolar ventilation increased, and more drugs were transported to alveoli to compensate for the uptake of drugs by the pulmonary circulation, which accelerated the increase of FA and FA/FI. The greater the blood/gas partition coefficient is, the more blood intake is. The more ventilation increases, the more obvious the effect of FA/FI will be.

(2) Concentration effect

FI can not only affect the level of FA, but also affect the speed of FA rising, that is, the higher the FI is, the faster the FA rises, which is called the "concentration effect".

(3) Cardiac output (CO)

Inhalation anesthetics are transferred from alveoli to blood by diffusion. When the volume of lung ventilation is constant, CO increases. The blood flow of the pulmonary circulation increases, and the anesthetics absorbed by the blood also increase. The FA increases slowly. The influence of cardiac output on alveolar drug concentration is also related to the blood/gas partition coefficient of the drug. The greater the blood/gas partition coefficient of drug is, the more blood intake is caused by the increase of CO, the more obvious the decrease of alveolar drug concentration.

(4) Blood/gas partition coefficient

The amount of dissolution of the drug in the unit volume of blood is balanced when inhaled anesthetics and blood are in equilibrium. The higher the blood/gas partition coefficient, the more anaesthetic drugs in the blood, the increase of the drug concentration in the alveoli decrease, the duration of anesthesia induction is prolonged, and the anesthetic recovery is delayed.

(5) The concentration gradient of anesthetics between alveoli and venous blood (F_{A-V})

The greater the F_{A-V}, the more the amount of drugs that the pulmonary circulation takes, that is, the more anesthetics that are taken from alveoli. At the early stage of induction, the anesthetics in mixed venous blood were close to zero, and F_{A-V} was very large, which promoted the intake of anesthetics by blood. As the anesthetic deepened and the time extended, the concentration of anesthetics in the venous blood increased, the F_{A-V} decreased, the intake speed slowed, and the intake decreased, and finally reached a relatively stable state.

Table 6-3-1　The Physiochemical Properties of Inhalation Anesthetics

Anesthetics	Molecular weight	Oil/gas	Blood/gas	Metabolic rate (%)	MAC
Diethyl Ether	74	65	12	2.1-3.6	1.9
Nitrous Oxide	44	1.4	0.47	0.004	105
Halothane	197	224	2.4	15-20	0.75
Enflurane	184	98	1.9	2-5	1.7
Isoflurane	184	98	1.4	0.2	1.15
Sevoflurane	200	53.4	0.65	2-3	2.0
Desflurane	168	18.7	0.42	0.02	6.0

3.1.1.3　Metabolism and toxicity

Most inhalation anesthetics are higher liposolubility, which is difficult to be discharged from the kidneys in prototype. Most of them are discharged from the respiratory tract. Only a small part of them are excreted in the urine after metabolism. The major metabolic sites are in the liver. Cytochrome P450 is the key drug metabolizing enzyme, which can accelerate the metabolism process of drugs. The process of drug metabolism and its metabolites have different effects on the function of liver and kidney. The toxicity of drugs is related to its metabolic rate, metabolic intermediates and final products. Generally speaking, the lower the metabolic rate, the lower its toxicity. From Table 6-3-1, we can see that the metabolic rate of desflurane and isoflurane is the lowest, and the toxicity is the lowest, which is followed by enflurane and sevoflurane, while halothane is the highest. The toxic product of halothane contains three fluoroacetic acid, which is easy to combine with protein and amino acid to induce hepatotoxicity. The main cause of nephrotoxicity is the increase of inorganic fluoride (F^-) concentration in blood. It is generally believed that when F^- concentration is less than 50 mol/L, no nephrotoxicity is observed, 50-100 mol/L has a certain nephrotoxicity, and higher than 100 mol/L must produce nephrotoxicity. For chronic renal failure, halogen inhalation anesthetics should be used carefully.

3.1.1.4 Inhalation anesthetics in common use

(1) Nitrous Oxide (N_2O)

Also known as laughing gas, colorless, tasteless, weak anesthesia performance, must be combined with other anesthetic drugs. When combined with other anesthetics, it can enhance the anesthetic strength and reduce the dosage of other inhalation anesthetics.

Nitrous Oxide is a less toxic inhalation anesthetic, which has no inhibitory effect on the circulation system, and has no significant influence on cardiac output, heart rate and blood pressure. It may be related to the exciting sympathetic nervous system. It has contraction effect on pulmonary vascular smooth muscle, which can increase pulmonary vascular resistance, but has no significant effect on peripheral vascular resistance. It can slightly inhibit respiratory system, reduce tidal volume and speed up respiratory rate, but it has no irritation on respiratory tract. The partition coefficient of blood/gas is low, the balance of concentration between alveoli and FI is fast, and the change of alveolar ventilation or cardiac output has no significant effect on the uptake rate of N_2O in the pulmonary circulation. The cerebral blood flow is increased, and the intracranial pressure is slightly elevated. Almost all N_2O is excreted by prototype through respiratory tract, and has no significant effect on liver and kidney function.

Clinical application: It is often used in combination with other anesthetics to maintain anesthesia, and it can be used for surgical operation, dental or obstetric analgesia. During anesthesia, the fraction of inspiration $O_2(FIO_2)$ must be maintained above 30%, so as to avoid hypoxemia. During anaesthesia recovery period, there may be diffused anoxia. After stopping N_2O inhalation, pure oxygen should be inhaled for 5 - 10 minutes. In addition, N_2O can increase the pressure of the closed cavity, such as the middle ear, intestinal cavity, etc. Therefore, the patients with intestinal obstruction should not be used.

(2) Enflurane

Colorless transparent liquid, stable property, strong anesthesia performance.

Enflurane inhibits the circulatory system, which leads to a decrease in blood pressure, cardiac output and myocardial oxygen consumption. Enflurane can increase the sensitivity of cardiac muscle to catecholamine, but it is not easy to cause arrhythmia. No irritation on respiratory tract, no increase in saliva and airway secretions. The inhibition of respiration is stronger, which is characterized by decreased tidal volume and increased respiration. It can enhance the effect of non-depolarizing muscle relaxant. It has inhibitory effect on central nervous system (CNS), but it can increase cerebral blood flow and intracranial pressure. When enflurane is used for deep anaesthesia, epileptic spike and explosive suppression can occur in electro-encephalogram(EEG). The metabolism of enflurane is low, which does not cause obvious changes in liver and kidney function.

Clinical application: It can be used for anesthesia induction and maintenance. Anesthesia induction is fast, and recovery is fast and stable. Enflurane reduces intraocular pressure and is beneficial for intraocular surgery. Electroencephalogram shows epileptic changes during deep anesthesia. The clinical manifestations are facial and muscle convulsions. Therefore, people with epilepsy should be cautious.

(3) Isoflurane

Colorless transparent liquid, stable property, strong anesthesia performance.

The inhibition of myocardial contractility is mild, but it can significantly reduce peripheral arterial resistance and reduce arterial pressure. It has a dilatation effect on coronary arteries and may cause coronary steal. It does not increase the sensitivity of myocardium to exogenous catecholamine. Mild inhibition of respiratory center, and can dilate bronchial smooth muscle. It can enhance the effect of non-depolarizing muscle relaxant. Low concentration has no effect on cerebral blood flow. high concentration can expand cerebral blood vessels, increase cerebral blood flow and increase intracranial pressure. The effect of increasing intracranial pressure is lighter than that of halothane or enflurane, and it can be counteracted by proper overventilation. The blood/gas partition coefficient is low, and alveolar concentration quickly balances with inhalation concentration. The metabolism is low, which does not cause obvious changes in liver and kidney function.

Clinical application: It can be used for anesthesia induction and maintenance. When inhaled by face mask, it is irritating and easy to cause cough and breath holding. Therefore, inhaled isoflurane was used to maintain anesthesia after frequent intravenous induction. The circulation is stable during anesthesia maintenance and the recovery is faster after the drug withdrew. Because of its slight inhibition of myocardial contractility and obvious peripheral vasodilatation, it can be used for controlled hypotension.

(4) Sevoflurane

Colorless and transparent. It has special aroma, no irritation and strong anesthetic performance. The anesthesia is quickly induced and revived.

The inhibition of myocardial contractility is mild, but it can reduce peripheral vascular resistance, reduce arterial pressure and cardiac output, and do not increase the sensitivity of myocardium to exogenous catecholamine. No irritation on respiratory tract, no increase in respiratory secretions. It has strong inhibitory effect on respiration and can expand bronchial smooth muscle. It can enhance the function of non-depolarizing muscle relaxant and prolong the time of action. It has inhibitory effect on CNS, diastolic blood vessels, and elevated intracranial pressure. It is mainly in the liver metabolism, the metabolic rate is low, and can react with the alkali lime in the carbon dioxide absorption tank in the respiratory circuit, mainly produce fluoromethyl-2-fluoroethylene ether and so on. The abnormal increase of fluoromethyl-2-fluoroethylene ether can damage the renal function.

Clinical application: It can be used for anesthesia induction and maintenance. The incidence of cough and breath holding was low when using face mask. The circulation is stable during the maintenance of anesthesia. After anaesthesia, the awakening is rapid and smooth and the incidence of nausea and vomiting is low.

(5) Desflurane

Colorless transparent liquid, stable property, weak anesthesia performance. The blood/gas partition coefficient is the lowest, and induction and recovery are very fast.

The inhibition of myocardial contractility is light, and has no significant effect on heart rate and blood pressure, and does not increase the sensitivity of myocardium to exogenous catecholamine. Mild inhibition of respiration, and it can inhibit the body's response to the increase of carbon dioxide partial pressure ($PaCO_2$) and stimulate the respiratory tract. It has inhibitory effect on neuromuscular junction and enhances the effect of non-depolarizing muscle relaxant. Inhibition of electrical activity in cerebral cortex and reduction of the rate of cerebral oxygen metabolism. Low concentration dose not inhibit central CO_2 response, but overventilation dose not reduce intracranial pressure; High concentration can make cerebral vasodilation and reduce its ability of self regulation. Almost all of them are excreted from the lungs. Their metabolic rate is very low, so their liver and kidney toxicity is low.

Clinical application: For induction and maintenance of anesthesia, it can be induced by mask alone. The incidence of coughing and breath holding is low when the concentration is less than 6%. The concentration of more than 7% can cause coughing, increased breath holding, airway secretion and even laryngospasm. Because of its small influence on circulatory function, it is beneficial for patients undergoing cardiac surgery or heart diseased patients undergoing non-cardiac surgery. Its induction and recovery is rapid, and it is also suitable for anesthesia in outpatient surgery, and the incidence of nausea and vomiting is significantly lower than other inhalation anesthetics. But special evaporator is needed, and the price is more expensive.

3.1.2   Intravenous anesthetics

The anesthetic is injected directly into the vein, which acts on the central nervous system through the blood circulation and produces a general anesthetic effect. It is called intravenous anesthetics. Its advantages are quick induction, no irritation to respiratory tract and no environmental pollution. Intravenous anesthetics are the main anesthesia induction drugs in clinical anesthesia, and they are also used for maintenance of anesthesia. However, the termination of intravenous anesthetics mainly depends on its pharmacokinetic characteristics, the individual differences are large, and the controllability is less than that of inhaled anesthetics, and it is difficult to fully meet the needs of the operation. Clinically, the combination of sedatives and analgesics as well as muscle relaxants can be used to provide satisfactory anesthesia. Commonly used intravenous anesthetics are as follows:

(1) Thiopental sodium

It was an ultra short effect barbiturate intravenous general anesthetic. The commonly used concentration is 2.5%, and the solution is strong alkaline. Thiopental can permeate blood-brain barrier, enhance the inhibitory effect of γ-aminobutyric acid (GABA) in the brain, and inhibit the ascending activation system of the network structure. 15-30 seconds after intravenous injection, the patient lose their consciousness and the action maintain 15-20 minutes.

Direct inhibition of cardiac and medullary vasomotor centers, peripheral vasodilatation, blood pressure lowering and its extent are closely related to the dose and speed of injection. The blood pressure of patients with low blood volume or heart failure is more significant. It has strong central respiratory inhibition, reduced tidal volume and respiratory rate, reduced the sensitivity of respiratory center to carbon dioxide, and even apnea. Thiopental inhibits the sympathetic nerve and make the parasympathetic function relatively enhanced, increases sensitivity of throat and bronchus. Local stimulation (oropharyngeal airway, tracheal tube, secretion and throat irritation) and surgical stimulation (irritation of the anus, bladder and peritoneum, etc.) are easy to induce laryngospasm and tracheal spasm. Thiopental sodium increased cerebrovascular resistance, reduced cerebral blood flow and cerebral metabolic rate, reduced cerebral oxygen consumption and intracranial pressure after intravenous injection. Thiopental can resist local anesthetic toxicity. Metabolism and degradation occur mainly in the liver. For patients with liver dysfunction, anesthesia recovery time prolonged.

Clinical application: ①Induction of general anesthesia. The usual dose is 4-6 mg/kg, supplemented by muscle relaxant can complete tracheal intubation. But it is not suitable for tracheal intubation alone, which can cause severe laryngeal spasm. ②Anesthesia for short operation: Abscess incision drainage, radiography,

2. 5% solution 3-5 mg/kg. ③Control convulsion：2. 5% solution 1-2 mg/kg. ④Basic anaesthesia in children：Intramuscular injection of 1. 5% -2% solution 15-20 mg/kg. Subcutaneous injection can cause tissue necrosis. Intra-arterial injection can cause arterial spasm and distal limb necrosis.

（2）Ketamine

It is a kind of fast working nonbarbiturate intravenous anesthetic. It selectively inhibits brain contact pathway and thalamic neocortex system，but has little effect on the reticular formation of brainstem. It has obvious analgesic effect. After 30-60 seconds of intravenous injection，consciousness disappears and the action time is 15-20 minutes. After intramuscular injection，it takes about 5 minutes to onset，and the effect is strongest in 15 minutes.

Ketamine can stimulate sympathetic nerve，increase heart rate，increase blood pressure and pulmonary artery pressure. However，for the hypovolemia and highly excited sympathetic nerve，ketamine is shown as myocardial inhibition. Therefore，it is not suitable for patients with coronary heart disease，hypertension and pulmonary hypertension. It has less effect on respiration. But when the dosage is too large or the injection speed is too fast，or when combined with other narcotic analgesics，it can cause significant respiratory depression and even apnea，which should be particularly vigilant. Ketamine can increase saliva and bronchial secretion and relax bronchial smooth muscle. It can increase cerebral blood flow，intracranial pressure and cerebral metabolic rate，increase extraocular muscle tension and increase intraocular pressure. Therefore，patients with intracranial hypertension and glaucoma patients should be cautious. Metabolism is mainly in the liver，and the metabolite，norketamine，still has certain biological activity and is excreted by the kidneys.

Clinical application：①Induction of anesthesia，intravenous injection of 1-2 mg/kg. ②Maintenance：Intravenous infusion of 15-45 μg/（kg · min）. ③Pediatric basic anesthesia：Intramuscular injection of 5-10 mg/kg，which sustains about 30 min. The main side effects include transient apnea，hallucinations，nightmares and other mental symptoms. Diazepam or midazolam can reduce or eliminate hallucinations or nightmares before anesthesia.

（3）Etomidate

It is a synthetic，non-barbiturate，quick and short acting intravenous anesthetic，and it has no analgesic effect. The patient's consciousness disappeared after about 30 seconds after intravenous injection，and the peak concentration in the brain within 1 minutes. It has little effect on blood pressure，heart rate and cardiac output. No increase in myocardial oxygen consumption and mild dilation of coronary artery. Little influence on breathing. It can reduce cerebral blood flow，intracranial pressure and metabolic rate. It is mainly metabolized in the liver，metabolites are not active，and has no significant effect on liver and kidney function.

Clinical application：①It is mainly used for general anesthesia induction，especially for elderly，weak and critically ill patients. The general dose is 0. 15-0. 3 mg/kg. The main side effects are myoclonus can occur after injection and irritation to the veins. It is easy to have nausea and vomiting after operation. It can inhibit the function of adrenal cortex. It is not suitable for long time and large dose application.

（4）Propofol

It is a chemically synthesized milky white liquid with sedative hypnotic effect. Propofol plays an anesthetic role by enhancing the inhibitory effect of GABA. The effect is quick. After 30-40 seconds of injection of 1. 5-2 mg/kg，the time of maintenance is only 3-10 minutes. After discontinuation，the recovery is fast and complete.

It has a significant inhibitory effect on the cardiovascular system，including the direct inhibition of the myocardium and the vasodilatation，the decrease of blood pressure，the slow rate of heart rate，the resistance of peripheral blood vessels and the decrease of cardiac output. High dose，rapid injection，or for hypovolemia and the elderly, can cause serious hypotension. There is a significant inhibition of respiration, which is manifested by reduced tidal volume and respiratory rate, even apnea. The degree of inhibition is closely related to the dose. It can reduce cerebral blood flow, intracranial pressure and cerebral metabolic rate. After liver metabolism, the metabolites have no biological activity. Repeated injection or continuous intravenous infusion had accumulation in the body but had no significant effect on liver and kidney. Intravenous injection can cause pain at injection site, and low dose lidocaine can be prevented.

Clinical application: ①Intravenou induction: 1. 5-2. 5 mg/kg. ②Maintenance: 6-10 mg/(kg · h) intravenous infusion alone or combined with other anesthetics. ③Outpatient anesthesia: 2 mg/(kg · h). The patient can answer the question 10 minutes after the drug is stopped. ④Adjuvant in block anesthesia, the dose is 1-2 mg/(kg · h). The side effect are venous irritation, and the strong respiratory inhibition. If necessary, assisted respiration should be done.

(5) Midazolam

It is a benzodiazepic drug, which enhances the effect of GABA and its receptor, thus producing sedative, hypnotic, antianxiety, anticonvulsant, reducing muscle tension and anterograde amnesia.

Small doses of midazolam have little influence on hemodynamics and respiration, and can reduce cerebral blood flow and brain oxygen consumption. When the dose is large, blood pressure drops, heart rate slows, and respiratory depression, especially when combined with other narcotic analgesics.

Clinical application: As a premedication and anesthetic adjuvant, it is also used for general anesthesia induction. Intravenous injection of 1-2 mg patients can fall asleep. The dosage of intravenous general anesthesia is 0. 15-0. 2 mg/kg.

3.1.3   Muscle relaxants

The muscle relaxant acts on the end of the motor nerve and the end plate of the skeletal muscle, and interferes with the conduction of normal impulse between the nerve and muscle, which is beneficial to surgical operation. But muscle relaxant can only make skeletal muscle paralysis, itself does not produce anesthetic effect, cannot make the patient's consciousness and feel disappear, nor does it produce forgetfulness. In the range of clinical dosage and normal ventilation, muscle relaxant has no significant effect on myocardium and vascular smooth muscle, nor does it interfere with the physiological function of the body. Muscle relaxant is not only conducive to operative operation, but also helps to avoid the harm of deep anesthesia.

3.1.3.1   The mechanism and classification of muscle relaxants

The neuromuscular junction includes presynaptic membrane, postsynaptic membrane and synaptic cleft between anterior and posterior membranes. In the physiological state, when the nerve impulse is transmitted to the motor nerve endings, the vesicle in the presynaptic membrane breaks down, releasing the neurotransmitter acetylcholine to the synaptic cleft and binding to the acetylcholine receptor in the postsynaptic membrane, causing the depolarization of the postsynaptic membrane to induce the contraction of the muscle fibers. Muscle relaxant plays a major role in the neuromuscular junction, which interferes with the conduction of nerve impulse. According to the different ways of interference, muscle relaxants are mainly divided into two kinds: depolarizing muscle relaxant and non-depolarizing muscle relaxant.

(1) Depolarizing muscular relaxants

It is represented by succinylcholine. The molecular structure of succinylcholine is similar to acetylcholine, which can bind to acetylcholine receptor, induce motor end plate depolarization and muscle fiber bundle contraction. Succinylcholine has a strong affinity with the receptor, and it is not easily decomposed by cholinesterase at the neuromuscular junction, so that the postsynaptic membrane can not repolarize but is in a continuous depolarization state that does not react to acetylcholine, thus producing muscle relaxation. When the concentration of succinylcholine in the binding site gradually decreases, the postsynaptic membrane repolarization and neuromuscular function can return to normal. Its characteristics are as follows: ①The postsynaptic membrane is in a state of continuous depolarization. ②For the first time, before the emergence of muscle relaxation, the organic fibers contract in bundles, which is due to the uncoordinated contraction of muscle fibers. ③Cholinesterase inhibitors can not only antagonize their muscle relaxant effect, but enhance muscle relaxant effect.

(2)Non-depolarizing muscular relaxants

With pancuronium, rocuronium and atracurium as the representative. They are combined with the acetylcholine receptor of postsynaptic membrane, but do not cause postsynaptic membrane depolarization. When the acetylcholine receptor over 75%-80% in the postsynaptic membrane is combined with a non-depolarizing muscle relaxant, the nerve impulses can cause the release of acetylcholine, but not enough receptors are combined. The muscle fibers can not depolarizing, and the conduction of the neuromuscular block is blocked. The muscle relaxant and acetylcholine competitive binding receptors have a dose-dependent manner. The use of cholinesterase inhibitors (e. g. , neostigmine) can slow down the decomposition of acetylcholine and repeatedly compete with muscle relaxants. The number of acetylcholine receptor binding reaches the threshold, which can cause muscle contraction. Therefore, the action of non-depolarizing muscle relaxant can be antagonized by cholinesterase inhibitors. Its characteristics are as follows: ①The blocking site is in the neuromuscular junction, occupying the acetylcholine receptor of the postsynaptic membrane. ②The number of acetylcholine released from the presynaptic membrane during nerve excitation is not reduced, but it is not effective. ③There is no fasciculation before muscle relaxation; ④It can be antagonized by cholinesterase antagonist.

3.1.3.2   Commonly used muscle relaxants

(1)Succinylcholine(scoline)

It is the most common depolarizing muscle relaxant. It works quickly and relaxes completely and shortly. Muscle relaxation occurs 15-20 seconds after intravenous injection. In 1 minute, muscle relaxant reaches its peak, and lasts for 8-10 minutes. If intravenous injection of low-dose non depolarizing muscle relaxant before intravenous administration, it can reduce or eliminate muscle tremor. Succinylcholine has no obvious effect on hemodynamics, but it can increase serum potassium level. Severe cases can lead to arrhythmia. It does not cause histamine release, so it does not cause bronchospasm. It can be hydrolyzed rapidly by plasma cholinesterase, and the metabolites are excreted with urine.

It is mainly used for tracheal intubation during general anesthesia induction, and the dosage is 1-2 mg/kg intravenous injection.

Side effects: it can cause bradycardia and arrhythmia; Extensive skeletal muscle depolarization can lead to elevated serum potassium; When tetanic contraction it causes elevation of intracranial, intraocular and intragastric pressure; Postoperative myalgia. Therefore, patients with hyperkalemia (severe trauma and burns, etc.), paraplegia, penetrating ocular injury, glaucoma should be forbidden to use.

(2)Pancuronium

It is a long-acting non-depolarizing muscle relaxant with strong muscle relaxant. The onset time is 3-6 minutes, and the clinical duration is 100-120 minutes. Panbrocurium can block cardiac muscarinic receptors, increase heart rate and even tachycardia. Inhibiting the reuptake of norepinephrine and causing the increase of blood drugs. Cholinesterase antagonist can antagonize its muscle relaxant. In the liver metabolism, after repeated medication, we should pay special attention to its postoperative residual effect. 40% of the drug is expelled from the kidney by the prototype, and the rest is excreted through biliary tract by prototypes or metabolites.

It is used for tracheal intubation during general anesthesia induction and intraoperative maintenance. The first dose of intravenous injection is 0.1-0.15 mg/kg. Intraoperative intermittent intravenous injection of 2-4 mg is performed to maintain muscle relaxation during general anesthesia. After the operation, cholinesterase antagonist can be used to antagonize the residual muscle relaxant effect.

Patients with hypertension, myocardial ischemia, tachycardia and liver and kidney dysfunction should be used cautiously, and patients with myasthenia gravis should be forbidden.

(3) Vecuronium

It is a non-depolarizing muscle relaxant with strong muscle relaxant, and its action time is shorter than pancuronium. The onset time is 2-3 minutes, and the clinical action time is 25-30 minutes. In the range of clinical dosage, vecuronium has little effect on the cardiovascular system, does not cause histamine release, nor does it resist the effect of vagus nerve. It is suitable for patients with ischemic heart disease. Mainly in the liver metabolism, 30% of it is expelled from the kidney by the prototype, and the rest is excreted through biliary tract by prototypes or metabolites.

It is used for tracheal intubation during general anesthesia induction and intraoperative maintenance. During operation, 0.02-0.03 mg/kg was given intermittently or continuous intravenous infusion at a speed of 1-2 μg/(kg·min) to maintain muscle relaxation during general anesthesia. In patients with severe liver and kidney dysfunction, the effect is prolonged and accumulated.

(4) Rocuronium

Non-depolarizing muscle relaxant, which is weak in muscle relaxant and short in acting time. It belongs to intermediate-acting muscle relaxant. Rocuronium is currently the fastest onset non-depolarizing muscle relaxant in clinic. When 1.2 mg/kg is used, it can be intubated in 60 seconds. Rocuronium has a specific antagonist-sugammadex, which can antagonize any degree of neuromuscular block caused by it. It has little effect on the cardiovascular system and does not cause histamine release. The metabolites of drugs are mainly excreted from bile and partly from the kidneys.

It is used for tracheal intubation during general anesthesia induction and intraoperative maintenance.

(5) Atracurium

Non-depolarizing muscle relaxant, with short action time. The onset time is 3-5 minutes, and the clinical action time is 15-35 minutes. Atracurium induced histamine release and the degree of release related to dosage, such as rash, tachycardia and hypotension. Severe bronchospasm can occur. Mainly through Hofmann degradation and plasma esterase hydrolysis, the metabolites excreted from the kidneys and biliary tract, and there was no significant accumulation effect.

It is used for tracheal intubation during general anesthesia induction and muscle relaxation during operation. 0.5-0.6 mg/kg is injected intravenously, and tracheal intubation is made after 2-3 minutes. During operation, 0.1-0.2 mg/kg is given intermittently or continuous infusion at a speed of 5-10 μg/(kg·min) to maintain muscle relaxation. Allergies and asthmapatients are used carefully.

(6) Cisatracurium

Non-depolarizing muscle relaxant. The onset time is 2-3 minutes, and the clinical action time is 50-60 minutes. Compared with atracurium, its advantages are not causing histamine release and hemodynamic stability in the clinical dose range. It is mainly degraded by Hofmann.

It is used for tracheal intubation during general anesthesia induction and muscle relaxation during operation. It has wide application and is suitable for elderly, heart, liver and kidney dysfunction patients.

0.15-0.2 mg/kg is injected intravenously, and tracheal intubation is made after 1.5-2 minutes. During operation, 0.02 mg/kg is given intermittently or continuous infusion at a speed of $1-2$ μg/ (kg · min) to maintain muscle relaxation.

3.1.3.3　Cautions in the application of muscle relaxants

①Tracheal intubation should be performed to assist or control breathing in order to maintain airway patency. ②Muscle relaxants are not sedative and analgesic, thus can not be used alone. They must be combined with general anesthetics. ③Succinylcholine can cause transient elevation of serum potassium, intraocular pressure and intracranial pressure. Therefore, succinylcholine is forbidden in patients with severe trauma, burns, paraplegia, glaucoma and elevated intracranial pressure. ④Low body temperature can prolong the effect of muscle relaxants, inhalation anesthetics, some antibiotics (such as streptomycin, gentamicin, polymyxin) and magnesium sulfate can enhance the effect of non-depolarized muscle relaxants. ⑤In patients with neuromuscular junctional disease (e. g. , myasthenia gravis) , the application of non-depolarizing relaxants is forbidden. ⑥Some relaxants is histamine-releasing, so they should be carefully used in asthmatic and anaphylactic patients.

3.1.4　Narcotic analgesics

Narcotic analgesics play an analgesic role in general anesthesia, combined with intravenous total anesthetics, sedative drugs and muscle relaxants to provide a perfect and comfortable anesthesia for the operation. But these drugs are addictive and belong to controlled drugs.

(1) Morphine

Acting on the limbic system of the brain can relieve tension and anxiety, increase pain threshold, relieve pain, cause euphoria, and become addictive. It has an obvious inhibitory effect on the respiratory center, and lightly slows the breathing, and the severe tidal volume decreases and even stops breathing, and it has the role of histamine release, thus causing bronchospasm. Morphine dilates arterioles and veins, reduces peripheral resistance, reduces returned blood and induces hypotension, but has no significant effect on myocardium. Other side effects are nausea and vomiting, skin pruritus, etc.

It is mainly used for analgesia, such as pain caused by trauma, operation, angina pectoris and so on. Because of its good analgesic effect, it is also used as a premedication and anesthetic adjuvant. Combined with sedative and muscle relaxant, general intravenous anesthesia is applied. The adult dosage is 5-10 mg subcutaneous or intramuscular injection.

(2) Pethidine

Pethidine has a role in analgesic, hypnotic and relieve muscle spasms. The myocardial contractility is inhibited, resulting in decreased blood pressure and decreased cardiac output. Mild inhibition of breathing, euphoria and addiction after medication. It is often used as a pre-anesthetic drug, the adult dosage is 50 mg, and the child is 1 mg/kg intramuscular injection. It is not suitable for child under 2 years old. Combined with promethazine or droperidol for adjuvant used in anesthesia. For postoperative analgesia, the adult dosage is 50 mg intramuscular injection, and the interval is 4-6 hours.

(3) Fentanyl

The synthetic opioid receptor agonist has a high fat solubility and a strong analgesic effect, which is 75-125 times higher than that of morphine. Fentanyl does not inhibit myocardial contractility, and has little effect on circulation and no histamine release. Respiration is inhibited, and respiratory depression is more obvious when combined with midazolam. Other side effects include muscle stiffness, nausea and vomiting, and itchy skin.

Clinical application：①Anesthesia induction：the common dose is 0. 1−0. 2 mg. ②Anesthesia mainte-nance：0. 05−0. 1 mg is usually added every 30−60 minutes before operation and during operation. ③Large dose of fentanyl combined anesthesia is commonly used in major cardiovascular anaesthesia. Fentanyl is in-duced by 20 μg/kg slow intravenous injections and combined with muscle relaxants to complete tracheal in-tubation. Fentanyl maintained anesthesia during the operation, and the total dosage of fentanyl reached 50−100 μg/kg. ④Monitored anesthesia care：It is used for outpatient surgery with little stimulation and short maintenance time, such as induced abortion, abscess incision and drainage, fentanyl dose for adult is 0. 1 mg.

(4) Sufentanil

The analgesic effect is the strongest opioid. The analgesic intensity is 5−10 times that of fentanyl, and the duration of analgesia is 2 times that of fentanyl, so it is commonly used for postoperative analgesia. Com-pared with equivalent dose of fentanyl, sufentanil has less effect on circulatory function, so it is also more suitable for anesthesia in cardiovascular surgery and elderly patients. The effect on respiratory system is dose−dependent, and the effect of inhibiting the stress reaction is better than that of fentanyl. The other side effects such as muscle stiffness, nausea and vomiting are similar to fentanyl.

Clinical application：①Anesthesia induction or outpatient anaesthesia：small doses of 0. 1−0. 2 μg/kg are used. ②Large dose combined anesthesia：Dosage of 2−50 μg/kg is commonly used for cardiovascular sur-gery and neurosurgical anesthesia. ③Postoperative analgesia：the postoperative analgesia pump was prepared.

(5) Remifentanil

For the ultra short effect opioid analgesics, the half−life of the analgesic is 9 minutes. Its elimination is not dependent on the function of the liver and kidney, and it is hydrolyzed by non−specific esterase in the blood and tissue to the inactive metabolite, so it has short time, rapid recovery and no accumulation. When used alone, the heart rate of the circulatory system was mainly slowed down；When combined with other an-esthetics, blood pressure and heart rate decrease；It can produce dose dependent respiratory depression. Af-ter 5−8 minutes of withdrawal, spontaneous breathing can be restored；the incidence of myotonia is high.

Clinical application：Used for induction and maintenance of anesthesia. The single dose of intravenous injection is 0. 5−1 μg/kg, and the recommended dosage for maintaining anesthesia is 0. 025−1. 0 μg/(kg · min). If target controlled infusion (TCI) is used to control remifentanil plasma concentration greater than 4 ng/mL, it can effectively inhibit the stress reaction during tracheal intubation. After stopping the in-fusion of remifentanil, the analgesic effect will soon disappear. Appropriate analgesic measures must be taken, such as giving small doses of fentanyl, epidural analgesia, etc.

3. 2　Basic Structure and Application of Anesthetic Ma-chine

Anesthesia machine provides oxygen, inhalation anesthetics and auxiliary respiration for patients. It is an indispensable device for clinical anesthesia and first aid. A good performance anaesthesia machine and correct skilled operation skills are essential for ensuring the safety of patients. Its main structures are as follows：

(1) Gas source

It mainly refers to the storage equipment for supplying oxygen, Nitrous Oxide (N$_2$O) and air, including compressed oxygen and liquid Nitrous Oxide, or central gas supply.

(2) Vaporizer

A device that effectively evaporates liquid volatile anesthetics into gases and accurately regulates the output concentration of anesthetics. The evaporator has drug specificity, such as sevoflurane evaporator, isoflurane evaporator, desflurane evaporator and so on.

(3) Breathing circuit system

Oxygen, air and inhalation anesthetics are transported to the respiratory tract of the patient through the respiratory loop, while the patient's exhaled air is discharged from the body.

(4) Ventilator

Respiratory devices are used to control the patient's breathing during anesthesia. Respiratory apparatus can be divided into constant volume and constant pressure. Respiratory parameters such as tidal volume, minute ventilation volume, pressure, respiratory frequency, ratio of inspiration to expiration time (I : E) and positive end-expiratory pressure (PEEP) can be set or adjusted according to patients'body weight and oxygen demand. The alarm limits of inhalation oxygen concentration, minute ventilation volume and airway pressure can also be set to ensure the safety of anesthesia.

3.3　Endotracheal Intubation

In order to ensure the patency of the patient's respiratory tract, the patient's breathing is managed effectively, and the special tracheal catheter is inserted into the patient's trachea through the mouth or the nasal cavity, that is, endotracheal intubation. This is a basic operative skill that anesthesiologists must master and is also an important part of clinical anesthesia. Its advantages are as follows: ①During the period of anesthesia, the patient's respiratory tract should be kept unobstructed, and foreign bodies should be prevented from entering the respiratory tract, and timely suction of tracheal secretions or blood. ②Effective artificial or mechanical ventilation is implemented to avoid hypoxia and carbon dioxide accumulation. ③It is safe, environmental protection and accurate inhalation of general anesthetics. Where general anesthesia is difficult to ensure the patient's respiratory tract unobstructed, such as intracranial surgery, thoracotomy, prone position surgery, etc. , patients whose respiratory tract is difficult to maintain unobstructed, such as tumor compression of trachea, general anesthetics to significantly inhibit breathing or use muscle relaxants, should be tracheal intubation. Tracheal intubation also plays an important role in the rescue of critically ill patients. Respiratory failure requires mechanical ventilation, cardiopulmonary resuscitation and severe neonatal asphyxia. Tracheal intubation is also necessary.

The commonly used methods for endotracheal intubation include direct vision orotracheal intubation and nasotracheal intubation. Generally speaking, orotracheal intubation is the first choice. A few patients require nasotracheal catheterization because of oral surgery or mandibular joint ankylosis and difficult mouth opening.

3.3.1　Direct vision orotracheal intubation

With laryngoscope exposing glottis under direct vision, the appropriate tube is inserted into the trachea through the oral cavity (Figure 6-3-1). The method of intubation: lift the head back and open the mouth. Laryngoscope which is hold in left hand is put into the oral cavity, it slowly pushed forward. First, the uvula was exposed. The epiglottis was brought up by the blade. If a curved blade is applied, the blade will be placed at the junction between epiglottis and the base of the tongue (epiglottis valley), and it will be raised forward and upward to reveal the glottis. If we use straight blade to intubate, we will directly raise the epiglottis and expose the glottis. In the right hand, the trachea tube is inserted into the mouth from the right mouth angle. At the same time, both eyes stare the direction of the tube advancing, accurately and gently the tube is inserted into the glottis. Inflating cuff. The depth of the tube inserted into the trachea is 4−5 cm for adult, and the distance between the tube tip and the middle inciso is 18−22 cm. After completion of intubation, make sure that the tuber has entered the trachea, and then it is properly fixed. The identified methods are as follows: ①When the chest is pressed, there is air flow in the orifice of the tube. ②During the artificial respiration, the bilateral chest symmetry fluctuate, and auscultation can hear clear and symmetrical breath sounds of both lungs. ③The transparent tube wall is clear when inhaling, and "white fog" changes can be seen on the exhalation. ④If the patient breathes spontaneously, the breathing bag can be expanded and compressed with breathing after connecting with the anesthesia machine. ⑤Monitoring end tidal carbon dioxide ($ETCO_2$): Correct graphics are confirmed.

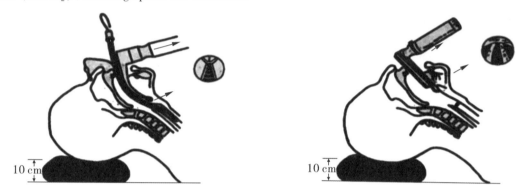

Figure 6−3−1   Orotracheal intubation with curved(left) and straight(right) blade laryngoscope

It's easier to judge if the end−of−expiratory CO_2 partial pressure($ETCO_2$) can be monitored, and it can be confirmed correcthy if the $ETCO_2$ is displayed.

3.3.2 Nasotracheal intubation

The endotracheal tube was inserted into the trachea through nasal cavity (Figure 6−3−2). Intubation method: First nasal mucosal surface anesthesia, and 3% ephedrine drip nasal mucosal vasoconstriction to reduce bleeding. Choose the appropriate diameter of the tube to insert into the nasal cavity. The intubation can be performed under visible light or by blind exploration under the condition of preserving the patient's spontaneous breathing.

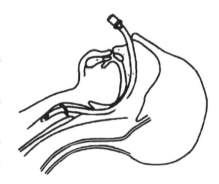

Figure 6−3−2   Nasotracheal intubation

3.3.3 Complications of endotracheal intubation

(1) During endotracheal intubation, the teeth were damaged or lost, the mucosa of the mouth, throat and nasal cavity were damaged and bleeding, and even the temporomandibular joint dislocation.

(2) Light anesthesia during tracheal intubation causes severe cough, choking, throat and bronchial spasm, tachycardia and sharp fluctuation of blood pressure, which leads to myocardial ischemia. Severe vagal reflexes lead to arrhythmia, bradycardia and cardiac arrest.

(3) Too small inner diameter of tracheal tube increases respiratory resistance; too large or too hard inner diameter of tracheal tube can easily damage respiratory mucosa, even cause acute laryngeal edema, or chronic granuloma. Respiratory obstruction can be caused by over-soft catheter which is easily deformed and twisted.

(4) The tube is inserted too deep into one side of the bronchus, leading to insufficient ventilation, hypoxia or atelectasis after operation. When the tube insertion is too shallow, it is easy for the patient to pull out because of the change of position, and serious medical incidents occur. Therefore, the position of the tube should be carefully checked after intubation and in the course of changing position, and the respiratory sounds of both lungs should be auscultated routinely.

3.3.4　Laryngeal mask

It is a kind of ventilation tool between the mask and endotracheal intubation. It has the advantages of simple operation, easy to master, small damage, well tolerated, and has been widely used in the opening of special emergency airway in clinical anesthesia. But laryngeal mask can not completely prevent aspiration, so it can not be used for patients with high risk of vomiting and reflux, and patients with subglottic airway obstruction are also prohibited.

3.4　The Implementation of General Anesthesia

3.4.1　Induction of general anesthesia

Induction of general anesthesia refers to the tracheal intubation from conscious state to mental disappearance and general anesthesia. This stage is called induction period of general anesthesia. Before induction, the anesthetic machine, tracheal intubation equipment, and aspirator should be prepared. Electrocardiogram, heart rate, blood pressure, SPO$_2$ should be monitored routinely. Vein and gastrointestinal decompression tube should be opened. The methods for induction of general anesthesia are as follows:

3.4.1.1　Inhalational induction

(1) Open drop method

With a metal mesh mask, a gauze is buckled to the patient's mouth and nose, and the volatile anesthetics are dripped on the gauze. The patient is inhaled by anesthetic and gradually into the anesthetic state when the patient is breathing. This method has great pollution to the environment, which is almost eliminated. In the past, it was mainly used for ether anesthesia.

(2) Mask inhalation induction

The anesthetic mask is buckled to the patient's mouth and nose, the anesthetic evaporator and oxygen is opened, and the concentration of inhaled anesthetics is gradually increased. When the patient's consciousness disappears and enters the anaesthetized state, the tracheal intubation is performed after the muscle relaxant is given.

3.4.1.2　Intravenous induction

Compared with inhalation induction, intravenous induction is rapid, comfortable and environmentally friendly. However, the depth of anesthesia staging is not obvious, which has great disturbance to the circulation of patients. Before induction, mask inhaled pure oxygen for 2-3 minutes, increased oxygen storage, and selected appropriate intravenous anesthetics such as propofol, etomidate, to inject slowly from the vein and closely monitor the changes of consciousness, circulation and respiration of patients. After the disappearance of consciousness, the patient is injected with muscle relaxant. The skeletal muscle and mandible gradually relaxed and the breathing stopped from shallow to complete. At this time, artificial breathing through a mask and then endotracheal intubation. Once the intubation is successful, it is immediately connected to the anesthesia machine and assisted by artificial respiration or mechanical ventilation.

3.4.2 Maintenance of anesthesia

(1) Inhalational anesthetic maintenance

At present the gaseous anesthetics is nitrous oxide, and volatile anesthetics are fluorides anesthetic agents which include enflurane, isoflurane, etc. Nitrous oxide is difficult to maintain anesthesia alone because its weak potency and risk to result hypoxia. Among these commonly used inhalation anesthetics, Nitrous Oxide is weak in anesthetic performance. When inhaled it with high concentration, anoxia is also dangerous and can not be used alone to maintain anesthesia. The anesthetic performance of volatile anesthetics is strong. Inhalation of certain concentration can make patients' consciousness and pain disappear and can be used alone to maintain anesthesia. But the muscle relaxant effect is not satisfied, and the higher the inhalation concentration, the more serious the physiological effects. Therefore, N_2O-O_2-volatile anesthetics are often used to maintain anesthesia, and when necessary, combined with muscle relaxant. Using Nitrous Oxide, should monitor the inhaled oxygen concentration and pulse oxygen saturation (SPO_2), inhaled oxygen concentration of not less than 30%. Volatile anesthetics use special evaporator to regulate their inhalation concentration. Meanwhile, continuous monitoring of inhalation anesthetics concentration makes the depth of anesthesia easier to control.

(2) Intravenous anesthetic maintenance

After anesthesia induction, the proper depth of anesthesia is maintained through intravenous administration. According to the needs of operation and the pharmacological characteristics of different intravenous anesthetics, a suitable intravenous drug delivery method was selected: single, sub dose or continuous injection. The present use of intravenous anesthetics, except ketamine, most of them belong to the hypnotic, no obvious analgesic effect. Some drugs such as thiopental, large doses have some analgesic effect, but very large physical interference. Therefore, short surgery uses single intravenous anesthetic, complicated or longer operation, tending to choose combined general anesthesia.

(3) Combined anesthesia

It refers to two or more than two kinds of general anesthetics and/or methods combined with each other, so as to achieve the best clinical anesthetic effect. According to the different routes of administration, combind anesthesia can be roughly divided into total intravenous anesthesia and combined intravenous-inhalation anesthesia.

1) Total intravenous anesthesia(TIVA): It refers to the combination of multiple short acting intravenous anesthetics after intravenous induction of anesthesia, and intermittent or continuous intravenous injection of drugs to maintain proper anesthetic depth. Total intravenous anesthesia is needed to achieve a stable anesthetic state. Intravenous anesthetics, narcotic analgesics and muscle relaxants are needed. In this way, we can give full play to the advantages of each drug and reduce its adverse effects. It has the advantages of fast induction and simple operation, and can avoid environmental pollution caused by inhalation anesthetics. If the medication is precise and appropriate, the anesthesia process is stable and the recovery is fast. But because it is a complex application of multiple drugs, how to choose the right time and dosage according to their respective pharmacological characteristics is very critical. Anesthetic signs and anesthetic staging are also difficult to distinguish accurately. Delayed recovery after anesthesia and residual effects of muscle relax-

ants can also cause serious complications. Therefore, the anesthesiologist must be proficient in a variety of pharmacological characteristics, flexible drug medication, in order to achieve good anesthetic effect. We should closely monitor the changes of vital signs of patients in clinical practice, and those who have conditions can be target controlled according to the characteristics of pharmacokinetics. There is not much dispute about the basic principles of TIVA. There are great differences between the specific methods, dosage size and timing of administration. The current intravenous anesthetics are propofol and midazolam. The anesthetic analgesics are sufentanil and fentanyl, while muscle relaxants use long or short effect drugs according to the needs of the operation.

2) Intravenous–inhalation combined anesthesia: The timing of total intravenous anesthesia is difficult to master. Sometimes anesthesia can be reduced suddenly, and a certain amount of volatile anesthetics can be inhaled to maintain the stability of anesthesia. On the basis of intravenous anesthesia, a suitable concentration of volatile anesthetics is inhaled. In this way, anesthesia can be maintained stable and simple, and it can reduce the dosage of inhalation anesthetics, and is conducive to rapid recovery after anesthesia. Intravenous–inhalation combined anesthesia is widely applied, and anesthesia operation and management are easy to master. The passive situation of abrupt reduction of anesthesia rarely occurs. However, if not mastered properly, it is also prone to delayed recovery after surgery.

3.4.3 The judgment of the depth of general anesthesia

Good general anesthesia should enable patients to have sufficient sedation, analgesia, satisfactory muscle relaxation and reasonable control of stress, which can meet the needs of surgery. It is especially important to determine the depth and maintain the best depth of anesthesia during the process of anesthesia. Improper anesthesia often leads to too deep or too shallow anesthesia, resulting in delayed recovery or awareness during the operation.

In 1930s, Guedel put forward the stage of ether anesthesia depth according to various clinical manifestations and signs of patients during the course of ether anesthesia. Despite the development of a variety of new anesthetics and the application of complex anesthesia techniques, the various indications of the depth of anesthesia in the anaesthesia are not completely changed, and can still be used as a reference for judging and mastering the depth of anesthesia in today's clinical anesthesia. The standard of the ether anesthesia depth staging is the level of consciousness, pain, reflex activity, muscle relaxation, respiration and circulation inhibition, that is, the inhibition of the central nervous system by general anesthetic.

The first phrase (forgetting period): From the induction of anesthesia to the disappearance of consciousness, the pain did not disappear during this period.

The second phrase (excitement period): The patient presents the excitement of struggle, breath holding, vomiting, cough, swallowing and so on. The response to the outside is enhanced and it is not suitable for any operation. Appropriate induction can make this period pass quickly.

The third phase (surgical anesthesia period): During this period, the anesthesia reached the required depth, breathing and circulation were stable. Pain stimulation could not cause somatic reflex and harmful autonomic nervous reflex (such as increased blood pressure and tachycardia). Further deepening of anesthesia aggravated the inhibition of breathing and circulation.

The fourth phase (bulbar paralysis period): respiratory arrest, pupil dilatation, blood pressure reduction to circulatory failure. This period needs to be avoided. If it appears, we should lighten the anesthetic as soon as possible and deal with it in time.

The application of combined anesthesia is difficult to predict the depth of general anesthesia. The use of powerful analgesics and muscle relaxants, the patient can not respond to pain, the muscles are completely relaxed, but know what is happening in the operation and can not be expressed, called "intraoperative awareness", causing serious mental injury to the patient. In order to avoid such adverse events, people have carried out a lot of exploration, but there is no reliable, convenient and effective method that can be used as a clinical routine. The analysis of Bispectrum index (BIS) electroencephalogram developed in recent years is considered to be of great value for judging the depth of sedation. The range of BIS is 0-100, the smaller the value, the deeper the sedation. Somatosensory evoked potentials, brainstem auditory evoked potentials and anesthetic entropy are hot topics, but they can not represent all aspects of anesthetic depth. In clinical practice, the depth of anesthesia should be judged according to the effects of compound drugs(including all kinds of anesthetics, analgesics, muscle relaxants, etc.)on consciousness, sensory, exercise, nerve reflex and the stability of the internal environment. When breathing spontaneously, breathing is enhanced and accelerated under a light anaesthesia. The stability of circulation is still an important sign to judge the depth of anaesthesia. The deep anesthesia should be taken into consideration when severe circulation inhibition, the increase of heart rate and the increase of blood pressure are the manifestations of light anesthesia. Volatile anesthetics have strong anesthetic performance. The high concentration inhalation of volatile anesthetics can make the patient's consciousness and pain disappear, but the muscle relaxant can not meet the requirements of the operation. For example, the blind pursuit of muscle relaxation will lead to deep anesthesia. Therefore, compound anesthesia is still based on rational drug compatibility and avoiding too light or deep anesthesia. It is important and complex to maintain the best depth of anesthesia. We should carefully observe the patients, make a reasonable judgement on the comprehensive indicators, and adjust the depth of anesthesia in time to meet the needs of the operation according to the strength of the stimulation. The depth of anesthesia is usually divided into light anesthesia stage, surgical anesthesia stage and deep anesthesia stage (Table 6-3-2). It has a certain reference value for evaluating the depth of anesthesia.

Table 6-3-2   The criterion of anesthetic depth under combined anesthesia

Stage	Respiration	Circulation	Ocular sign	Others
Light	irregular, cough airway resistance ↑ laryngeal spasm	BP ↑ HR ↑	ciliary reflex (−) eyeball movement(+) eyelid reflex(+) lacrimation	swallowing reflex (+) sweating secretion ↑ bodymovement
Surgical	regular, airway resistance ↓	BP mild lower but stable	eyelid reflex(−) fixed eyeball	no body movement
Deep	regular, airway resistance ↓	BP ↓	light reflex(−) enlarged pupil	

3.5   Complications and Treatment of General Anesthesia

3.5.1   Regurgitation and aspiration

Patients with full stomach, ileus, obstetrics and pediatric surgery are prone to vomiting and aspiration during general anesthesia, resulting in suffocation or aspiration pneumonia. Vomiting can occur during anesthesia induction, anesthesia and recovery period. The nature and quantity of reflux or aspiration are different, and the consequences are different. For example, the mortality rate of aspiration of large amount of gastric contents is high. No matter aspiration is solid food or gastric juice, it can cause acute respiratory obstruction. Complete airway obstruction can instantly suffocate and anoxia. If the obstruction can not be relieved in time, it can immediately endanger the life of the patient. Aspiration of gastric juice can cause lung injury, bronchial spasm and increased capillary permeability, further leading to pulmonary edema and atelectasis. The degree of lung injury is related to gastric juice volume and pH. The larger the volume of inhalation, the lower the pH is, the more serious the lung injury is. During anesthesia, various measures to prevent reflux and aspiration are necessary. The main measures include reducing gastric contents, promoting gastric emptying, elevating pH in gastric juice and enhancing airway protection. Before elective surgery, patients should strictly forbid drinking and fasting. Those who have full stomach must undergo surgery should choose local anesthesia or intraspinal anesthesia as far as possible and keep the patient awake. If general anesthesia is necessary, anesthesia should be performed according to the full stomach, and tracheal intubation should be awake if necessary.

3.5.2 Airway obstruction

With glottis as the boundary, airway obstruction can be divided into upper airway obstruction and lower respiratory tract obstruction or both.

(1) Upper airway obstruction

The most common causes are glossoptosis (Figure 6-3-3), oral secretions and foreign body obstruction, laryngeal edema, laryngeal spasm and so on, mainly manifested as difficulty in breathing. When the tongue falls back, the head is back and the mandible is taken up (Figure 6-3-4). Placement of oropharynx or the nasopharyngeal airway (Figure 6-3-5, Figure 6-3-6), the secretion and foreign body of the throat section can be cleaned up in time, and the obstruction can be relieved. Laryngeal edema is commonly seen in infants and difficult tracheal intubation, and can also be caused by pulling or stimulating larynx. Mild intravenous injection of corticosteroids or inhalation of epinephrine can relieve; immediate emergency tracheotomy is needed for a serious person. Laryngeal spasm, patients showed difficulty breathing, inspiratory crowing sound. Laryngeal spasm, patients showed difficulty breathing, inspiratory crowing sound, may be hypoxia and cyanosis due to hypoxia. For mild laryngeal spasms, it can relieve the inducements and relieve the pressure, and severe cases need tracheal intubation or first aid through the thyrocricocentesis cannulation. To prevent laryngeal spasm, we should avoid larynx stimulation during shallow anesthesia.

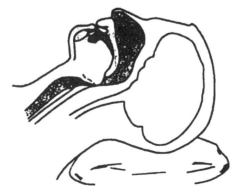

Figure 6-3-3　Glossoptosis caused by airway obstruction

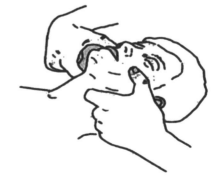

Figure 6-3-4　Jaw thrust method

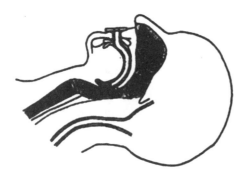
Figure 6-3-5　Oropharyngeal airway

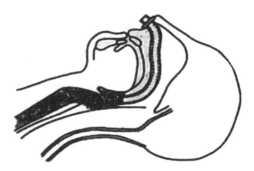
Figure 6-3-6　Nasopharyngeal airway

(2) Lower airway obstruction

The common cause is trachea, bronchial secretion or vomitus, obstruction not serious person can have noobvious symptom; The patients with severe obstruction are dyspnea, low tidal volume, high airway resistance, anoxic cyanosis, fast heart rate and hypotension, which can jeopardize the patient's life if not treat in time. Lower respiratory tract obstruction can also be caused by bronchial spasm, mostly in patients with asthma or chronic bronchitis. Lung auscultation can hear wheezing, and respiratory sounds disappear in severe case. The maintenance of appropriate depth of anesthesia and good oxygenation is an important measure to alleviate bronchospasm. When necessary, aminophylline 0.125-0.25 g or hydrocortisone 100 mg can be injected.

3.5.3　Hypoventilation

Hypoventilation can occur during and after anesthesia, showing hypoxemia and/or CO_2 retention. The injury of craniocerebral operation and the remnants of narcotic drugs are the main causes of respiratory depression. Mechanical ventilation should be used to maintain the respiration until the respiratory function is completely restored, and the antagonist should be used to reverse when necessary.

3.5.4　Hypoxemia

When inhaling air, when $SpO_2 < 90\%$, $PaO_2 < 60$ mmHg or pure oxygen, $PaO_2 < 90$ mmHg can be diagnosed as hypoxemia. The clinical manifestations are shortness of breath, cyanosis, dysphoria, tachycardia, arrhythmia, high blood pressure, et al. The common causes and principles of treatment are as follows: ①The malfunction of the anesthetic machine, the insufficient supply of oxygen, the insertion of tracheal tube into the bronchial tube, the prolapse of trachea tube and the obstruction of the respiratory tract can cause hypoxemia, and the respiratory circuit and tracheal tube are checked in time. ②Diffuse anoxia: it can be seen in N_2O inhalation anesthesia, stop inhaling N_2O, inhaling pure oxygen. ③Atelectasis: oversecretion or hypoventilation can result in decreased lung capacity. It can be improved by sputum suction, ventilation and lung recruitment. ④Aspiration: the severity depends on the amount of inhalation and pH. Light is effective for oxygen therapy. Severe mechanical ventilation is necessary. ⑤Pulmonary edema: it can occur in acute left heart failure or increased capillary permeability, increase the concentration of inhaled oxygen, and actively treat the primary disease.

3.5.5　Hypotention

During the period of anesthesia, the decreased systolic blood pressure exceed 30% of the basic value or the absolute value is lower than 80 mmHg, we should deal with it in time. Severe cases may suffer from inadequate organ perfusion, such as myocardial ischemia and central nervous system dysfunction. Common causes and treatment: ①Anesthesia is too deep. If the volume of blood is insufficient before anesthesia, it will be more obvious. Adjust the appropriate depth of anesthesia while supplementing the volume. ②Excessive intraoperative blood loss can cause hypovolemic shock, and timely transfusion. ③Anaphylaxis, hypoadrenocortical hypofunction and rewarming can cause hypotension and tachycardia due to the decrease of blood vessel tension. Treatment includes etiological treatment, supplementation of blood volume and proper use of vasoconstrictor. ④During operation, the reflex blood pressure decreased and bradycardia was induced when pulling the internal organs. Timely relief of irritation, if necessary, atropine symptomatic treatment.

3.5.6 Hypertension

During anesthesia, the diastolic blood pressure is higher than 100 mmHg or the systolic blood pressure is 30% higher than the basic value. It should be treated according to the causeof disease. Common causes: ①It is associated with comorbidities, such as essential hypertension, pheochromocytoma and intracranial hypertension. ②It is related to operation and anesthesia manipulation, such as surgical exploration and endotracheal intubation. ③Insufficient ventilation leads CO_2 accumulation. ④Drug induced hypertension, such as ketamine. Treatment principle: intravenous anesthesia with fentanyl during induction of general anesthesia can relieve cardiovascular responses during tracheal intubation. Treatment principle: intravenous injection of fentanyl during induction of general anesthesia to reduce the cardiovascular response to tracheal intubation; to adjust the depth of anesthesia in the operation according to the extent of the surgical stimulation; to control blood pressure and maintain circulation stability for those with intractable hypertension.

3.5.7 Arrhythmias

Sinus tachycardia and hypertension occur at the same time, often for the performance of shallow anesthesia, and properly deepen anesthesia. Hypoxemia, anaemia and anoxia can also be seen as faster heart rate and treatment for etiological factors. When the operation pulls the viscera (such as gallbladder) or the oculocardiac reflex, for the stimulation of vagus leads to bradycardia, a serious person can cause sudden cardiac arrest. It should be stopped immediately, and atropine is intravenously administered if necessary. When premature beat occur, we should first clarify its properties and observe its effect on hemodynamics. Occasional premature ventricular contractions during anesthesia need no special treatment. Due to shallow anaesthesia or CO_2 accumulation, ventricular premature contraction can be alleviated if anesthesia is deepened or CO_2 is released. If ventricular premature contraction is multisource, frequent or accompanied by R−on−T phenomenon, it indicates myocardial perfusion is insufficient. We should treat the primary disease actively.

3.5.8 Hyperthermia, twitch and convulsion

It is common in pediatric anesthesia. Because the temperature regulation center of infants is not yet developed well, the temperature is easy to change with the ambient temperature. If not treated with high fever, it can cause twitch or even convulsion. Once the body temperature is elevated, physical cooling should be actively done. The temperature rises in the anaesthesia, also should be vigilant to the occurrence of malignant hyperthermia, which shows a sharp rise in body temperature, can exceed 42 ℃, continuous muscle contraction, the $PaCO_2$ rises rapidly, and the mortality is very high. The drugs that are most likely to induce malignant hyperthermia are succinylcholine and halothane. The incidence of European and American countries is slightly higher than that of Chinese.

Chapter 4

Local Anesthesia

4.1 Pharmacology of Local Anesthetics

4.1.1 Chemical structure and classification

The chemical structure of commonly used local anesthetics is made up of three parts: aromatic (lipophilic), amine (hydrophilic) and intermediate chain. The intermediate chain may be an ester or an amide one. According to the difference in the middle chain, it can be divided into two types: ester anesthetics, such as procaine and tetracaine; amides anesthetics, such as lidocaine, bupivacaine, levobupivacaine, ropivacaine. According to the intensity and time of action, low efficacy and short effect local anesthetics, such as procaine; medium efficacy and medium effect anesthetics, such as lidocaine; high efficiency, long effect anesthetics, such as tetracaine, bupivacaine, levobupivacaine, and ropivacaine.

4.1.2 Physicochemical properties and anesthetic performance

The physical and chemical properties of local anesthetics can affect the anesthetic effect, mainly including dissociation constant, liposolubility and plasma protein binding rate.

(1) Dissociation constant(pK_a)

The local anesthetic solution contains two parts, the undissociated base (B) and the dissociated cation (BH$^+$). The degree of dissociation depends on the pH of the solution. The larger the pH is, the less [BH$^+$] is and the more dissociated base (B) is. When the concentration of [B] and [BH] in solution is exactly the same, the pH is called pK_a of the local anesthetic. After the administration of local anesthetic, the pH of the tissue fluid is closer to 7.4, the greater the pK_a of the drug, the smaller the nonionic part, the nonionic part with lipophilic and easy to pass through the tissue, so the pK_a of the local anesthetic can affects: ①Onset time: the larger the pK_a is, the more ionic parts are, and it is not easy to penetrate neural sheath and membrane the onset time is prolonged. ②Diffusability: the larger the pK_a, the worse the diffusability. The pK_a of lidocaine is close to normal pH, so it works quickly.

(2) Liposolubility

The liposolubility of local anesthetics is the main physicochemical property determining the strength of local anesthetics. The higher the Liposolubility, the stronger the anesthetic effect of local anesthetics. Bupivacaine and tetracaine are high fat soluble, lidocaine is medium, procaine is the lowest. According to this rule, the anesthetic effect of bupivacaine and tetracaine is the strongest, lidocaine is the middle, procaine is the weakest, and ropivacaine is slightly lower than that of bupivacaine in liposolubility.

(3) Protein binding rate

The protein binding rate of local anesthetics is positively correlated with the time course of local anesthetics, with high binding rate and longer action time. After injection of local anesthetics in the body, the free part of the anesthetic is effect and the other part is combined with the protein of the local tissue. The drug combined with the state will temporarily lose its pharmacological activity. The protein binding rate of bupivacaine is high and the aging is long.

4.1.3   Absorption, distribution, biotransformation and clearance

(1) Absorption

The local anesthetic drug is absorbed into the blood circulation after its absorption, and its absorption quantity and speed determine the blood drug concentration. Influencing factors: ①Drug dose: The peak concentration of the blood drug is proportional to the dose of the one injection. In order to avoid toxic reaction caused by excessive concentration, the limit of single medication is prescribed for every local anesthetic. ②The location of administration is directly related to the blood supply of the place. Generally, intercostal nerve block is absorbed faster and subcutaneous injection is slower. If it is directly administered to the throat, tracheal mucosa or inflammatory tissue, the absorption rate will be very fast. ③Performance of local anesthetics: Procaine and tetracaine dilate the blood vessels in the injection area and accelerate the absorption of drugs. Ropivacaine and bupivacaine are easy to bind to protein, so the absorption rate is slowed down. ④Vasoconstrictors: For example, adding some adrenalin in local anesthetic solution can make vasoconstriction, delay the absorption of the solution, prolong the time of action, and reduce the occurrence of toxic reaction.

(2) Distribution

After local anesthetics are absorbed into the blood circulation, they are first distributed into the rich blood perfusion organs, such as heart, brain and kidney. Then, it was redistributed at a slower rate to muscle, fat and skin with poor perfusion.

(3) Biotransformation and clearance

The local anesthetic is cleared and transformed in blood, and its metabolites are more water-soluble and excreted from the kidneys. Amide local anesthetics are metabolized in the liver by mitochondrial enzyme hydrolysis, so the dosage of drug in patients with liver failure should be reduced. The ester local anesthetics are mainly hydrolyzed by plasma pseudocholinesterase. If there is a congenital pseudocholinesterase, or the decrease in the amount of the enzyme caused by liver cirrhosis, severe anemia, cachexia, and late pregnancy, the dosage of ester anesthetics should be reduced.

4.1.4   Adverse reactions of local anesthetics

(1) Toxic reaction

When the local anesthetic is absorbed into the blood, when the blood concentration reaches a certain threshold, it will cause systemic toxicity of local anesthetics, and severe cases can be fatal. There is a direct relationship between the severity and the concentration of blood. The common causes of toxic reactions are as follows: ①The single dose exceeded the patient's tolerance. ②Inadvertent intravacular injection. ③The injection site is rich in blood supply and is absorbed too fast. ④The patient's body weakness and other reasons led to a decrease in local anesthetics tolerance and a small dose of local anesthetics can cause toxic reaction, which is called hypersusceptibility.

Toxicity is mainly manifested in central nervous system and cardiovascular system. Mild toxic reactions often occur in patients with numbness around the mouth, vertigo, chills, panic disorder and disorientation. At this time, if discovered in time, symptoms usually disappear in a short time. If it continue to develop, patient will lose consciousness and develop tremors of the facial muscles and limbs. Once twitch or convulsion happens, it can cause anoxia and further development, resulting in death of respiratory and circulatory failure. The descending system of the central nervous system is more likely to be inhibited than the excited system neurons, so it is first manifested in the excitement, such as the rise of blood pressure and heart rate, etc. When blood concentration continues to increase, total inhibition will appear. The main cardiovascular toxicity of local anesthetics is to inhibit cardiac muscle, conduction system and peripheral vascular smooth muscle, reduce myocardial contractility, reduce cardiac output and blood pressure. When the blood concentration of the anesthetic is very high, the peripheral vasodilation are extensive, atrioventricular block, bradycardia, and sudden cardiac arrest.

The measures to prevent the toxic reaction of local anesthetics include the dosage of single dose is not more than the limit, the blood is free before injection, the dosage of the drug is reduced according to the specific situation and the location of the drug, adrenaline is added in the solution, and the drugs such as diazepam or barbiturate are given as premedication.

Once toxic reaction occurs, it is necessary to stop giving drugs immediately and mask oxygen inhalation. Moderate toxicity can be prevented and controlled by giving midazolam or diazepam. If convulsions or seizures occur, general intravenous thiopental $1-2$ mg/kg is advocated administering. For recurrent seizures, the authors can also receive tracheal intubation after intravenous injection of succinylcholine 1mg/kg. If hypotension occurs, ephedrine or hydroxylamine can be used to maintain blood pressure. When the heart rate is slow, atropine is injected intravenously. Once the respiratory and cardiac arrest occurs, cardiopulmonary resuscitation should be carried out immediately.

(2) Anaphylaxis

Clinically, there are more allergic reactions to ester local anesthetics, and amide is very rare. Sometimes, it is easy to mistake the toxic reaction of local anesthetics or the adverse reaction of adrenaline for anaphylaxis. Anaphylaxis refers to the emergence of urticaria, laryngeal edema, bronchial spasm, hypotension and neurovascular edema after a small amount of local anesthetics, even jeopardizing life. If anaphylaxis is found, first stop using local anesthetics and use glucocorticoids and antihistamines. Its preventive measures are still difficult to be affirmed. The traditional local anesthetic skin test predicts the local anesthetic allergy is not credible, because the false positive rate is as high as 40% . Therefore, there is no need for routine local anesthetic skin test. If the patient has allergic history of local anesthetics, it can be converted to amide local anesthetics.

4.1.5   Common used local anesthetics

(1) Procaine or Novocaine

A commonly used ester local anesthetic is less effective and shorter time but safer. Its anesthesia efficiency is weak, and its mucosal penetration is poor, so it is not suitable for topical anesthesia and epidural block. Because of small toxicity, it is suitable for local infiltrational anesthesia. A single limit of 1 g for adults.

(2)Tetracaine

A strong,long-aging ester local anesthetic. Tetracaine has high liposoluble and strong penetrability. It is suitable for topical anesthesia,nerve block and epidural block. The single maximum dose of adult is not more than 100 mg.

(3)Lidocaine or xylocaine

It is an amidic anesthetic with medium efficacy and time. The blocking performance of diffusion and mucosal penetration is good,and can be applied to various local anesthetic methods,but the concentration is different. The single maximum dose of adult is not more than 400 mg.

(4)Bupivacaine

A strong and long aging amidic anesthetic. It is commonly used in nerve block,epidural block and spinal anesthesia,seldom with local infiltration. It has high plasma protein binding rate,so it can be used for labor analgesia with less amount penetrating placenta. The concentration is 0. 125% -0. 25%. The time of action is 4-6 hours. The single maximum dose of adult is not more than 150 mg. Attention should be paid to the toxicity of the heart. The basic pharmacological properties and clinical use of levobupivacaine are similar to those of bupivacaine,but the cardiotoxicity is less than that of bupivacaine.

(5)Ropivacaine

It is a new amide type local anesthetic. Its intensity and pharmacokinetics are similar to those of bupivacaine,but its cardiotoxicity is small. With low concentration and low dose,it can only block the sensory nerve,and it has obvious sensation and movement separation;it has high binding rate with plasma protein, so it is especially suitable for epidural analgesia,such as labor analgesia. The concentration of epidural block is 0. 25% -0. 75% ,while 0. 75% -1% concentration can produce better motor nerve block. The maximum net amount of adult in adult is not more than 200 mg.

4. 2　Methods of Local Anesthesia

4. 2. 1　Surface anesthesia

It is called the surface anaesthesia to apply the strong penetrating anesthetic to the mucous surface,to block the nerve endings through mucous membrane,and to make the mucosa anaesthetized. It is suitable for superficial surgery or endoscopy in eyes,nose,throat,trachea,urethra and so on. Commonly used drugs for anesthesia are 1% -2% tetracaine or 2% -4% lidocaine.

4. 2. 2　Local infiltration anesthesia

Local anesthetics were injected into various tissues,including intradermal,subcutaneous,and sarcolemma,so as to achieve local anesthetic effect. That is called local infiltration anesthesia. Basic operation methods:first,the needle is inserted into the skin at the end of the operative incision,and then the needle tip is pushed downward into the skin. After injection,the orange peel uplift is formed,called the dermal mound. The needle is pulled out,and then inserted into the edge of the first mound. The dermal mound line is formed by the same operation. After subcutaneous injection of a local anesthetic to the skin,you can cut the skin and subcutaneous tissue. If operation is performed to deep tissue,it can be injected into the sub-sarcolemma and the intra-sarcolemma. If the muscle layer is separated,peritoneal infiltration should be performed. So infiltrate a layer,cut a layer,in order to anesthetic effect is exact,reduce the pain of patients.

Commonly used drugs are 0.5% procaine or 0.25% –0.5% lidocaine.

Attention should be paid to local infiltration anesthesia:①Injection of drug solution into the tissue requires a certain volume to make the solution contact with nerve terminals and enhance the anesthetic effect. ②In order to avoid more than a single limit, it can be diluted to reduce the concentration of solution. ③Before each injection, it is necessary to return to avoid injecting blood vessels. ④There is no pain in the solid organ, and no drug is used. ⑤The addition of adrenalin concentration (1 : 200 000–1 : 400 000, 2.5–5 g/mL) can delay the absorption of local anesthetics and prolong the time of action.

4.2.3   Regional anesthesia

Local anesthetics were injected around the bottom of the operative area to block nerve fibers in the operative area, called regional block. It is suitable for excision of lumps and cysts, such as excision of benign breast tumor and scalp operation. The method and dosage are similar to those of local infiltration anesthesia. Its advantages are as follows:①Avoid pricking into the tumor tissue. ②To avoid local infiltration of some liquid, some tiny masses are not easy to be palpated. ③No influence on the local anatomy of the surgical area.

4.2.4   Nerve blockade

Local anesthetics are injected around the nerve trunk, plexus and nodes, blocking the impulse conduction in these innervated areas, and producing anesthetic effect, called nerve block. The common nerve blocks are intercostal, suborbital, sciatic, finger (toe) nerve block, cervical plexus and brachial plexus block, as well as stellate ganglion and lumbar sympathetic ganglion block.

4.2.4.1   Intercostal nerve block

The anterior branch of the T_{1-12} spinal nerve is circled around the trunk, and it extends into the ribs of the costal angle at the lower edge of the ribs and closely to the inferior direction of the artery. Over the anterior axillary line, nerves and blood vessels locate between internal and external intercostal muscles, and seperates lateral cutaneous nerve at the anterior axillary line. The intercostal nerves innervating the intercostal muscles, abdominal muscle and the corresponding skin areas.

Because the lateral cutaneous nerve has been seperated at the anterior axillary line, the block point should be selected at the costal angle or posterior axillary line. The patient waslying on the side or prone position, the upper limb abduction and the forearm lifting. The ribbed angle is 6–8 cm from the middle line. The above rib angle is near the midline, the below angle is far from the midline. Feel clear the rib which the blocked nerve located, holding the syringe at the lower edge of the ribs, piercing the skin perpendicular to the lower edge of the ribs to touch the bone of the ribs, and then thrust the needle down into the inside, slid through the lower edge of the rib and then go deep into 0.2–0.3 cm, and then injecting the local anesthetic 3–5 mL with withdraw no blood and air. The posterior axillary line injection is the same except for the location of puncture point.

Complication:①Pneumothorax. ②The toxic reaction of local anesthetics is that:the drug is accidentally injected into the intercostal vessels or blocks many intercostal nerves, which is caused by excessive dosage and excessive absorption.

4.2.4.2   Finger (toe) nerve block

For a finger or toe operation. The dorsal side of nerve finger is the branch of the radial and ulnar nerve. The palmar side of the palm and fingers is the branch of median and ulnar nerve. There are four digital nerves innervate in each finger, that is, the left and right sides of the palmar digital nerves and the dorsal digital nerves. The digital nerve block is carried out between the base of the fingers or the metacarpal bones. The method nerve block of toe is similar to that of digital nerve block. When using local anesthetics in fingers, toes and penis, the adrenaline is forbidden, and the dosage should not be too much, so as to avoid tissue necrosis caused by strong contraction of blood vessels.

(1) Finger root block

In the dorsal part of the finger, enter the needle and slide forward through the phalanges to the subcutaneous part of the palmar, injecting 1% lidocaine 1 mL. Then withdraws the needle to subcutaneous entry poin percutaneous injection of 0.5 mL. The other side of the finger is injected by the method.

(2) Intermetacarpal injection

From the back of the hand into the bone between the metacarpal bones, directly to the subcutaneous part of the palmar surface. With the needle advancing and pulling out, 1% lidocaine 4−6 mL was injected.

4.2.4.3   Brachial plexus block

The brachial plexus is mainly composed of the anterior branches of C_{5-8} and T_1 spinal nerves, which innervate the sensation and movement of the upper limbs. These nerves are released from the intervertebral foramen and pass through the intermuscular sulcus between the anterior and middle scalene muscles to form brachial plexus in the intermuscular groove. Then cross the first rib surface above the clavicle to enter the armpit, forming the main terminal nerve, namely the median, radial, ulnar and musculocutaneous nerves. In the intermuscular groove, the brachial plexus is wrapped by the tunica vaginalis formed by the anterior and oblique fascia of the vertebra, which extends over the clavicle to the subclavian artery sheath and the axillary sheath in the armpit. The intermuscular groove, supraclavicular or axillary fossa can be selected as the blocking points of brachial plexus. They are called intermuscular groove, supraclavicular and axillary pathways, respectively (Figure 6−4−1). Local anesthetics must be injected into the tunica vaginalis during block.

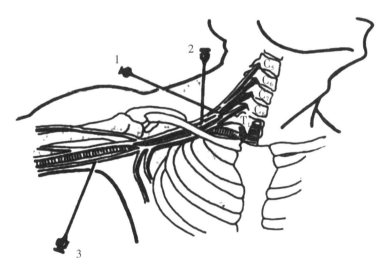

Figure 6−4−1   **Brachial plexus block**
1. Intermuscular groove pathway; 2. Supraclavicular pathway; 3. Axillary pathway.

(1) Intermuscular groove pathway

The patient lies supine on their back, head bias to contralateral, arm side down and shoulder drop. Let the patient slightly raise the head, expose the clavicular end of sternocleidomastoid muscle, slide with fingers on the rear edge, and touch a small muscle, the anterior scalene muscle. The depression between the anterior and middle scalene muscles is the intermuscular groove, which runs down the intermuscular groove and is about 1 cm above the clavicle, a thin transverse muscle can be touched, namely the musculi omohyoideus which with the anterior and middle scalene muscles consist of a small upper and lower big scalene triangle. The the puncture point is located at scalenus triangularis adjacent to the omohyoid muscle, where is equivalent to the level of C_6 transverse process. Needle perpendicular to the skin, puncture the anterior fascia, a sense of breakthrough, and then advance medially and foot direction a little. When the needle reaches the brachial plexus, the patient may feel paresthesia or muscle twitch, withdraw no blood or cerebrospinal fluid, and slowly inject local anesthetic. Generally, 1% lidocaine 25 mL is used or can also be combined with long-acting local anesthetic bupivacaine or ropivacaine.

(2) Supraclavicular pathway

The position of the patient is the same as the intermuscular groove pathway, so as to fully expose the neck, a small pillow can be placed underside of the affected shoulder. At 1 cm above the midpoint of the clavicle, the needle is entered, backward, inside and down. When the patient complained of the paresthesia radiating to the finger, wrist, or forearm or the muscle twitching, stop advancing needle, and after withdraw no blood, the patient is injected with the appropriate 25–30 mL local anesthetic solution. If there is no paresthesia, the first rib will be touched when the tip of the needle enters 1–2 cm, which can be explored along the longitudinal axis of the first rib, leading to the paresthesia, or as a fan block along the ribs, and can also block the brachial plexus, so as to achieve the anesthetic effect.

(3) Axillary pathway

On the supine position, the upper extremity is abducted 90°, and the forearm is flexion upward. The highest point of the axillary artery pulsation is found at the top of the axilla. The right hand holding the needle, index and middle fingers of the left hand fixes skin and artery, at the side edge of the artery needle vertically enter the skin. When piercing the sheath, there is a clear sense of breakthrough, that is, stop moving. Loosening the fingers, the tip of the needle oscillates with the pulse of the artery, indicating the tip of the needle is in the axillary sheath. After withdraw no blood, the patient is injected with the appropriate 25–30 mL local anesthetic solution. The musculocutaneous nerve leaves axillary sheath at the level of coracoid process entering into the coracobrachialis muscle. Therefore, this nerve is often not easy to block completely. Its dominant forearm lateral and thumb base often have poor anesthetic effect.

Indication: Brachial plexus block is suitable for upper limb surgery. Intermuscular ditches can be used in the operation of clavicle, shoulder and proximal humerus. Axillary path is more suitable for forearm and hand surgery.

Complication: Brachial plexus block is the risk of local anesthetic toxicity. The intermuscular groove pathway and supraclavicular approach are also prone to phrenic palsy, recurrent laryngeal nerve palsy and Horner's syndrome. Horner's syndrome is due to the blockage of stellate ganglion, including ipsilateral pupil reduction, blepharoptosis, nasal mucosal congestion and facial flushing. If the puncture is improper, the supraclavicular path is more likely to occur pneumothorax, the intermuscular ditches can cause high epidural block, or the drug solution is misplaced into the subarachnoid cavity to cause the whole spinal anesthesia.

4.2.4.4　Cervical plexus block

The cervical plexus is composed of the anterior branch of the C_{1-4} spinal nerve. After the spinal nerve passes through the intervertebral foramen, it reaches the tip of the transverse process through the back of the vertebral artery, and the branches anastomose with each other after the transverse process, forming the cervical nerve. The cervical plexus is divided into deep plexus and superficial plexus, which dominates the muscle tissue and skin of neck. The deep plexus is at the same level with the brachial plexus at the scalene muscle, and is covered by the anterior fascia, which dominates the deep tissue of the anterior and lateral sides of the neck. The superficial plexus is radially distributed in the middle posterior border of the sternocleidomastoid muscle. Forward is the anterior cervical nerve, down to the supraclavicular nerve, and back to the large ear nerve. It distributes in the submaxillary, clavicle, the whole neck and the occipital skin, and the sense of the shawl shape dominates this area.

(1) Deep plexus block

There are two kinds of blocking methods commonly used. ①Anterior cervical block: The C_4 transverse process is often used. The patient lies supine, head turn to the opposite side, and from the mastoid tip to the C_6 transverse process line is drwan. The puncture point is on this line. C_4 transverse process is located near the crossing point between sternocleidomastoid muscle and external jugular vein. Fingers can be used to press the transverse process. At this level, 2-3 cm can pierce to touch the transverse process bone, withdraw no blood and cerebrospinal fluid, and inject local anesthetic 10 mL. ②Intermuscular blockade: The method is same of intermuscular groove for brachial nerve block, but the puncture point is at the tip of the intermuscular groove, after piercing of the anterior fascia of the vertebra, it does not need to find the paresthesia, injecting the local anesthetic 10 mL and oppressing the lower part of intermuscular groove to prevent blocking the brachial plexus.

(2) Superficial plexus block

The position is the same to above. At the midpoint of the posterior margin of the sternocleidomastoid muscle, 1% lidocaine 6-8 mL is injected subcutaneously, or 3-4 mL was injected at this point, and then the posterior margin of the sternocleidomastoid muscle is injected to the cephalic and caudal side 2-3 mL respectively.

Indication: It is suitable for neck surgery, such as thyroid, tracheotomy and carotid endarterectomy, etc.

Complication: The complications of superficial plexus block are rare. The complications of deep plexus block are as follows: ①The toxic reaction of local anesthetic: rich blood vessels in neck. If entering vertebral artery inadvertently, a small dose of local anesthetics may cause central neurotoxicity. ②The solution is entered into the subarachnoid or epidural cavity by mistake. ③Phrenic paralysis. ④Recurrent laryngeal nerve palsy: hoarseness or even loss of voice. Therefore, bilateral deep plexus block can not be done at the same time. ⑤Horner's syndrome.

In recent years, nerve blockade under the guidance of neurostimulator and (or) ultrasound apparatus has changed the past dependence on "paresthesia" to locate the nerve and helps to achieve a better anesthetic effect.

Chapter 5

Intravertebral Anesthesia

5.1 Anatomic Basis of Intravertebral Anaesthesia

5.1.1 Spine and vertebral canal

The spine is composed of various vertebrae (including sacrum and coccyx) and connecting devices such as intervertebral disc, intervertebral joint and ligament. The typical vertebrae consists of two main parts, the vertebral body and the vertebral arch, vertebral body and bilateral vertebral arch forming vertebral foramen. All the vertebral foramen and sacral canal superposition constitute the spinal canal. The vertebral canal starts from the upper foramen magnum and end at the lower sacral hiatus. The canal contains the spinal cord and its membrane and other structures. The adult spine presented four curvatures, neck flexion and waist flexion forward, chest flexion and sacral flexion backward (Figure 6-5-1). When patient is supine, the location of C_3 and L_3 are the highest, and T_5 and S_4 are the lowest, which has an important influence on the distribution of anesthetic solution during spinal anesthesia.

5.1.2 Ligament

The three ligaments connecting the adjacent vertebrae are supraspinous ligament, interspinous ligament and ligamentum flavum from outside to inside, respectively (Figure 6-5-2). The supraspinous ligament is thin and tough, connected to the tips of the spine. With the increase of age, the calcification of the ligament is obvious, the supraspinous ligament is hard as bone, then the paramiddle approach should be taken to avoid the ossific supraspinous ligament. The interspinous ligament is relatively weak, connecting two upper and lower spinous processes, anterior ligamentum flavum and subsequent supraspinous ligament. Theligamentum flavum is connected from the lower edge and the inner surface of the upper vertebral arch to the upper edge and outside of the lower vertebral arch plate. It is almost all composed of elastic fibers. The tissue is tight and tough. The sudden increase of resistance and the feeling of falling through the ligament are significant. During intraspinal anesthesia, the puncture needle passes through the skin, subcutaneous tissue, supraspinal ligament, interspinous ligament, and ligamentum flavum, reaching the epidural cavity and continues through the dura and arachnoid, that is subarachnoid cavity.

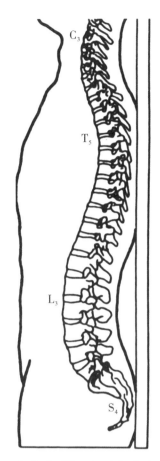

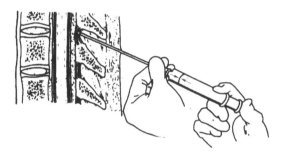

Figure 6-5-1　The physiological curva-　Figure 6-5-2　The elasticity of the ligamentum flavum
ture of the spine

5.1.3　Spinal cord, spinal membrane and space

There are spinal cord, spinal cord capsule, spinal nerve and other structures in the spinal canal. The upper part of the spinal cord is connected to the brain at the foramen magnum, and the lower end terminates on the lower edge of the L_1 vertebral body or the upper edge of the L_2 vertebral body. It is downwordly attached to the back of the coccyx with filum terminale. The lower end of the spinal cord is located at the lower edge of L_3 and moves up with age. Therefore, adult lumbar puncture should be done below L_2 lumbar intervertebral space while children under L_3.

The membranes of spinal cord are pia mater spinalis, arachnoid and dura mater spinalis from inside to outside. The spinal pia mater is closely related to the surface of the spinal cord and deeper into the spinal cord fissure. The lacuna between the spinal pia mater meninges and the arachnoid is called the subarachnoid cavity. It is connected to the subarachnoid cavity of the brain. It has a blind end at the level of S_2 and containing cerebrospinal fluid inside. The dura mater is composed of dense connective tissue and less blood supply. It is difficult to heal after puncturing. The space between the spinal dura mater and the inner wall of the spinal canal (the ligamentum flavum and the periosteum) is epidural space containing fat, lymphoid tissue and epidural vein (Figure 6-5-3). The epidural cavity closed upwards into the foramen magnum, and cranial cavity impassability, down in the S_2 level closed into the dural sac. There is a potential lacuna between the dura mater and the arachnoid membrane, known as the subdural space.

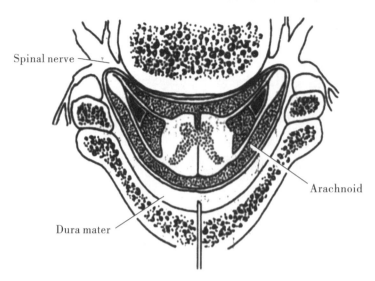

Figure 6-5-3　Transverse section of the spinal canal

5.1.4　Root dura mater, root arachnoid and root pia mater

When the spinal nerve is away from the spinal cord, the spinal cord is covered by the pia mater, arachnoid and dura mater, and extends to both sides. Among them, the pia mater extends to the root pia mater, the arachnoid membrane extends to the root arachnoid membrane, and the dura mater extends to the root dura mater. The lacuna between the root pia mater and the root arachnoid membrane is called the root subarachnoid space. It is the same as the spinal subarachnoid space, and the blind capsule is closed at the intervertebral foramen. The root dura mater is thinner and thinner as it approached the foramen intervertebralis. The proliferation of root arachnoid cells can form or penetrate the root dural villi, and increase with age. Arachnoid villi are beneficial for draining cerebrospinal fluid and clearing particulate matter in subarachnoid space.

5.1.5　Sacral canal

The sacral canal is the lumen of the vertebral canal in the sacrum. Through sacral foramen puncture, local anesthetic is injected into the sacral canal to block the sacral spinal nerve, which is called sacral block which is a kind of epidural block. The volume of the sacral canal is 25-30 mL, which contains loose connective tissue, fat and abundant venous plexus. Because the dura mater and arachnoid membrane are closed to the dural sac at the level of S_2, sacral canal is part of epidural space and communicates with lumbar epidural space. The lower sacral canal terminates in sacral hiatus, sacral hiatus is "V" or "U" shape, on both sides there are large bony protuberances, called sacral cornu. Sacral hiatus and sacral cornu are important anatomical markers for sacral puncture. The average distance from the dural sac to the sacral hiatus is 47 mm. In order to avoid intruding into the subarachnoid space, the insertion needles should not be too deep when the sacral canal is punctured. Because there are many variations in the structure of the sacral canal, puncture may be difficult or failed.

5.1.6　Spinal nerves

There were 31 pairs of spinal nerves, including 8 pairs of cervical nerves (C), 12 pairs of thoracic nerves (T), 5 pairs of lumbar nerves (L), 5 pairs of sacral nerves (S), and 1 pairs of caudal nerves (Co).

Each spinal nerve is made up of the anterior root which dominate movement and the posterior root which dominate sensation. The anterior root is emitted fromanterior horn of spinal cord, consisting of motor nerve fibers and sympathetic efferent fibers (sacral part is parasympathetic efferent fibers) , also known as ventral roots. The posterior root is composed of sensory nerve fiber and sympathetic nerve afferent fiber (sacral part is parasympathetic afferent fiber) , and enters the posterior horn of spinal cord, also known as dorsal root. According to thickness, all kinds of nerve fibers are motor fibers, sensory fibers, sympathetic and parasympathetic fibers. The latter is blocked by contact with low concentration of local anesthetics.

5.2　The Mechanism and Physiology of Intravertebral Anesthesia

5.2.1　Cerebrospinal fluid

The adult cerebrospinal fluid(CSF) volume is 120–150 mL, and the spinal subarachnoid space is only 25–35 mL. CSF is transparent and clear, pH is 7.4, specific gravity is 1.000 3–1.000 9. Cerebrospinal fluid pressure is not more than 100 mmH$_2$O at supine position, 70–170 mmH$_2$O at lateral position, 200–300 mmH$_2$O at sitting time. CSF plays a role in diluting and spreading local anesthetics during lumbar anesthesia.

5.2.2　Site of action

In spinal anesthesia, local anesthetics directly affect the anterior root, posterior root and spinal cord. Local anesthetics have little effect on the surface block of the spinal cord itself, mainly through blocking the spinal nerve roots and completing the spinal anesthesia. However, there may be some ways for the effect of epidural anesthesia : ①The solution exudates the intervertebral foramen, produces paravertebral nerve block, and distributes along the perineurium and soft membrane, and acts on the spinal nerve roots. ②Through the arachnoid villi enter the subarachnoid space of the root, acting on the spinal nerve roots. ③Through the spinal dura mater and arachnoid space, it enters the subarachnoid space and enters cerebrospinal fluid. It acts on the spinal nerve root and spinal cord as same as spinal anesthesia. Because the spinal nerve roots away from the spinal cord are not covered by epicardium, and are easily blocked by local anesthetics. The local anesthetics entering the subarachnoid space will be diluted by CSF. Therefore, compared with epidural block, spinal anesthesia has higher drug concentration but smaller volume and dose, and the concentration after dilution is much lower than epidural block. Local anesthetics in epidural anesthesia requires multiple diffusion distribution in the epidural cavity, which requires more volume than lumbar anesthesia to achieve a perfect epidural block effect.

5.2.3　Anesthesia level and block effect

The anesthetic level is the extent of the skin pain loss by the pinprick method after the sensory nerve is blocked. Blocking the sympathetic nerve can relieve the visceral distraction, block the sensory nerve can block the pain conduction of the skin and muscles, block the motor nerve can produce muscle relaxation. Both sympathetic and sensory nerves are myelinated, but the thickness is different. The sympathetic nerve is first blocked, and the level is generally 2–4 segments higher than the sensory nerve; the motor nerve was myelin nerve and is less sensitive to local anesthetics, so it is blocked at the latest, and its level was

1-4 lower than that of the sensory nerve. The distribution of spinal dermatomal level on the body surface is shown in Figure 6-5-4. According to the surface anatomic markers, spinal nerve innervation in different sites is as follows: T_2—Superior border of manubrium of sternum; T_4—Connecting line of bilateral nipples; T_6—Region below xiphoid process; T_8—Hypochondrial border; T_{10}—umbilical part; T_{12}—2-3 cm above symphysial surface; L_{1-3}—anterior part of thighs; L_{4-5}—Posterior crural region and feet back; S_{1-5}—back of thighs and legs and perineoanal region. If the pain disappeared up to xiphoid level, lower to 2-3 cm above pubic symphysis, is expressed as a T_{6-12} level of anesthesia.

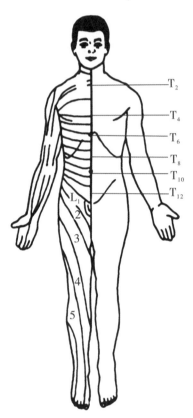

Figure 6-5-4   The segmental distribution of the spinal nerve on the surface of the body

5.2.4   The effect of intravertebral anesthesia on physiology

5.2.4.1   Respiration

The key to affect respiratory function is the height of block level, especially the range of motor level. In the case of subarachnoid block or upper thoracic epidural block in high height, the block of motor nerve can cause intercostal paralysis, affect the contraction of the respiratory muscles, breathing weaken or even disappear, but the basic ventilation can still be maintained as long as the phrenic nerve (C_{3-5}) is not blocked. But if the diaphragm is paralyzed at the same time, abdominal respiration will weaken or disappear, which will lead to insufficient ventilation or even respiratory arrest. Therefore, when using high epidural block, the concentration of local anesthetics should be reduced, so that the motor nerve will not be blocked or slightly blocked, so as to avoid serious impact on breathing.

5.2.4.2   Circulation

Hypotension: When intravertebral blocking, local anesthetics block the sympathetic vasoconstrictor fibers of the thoracic and lumbar segments (T_2–L_2), the diastole of the arterioles decrease peripheral resistance, the dilation of the veins increases the volume of blood in the venous system, the returned blood volume decrease and the the cardiac output decrease, which leads to the decrease of blood pressure. If the block level is below T_5, the circulatory function can be compensated by the vasoconstriction in the upper half of the body, but it is still not enough to maintain the blood pressure at the original level. In particular, inadequate preoperative preparation, insufficient blood volume, atherosclerosis or heart failure, high anesthesia level, and a wide range of block are likely to be more obvious. The heart rate slows down; the excitability of the vagus nerve is relatively enhanced when the sympathetic nerve is blocked in the intraspinal block, and the venous blood flow is reduced and the right atrial pressure drops, resulting in the venous cardiac reflex. When high height block occurs, cardiac acceleration nerve (T_{1-4}) is inhibited and bradycardia is also induced.

5.2.4.3 Others

When intraspinal block, vagal nerve excitability is relatively enhanced, causing gastrointestinal hypermotility, which is easy to induce nausea and vomiting. It also has certain effect on liver and kidney function, and also can inhibit bladder micturition function and cause urinary retention.

5.3 Subarachnoid Block

Subarachnoid block, also known as spinal anesthesia or lumbar anesthesia, is injected the local anesthetics into the subarachnoid space, blocking the function of some spinal nerve and causing the anesthetic effect of the corresponding control area. The blocking range of the subarachnoid block is limited to the anus and perineum, also known as saddle anesthesia.

5.3.1 Classification

It can be classified according to the way of administration, the level of anesthetic plane and the specific gravity of local anesthetics solution.

(1) The way of administration: Single and continuous methods.

(2) Level of anesthesia: The plane reaches T_{10} and below is low plane spinal anesthesia, higher than T_{10}, but lower than T_4 for middle plane spinal anesthesia, reaching T_4 and above for high plane spinal anesthesia.

(3) Specific gravity of local anesthetic solution: When the specific gravity of the soulution is higher than or equal to or less than that of CSF, it is also called hyperbaric, isobaric and hypobaric spinal anesthesia.

5.3.2 Subarachnoid block technique

When the subarachnoid space is punctured, the patient usually takes the lateral position, the back is perpendicular to the edge of the operation table, both hands holding knees, the thighs attaching to the abdominal wall, the back and waist is curved like arch, the gap between the spinous process is open and the puncture is easy to be done. The choice of puncture site in adults is generally in the L_{3-4} gap, where the subarachnoid space is the widest, the spinal cord has been formed the filum terminale, and can move up or down a gap as appropriate. On the two sides, the highest point of iliac spine is connected. The intersection of this line and spine is L_4 spinous process or L_{3-4} spinous process space. When puncture is done by straight method,1% lidocaine is used to make pips at the puncture site,and infiltrate the subcutaneous tissue and the ligament of the spine. The puncture needle should be entered at the midpoint of lumbar spinous process space. The direction of the needle should be perpendicular to the back of the patient,and slowly enter the needle,and carefully feel the resistance change at the tip of the needle. When the needle passes through the ligamentum flavum,there will be a significant sense of fall,continuing entering the needle to puncture the dura mater and arachnoid,there will be a second fall. Pull out the needle core to see the cerebrospinal fluid drop out,that is to say puncture success. Sometimes the patient's cerebrospinal fluid pressure is low,no free flow of cerebrospinal fluid after puncture,the patient's jugular vein can be compressed by the assistant or let the patient hold breath,in orderto raise the pressure of cerebrospinal fluid to make it flow out freely. After the puncture is successful,the prepared syringe with local anesthetic is connected with the puncture needle. After injection,the puncture needle and syringe will be pulled out together. The lateral approach is the puncture needle entering at 1−1.5 cm lateral to the midline of the spinous process,and the needle incline to the middle line. It is about 75°to the skin,avoiding the supraspinal ligament,and through the ligament flavum,the dural mater and the arachnoid to reach the subarachnoid space. It is suitable for elderly patients with calcification of supraspinal ligament,obese patients or those who have difficulty in direct approch.

5.3.3　Local anesthetics of common use

(1)Procaine

The dosage of procaine in adults is 100−150 mg,the highest dose is 200 mg,and only 50−100 mg is needed in saddle anesthesia. A commonly used 5% procaine is hyperbaric solution which is formulated as follows:Procaine 150 mg (white powder) is dissolved in 5% glucose solution or cerebrospinal fluid 2.7 mL,plus 0.1% adrenaline 0.3 mL. The onset time is 1−5 minutes,so the anesthetic level should be adjusted within 5 minutes. The duration of action is only 45−90 minutes,which is suitable for short time operation. If procaine 150 mg is dissolved in 10 mL of injection water,it is made up of 1.5% hypobaric solution. .

(2)Tetracaine

The dose of tetracaine in adults is 10−15 mg and the highest dose is 20 mg. A commonly used 0.33% tetracaine is hyperbaric solution which is formulated as follows:1% tetracaine 1 mL,10% glucose solution and 3% ephedrine solution each 1 mL,the so−called 1 : 1 : 1 hyperbaric solution. Tetracaine hyperbaric solution is slow onset. It usually takes 5−10 minutes,and it takes 20 minutes to fix the block plane. The duration of anesthesia is longer,and the time of action is 2−3 hours. If tetracaine 10 mg is dissolved in 10 mL of injection water,it is made up of 0.1% hypobaric solution.

(3)Bupivacaine

The usual dose of bupivacaine is 8−15 mg,and the maximum dose should not exceed 20 mg. The common concentration is 0.5%−0.75%,which can be prepared by 10% glucose solution to hyperbaric solution. The onset time and action time are all similar to tetracaine. If bupivacaine is diluted to 0.25% concentration by injecting water,it is a hypobaric solution.

5.3.4　Adjustment of anesthesia level

When the anesthetic is injected into the subarachnoid space,the anesthetic level must be adjusted and controlled for a short time to reach the scope of operation and avoid excessive level. Once the time needed for the combination of anesthetic with nerve tissue is exceeded,the adjustment of the level becomes difficult. If the anesthesia level is too low to meet the needs of the operation,the anesthetic failure is caused,and the too high level of anesthesia has a greater impact on the patient's physiology, such as the weakening of respiration, bradycardia, and even jeopardize the patient's life. Many factors affect the subarachnoid space block level, such as the dose and specific gravity of the local anesthetic solution, the higher the dose, the higher the level; the hyperbaric solution moving to the lower, the hypobaric solution moving to the high place, and the isobaric solution staying near the injection point. Besides, the selection of puncture space, the posture of patient and the speed of injection are also important factors for adjusting the level.

(1) Puncture space

Because of physiological curve of spine, L_3 is at the highest point while T_5 and S_4 at the lowest in supine. When the hyperbaric solution is injected at L_{2-3} space, after patient's posture converting to supine, the solution flows to thoracic segment which make the level easy to higher; When the solution is injected at L_{4-5}, most drug flows to sacral segment which cause lower level.

(2) Posture of patient

The change of patient's posture is very important for the adjustment of anesthetic level. The supine position is changed after injection. According to the need of surgery, the position of the patient can be adjusted to adjust the anesthetic level. When the level is too low, the operating table can be transferred to the head low foot high position, and the level will be raised because of the diffusing of the hyperbaric solution in the CSF. Once the level is enough, the operating table is immediately transferred to the horizontal position, and the changes of respiration and blood pressure of patient are closely observed. The adjustment level is completed within 5–10 minutes after the injection. If the operative site is in the lower extremities, the patient's limbs should be placed on the lower side when puncturing, and the lateral position should be kept for 5–10 minutes after injection. The anesthetic effect is on the affected side. If anus and perineal area are needed, saddle anesthesia is needed. The patients can be seated and punctured with a small dose of solution (approximate 1/2 of general dose) at the L_{4-5} interval. The local anesthetic only block the caudal caudal nerve.

(3) Speed of injection

In general, the injection speed faster, more wide range of anesthesia; speed is slow, the drug is more concentrated, more limited range of anesthesia. The general injection rate is suitable for 1 mL solution per 5 seconds.

5.3.5   Complications

5.3.5.1   Intraoperative complications

(1) Blood pressure drops and heart rate slows down

After spinal anesthesia, the decrease of blood pressure is due to the spinal nerve block, the dilation of the arteriole decreases peripheral vascular resistance, and the venous dilatation increases the volume of blood in the venous system, while the amount of the returned blood is reduced and the volume of cardiac output drops, which leads to the decrease of blood pressure. The higher the level of anesthesia, the wider the scope of block, the greater the range of vasodilatation, and the smaller the range of compensatory vasoconstriction, the more obvious the blood pressure drop. In general the lower the block level, the blood pressure decrease is not obvious, the combination of hypertension, heart disease or insufficient blood volume, self compensatory ability is low, more prone to hypotension. Once the anesthesia level is over T_4, the cardiac accelerating nerve fiber (T_{1-4}) is blocked and the vagus nerve is relatively hyperactive, which is likely to cause bradycardia. The first treatment of blood pressure drops is to expand the blood volume, and can be used for intravenous infusion of 200–300 mL quickly. If there is no obvious effect, intravenous injection of ephedrine and other vasoactive drugs until the blood pressure rises. Bradycardia can be treated by intravenously injected with atropine to reduce vagal tension.

(2) Respiratory depression

When the spinal anesthesia level exceeds T_4, the thoracic spinal nerve blocked, the intercostal muscle paralysis, the patient feel chest tightness and cough weakness, inability to sound, chest breathing weakened, and even cyanosis. When all spinal nerves are blocked, total spinal anaesthesia occurs, respiratory arrest, blood pressure drop or even cardiac arrest. Tracheal intubation should be performed immediately, artificial respiration and maintenance of circulation should be carried out. High level of the plane can also cause ischemia and anoxia of the respiratory center, which is also the cause of respiratory depression. Oxygen inhalation or assisted respiration should be given to patients with respiratory insufficiency.

(3) Nausea and vomiting

The reasons include the following: ①When the anesthesia level is too high, hypotension and respiratory depression can cause cerebral ischemia and hypoxia, and stimulate the vomiting center. ②When the anesthesia level is too high, hypotension and respiratory depression can cause cerebral ischemia and hypoxia, and stimulate the vomiting center. ③The abdominal viscera was pulled during operation. ④The patient is sensitive to the drugs used in the operation. To deal with nausea and vomiting, we should look for the cause and symptomatic treatment, such as raising blood pressure, oxygen inhalation, atropine before anesthesia, and suspending operation traction. Droperidol, ondansetron and other drugs also have a certain role in the prevention and treatment.

5.3.5.2　Postoperative complications

(1) Headache

Headache is one of the common complications after spinal anesthesia, and the incidence is 3% -30%. Typical headache occurrs at 6-12 hours after puncture, most of which occurrs on the 1-3 day after spinal anesthesia, and it is more common in obstetrics and gynecology department. A feature is the headache is aggravated when raise head or sit up, and reduced or disappeared after supine. About 75% of the patients' syndrome can disappear within 4 days, usually less than a week, but there are also longer course. The main reason for headache after spinal anesthesia is cerebrovascular fluid leakage through the puncture hole, resulting in intracranial pressure decrease and intracranial vascular dilatation, causing vascular headache. Due to the poor blood supply of spinal dura mater and arachnoid membrane, the puncture hole is difficult to heal, so the occurrence of headache is directly related to the thickness of puncture needle. The incidence is relatively higher in thicker puncture needle or repeated puncture. In order to prevent headache after spinal anesthesia, we should try to use fine puncture needles, avoid repeated puncture, infuse enough liquid to prevent insufficient blood volume. Before anesthesia, we should give patients the necessary explanation, eliminate their concerns, and avoid the possibility of headache after spinal anesthesia. Patients with headache after spinal anesthesia must lie in bed and rest. They can take analgesic or antipsychotic drugs. Acupuncture or abdominal banding is also effective. Patients with severe headache can be injected with normal saline, 5% glucose solution or dextran 15-30 mL in the epidural cavity. The curative effect is better. It is possible to use the epidural autologous blood filling therapy when necessary.

(2) Urinary retention

Urine retention after spinal anesthesia is more common. Due to block of S_{2-4}, bladder tension can be lost and bladder can be overfilled, especially in male patients. Especially for the incision pain after the lower abdominal, anus or perineal operation, and the patient's inability to urinate in bed which can cause urinary retention. For treatment, hot compress, acupuncture and intramuscular injection of parasympathetic nerve stimulant carbachol can be used, , and urinary catheterization can be used if necessary.

（3）Suppurative meningitis

Direct or indirect causes, such as skin infection and sepsis, can cause purulent meningitis after spinal anesthesia. Severe patients can be life-threatening, so prevention is the key.

（4）Neurological complications after spinal anesthesia

The causes of nerve damage caused by lumbar anesthesia are the tissue toxicity of local anesthetics, accidental exposure to harmful substances and puncture injury, and so on. Common neuropathic complications include the following. ①Cerebral nerve paralysis: One week after spinal anesthesia, severe headache and vertigo often occur, followed by strabismus and diplopia. The pathogenesis is similar to the headache after the spinal anesthesia. The cerebrospinal fluid is overflowing from the puncture hole of the cerebrospinal meninges, and the brain tissue loses the support of the cerebrospinal fluid. When the patient is sitting or standing, the brain tissue is drooping to the foot by gravity and oppresses the cranial nerve. The abducens nerve is longer and easier to be pulled or compressed. Treatment measures: Correct intracranial hypotension after spinal anesthesia, give vitamin B and symptomatic treatment. Most patients are able to heal themselves within 6 months. ②Adhensive arachnoiditis: This course of disease develops slowly. It often starts with sensory disturbance, and then develops into sensory loss and paralysis. The pathological changes are chronic proliferative inflammatory reactions of the pia mater and arachnoid. The subarachnoid and epidural cavities are all adhesion and atresia, and the blood vessels are also blocked by the pathogenesis of inflammation, resulting in the degeneration of the spinal cord and the spinal nerve root. ③Cauda equina syndrome: The cause is basically the same as Adhensive arachnoiditis. Its characteristics are limited to the sensory and motor disorders in the perineal region and the distal part of the lower extremities. Light patient is only manifested as urinary retention, and severe is urine and fecal incontinence. In the case of chemical damage, the recovery is very slow. If it is injured by puncture of the nerve fiber of cauda equine, it will be healed in a few weeks or months.

5.3.6　Indications and contraindications

Indications: Lumbar anesthesia is suitable for operation in hypobelly, pelvic cavity, lower limbs and anoperineal region. which last short than 3 hours, such as appendectomy, repair of hernia, hemorrhoidectomy.

Contraindications: ①Disease in central nervous system, such as meningitis, anterior poliomyelitis, intracranial hypertension. ②Sepsis, shock. ③Skin infection at or near puncture site. ④Spinal trauma and tuberculosis. ⑤Acute heart failure and onset of coronary heart disease. In addition, the dosage and the level of anesthesia should be strictly controlled for the elderly, heart disease and hypertension. Those who can not cooperate, such as children, severe neurosis and psychotic patients, usually do not need spinal anesthesia.

5.4　Epidural Block

The epidural block is injected of the local anesthetics into the epidural cavity, blocking the conduction function of the spinal nerve and making a temporary paralysis of the corresponding area, also known as epidural anesthesia. There are two kinds of methods, one is single and the other is continuous. In clinic, continuous method is common.

5.4.1 Epidural puncture

(1) Posture

The posture of epidural puncture has two kinds: lateral position and sitting position. The lateral position is mainly used in clinic. The method of lateral position is the same as that of lumbar anesthesia.

(2) Selection of puncture sites

Epidural puncture can be carried out in the space of neck, chest, waist and sacrum. Because of no cerebrospinal fluid in the epidural space, the diffusion of local anesthetic solution is mainly dependent on their volume to the two ends. Therefore, the puncture site is generally chosen at the corresponding spinous process in the center of the surgical area. The selection of puncture sites of various operation can be referred to Table 6-5-1.

Table 6-5-1   Intervertebral space for different operation

Surgical site	Operation name	Puncture space
Cervical part	Operation of thyroid gland and thyroid lymphatic system	C_{5-6} or C_{6-7}(cephalad)
Upper limbs	Operation on both hands	$C_7 T_1$(cephalad)
Chest wall	Breasts	T_{4-5}(cephalad)
Epigastrium	Operation on stomach, bile duct, spleen, liver and pancreas	T_{8-9}(cephalad)
Midgastrium	Operation on intestine	T_{9-10}(cephalad)
Lumbar part	Operation on kidney, adrenal gland and ureter	T_{10-11}(cephalad)
Subgastrium	Operation on appendix	T_{11-12}(cephalad)
Pelvic cavity	Operation on uterus and rectum	$T_{12} L_1$, L_{4-5}(both cephalad)
Inguinal region	Operation of inguinal groove or hip joint	L_{1-2}(cephalad)
Lower limbs	Operation of thighs	$L_{2\ 3}$(cephalad)
	Operation of crus	L_{3-4}(cephalad)
Perineum	Operation on anus and perineum	L_{3-4}(caudalad)or sacral block

(3) Puncture technique

Epidural puncture can be classified into straight approach and lateral approach. Epidural space is achieved when the needle passes through the ligamentum flavum when epidural puncture. The key to successful epidural puncture is not puncturing the spinal dura mater. Therefore, we should emphasize the sense of breakthrough when the needle pierced the ligamentum flavum. The following methods can be used to determine whether the needle reaches the epidural space: ①When the needle reaches the ligamentum flavum, pushes the core rod of the syringe to rebound and drag, and the bubble is pressed down. Continue to enter the needle slowly. Once the ligamentum of the ligamentum flavum is broken, there is a sense of loss. The liquid and small bubbles can be injected without resistance, and there is no flow of cerebrospinal fluid back, indicating the tip of the needle reaching the epidural cavity. ②Capillary negative pressure method: When sensing puncture needle arrives at the ligamentum flavum, connects it with the liquid filled capillary tube, and continues to enter the needle slowly. When the puncture needle enters the epidural space, it suddenly feels empty. At the same time, the fluid in the tube is inhaled into the epidural space, which is a specific negative pressure phenomenon in the epidural space. After the needle tip in the epidural cavity is determined, the epidural catheter can be inserted through the puncture needle. In order to prevent the catheter from knot in the epidural cavity, the length of the catheter in the epidural cavity is not too long, usually 3 – 4 cm. Withdraw the puncture needle and fix the catheter for continuous injection.

5.4.2   Common local anesthetics and injection methods

The commonly used local anesthetics in epidural block include lidocaine, tetracaine, bupivacaine and ropivacaine. Lidocaine is commonly used in 1.5% –2% solution. The onset time is 5–8 minutes, and the duration of action is about 1 hour. The maximum dosage for adult is 400 mg. Tetracaine is commonly used in 0.25% –0.33% concentration, the onset time is 10–20 minutes, the maintenance time is 1.5–2 hours, the maximum dosage is 60 mg. Bupivacaine is generally used in 0.5% –0.75% concentration, the onset time is 7–10 minutes, and maintain for 2–3 hours. The commonly used concentration of ropivacaine is 0.75% , which is slightly weaker than bupivacaine, and the cardiovascular toxicity is less than that of bupivacaine. If the patient has no hypertension, adrenaline can be added in the solution (the concentration is 5 g/mL) to postpone the absorption rate of local anesthetic, prolong the time of action and reduce the toxic reaction of local anesthetic. After successful catheterization, a test dose of 2% lidocaine 3–5 mL is injected and observe for 5–10 minutes. Because the volume and dose of epidural block are 3–5 times larger than that of spinal anesthesia, if all the solution is injected into the subarachnoid space, the serious consequences of total spinal anaesthesia will be produced. If the pain and motor function of the lower extremities disappear within 5 minutes after injection, and the blood pressure drop and so on, it is suggested that the local anesthetic has been entered into the subarachnoid space, and the drug injection should be stopped immediately. If the blood pressure drop sharpply or breathing difficulties, emergent rescue should be carried out. After confirming no the spinal anesthesia phenomenon, the additional dose can be determined according to the effect of test dose. The sum of the test dose and the additional dose is called the initial dose. When the action of initial dose is going to disappear, the second dose injected is 1/2–2/3 the of initial dose.

5.4.3   Adjustment of anesthesia level

The anesthesia level of epidural block is segmental, which is different from spinal anesthesia. The main factors affecting the level are as follows:①the larger the volume, the faster the injection speed is, the wider the block scope is. On the contrary, the drug solution is relatively concentrated, and the blocking scope is narrow. ②The choice of the puncture space is most important. If the space is not properly selected, it may appear that the upper or lower level can not meet the operation requirements, cause the failure of anesthesia, or inhibit the respiratory and circulatory function due to the high level. ③Catheter placement and direction:the catheter is placed cephaladly, and the anesthetic solution is easily diffused to the thoracic and cervical segments. The catheter is toward the caudal side, and the solution is easily diffused to the lumbar and sacral segments. If the catheter is on the one side, there may be a block on one side. ④The way of injection:when the dosage is the same, the block level of the single injection is usually wider than that of multiple injection. The range of anesthesia in the cervical segment is wider than that in the thoracic part, and the thoracic one is wider than the lumbar segment. ⑤Patient's condition:infants, elderly, arteriosclerosis, pregnancy, dehydration, cachexia, and other patients, the anesthetic range is often wider than the general, so it should be injected multiply and reduce the dose. Besides, the concentration of solution and the posture of patients can also affect the range of anesthesia.

5.4.4 Complications

5.4.4.1 Intraoerative complications

(1)Total spinal anesthesia

When epidural block, if the puncture needle or the epidural catheter, is not found in the subarachnoid cavity in time, most or all of the local anesthetics are injected into the subarachnoid cavity, which can produce an abnormally extensive block, known as total spinal anesthesia. Patients can suffer from dyspnea, decreased blood pressure, confusion or loss of consciousness within a few minutes after injection, and then stop breathing. The principle of treatment to total spinal anesthesia is to maintain patient's circulatory and respiratory function. Once total spinal anesthesia occurs, it should be pressurized to oxygen with a mask and emergent tracheal intubation for artificial respiration, accelerate the infusion and maintain the circulation stability with vasopressin. If handled in a timely and correct way, serious consequences can be avoided, otherwise cardiac arrest can be induced. Measures for the prevention of total spinal anesthesia include the following: It is necessary to strictly comply with the operating procedures, careful puncturing in case of puncturing the dural mater; after the catheter is placed into the epidural space, no cerebrospinal fluid should be sucked back. The test dosage must be observed for 5−10 minutes during the course of drug use, and no spinal anesthesia should be identified before continuing administration.

(2)Toxic reaction of local anesthetics

There are abundant venous plexus in epidural space, and the absorption of local anesthetics is very fast. Even the catheter accidentally enters the blood vessels, so that local anesthetics can be directly injected into the blood vessels. The vascular injury by catheter can also accelerate the absorption of anesthetics. All these factors can cause different degrees of toxic reactions. In addition, a dose of more than the largest dose is also a common cause of toxic reactions.

(3)Blood pressure drop

Mainly due to the blockage of sympathetic nerve, arterioles and vein dilate, resulting in reduced returned blood volume and decreased blood pressure. Especially for the upper abdominal surgery, the thoracolumbar block has a wide range of sympathetic nerve block, and block cardiac sympathetic nerve which lead to bradycardia is prone to cause hypotension. Characteristics: ①Epidural onset is slow, so the decrease of blood pressure appears later. ②Some operations require an epidural block with a higher level of anesthesia, and the decrease in blood pressure is smaller if the upper and lower levels are controlled in a limited range. ③The dosage of local anesthetics for epidural block is large. Attention should be paid to avoid the direct inhibition to cardiovascule by local anesthetics absorbed into circulation and aggravate the decrease of blood pressure.

(4)Respiratory depression

Epidural block has little effect on resting ventilation volume, but it can inhibit the movement of intercostal muscles and diaphragm, resulting in reduced respiratory reserve function. When the level of anesthesia is below T_8, it has little effect on respiratory function. If the anesthesia level is above T_2, the ventilation reserve function will decrease significantly. Reducing the concentration of drugs can reduce the block of motor nerve and reduce the inhibition of respiration, such as the commonly used low concentration (1% −3%) lidocaine in clinical cervical epidural block, lidocaine, which is commonly used in the upper thoracic segment of 1.3% −1.6%, although the anesthesia level is high, but it has little effect on the respiratory function.

（5）Nausea and vomiting

The causes of nausea and vomiting in epidural block are similar to that of spinal anesthesia.

5.4.4.2   Postoperative complications

Complications after epidural block are not common. A few patients developed low back pain or transient urinary retention, which generally recovered quickly. However, severe neurological complications, even paraplegia, were caused by operation injury, anterior spinalartery embolization, adhesiveness arachnoid, and intraspinal occupying lesions. Strict and standardized operation is very important for preventing these complications. In order to avoid the risk of complications, we should change the anesthetic method in time.

（1）Nerve injuries

It shows partial sensory and/or motor dysfunction related to nerve distribution. It is usually caused by puncture needle and epidural catheter directly injuried the spinal cord. The neurotoxicity of local anesthetics should also be considered. If patient feels pain or electric shock, the nerves must be touched when puncturing or placing catheter. The longer duration of abnormal sensation may lead to persistent neuropathy and should be replaced by other anaesthesia, and the symptoms of most patients, such as paraplegia, pain, and numbness, can be relieved within a few weeks.

（2）Epidural hematoma

The bleeding rate of epidural puncture is 2% –6% , but the incidence of paraplegia caused by hematoma is only 1 : 20 000. Coagulation disorders or anticoagulant drugs are easy to cause bleeding. The prognosis depends on the early diagnosis and the timely operation. After epidural block, there is no withdrawal of the anesthesia, or the myasthenia and paraplegia after the withdrawal, which are the signs of the formation of the hematoma to oppress the spinal cord. Early diagnosis, laminectomy can be done for decompression of hematoma within 8 hours after hematoma formation. If it is more than 24 hours, it is usually difficult to recover. Epidural block is forbidden for coagulant dysfunction and anticoagulant drugs are being used.

（3）Anterior spinal artery syndrome

The anterior spinal artery embolization, long time of insufficient blood supply, can cause ischemic changes and even necrosis of the spinal cord, which is characterized by the symptoms of motor disorders, called the anterior spinal artery syndrome. Patients generally have no sensory impairment, complaints of heavy body, difficulty in turning over, some patients can gradually recover, and some patients have permanent painless paraplegia. The inducing factors are as follows：①Arteriosclerosis and vascular stenosis are common in the elderly. ②The too high concentration of epinephrine in local anesthetics causes persistent spasm of the anterior spinal artery. ③Severe hypotension during anesthesia.

（4）Epidural abscess

The reason is aseptic operation is not strict, or puncture needle passes infected tissue, cause epidural cavity infection and gradually form abscess. Clinical symptoms of spinal cord and nerve root are stimulated and oppressed such as radiation pain, myasthenia and paraplegia, accompanied by signs of infection. Treatment should be given large dose of antibiotics, and early laminectomy drainage.

（5）Difficulty of pulling out or catheter fracture

Because of the reasons such as laminae, ligaments and paraspinal muscles rigidity, it is difficult to pull out the catheter. If the compression is too tight or forced to pull out, it will lead to the fracture of the catheter. The patient can be placed in the original puncture position, and it can usually be successfully pulled out. If it is still difficult, hot compress or local anesthetic should be injected around the catheter, and then pull out evenly and slowly. If the catheter broken residue left in body, no infection or nerve irritation symptoms, the residual catheter ends need not to be removed, but should be observed closely.

5.4.5　Indications and contraindications

5.4.5.1　Indications

It is suitable for the operation in abdomen, waist, and lower limbs under diaphragm, and no operative time limit. It can also be used in surgery in neck, upper limbs and chest wall, but anesthesia operation and management technology are more complex. We must carefully monitor blood pressure, heart rate and other vital signs. We should be cautious when using them.

5.4.5.2　Contraindications

Contraindications are similar with those of lumbar anesthesia. Any skin infection, coagulation disorder, shock, spinal tuberculosis or severe malformation and central nervous system diseases should be taboo. For elderly patients, pregnancy, anemia, hypertension, heart disease, low blood volume and other patients, we should be very careful, reduce the dosage and strengthen the management of patients in anesthesia.

5.5　Sacral Block

The local anesthetic is injected into the sacral canal (sacral epidural space) through sacral hiatus to block the sacral spinal nerve, which is called sacral block. Sacral canal block is a part of epidural block. Sacral block is suitable for operation in rectum, anus and perineum.

5.5.1　Sacral canal puncture

The patient took the lateral or the prone position. In the lateral position, the back is arched, and the two knees close to the abdomen. At the prone position, the hip is underlied by a little pillow, with two legs slightly separated, tiptoe to the inside, and the heel to spin to relax the buttocks muscles. Before the puncture, touche the tip of the caudal bone, and then along the middle line, 3-4 cm can touch a "V" or "U"-shaped opening to caudal cave, both side of each has a bony bulge of the sacral horn, which is the sacral hiatus. 1% lidocaine is used in the center of the sacral fissure to make the skin infutration. The needle pierced vertically the sacrocaudal ligaments which cover the sacral hiatus. When the ligament is penetrated, there was a sudden disappearance of the resistance. At this time, the needle is entered into the caudal cavity with 30° angles with skin. If the angle is too large, the needle touches the anterior wall of the sacral canal or directly penetrated into the skin tissue. If the angle is too small, the needle touches the posterior wall of the sacral canal and dose not enter the caudal cavity. After insertion of the needle into the sacral canal, the advanced depth is about 2 cm. The bony sign on the upper edge of sacral canal is connected line of the posterior superior iliac spine. The puncture needle should not go too deeply, otherwise, it will be dangerous to enter the subarachnoid space. When the simplified sacral canal vertical needle insertion is used, the patient is taken lateral position, the sacrococcygeal ligament is vertically puncturing through the upper end of the sacral hiatus with a 7 gauge short needle. After the successful puncture, the syringe should be connected. Withdrawing no blood and cerebrospinal fluid, the local anesthetic can be injected. There should be no obvious resistance when injected, and no local subcutaneous swelling after injection. This method is safer.

5.5.2　Commonly used local anesthetics

1%-1.5% lidocaine or 0.25%-0.5% bupivacaine (all add appropriate amount of adrenaline) is used in adults with a general volume of 20 mL, and the anesthetic time was 1.5-2 hours and 4-6 hours, respectively. After a successful injection, the dose of 5 mL is first injected. After 5 minutes, no adverse reaction is observed, and the remaining 15 mL is injected.

5.5.3　Complications

There are abundant venous plexus in the lumen of sacral canal. If the blood vessel is punctured and the absorption of local anesthetics is accelerated, local anesthetic toxicity will be produced. If the puncture needle is too deep, perforating dural sac and arachnoid and puncture into the subarachnoid space will result in wide level block or total spinal anesthesia. In addition, the postoperative urine retention is also more common. In case of sacral canal malformation, puncture point infection, puncture difficulty or blood return, saddle anesthesia or epidural anesthesia can be switched to.

5.6　Combined Block of Subarachnoid and Epidural Space

The combination of subarachnoid and epidural block, also known as combined spinal–epidural anesthesia, has been widely used in lower abdomen and lower limb surgery in recent years. Its advantages are as follows: ①It has the characteristics of spinal anesthesia onset fast, perfect analgesia and muscle relaxation. ②When epidural block is used, we can control the anesthesia level and meet the needs of long time operation. There are two kinds of puncture method: two point method and one point method. Two point method: the position of the patient is the same as that of the spinal anesthesia. Generally, T_{12}–L_1 is first selected for epidural puncture and placement of catheter. Then subarachnoid puncture is performed at L_{3-4} interval. One point method: a special combined puncture needle is used for epidural puncture through the L_{2-3} spinous process. After the puncture is successful, the subarachnoid puncture is performed with a matching lumbar puncture needle through the epidural puncture needle. Local anesthetic can be injected into (lumbar anesthesia) when CSF outflow. After withdrawal of lumbar puncture needle, epidural catheter is placed cephalad and epidural catheter is fixed. Because the lumbar puncture needle is very thin, the damage to the dura mater is very small, the incidence of postoperative headache is significantly reduced, but the time for injection is 45–60 seconds. At present, the clinical one point method is used more.

Chapter 6

Monitoring and Mannagement During Anesthesia and Recovery Period

6.1 Monitoring and Management During Anesthesia

The patient's vital organ may be affected by operation and anesthesia. If the influences are not discovered and corrected in time, temporary or permanent damage may beresulted. So the vital signs and early changes of physiology must be monitored rigorously to find out and correct the changes as early as it can to avoid serious complication.

6.1.1 Monitoring and treatment of anesthesia depth

Anesthesia depth refers to the status of central nerve system when the control effect of general anesthetics and counter-action of operative stimulus reach to an equilibrium. An ideal anesthesia should ensure patient painlessness, unconsciousness and stabilization in hemodynamics during operation and recovery complete and non-recall after operation. So far no available technique can judge anesthesia depth accurately and effectively. In clinic, the judgement of aesthesia depth is mainly depended on the patient's presentation, such as blood pressure, heart rate, respiratory amplitude and rhythm, eye sign and muscle relaxation, etc. , and guided by the modern anesthetic monitoring technique. Now the available anesthetic monitoring techniques include quantitative-EEG, evoked potential(EP), low esophageal contraction(LEC) and heart rate variability(HRV), etc.

The methods of regulating anesthesia depth include the following: ①Guided by MAC in inhalation aesthesia. ②Application of combined anesthesia. ③Using local anesthesia or deepening anesthesia to reduce the influence of circulation by nerve reflex during traction of nerves and vessels and periosteal stimulus as well as visceral exploration.

6.1.2 Monitoring and treatment of cardiovascular function

6.1.2.1 Monitoring

①Pulse. ②Arterial pressure. ③Electrocardiogram. ④Microcirculation. ⑤Central venous pressure. ⑥Hemodynamic monitoring.

6.1.2.2   Etiology and treatment of circulation disorder

(1) Reasons and treatments of hypotension

Hypotension is diagnosed by blood pressure lower than 20% of preanesthetic value or <80/60 mmHg. The cause has three aspects: ①Patient's condition, such as imbalance of water, electrolytes, cardiovascular disease, adrenocortical insufficiency or catecholamine deficiency. ②Anesthesia: some anesthetic agents as pethodine and technique as intravertebral anesthesia may decrease blood pressure; hyperventilation during controlled or assistant ventilation which increases intrathoracic pressure may also cause hypotension by reducing returned blood. ③Operation: blood loss, traction, anaphylaxis, transfusion, etc., may lead to hypotension.

Treatment: ①Lighten the depth of anesthesia for too deep anesthesia. ②Volume expansion: As for insufficient blood volume, maintaining normal blood volume by reasonalbe rehydration and transfusion. ③Neuroreflexive hypotension: The operation should be suspended for several minutes. Sufficient oxygen supply and carbon dioxide accumulation should be avoided and regional block with local anesthetics. ④Proper use of vasoactive agents: Commonly use ephedrine 5–10 mg to increase vascular resistance or dopamine 2–4 mg to increase cardiac output. If accompanied by bradycardia, atrapine should be administered. ⑤Correction of mechanical factors: chest drainage, such as pneumothorax, decrease or stop positive expiratory pressure ventilation (PEEP) in general anesthesia; relieve the compression of the vena cava (such as move uterus of the pregnant woman to left).

(2) Reasons and treatments of hypertension

Blood pressure in anaesthesia is higher than basic value of 20% or >170/100 mmHg, hypertension can be diagnosed. Reasons: ①Too shallow anesthesia or uncomplete analgesia. ②Tracheal intubation or extubation stimulation, etc. ③Adrenaline in local anesthetics is absorbed too fast or too much. ④Hypoxia or CO_2 retention. ⑤Mass secretion of catecolamine, such as pheochromocytoma is stimulated during surgery. ⑥Increased intracranial pressure, such as craniocerebral trauma, can increase blood pressure and slow heart rate. ⑦Concomitant diseases such as essential hypertension, gestational toxicosis, pregnancy induced hypertension.

Treatment: ①Remove the cause of the disease. ②Application of vasoactive drugs: The principle of vasoactive drugs is small dose, close observation and avoidance of excessive blood pressure, resulting in reduced perfusion and new damage to heart, brain and kidney. The common drugs include Urapidil, calcium bloker, α-receptor blocker, etc.

(3) The causes and prevention of myocardial ischemia

①Stress reaponse: such as light anesthesia, incomplete analgesia, nervous, dread, intubation response, and hypoxia, etc. ②Severe fluctuation of blood pressure during operation: Continuous long time hypotension can reduce the blood flow of coronary artery obviously. Long term hypertension is the increase of cardiac work and the increase of oxygen ventilatory dysfunction.

Prevention: ①Prevention of myocardial oxygen supply reduction, positive correction of hypotension; maintain close to normal blood volume and moderate ventilation to prevent hypoxia; prevention of excessive inhibition on circulation function by anesthetic drugs. ②Avoid the increase of myocardial oxygen consumption: such as avoiding tachycardia and hypertension. ③Minimize perioperative stress response: such as maintaining the appropriate depth of anesthesia, reducing the intubation response.

(4) Reasons and treatments of arrhymia

①Anesthetic drugs: related to the dose and concentration of anesthetics. ②Factors of anesthesia or operation: such as bronchial intubation and extubation, tracheoscopy and esophagoscopy, traction of hilum of lung may cause bradycardia, sinus arrhythmia, and even atrioventricular block or cardiac arrest; tracheal intubation may cause sinus tachycardia, especially under hypoxia and CO_2 retention. ③Hypoxia and CO_2 retention. ④The effect of preoperative arrhythmia. ⑤Electrolyte disturbance: acute hypokalemia increases myocardial ecxitability and incline to induce atrial premature beat, ventricular tachycardia, ventricular fibrillation; and that hyperkalemia may cause sinoauricular block, atrioventricular block and even cardiac arrest. ⑥Hypothermia anesthesia.

Treatment: ①Finding and eliminating the inducing factors of arrhythmia. Focus the therapy on primary disease. ②For different types of arrhythmia, we should apply antiarrhythmic drugs appropriately. ③Immediate direct current conversion of ventricular fibrillation and malignant ventricular; chronic arrhythmias with symptoms, such as Ⅲ atrioventricular block, should be fitted with pacemakers; supraventricular tachycardia, such as preexcitation syndrome, caused by congenital anomalous conduction and bypass, should be treated by radiofrequency radical operation.

6.1.3 Monitoring and management of respiration

6.1.3.1 Monitoring

①Clinical symptoms and signs: observe the fashion of respiratory movement, frequecy, rhythm and amplitude. ②Monitoring of respiratory function: include tidal volume, minute ventilation, airway pressure and peak pressure, respiratory frequency, I : E ratio, PEEP and oxygen concentratjion, etc. ③Monitoring of pulse, blood oxygen saturation. ④Monitoring of blood gas analysis and end-expiratory CO_2 concentration (PetCO₂) when necessary.

6.1.3.2 Representation and treatment of respiratory abnormalities

①Breath-hold: most occur during the induction of anesthesia under too shallow anesthesia, surgical stimulation of periosteum and visceral nerve and other conditions. We should suspend surgery and deepen anesthesia. ②Tachypnea: respiratory frequency >40 BPM. The amplitude is deep or shallow. It is most commonly seen in hypoxia and carbon dioxide accumulation. Carbon dioxide accumulation is the most obvious manifestation of deep and fast breathing. The gas exchange area caused by tracheobronchial tube or bronchial anaesthesia is insufficient, airway obstructed, soda lime failure, machine valve malfunction, pulmonary edema, atelectasis, shock, and heart failure and too shallow anesthesia may all occur. It is necessary to check the causes immediately and adjust the process. ③Bronchial spasm: It is characterized by respiratory dyspnea, wheezing, and widespread dry rale of two lung; if an artificial airway has been built, the anesthesia machine can show increased airway resistance, accompanied by increased heart rate and even arrhythmia; the drugs such as ketamine, isoflurane and vecuronium, which have the dilatation effect on the bronchus and the histamine free release can be used to prevented. At the same time, we should pay attention to prevent mistaken aspiration and remove the secretions in time, and the anesthesia should not be too shallow. Once it occurs, we should give antispasmodic and antiasthmatic treatment in addition to eliminating the inducements and fully inhaling oxygen. ④Apnea: Anesthetics, muscle relaxants, surgical stimulation, artificial or mechanical ventilation can all cause, stopping medication and stimulation, and most of them can recover by themselves. ⑤Larynx spasm: Drugs, too shallow anesthesia or low oxygen, secretions, laryngoscope which induced throat hypersensitivity may lead to laryngeal spasm. Mild laryngospasm, only show larynx stridor during inhalation, can be alleviated by relieving local stimulation; moderate laryngeal spasm has larynx stridor during inhalation and exhalation. The mask should be pressurized immediately to inhale oxygen and relieve the cause of the disease. Severe laryngospasm which airway is completely obstructed, has strong breathing action and no larynx stridor. Postive pressure ventilation can not be carried out. Tracheal intubation after intravenous injection of succinycholine and artificial ventilation should start immediately, thyrocricoid puncture or tracheotomy may be done in emergency.

Anesthesia and surgery can weaken the self regulating ability of the body, including the regulation of body temperature. The change of temperature also causes some stress reactions to the body, which can affect the recovery of patients, and it can also endanger the lives of patients. Temperature detection during anesthesia is very necessary for some patients.

(1) Temperature monitoring equipment

At present, various electronic thermometers are mainly used during operation, thermistor thermometer and thermocouple thermometer are most commonly used.

(2) Monitoring sites

The temperature of different parts of the body is different. The body temperature at the deep part, that is core temperature, is relatively constant. The organs which have rich blood perfusion such as brain, heart and kidney have higher temperature, near 38 ℃. However other organs which are less perfusion have a lower temperature. Blood temperature can been seen as the mean of visceral temperature. The following site can be choosen to measure temperature: axilla, nasopharynx, oral cavity, esophagus, rectum, tympanic membrane, urinary bladder, blood, trachea, muscle, skin, etc.

(3) The methods of control body temperature during anesthesia and operation

①Regulate the temperature of operation room and reduce the stress reaction of patients to environmental temperature. ②The installation and use of the gas heating humidifier on the anesthesia machine can reduce the heat loss of the body. ③The variable temperature water tank used in cardiopulmonary bypass can satisfy the requirement of body temperature during operation by regulating blood temperature directly. ④Radiant heater is mainly used for warming up after operation to prevent shivering. ⑤Esophageal heater: raise the body temperature through the heat exchange between the esophagus and the hot water.

6.2 Monitoring and Management Recovery Period

For most surgical patients, anesthesia recovery is a process of recovery from anesthesia. But some patients may be fatal in this process, only when skilled doctors and nurses are rescued, can they quickly turn the corner. The purpose of setting up the anesthesia recovery room is to provide the patient with a stable recovery after anesthesia and the space for rescue in critical situations.

6.2.1 Monitoring

The contents are as follow: ①Pulse blood oxygen saturation. ②At least every 15 minutes, vital signs were observed, including blood pressure, heart rate, respiratory rate, airway resistance and patient's wakefulness. ③ECG. ④Body temperature. ⑤For those who need ventilator assisted ventilation for the delay of recovery and not fully recovering the respiratory function, the tidal volume and spontaneous breathing frequency should be measured regularly and the arterial blood gas analysis should be carried out when necessary.

6.2.2 Management

(1) Management of respiratory system

Hypoxemia should be prevented. The main causes of hypoxemia in recovery rooms are airway obstruction, respiratory depression and lung lesions. Airway obstruction should be unblocked or adjusted head position; for respiratory suppression, we must first relieve the cause, and respiratory support is safer; for pulmonary lesions, only oxygen inhalation dose not solve the problem. The fundamental method is to expand the alveoli, so PEEP 0.49 kPa(5 cmH$_2$O) is used as much as possible except for the use of a larger tidal volume in the ventilator.

(2) Management of circulative system

The common symptom are hypotension and hypertesion. ①The most common cause of hypotension is lack of blood volume, which may be insufficient relative to blood transfusion or vasodilatation. The measurement of central venous pressure often contributes to the correct conclusion. In addition, postoperative intracavity hemorrhage continues to be a particular problem. Other special reasons such as cardiogenic shock, tension pneumothorax, severe hypoglycemia have corresponding symptoms and medical history can be used as reference, as long as careful, diagnosis is generally not difficult, should be dealt with in the cause of the disease. ②Hypertension: Common causes include pain, hypoxia, tracheal stimulation, bladder distention, hypercapnia and intracranial hypertension, etc. Preoperative arteriosclerosis or early hypertension in patients is associated with increased blood pressure after operation. The causes of should be relieved, followed by symptomatic treatment to reduce blood pressure.

(3) Nausea and vomiting

Patients often occur after general anesthesia, especially women and children. Nausea and vomiting are often the result of narcotic drugs on chemoreceptor stimulation. Nausea and vomiting can cause discomfort, and autonomic nervous responses such as high blood pressure and rapid heartbeat which can also cause some complications, such as cerebral hemorrhage and cardiovascular accident. Although there are no well recognized preventive and therapeutic methods, some measures can be considered. Intraoperative application of droperidol can reduce the incidence.

(4) Waking delay

Reasons: ①Continuous anaesthesia. ②Respiratory dysfunction. ③Serious accident occurred during the operation: such as massive bleeding, myocardial ischemia or infarction, intracranial hypertension caused by rupture of intracranial aneurysm. ④Abnomal body temperature: The inhibitory effects of all the anesthetics were enhanced when the body temperature decreased which delay awakeness. The patients were all coma for a long time when the malignant hyperthermia induced by anesthesia or postoperative wound pain occur. We should maintain stable circulation, normal ventilation and adequate oxygen supply. Then we will further find out the causes and treat them according to the etiology.

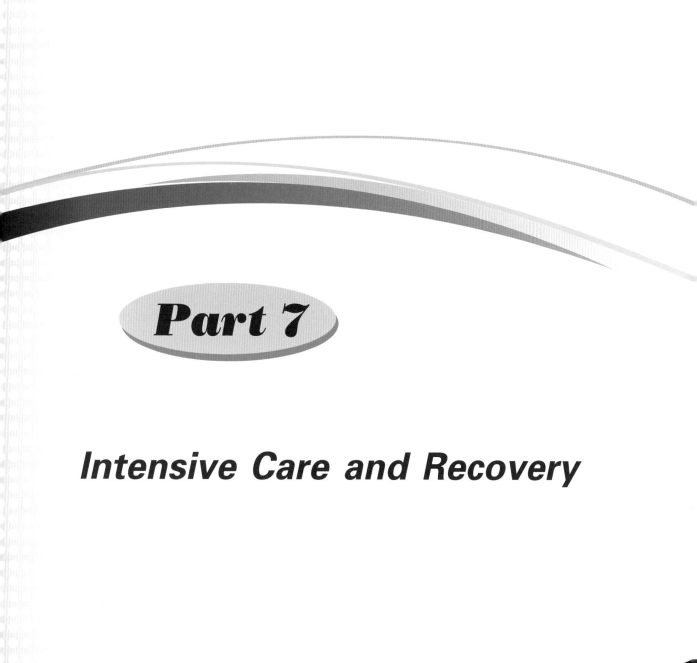

Part 7

Intensive Care and Recovery

7.1　Introduction

The intensive care unit (ICU) is the hospital facility within which the highest level of continuous patient care and treatment is provided. It comes from the recovery room and the shock therapy unit. The way of collecting critically ill patients is helpful to decrease mortality and/or deformity and improve medical quality. So the ICU is an importance portion in the modern hospital.

7.1.1　The establishment of ICU

The establishment of ICU is based on the hospital scale, disease category, technique and equipments. 3% –6% of the hospital total beds are used for this purpose and are organized usually into units of 6–8 beds, as this is considered to be the optimal size. A much greater area needs to be allocated to each bed than in ordinary wards because several nurses must treat patients simultaneously and bulky items of equipment often need to be accommodated. Each bed area is supplied with oxygen and piped suction, medical compressed air and sometimes nitrous oxide. Sufficient local storage space is required to make the nurse self –sufficient for common procedures such as administration of drugs and tracheal aspiration. Each bed area should be equipped with a self–inflating resuscitation bag to enable the staff to maintain artificial ventilation in case the mechanical ventilator fails. The department that provides the unit staff differs from hospital to hospital; units serving primarily a single specialty (e. g. , cardiac surgery or neurosurgery units) are usually staffed by the specialty involved, whereas most general ICUs are staffed by the anesthetic department, which is well used to providing round–the–clock emergency services.

7.1.2　Patients admitted to the unit

Patients admitted to the unit should be those whose lives are in imminent danger but in whom, it is believed, the immediate risk may be averted by active and often invasive therapeutic efforts. A wide range of pathological conditions may lead to such a state but all involve failure, or the threat of failure, of the respiratory and/or circulatory systems. In addition, dysfunction of one or more of the renal, gastrointestinal, hepatic, hematological and neurological systems may be present, but involvement of one of these systems alone is rarely a reason for admission to the ICU. There are two receiving standards. One is to divide the case condition into four grades: grade Ⅰ, patients needn't regular observation or invasive monitoring; grade Ⅱ, the case condition is unsteady, patients need monitoring in case of accident; grade Ⅲ, patients may take place the accident at any time and need invasive monitoring; grade Ⅳ, the case condition is so severe that patients must proceed complicated monitoring and special treatment measure. Grade Ⅲ and grade Ⅳ cases must be admitted to the ICU. The other is therapeutic intervention scoring system (TISS), patients whose score is more than four are admitted to the ICU.

Patients admitted to the ICU require active and aggressive therapy for either appropriate management of a diagnosed condition or resuscitation while a definitive diagnosis is made. Critically ill patients usually benefit from prompt rather than delayed admission to the unit and early notification of such patients elsewhere in the hospital is to be encouraged.

The ICU is not an appropriate place for patients whose death is judged inevitable because of their acute illness or underlying pathology, e. g. , the severe chronic bronchitis on maximum treatment or the terminal cancer patient. There is often pressure to admit such patients because they require high levels of nursing care. It is easier to initiate complex therapeutic and supportive effort than it is to withdraw it. Critically ill patients can rarely discuss details of their care and their relatives may also find it difficult to make an objective judgment. It is a moral responsibility of ICU staff to inform patients' relatives if it becomes clear that restoration of a patient's ability to lead an independent existence is impossible. It should be noted that it is unethical and unlawful to treat a patient against his or her volition.

7.2 Respiratory Monitoring and Respiratory Care

7.2.1 Respiratory monitoring

Monitoring the respiratory function of critically ill patients is important to instruct clinical treatment. It not only is helpful to judge the damage degree of the respiratory function and evaluate the effect of respiratory care, but also can predict the ventilator weaning. Common respiratory function monitoring parameters are listed in Table 7-1-1.

Table 7-1-1 Common respiratory function monitoring parameters

Parameters	Normal data	Artificial ventilation sign
V_T(mL/kg)	5-7	—
RR	12-20	>35
V_D/V_T	0.25-0.40	>0.60
$PaCO_2$(mmHg)	35-45	>55
PaO_2(mmHg)	80-100	<70(Oxygen assistance)
SaO_2(%)	96-100	—
Q_s/Q_T(%)	3-5	>20
VC (mL/kg)	65-75	<15
MIF (cmH$_2$O)	75-100	<25

7.2.2 Oxygen therapy

The clinical goal of oxygen therapy is to increase the alveolar oxygen content (C_{AO_2}), which is essentially equivalent to increasing the alveolar PO_2(P_{AO_2}). An increase in the C_{AO_2} may result in an increase in the C_{AO_2}, thereby decreasing the work of breathing and myocardial work required to attain a given arterial oxygen content.

7.2.2.1 Oxygen delivery systems

Oxygen therapy is provided by either partial rebreathing or nonrebreathing delivery systems that do not require a CO_2 absorber. A partial rebreathing system allows for the initial portion of the expired gases containing little or no CO_2 to be collected in a reservoir while the remaining expiratory gases are vented to the atmosphere. Most oxygen delivery systems are intended to function as nonrebreathing systems in which all exhaled CO_2 is vented to the atmosphere and only fresh inspiratory gases are inhaled. Nonrebreathing systems are divided into high-flow (fixed performance) and low-flow (variable performance) systems.

A high-flow oxygen delivery system provides the total inspired atmosphere so that a premixed F_iO_2 is consistently and predictably delivered. To accomplish this goal, the inspiratory gas flows must be 3-4 times the measured minute ventilation. So-called venture devices are the most commonly used high-flow oxygen devices for nonintubated patients.

A low-flow oxygen delivery system requires that the patient inspire some room air to meet inspiratory demands. These systems are popular because of their simplicity, patient comfort, and economics. F_iO_2 is unstable and is determined by the size of the oxygen reservoir, the oxygen flow rate, and the breathing pattern. Face mask and nasal cannula are the most commonly used low-flow oxygen devices.

7.2.2.2　Clinical application of artificial ventilation

(1) Indications for artificial ventilation

Patients who are unable to maintain adequate levels of oxygenation or who develop hypercapnia may be candidates for mechanically assisted ventilation, provided that their pulmonary pathology is potentially reversible.

(2) Common ventilation mode

Control-mode ventilation (CMV) is a volume-preset mode in which the patient is not allowed to participate in any phase of breathing cycle.

Assist/control-mode ventilation (AMV) is a volume-preset mode in which the ventilator frequency is determined by the patient's inspiratory efforts.

Intermittent mandatory ventilation (IMV) is a ventilator system that allows spontaneous breathing via a continuous-flow device. Machine breaths are delivered at preset time intervals.

Pressure support ventilation (PSV) is a volume-variable mode in which the ventilator frequency is determined by the patient's inspiratory efforts; a preset system pressure is rapidly achieved and is maintained throughout inspiration by adjustment of machine inspiratory flow, and inspiration ends when the inspiratory flow falls below a preset minimal value.

Positive end-expiratory pressure (PEEP) in conjunction with positive pressure breaths (CMV+PEEP, A/CMV+PEEP).

(3) Adjusting the ventilator

There are two main types of ventilator in common use: those which deliver a preset tidal volume and those which develop a set pressure during each inspiration. In most units, volume-preset machines predominate. The ICU resident should become familiar with the controls and facilities of ventilators available in the unit-preferably with an experienced colleague when the machine is not attached to a patient. The characteristics of the ventilatory cycle may be altered to suit the patient and reduce influence on other organs.

The ventilator should be adjusted initially to deliver a tidal volume of 10-15 mL/kg (approximately 1000 mL for a 70 kg patient) and a minute volume of 8-10 L/min. An initial inspired oxygen concentration of 40% is appropriate for most patients, but an initial concentration of 50% or more should be selected in patients who are already hypoxemic despite oxygen therapy. If controllable, the inspiratory time should be approximately half the expiratory time. After approximately 10 min, arterial blood gases should be measured and the inspired oxygen concentration adjusted if necessary. Adjusting respiratory parameters are listed in Table 7-1-2.

Table 7-1-2　Respiratory parameters adjusting

Ventilation mode	IMV, A/CMV
V_T (mL/kg)	10-15
RR (BPM)	8-12
FiO_2	0.4-1.0
I : E	1 : (1.5-2.0)
Aspiratory time	1-2
Aspiratory stopping time	0-0.6
PEEP (cmH_2O) (kPa)	2-5(0.2-0.5)

(4) Weaning from the ventilator

Mechanical ventilation should be prolonged only for specific reasons. It should be routine to consider weaning the patient each day. Patients who are otherwise stable should be weaned as soon as possible: ①Pulmonary function seems likely to be adequate during spontaneous ventilation. ②Neuromuscular strength and co-ordination seem to be sufficient to maintain an adequate minute volume and to permit coughing.

The indications for weaning, extubation are shown in Table 7-1-3. It is probably safer to wean patients from IPPV and to extubate the trachea early in the day rather than in the late afternoon or evening, as less medical and nursing supervision tends to be available at night. In general, the shorter the period of ventilation, the simpler the weaning procedures; weaning over a period of several days may be necessary after prolonged IPPV, particularly for neuromuscular disorders.

Table 7-1-3　Guidelines for weaning, extubation

Respiratory parameter	Start weaning	Extubation sign
VC (mL/kg)	≥5	≥10-15
MIF (cmH_2O)	≥10	≥25
PEEP (cmH_2O)	≤10	≤5
PaO_2(mmHg) , inhaling O_2	≥60	≥60
pH	≥7.30	≥7.30
RR (BPM)	<45	<35
MV (L/min)	<18	<10

7.3　Clinical Application of Cardiovascular Monitoring

7.3.1　Use of monitoring parameters to estimate circulation function

Maintenance of perfusion of vital organs is one of the principal tasks of the anesthetist during surgery. Adequate perfusion is dependent on adequate venous return to the heart, cardiac performance and arterial pressure.

Direct measurements of cardiac output and blood volume are difficult during anesthesia and require invasive procedures which are inappropriate in many situations. Adequacy of cardiac output and circulating blood volume may be inferred indirectly from observation of the cardiovascular variables such as BP and CVP (Table 7-1-4).

Table 7-1-4   Clinical meaning of the relationship between CVP and BP

CVP	BP	Clinical meaning
Down	Down	Blood volume down
Down	Normal	Blood volume little down
Up	Down	Heart dysfunction, blood volume more
Up	Normal	Volume blood vessel contraction, pulmonary circula-tion resistance increasing
Normal	Down	Cardiac output down, volume blood vessel contraction

7.3.2   Use of monitoring results to decide the primary treatment principle

We can judge heart preload, heart afterload and myocardial constriction according to the results of hemodynamic monitoring and calculation. When PCWP (pulmonary capillary wedge pressure) is below 10 mmHg, it implies low heart preload and hypovolemia and needs blood or fluid replacement. To a certain extent, preload increment can increase CO (cardiac output). When PCWP is higher than 18 mmHg, it need diuretics or blood vessel extending medicine to decrease it and protect myocardium, increase CO. When total peripheral resistance (TPR) is below 100 kPa · s/L, it implies low heart afterload and needs blood or fluid replacement and vessel contracting medicine if necessary; when TPR is higher than 200 kPa · s/L, heart afterload increases. It needs blood vessel extending medicine to increase stroke volume (SV) and CO. When myocardial contractility decreases, it indicates cardiac index (CI) and left ventricular stroke work index (LVSWI) decrease, it needs positive inotropic medicine to cure. While myocardial contractility increases, heart rate is quicker; the blood pressure is higher; the myocardial consuming oxygen is more, it needs β-adrenoceptor blocking drugs to cure.

7.3.3   Use of monitoring results to instruct fluid treatment

Measurement of CVP is performed frequently in patients with advanced cardiovascular diseases and those undergoing major operations. Measurement of CVP is a valuable aid to blood and fluid replacement. If CVP increases above normal and remains high with no improvement in arterial pressure, it is likely that myocardial failure has occurred and inotropic support may be required.

Measurement of PCWP is performed frequently in patients with advanced cardiovascular diseases and critically illness. When PCWP pressure is extremely high or low, it is easy to recognize that this value must be adjusted to avoid pulmonary edema or improve cardiac output. However, things are rarely so clear-cut in critically ill patients, and the target value for optimal wedge pressure is uncertain and often decided empirically. Under these circumstances, a rapid fluid challenge may be a useful method to determine whether the PCWP is optimal for the patient in that setting. An intravenous bolus of crystalloid solution (200 mL) is given rapidly over 15 minutes, and the change in PCWP is measured, along with other pertinent hemodynamic variables. If the baseline wedge pressure is high or if a severe pulmonary capillary injury is present, a reduced volume may be used. Small increases in PCWP following the fluid challenge (less than 3 mmHg) suggest that the ventricle is operating on the flat portion of its diastolic filling curve, whereas large increases in wedge pressure (7 mmHg or greater) suggest that the steep portion of the curve has been reached and that little further increase in stroke volume and cardiac output can be achieved without a substantial risk of producing hydrostatic pulmonary edema.

7.4 Cardiopulmonary Resuscitation

Cardiopulmonary resuscitation (CPR) is required when supply of oxygen to the brain is insufficient to maintain function. Oxygen delivery is dependent upon cardiac output, hemoglobin concentration and saturation of hemoglobin with oxygen. CPR is required most commonly after cardiac arrest, respiratory arrest or a combination of two. A successful CPR is not only recover cardiopulmonary function but also cental nerve function. Brain is the most susceptible organ to hypoxia, so the key point during CPR is maintain the perfusion of brain. Now CPR has expanded to CPCR (cardiopulmonary cerebral resuscitation). The whole CPCR can be divided into three stages, which are basic life support, advanced life support and aftercare.

7.4.1 Cerebral hypoxia

Brain has a limited facility for anaerobic metabolism and can not store oxygen. Hypoxemia is tolerated remarkably well in normal individual, as cerebral blood flow (CBF) increases substantially to compensate for reduced oxygen carriage in blood. In contrast, ischemia (e. g. , circulatory arrest) or hypoxemia in a patient unable to increase CBF(e. g. , cerebrovascular atherosclerosis or a low cardiac output) results in the rapid onset of anaerobic metabolism. The cerebral cortex is damaged permanently by ischemia of more than 3–4 min duration. Thus, although a patient may survive an episode of circulatory arrest, permanent impairment of cerebral function may result if cerebral oxygen delivery is not restored within 3–4 min of the initial cessation of blood flow. The commonest cause of brain damage after cardiac arrest is delay in starting resuscitation. Therefore, when circulatory arrest has occurred, it is essential to start CPR as rapidly as possible.

7.4.2 Signs of cardiac arrest

Sudden deep unconsciousness, dilated pupils(unreliable) , ashen cyanosis, absent of carotid and femoral pulse apnea or gasping are the most common signs.

Here sudden deep unconsciousness and absent of major pulses are sufficient to justify diagnosis.

Guidelines to guide the performance of cardiopulmonary resuscitation have been developed by the Euorpean Resuscitation Council and the American Heart Association. These guidelines are based on the concept of the "chain of survival". The chain of survival requires that following an initial clinical assessment of the patient's condition, a telephone call for help is made before starting basic life support. This early call for help decreases the time to the first defibrillation, shorten the time to the delivery of advanced life support, decreases the length of time of performance of basic life support and improves survival from the initial resuscitation.

7.4.3 Assessment

Approach the patient ensuring that there is no further danger from the surrounding environment. Assess the level of responsiveness by gently shaking and shouting "Are you all right?"

(1) Airway

In the unresponsive patient, open the airway by tilting the head back and lifting the jaw forwards. This displaces the tongue, the most common cause of airway obstruction, from the back of the pharynx. In case of suspected cervical spine injury, the airway should be opened by using the jaw thrust manoeuvre only whilst maintaining inline cervical spine immobilization. Head tilt and neck extension must never be used in this situation.

(2) Breathing

Look—to see the chest wall is moving or if the abdominal wall is indicating an obstructed airway by see-saw movement.

Listen—over the mouth for sounds of air movement or for sounds indicating an obstructed airway.

Feel—over the mouth with the side of the face for sign of air movement indicating effective breathing.

(3) Circulation

Check the rate and rhythm of the carotid pulse.

(4) Call for help

It is essential to telephone for help as soon as the assessment has been completed.

7.4.4   Basic life support

7.4.4.1   Cardiac arrest

If breathing and pulse are absent commence basic life support, which is combination of chest compression and ventilation.

(1) Chest compression

Chest compression are performed on the lower third of the sternum, two fingers breadth above the xiphisternum. The overlapping heels of both hands are used to compress the chest by depressing the sternum 4–5 cm at a rate of 80 compressions per minute (range 60–100 compression per minute). After 15 compressions open the airway by tilting the head and lifting the chin and give two expired air breaths.

(2) Breathing

This is achieved by expired air ventilation. With the airway held open, pitch the nostrils closed. Take a full breath and seal your lips over the patient's mouth. Blow steadily into the patient's mouth, watching the chest rise as if the patient was taking a deep breath. Each breath should take approximately 2 s for a full inflation. Maintaining the airway, take your mouth off the patient and allow the chest to fall in expiration. Repeat this maneuver to give two ventilations.

Continue basic life support, 15 chest compressions with 2 expired air ventilations, until advanced life support to perform further assessments of the patient unless the patient show signs of recovery.

7.4.4.2   Respiratory arrest

If the patient is not breathing but has a pulse, perform 10 expired air breaths before leaving for help. On returning to the patient, recheck the breathing and the pulse rate. If a pulse is present continue expired air breathing at a rate of 10 breaths per minute but recheck the pulse after every 10 breaths. Commence full basic life if the pulse stops.

Mechanism of action of chest compression: The original theory of the action of chest compressions was that the heart was squeezed between the sternums superiorly and vertebral column posteriorly with each depression of the sternum. Each compression of the heart pumped blood around the circulation (the heart pump theory).

A later theory, the chest pump theory, is based on the concept that each chest compression raises the intrathoracic pressure. This raised pressure is transmitted to the intrathoracic vessels; the arteries, being thickwalled, retain and transmit this pressure whereas the veins, being thin-walled collapse. The result is a pressure gradient between the arterial and venous system and thus a forward flow of blood around circulation. Basic life support only provides 10% –15% of normal cardiac output and should be regarded as "buying time" until the commencement of advanced life support.

7.4.4.3　Advanced life support

The performance of advanced life support needs some special equipment and drugs. In adult resuscitation, the early use of a defibrillator in ventricular fibrillation has a definitive effect on eventual survival. In specialized in-hospital areas, for example the operating theatre, the intensive care unit, the time to defibrillation is negligible. In these situations it is recommended that if defibrillation is immediately to hand, basic life support is not initiate until defibrillation has been attempted.

There are four underlying disorders of cardiac rhythm associated with cardiac arrest:

(1) Ventricular fibrillation.

(2) Ventricular tachycardia.

(3) Asystole.

(4) Electromechanical dissociation (pulseless electrical activity).

Ventricular fibrillation and ventricular tachycardia have identical treatment protocols, thus only three treatment schedules are presented. Of these, the protocol for ventricular fibrillation is the most important as this arrhythmia is the commonest cause of sudden cardiac death, and it is also the most amenable to treatment.

7.4.4.4　Ventricular fibrillation

In a witnessed or mornitored of cardiac arrest, precordial thumb should be administered immediately. Early defibrillation is recommended and if the first three defibrillation shocks can be delivered quickly, then this initial defibrillation sequence should not be interrupted for basic life support procedures.

An initial DC shock at 200 J probably cause minimal myocardial damage and is adequate to achieve success in most recoverable situations. This first DC shock decrease the thoracic impedance, thus increasing the amount of energy from the second DC shock at 200 J that reaches the heart. Following two 200 J shocks, one defibrillation is attempted at the maximum delivered energy level of 360 J. If all three initial defibrillation attempts are unsuccessful, the prospects of recovery are poor.

Resuscitation should continue with tracheal intubation and lung ventilation with 100% oxygen. Where intubation is not achieved, ventilation with a high inspired oxygen level can be carried out using a self-inflating bag valve and mask, together with an oxygen reservoir system. Alternatively, a laryngeal mask airway can be inserted, which provide a more secure airway and more effective ventilation compared with an oral Guedel airway and a bag-valve mask system.

At the same time as intubation is being established, Peripheral venous access should be established and attempts should be made to cannulate a large peripheral vein with a 14G or 16G cannula.

Adrenaline 1 mg (10 mL of 1 in 10 000 solution or 1 mL of 1 in 1000 solution) is next action in the protocol. If intravenous access has not been established then 2–3 mg can be given via the tracheal route. Adrenaline is used in resuscitation mainly for its α-adrenergic receptor stimulant effects. This α-adrenergic action causes peripheral vasoconstriction, raises the systemic vascular resistance, raises the end-diastolic filling pressure and improves coronary perfusion. In addition, adrenaline is believed to "harden" the major vessels leading away from the heart thus aiding in the transmission of the raised intrathoracic pressure and the forward flow of blood. Adrenaline has a β-adrenergic stimulant activity on the chronotropic and inotropic activity of the myocardium.

Ten sequence of basic life support in the ratio of five compression to one ventilation should follow the administration of adrenaline. The further three defibrillation at 360 J are then given. Resuscitation in the form of basic life support should not be interrupted for more than 15 s to perform any of the above maneuvers. Furthermore, there should be no more than a 2 min delay between the third and fourth shock in the algorithm.

If the second set of defibrillation attempts is still unsuccessful the loop, via intubation and intravenous access, should be repeated. Therefore in any 2 min cycle of resuscitation three defibrillation attempts (360 J), 1 mg of intravenous adrenaline and 10 cycles of basic life support (five compressions; one ventilation) is applied to the patient. The chance of a successful resuscitation decreases with an increasing number of shocks and with a prolonged resuscitation time.

7.4.4.5   Asystole

Asystole is a flat electrocardiographic trace indicating no ventricular activity. Occasionally, there may be P wave electrical activity only.

The results of resuscitation from asystole are extremely poor. It is therefore essential that ventricular fibrillation is not missed. Unless ventricular fibrillation can be definitely be excluded the treatment of asystole is started as ventricular fibrillation until an appropriate endpoint. Atropine 3 mg intravenously may be given once during the first cycle of asystole resuscitation, which is used to counter any excess vagal tone.

Electrical pacing of the heart can be attempted where there is P wave activity evident. Percutaneous or pervenous pacing can be attempted depending on the local skill and available equipment. Pacing has not been a great success in the asystole resuscitation situation. This may be a failure in technique or alternatively it may be that pacing is only considered at too late a stage in the resuscitation sequence, probably when the myocardium is beyond electrical situation.

7.4.4.6   Electromechanical dissociation

Electromechanical dissociation(EMD) or pulseless electrical activity (PEA) has the worst prognosis of all rhythm associated with cardiac arrest. It is diagnosed when the electrocardiogram shows electrical activity but there is no palpable peripheral pulse.

EMD is usually associated with a specific cause (hypovolemia, tension pneumothorax, pulmonary embolism, drug overdose, hypothermia, and electrolyte imbalance) and this should be diagnosed and treated as a priority. In some cases cardiac arrest may not be absolute and the circulation may need support by chest compression. The algorithm for EMD follow the same pattern as previously, only in EMD the cause is diagnosis and treated followed by establishing tracheal intubation and venous access, the administration of adrenaline 1 mg and basic life support at five compressions to one ventilation before the cycle id repeated.

In the EMD situation other additional pressure agents may be considered more advantageous; calcium chloride may be used especially in the diagnosis of an overdose of calcium channel blocking drugs. Adrenaline may be given in a high dose of 5 mg, but this high dose has been associated with post resuscitation renal failure.

7.4.4.7   Alklinizing agents

In prolonged resuscitation the patient may become increasingly acidosis. This is especially so when initial basic life support has been delayed, ventilation has not been performed effectively (respiratory acidosis) or chest compressions have not been successful in achieving a satisfactory flow of blood (metabolic acidosis). In most cases, establishing effective basic life support will maintain the acid-base status quo without further intervention.

The associated acidosis may be reversed pharmacologically by administration of sodium bicarbonate. It is best titrated into the circulation in response to the arterial blood gas result by the formula: Base deficit ÷ 3×body weight (kg). The result is in mmol of HCO_3 solution. (1 mL of 8.4% $NaHCO_3$ = 1 mmol HCO_3).

Sodium bicarbonate should not be administered without considering the following:

It dose not improve ability to defibrillate the heart.

It shifts the oxyhemoglobin dissociation curve and inhibits the release of oxygen.

It causes hyperosmolality and hypernatremia.

It produces paradoxical acidosis.

It exacerbates central nervous acidosis.

7.4.5 After care

Following resuscitation, all patents should be cared for on a specialized unit, e. g. , an intensive or coronary care unit. Careful monitoring of vital functions should be established and abnormalities in serum electrolyte concentrations corrected to prevent reoccurrence of event. The majority will require further circulatory and respiratory support.

7.4.5.1 Cardiovascular system

Cardiac output may remain unsatisfactory as a result of cardiogenic shock and may be so poor that unconsciousness persists. A low cardiac output may result from the following:

(1) Poor myocardial contractility, e. g. , after myocardial infarction or pulmonary embolus. Dopamine 2–10 μg/ (kg · min) by infusion is the treatment of choice. In this dose range, it has little vasoconstrictor effect and cause a preferential increase in renal blood flow. The optimal preload for the failing heart should be ensured by cautious administration of colloid as guided by the CVP. A normal CVP does not exclude the possible development of pulmonary edema.

(2) Hypovolemia. This requires further transfusion guided by CVP measurement.

(3) Arrhythmias. These require treatment if cardiac output is compromised or they are electrically unstable and therefore predispose to a further episode of circulatory arrest.

7.4.5.2 Respiratory system

Lung dysfunction id produced during resuscitation for reasons which may include inhalation of vomit, lung contusion, fracture ribs and pueumothorax. Pulmonary edema may occur in the presence of heart failure and after head injury, drowning or smoke inhalation. Oxygen therapy for 24 hours should follow any episode of circulatory arrest. If overt respiratory failure supervenes, more intensive treatment is required, including possibly a period of artificial ventilation. All patients should have a chest X-ray and blood gas analysis after resuscitation.

7.4.5.3 Central nervous system

Efficient cardiac massage and ventilation provide sufficient oxygen delivery to protect the brain from damage, although not to prevent depression of function. If efficient resuscitation was started immediately after circulatory arrest occurred and was continued until restoration of an adequate spontaneous cardiac output, the patient should regain consciousness fairly quickly. Recovery tends to be delayed after prolonged arrest or when general anesthesia is involved. The failure of recovery may be caused by low cardiac output and brain damage.

7.4.5.4 Management of brain damage

The aim of treatment is to provide optimal condition for recovery of cerebral cells and prevention of secondary neuronal damage.

(1)General measures

If airway obstruction is in presence, continued tracheal intubation protects the lungs, secure the airway and renders it easy to institute mechanical ventilation if respiration becomes inadequate. With the airway secure, epileptiform fits which increase $CMRO_2$ may be treated safely with anticonvulsants. The unconscious patient whose trachea is not intubated should be nursed in the lateral position to assist drainage of oral secretions. Arterial pressure should be maintained in the normal range to ensure adequate cerebral perfusion pressure and hematocrit in the low normal range to optimize oxygen delivery. Tissue hydration and blood biochemistry should be maintained as normal. An increase in body temperature increases $CMRO_2$ and should be avoided. Depth of coma should be assessed regularly.

(2)Specialized treatment

1)Hyperventilation: Mild passive hyperventilation to a $PaCO_2$ of 4 kPa helps to minimize increases in intracranial pressure secondary to cerebral edema, although there is no evidence that cerebral damage after cardiac arrest is reduced by hyperventilation if the patient is able to achieve adequate gas exchange when breathing spontaneously. Control of ventilation may be achieved with the aid of muscle relaxants or cerebral depressants. A head-up tilt assists cerebral drainage.

2)Osmotherapy: Increasing the plasma osmolality decreases intracranial water content and thus ICP. Mannitol (0.25 g/kg initially) is often used. Mannitol increases the circulating blood volume and may be dangerous in the presence of pulmonary edema or a high CVP. In this situation, fusemide or bumetanide may be more appropriate.

3)Steroid: No evidence that steroids are beneficial after cardiac arrest.

4)Barbiturates and CNS depressant: Thiopentone and diazepam are often used in conventional doses to provide sedation, facilitate control of ventilation and suppress seizures. Both of these drugs must be used with care after circulatory arrest. In particular, large loading doses of barbiturate are contraindicated, as they produce profound cardiovascular depression.

5)Calcium antagonists: The role of these drugs after cardiac arrest still awaits clarification. At present time, there is no evidence that they are of value when administered in the post-resuscitation period.

(3)Initiating and terminating CPR

In the first instance, all patients should be resuscitated unless the medical or nursing notes indicate that contrary decision has been reached. If it is becomes apparent when resuscitation has started that CPR would be inappropriate (terminal stage of an incurable disease), it should ceased.

Further cerebral function can not be predicted accurately during CPR and suspicion of brain damage is no justification for terminating resuscitation, When in doubt, CPR should be continued until there is no doubt that the patient will fail to recover. Good recovery has taken place after 1-2 h of continuous CPR.

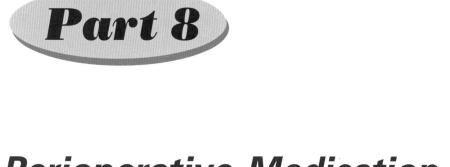

Part 8

Perioperative Medication Management

Chapter 1

Preoperative Preparation

The preoperative management of any patient is part of a continuum of care that extends from the surgeon's initial consultation through the patient's full recovery. Surgeons lead the effort to assure that correct care is provided to all patients, and is responsible for balancing the hazards of the natural history of the condition if left untreated versus the risks of an operation. A successful operation depends upon the surgeon's comprehension of the biology of the patient's disease and keen patient selection.

1.1 Preparation of the Patient

A systemic approach to patient preparation focuses upon risk assessment and reduction, as well as education of the patient and family.

1.1.1 History and physical examination

The surgeon and team should obtain a proper history from each patient. The history of present illness includes details about the presenting condition, including establishing the acuity, urgency, or chronic nature of the problem. Inquiries will certainly focus on the specific disease and related organ system.

The past medical history should include prior operations, especially when germane to the current situation, medical conditions, prior venous thromboembolism (VTE) events such as deep vein thromboses (DVT) or pulmonary emboli (PE), bleeding diatheses, prolonged bleeding with prior operations or modest injuries (e. g. , epistaxis, gingival bleeding, or ecchymoses), and untoward events during surgery or anesthesia, including airway problems. One must secure a list of active medications, with dosages and schedule. Moreover, it is beneficial to inquire about corticosteroid usage within the past 6 months, even if not current, to avoid perioperative adrenal insufficiency. Medication allergies and adverse reactions should be elicited, although knowledge about environmental and food allergies is also valuable and should be recorded so that these exposures are avoided during the hospital stay.

A thorough physical examination is also an essential part of the patient assessment. Even if the surgeon already knows from imaging that there will be no pertinent physical findings, human touch and contact are fundamental to the development of a trusting physician–patient relationship. In addition to the traditional vital signs of pulse, blood pressure, respiratory rate, and temperature, for many operations it is also important to record the patient's baseline oxygen saturation on room air, weight, height, and body mass index (BMI). The physical examination includes an assessment of general fitness, exercise tolerance, cachexia, or obesity, as well as focusing on the patient's condition.

1.1.2   Preoperative testing

Laboratory and imaging investigations are tailored to the individual patient's presenting condition. There should be no "routine" battery of preoperative laboratory studies for all patients. In fact, published data do not support an association between routine studies and outcome. Tests should be selected based upon the patient's age, comorbidities, cardiac risk factors, medications, and general health, as well as the complexity of the underlying condition and proposed operation.

1.1.3   Risk assessment and reduction

The essence of preparing a patient for an operation regards considering whether the benefits of the operation justify the risks of doing harm, along with deciding how to minimize or eliminate those hazards. The most universally used classification system is the one developed by the American Society of Anesthesiologists (ASA), which is based on the patient's functional status and comorbid conditions (e. g. , diabetes mellitus, peripheral vascular disease, renal dysfunction, and chronic pulmonary disease). This classification system stratifies the degree of perioperative risk for patients(Table 8−1−1). While somewhat rudimentary, this system has faithfully served anesthesiologists and surgeons in predicting how well patients might tolerate operations.

Table 8-1-1   ASA Classification

ASA classification	Preoperative health status	Example
ASA 1	Normal healthy patient	No organic, physiologic, or psychiatric disturbance; excludes the very young and very old; healthy with good exercise tolerance
ASA 2	Patients with mild systemic disease	No functional limitations; has a well−controlled disease of one body system; controlled hypertension or diabetes without systemic effects, cigarette smoking without chronic obstructive pulmonary disease (COPD); mild obesity, pregnancy
ASA 3	Patients with severe systemic disease	Some functional limitation; has a controlled disease of more than one body system or one major system; no immediate danger of death; controlled congestive heart failure (CHF), stable angina, former heart attack, poorly controlled hypertension, morbid obesity, chronic renal failure; bronchospastic disease with intermittent symptoms
ASA 4	Patients with severe systemic disease that is a constant threat to life	Has at least one severe disease that is poorly controlled or at end stage; possible risk of death; unstable angina, symptomatic COPD, symptomatic CHF, hepatorenal failure
ASA 5	Moribund patients who are not expected to survive without the operation	Not expected to survive > 24 h without surgery; imminent risk of death; multiorgan failure, sepsis syndrome with hemodynamic instability, hypothermia, poorly controlled coagulopathy

Continue to Table 8-1-1

ASA Classification	Preoperative health status	Example
ASA 6		A declared brain-dead patient whose organs are being removed for donor purposes

The ASA index generally associates poorer overall health with increased postoperative complications, longer hospital stay, and higher mortality. ASA classes I and II correspond to low risk, class III to moderate risk, and classes IV and V to high risk.

Cardiovascular

(1) Factors affecting cardiac risk

Significant cardiovascular risk factors include angina pectoris, dyspnea and evidence of right-side or left-side heart failure, any cardiac rhythm other than sinus rhythm, more than five ectopic ventricular beats per minute, aortic stenosis with left ventricular hypertrophy, mitral regurgitation, and previous myocardial infarction(MI). The risk of intraoperative or postoperative MI is much higher in patients who have suffered heart muscle damage within the preceding 6 months.

1) Functional capacity

Patients who are able to exercise on a regular basis without limitations generally have sufficient cardiovascular reserve to allow them to withstand stressful operations. Those with limited exercise capacity often have poor cardiovascular reserve, which may become manifest after noncardiac surgery. Poor functional status (and exercise capacity) is associated with worse short-and long-term outcomes in patients undergoing noncardiac operations, as well as with shorter nonoperative lifespans. Functional capacity is readily expressed in terms of metabolic equivalents (METs). Multiples of the baseline MET value can then be used to quantify the aerobic demands posed by specific activities, as in the Duke Activity Status Index(Table 8-1-2).

Table 8-1-2 MET scores for selected activities (Duke Activity Status Index)

MET Score	Activity
1-4	Light activities of daily home life (e. g. , eating, getting dressed, using the toilet, cooking, washing dishes) Walking 1-2 blocks on level ground at 2-3 mph
5-9	Climbing one flight of stairs Walking up a hill Walking on level ground at rate > 4 mph Running a short distance More strenuous household chores (e. g. , scrubbing floors, moving furniture) Moderate recreational activities (e. g. , hiking, dancing, golf)
>10	Strenuous athletic activities (e. g. , tennis, running, basketball, swimming) Heavy professional work

It has been established that perioperative cardiac and long-term risks are increased in patients unable to meet the 4-MET demand associated with most normal daily activities. Thus, the surgeon's assessment of the patient's exercise capacity is a practical, inexpensive, and gratifyingly accurate predictor of that patient's ability to tolerate a surgical stress.

2) Type of surgical procedure

The procedure–specific cardiac risk associated with a noncardiac operation is related almost exclusively to the duration and intensity of the myocardial stressors involved. Procedure–specific risk for noncardiac surgery can be classified as high, intermediate, or low(Table 8–1–3).

Table 8–1–3　Selected surgical procedures stratified by degree of cardiac risk

Degree of cardiac risk	Type of procedure
Low(<1%)	Endoscopic procedures Ambulatory procedures Ophthalmic procedures Aesthetic procedure
Intermediate(1% –5%)	Minor vascular procedures(e. g. ,carotid endarterectomy) Abdominal procedures Thoracic procedures Neurosurgical procedures Otolaryngologic procedures Urologic procedures
High (>5%)	emergency procedures (intermediate or high risk) Major vascular procedures (e. g. ,peripheral vascular surgery, AAA repair) Extensive surgical procedures with profound estimated blood loss, large fluid shifts, or both Unstable hemodynamic situations

3) ACC/AHA guidelines

Comprehensive identification of patients who are at substantial risk for perioperative cardiac morbidity remains a difficult task. An evaluation strategy that avoids these limitations has been proposed by combined task forces from the American College of Cardiology and the AHA. These guidelines are evidence based, include an explanation of the quality of the data, and provide comprehensive algorithms for the propriety of testing, medications, and revascularization to assure cardiac fitness for operations. The ACC/AHA guidelines take the form of an eight–step algorithm for patient risk stratification and subsequent determination of appropriate cardiac evaluation; this algorithm is available on the ACC's web site (www. acc. org/clinical/guidelines/perio/update/ fig1. htm).

As important as preoperative cardiac risk stratification is, a cardiology consultation also lays the groundwork for postoperative risk assessment and later modifications of coronary risk factors.

Preoperative aspirin usage should continue among patients at moderate to high risk for coronary artery disease, unless the risk of resultant hemorrhage definitely outweighs the likelihood of an atherothrombotic event.

4) Pulmonary

Postoperative pulmonary complications (PPC), such as the development of pneumonia and ventilator dependency, are debilitating and costly. They are associated with prolonged lengths of hospital stay, an increased likelihood of readmission, and increased 30–day mortality. Therefore, it is critical to identify patients at greatest risk for PPC. Established risk factors for PPC include advanced age, elevated ASA class, congestive heart failure, functional dependence, known chronic obstructive pulmonary disease, and perhaps malnutrition, alcohol abuse, and altered mental status. In addition, hazards are greater for certain operations (e.

g. , aortic aneurysm repair, thoracic or abdominal, neurosurgery, head and neck, and vascular), prolonged or emergency operations, and those done under general anesthesia. A risk calculator was devised to predict the likelihood of PPC occurrence, indicating seven independent risk factors. These include low preoperative arterial oxygen saturation, recent acute respiratory infection, age, preoperative anemia, upper abdominal or thoracic operations, duration of operation over 2 hours, and emergency surgery.

A multivariable logistic regression has affirmed that active smoking is significantly associated with postoperative pneumonia, SSI, and death, when compared to nonsmokers or those who have quit smoking. The benefits of preoperative smoking cessation seem to be conferred a er an interval of at least 4 weeks. Conversely, the risk of developing PPC is the same for current smokers versus those who quit smoking for less than 4 weeks before an operation. Smoking cessation also confers favorable effects on wound healing. Therefore, patients should be encouraged to stop smoking at least 1 month before operations, ideally with programmatic support through formal counseling programs and possibly smoking cessation aids such as varenicline or transdermal nicotine.

Patients identified as being at highest risk for the development of PPC may benefit from preoperative consultations with respiratory therapy and pulmonary medicine experts.

Patient education focuses upon inspiratory muscle training (including the usage of incentive spirometry), the concepts of postoperative mobilization, deep inspiration, and coughing, along with oral hygiene (tooth brushing and mouth washes).

Diabetes mellitus

Patients with diabetes mellitus are more likely to undergo operations than are those without diabetes, and their care is associated with longer lengths of hospital stay, increased rates of postoperative death and complications, and relatively greater utilization of health care resources. Increased perioperative glucose levels have correlated with a higher risk of SSIs in general surgery, cardiac surgery, colorectal surgery, vascular surgery, breast surgery, hepatobiliary and pancreas surgery, orthopedic surgery, and trauma surgery. The relative risk of an SSI seems to incrementally increase in a linear pattern with the degree of hyperglycemia, with levels greater than 7.8 mmol /L being the sole predictor of SSI upon multivariate analysis.

Current recommendations for desirable glucose ranges in critically ill patients are commonly about 6.7–10 mmol /L, but the best range for perioperative glucose levels is not yet established, and low levels may result in harm when clinicians try to achieve "tight" control of blood sugars. Although preoperative blood sugar and hemoglobin A1c levels have not clearly correlated with adverse outcomes, good control of glucose before operations likely facilitates blood sugar management during and after operations. An abundance of data support postoperative glucose control as a major determinant of postoperative complications, with emerging data also indicating an adverse effect of intraoperative hyperglycemia.

Patients having operations that require fasting status are advised about oral antihyperglycemic medications on the day of surgery in accordance to Table 8-1-4. Injectable medications such as exenatide and pramlintide are not administered on the day of surgery, and insulin therapy is determined by the duration of action of the particular preparation, as outlined in Table 8-1-5. Patients with type 1 diabetes require basal insulin at all times. Patients with insulin pumps may continue their usual basal rates.

Table 8-1-4　Instructions for preoperative management of oral antihyperglycemic medications

Medication	Prior to procedure	Afer procedure
Short-acting sulfonylureas: Glipizide (Glucotrol), glyburide (DiaBeta, Glynase, Micronase)	Do not take the morning of procedure	Resume when eating
Long-acting sulfonylureas: Glimepiride (Amaryl), glipizide XL (Glucotrol XL)	Do not take the evening prior to or the morning of procedure	Resume when eating
Biguanides: Metformin (Glucophage), metformin ER (Glucophage XL)	Do not take the morning of procedure; do not take the day prior to procedure if receiving contrast dye	Resume when eating. After contrast dye wait 48 h and repeat creatinine prior to restarting
Thiazolidinediones: Pioglitazone (Actos), rosiglitazone (Avandia)	Do not take the morning of procedure	Resume when eating
Alpha-glucosidase inhibitors: Acarbose (Precose), miglitol (Glyset)	Do not take the morning of procedure	Resume when eating
DPP-4 Inhibitors: Sitagliptin (Januvia)	Do not take the morning of procedure	Resume when eating
Meglitinides: Nateglinide (Starlix), repaglinide (Prandin)	Do not take the morning of procedure	Resume when eating

Table 8-1-5　Instructions for preoperative management of injectable antihyperglycemic medications and insulin

Medication	Prior to procedure	Afer procedure
Injectable Medications		
Exenatide (Byetta)	Do not take the morning of procedure	Resume when eating
Symlin (Pramlintide)	Do not take the morning of procedure	Resume when eating
Insulins		
Glargine (Lantus)	Take usual dose the night before or the morning of procedure	Resume usual schedule after procedure
Detemir (Levemir)	Take usual dose the night before or the morning of procedure	Resume usual schedule a er procedure
NPH (Humulin N, Novolin N)	Take 1-2 of usual dose the morning of procedure	Resume usual schedule when eating, 1-2 dose while NPO
Humalog mix 70/30, 75/25, Humulin 70/30, 50/50, Novolin 70/30 (all mixed insulins)	Do not take the morning of procedure	Resume usual schedule when eating
Regular insulin (Humulin R, Novolin R)	Do not take the morning of procedure	Resume when eating
Lispro (Humalog), Aspart (Novolog), Glulisine (Apidra)	Do not take the morning of procedure	Resume when eating
Subcutaneous insulin infusion pumps	Requires tailored recommendations. In general, most patients may continue their usual basal rate and correction doses, and resume meal-time boluses when eating again	

Generally before an operation, glucose values ≤ 180 mg/dL are satisfactory and require no treatment. Glucose levels of 181–300 mg/dL prompt to begin an infusion of intravenous (IV) insulin before the operation, along with a 5% dextrose solution to minimize the chances of hypoglycemia. Intravenous insulin is best for perioperative glucose control due to its rapid onset of action, short half–life, and immediate availability (as opposed to subcutaneous absorption). Insulin may be administered with an IV bolus technique or via continuous IV infusion, but regular glucose monitoring (e. g., hourly for continuous insulin infusions) is necessary in either system to assure adequate control and to avoid hypoglycemia.

(2) Fluid and blood volume

Surgeons and anesthesiologists have traditionally advocated liberal perioperative fluid resuscitation during recent decades, often overestimating insensible and "third space" fluid losses. As a result, patients can develop significant volume overload that is associated with serious complications. Recent data instead support goal–directed (or protocol–based) fluid restriction as likely resulting in a decreased incidence of cardiac and renal events, pneumonia, pulmonary edema, ileus, wound infections, and anastomosis and wound healing problems, as well as shorter durations of hospital stay. Unfortunately, traditional vital signs, including even central venous pressure, do not reliably correlate with intravascular volume or cardiac output. Newer, minimally invasive modalities for monitoring cardiac output offer promise to determine optimal preload volume and tissue oxygen delivery before and during operations, including esophageal Doppler and analyses of stroke volume variation and pulse pressure variation. The precise standards of goal–directed volume resuscitation remain elusive, but surgeons and anesthesiologists should prospectively collaborate regarding plans for both volume resuscitation and the selection.

Blood transfusions may be necessary before operations, especially in the setting of active hemorrhage or profound anemia. However, transfusions have been associated with increased operative mortality and morbidity, decreased long–term survival, greater lengths of hospital stay, and higher chances of tumor recurrence due to immunosuppressive effects imparted by transfused blood. The benefits of transfusions must be balanced against their hazards. Of course, bleeding diatheses require preoperative correction, including transfusions of blood products such as fresh frozen plasma, specific clotting factors, or platelets. Hematology consultations are invaluable when blood incompatibilities or unusual factor deficiencies are present.

(3) Nutrition

Preoperative nutritional status bears a major impact on outcome, especially with respect to wound healing and immune status. A multivariate analysis recognizes hypoalbuminemia (albumin < 3.0 mg/dL) as an independent risk factor for the development of SSIs, with a fivefold increased incidence versus patients with normal albumin levels. Among moderately to severely malnourished patients, e orts may be focused upon preoperative feedings, ideally via the gut, although at least 1 week of the regimen is necessary to confer benefit. Total parenteral nutrition is an option for select patients in whom the gut can not be used, but it conveys potential hazard.

At the other end of the spectrum, investigators have demonstrated that severe obesity is associated with increased rates of postoperative mortality, wound complications, renal failure, and pulmonary insufficiency, as well as greater durations of operative time and hospital stays. Unfavorable prognostic elements include BMI ≥ 50 kg/m^2, male sex, hypertension, PE risks (e. g., presence of a VTE event, prior inferior vena cava filter placement, history of right heart failure or pulmonary hypertension, findings of venous stasis disease), and age ≥ 45 years.

(4) Endocrine

Endocrine deficiencies pose special problems. Patients may have either primary adrenal insufficiency or chronic adrenal suppression from chronic corticosteroid usage. Inadequate amounts of perioperative steroids can result in an Addisonian crisis, with hemodynamic instability and even death. The need for perioperative "stress" steroid administration is a function of the duration of steroid therapy and the degree of the physiologic stress imposed by the operation. Supplemental corticosteroids should definitely be administered for established primary or secondary adrenal insufficiency, for a current regimen of more than the daily equivalent of 20 mg of prednisone, or for those with a history of chronic steroid usage and a Cushingoid appearance. Perioperative steroids should be considered if the current regimen is 5-20 mg of prednisone for 3 weeks or longer, for a history of more than a 3-week course of at least 20 mg of prednisone during the past year, for chronic usage of oral and rectal steroid therapy for inflammatory bowel disease, or for a significant history of chronic topical steroid usage (> 2 g daily) on large areas of affected skin. Increased amounts of corticosteroids are not necessary for patients who have received less than a 3-week course of steroids. Patients having operations of moderate (e. g. , lower extremity revascularization or total joint replacement) and major (e. g. , cardiothoracic, abdominal, central nervous system) stress should receive additional corticosteroids as outlined in Table 8-1-6. Minor or ambulatory operations, including those under local anesthesia, do not require supplemental steroids. Excessive amounts of steroids can have adverse consequences, including increased rates of SSIs, so hydrocortisone should not be indiscriminately prescribed. Of course, glucose levels should be closely monitored while patients receive steroids. Conversely, patients with advanced Cushing syndrome require expeditious medical and perhaps surgical treatment due to the potential for rapid deterioration, including fungal sepsis.

Table 8-1-6　Recommendations for perioperative corticosteroid management

Type of operation	Corticosteroid administration
Minor/ambulatory operation Example: inguinal hernia repair or operation under local anesthesia	Take usual morning steroid dose; no supplementary steroids are needed
Moderate surgical stress Example: lower extremity revascularization, total joint replacemen	Day of surgery: Take usual morning steroid dose Just before induction of anesthesia: Hydrocortisone 50 mg IV, then hydrocortisone 25 mg IV every 8 h × 6 doses (or until able to take oral steroids) When able to take oral steroids, change to daily oral prednisone equivalent of hydrocortisone, or preoperative steroid dose if that dose was higher On the second postoperative day: Resume prior outpatient dose, assuming the patient is in stable condition
Major surgical stress Example: major cardiac, brain, abdominal, or thoracic surgery Inflammatory bowel disease	Day of surgery: Take usual morning steroid dose Just before induction of anesthesia: Hydrocortisone 100 mg IV, then hydrocortisone 50 mg every 8 h × 6 doses (or until able to take oral steroids) On the second postoperative day: Reduce to hydrocortisone 25 mg q8h if still fasting, or oral prednisone 15 mg daily (or preoperative steroid dose if that was higher) Postoperative day 3 or 4: Resume preoperative steroid dose if the patient is in stable condition

For patients who have a complicated postoperative course or a prolonged illness, consider endocrinology consultation for dosing recommendations. If the steroid-requiring disease may directly impact the postoperative course [e. g. , autoimmune thrombocytopenia (ITP) or hemolytic anemia], specific dosing programs and tapers should be advised prior to surgery and in consultation with the appropriate service (e. g. , hematology for ITP patients) during hospital stay.

For patients with inflammatory bowel disease in whom all affected bowel was resected, taper to prednisone 10 mg daily (or IV equivalent) by discharge (or no later than postoperative day 7), followed by an outpatient taper over the next 1 - 3 months, depending on the duration of prior steroid usage and assuming that there are no concurrent indications for steroids (e. g. , COPD).

Thyrotoxicosis must be corrected to avoid perioperative thyroid storm. Management includes antithyroid medications (e. g. , methimazole or propylthiouracil) and beta-blockers; saturated solution of potassium iodide controls hyperthyroidism and reduces the vascularity of the gland in patients with Graves disease. On the other hand, significant hypothyroidism can progress to perioperative hypothermia and hemodynamic collapse and thus requires preoperative hormone replacement. This is normally accomplished with daily oral levothyroxine, but greater doses of IV thyroid hormone may be necessary to acutely reverse a significant deficit. Large goiters can affect the airway and require collaboration between surgeon and anesthesiologist, possibly including a review of imaging to demonstrate the extent and location (e. g. , substernal) of the goiter. When possible, computed tomography contrast should be avoided in patients with significant goiters as the iodine load may provoke thyrotoxicosis.

Geriatric patients

As the elderly demographic expands, surgeons are confronted with increasingly frail patients who have multiple comorbidities. The frailty index (FI) is used to measure the health status of older individuals—as a proxy measure of aging and vulnerability to poor outcomes. It is defined as the proportion of deficits present in an individual out of the total number of age-related health variables considered. An frailty index can be created in most secondary data sources related to health by utilizing health deficits that are routinely collected in health assessments. These deficits include diseases, signs, symptoms, laboratory abnormalities, cognitive impairments, and disabilities in activities of daily living.

Frailty Index (FI) = (number of health deficits present) ÷ (number of health deficits measured)

A recent multivariate analysis demonstrated that among more than 58,000 patients undergoing colon resection, independent predictors of major complications were an elevated frailty index, an open (vs laparoscopic) operation, and ASA Class 4 or 5, but interestingly not wound classification or emergency status. The care of the elderly requires thoughtful considerations of their diminished physiologic reserve and tolerance of the insult of an operation. Interventions may include preoperative and early postoperative physical therapy, prospective discharge planning, and the introduction of elder-specific order sets. Simple scoring systems can provide valuable information for the surgeon to present to the patient and family so that they can anticipate the nature of the postoperative care and recovery, including potential transfer to a rehabilitation facility and long-term debility.

(5) Cancer therapy

Many patients undergo neoadjuvant therapy for malignancies involving the breast, esophagus, stomach pancreas rectum, so tissues, and other sites. The surgeon is responsible for restaging the tumor before proceeding with a resection. In general, the interval between the completion of the external beam radiation and the operation is commensurate with the duration of the radiation therapy. Similarly, a reasonable amount of time should elapse a er systemic therapy to permit restoration of bone marrow capacity and nutrition, to the extent possible. Angiogenesis inhibitors such as bevacizumab disrupt normal wound perfusion and healing. The duration of time between biological therapy and an operation is not firmly established. However, it is probably best to allow 4 - 6 weeks to elapse a er treating with bevacizumab before proceeding with an operation, and the therapy should not be resumed until the wound is fully healed, perhaps 1 month later.

1.2 Prevention of Surgical Site Infections

A surgical site infection(SSI)is an infection that occurs after surgery in the part of the body where the surgery took place. SSIs can be classified into three categories: superficial incisional SSIs (involving only skin and subcutaneous tissue), deep incisional SSIs (involving deep soft tissue), and organ/space SSIs (involving anatomic areas other than the incision itself that are opened or manipulated in the course of the procedure).

Surgical site infections (SSIs)are major contributors to postoperative morbidity and can be monitored and reduced by multiple complex interventions that are institution-specific. Excellent surgical technique is obviously a major factor in eliminating SSIs, and this involves limiting wound contamination, blood loss, the duration of the operation, and local tissue trauma and ischemia (e. g. , using sharp dissection rather than ex-cessive electrocoagulation). However, a variety of adjuvant preoperative measures, beyond glycemic control described above, also contribute to the prevention of SSIs. Antibiotics should be administered within the 1-hour period before incision for certain clean operations and for all clean-contaminated, contaminated, and dirty operations. In addition, further dosages of the antibiotics should be infused about every two half-lives during the operation (e. g. , every 4 hours for cefazolin). Correct antibiotic selection is determined by sever-al factors, such as the bacterial flora that are most likely to cause an infection, local bacterial sensitivities, medication allergies, the presence of MRSA, and the patient's overall health and ability to tolerate an infec-tion. When antibiotics are administered for SSI prophylaxis rather than for treatment of an established or suspected infection, they are typically not continued after surgery, except in special circumstances such as vascular grafts, cardiac surgery, or joint replacements. Even then, prophylaxis should expire within one to two days.

Wound perfusion and oxygenation are also essential to minimize the likelihood of SSIs. A sufficient in-travascular blood volume provides end-organ perfusion and oxygen delivery to the surgical site. The mainte-nance of perioperative normothermia also has salutary effects on wound oxygen tension levels and can conse-quently reduce the incidence of SSIs. Therefore, the application of warming blankets immediately prior to the operation may support the patient's temperature in the operating room, especially for high-risk operations such as bowel resections that o en involved a prolonged interval of positioning and preparation when a broad surface area is exposed to room air. Similarly, some data support hyperoxygenation with $FiO_2 \geqslant 80\%$ during the first 2 hours after a major colorectal operation.

Preoperative preparation of the operative site

The sole reason for preparing the patient's skin before an operation is to reduce the risk of wound infec-tion. A preoperative antiseptic bath is not necessary for most surgical patients, but their personal hygiene must be assessed and preoperative cleanliness established. Multiple preoperative baths may prevent postop-erative infection in selected patient groups, such as those who carry Staphylococcus aureus on their skin or who have infectious lesions. Chlorhexidine gluconate is the recommended agent for such baths.

Hair should not be removed from the operative site unless it physically interferes with accurate anatom-ic approximation of the wound edges. If hair must be removed, it should be clipped in the OR. Shaving hair from the operative site, particularly on the evening before operation or immediately before wound incision in the OR, increases the risk of wound infection. Depilatories are not recommended, because they cause serious irritation and rashes in a significant number of patients, especially when used near the eyes and the genitalia.

In emergency procedures, obvious dirt, grime, and dried blood should be mechanically cleansed from the operative site by using sufficient friction. In one study, cleansing of contaminated wounds by means of ultrasound debridement was compared with high-pressure irrigation and soaking. The experimental wounds were contaminated with a colloidal clay that potentiates infection 1000 – fold. The investigators irrigated wounds at pressures of 8–10 psi, a level obtained by using a 30 mL syringe with a 1.5 in. long 19-gauge needle and 300 mL of 0.85% sterile saline solution. High-pressure irrigation removed slightly more particulate matter (59%) than ultrasound debridement (48%), and both of these methods removed more matter than soaking (26%). Both ultrasound de-bridement and high-pressure irrigation were also effective in reducing the wound infection rate in experimental wounds contaminated with a subinfective dose of S. aureus.

For nonemergency procedures, the necessary reduction in microorganisms can be achieved by using povidone-iodine (10% available povidone-iodine and 1% available iodine) or chlorhexi-dine gluconate both for mechanical cleansing of the intertriginous folds and the umbilicus and for painting the operative site. Which skin antiseptic is optimal is unclear. The best option appears to be chlorhexidine gluconate or an iodophor. The patient should be assessed for evidence of sensitivity to the antiseptic (particularly if the agent contains iodine) to minimize the risk of an allergic reaction. What some patients report as iodine allergies are actually iodine burns. Iodine in alcohol or in water is associated with an increased risk of skin irritation, particularly at the edges of the operative field, where the iodine concentrates as the alcohol evaporates. Iodine should therefore be removed after sufficient contact time with the skin, especially at the edges. Iodophors do not irritate the skin and thus need not be removed.

Chapter 2

Postoperative Care

The recovery from major surgery can be divided into three phases: ①An immediate, or postanesthetic phase. ②An intermediate phase, encompassing the hospitalization period. ③A convalescent phase.

During the first two phases, care is principally directed at maintenance of homeostasis, treatment of pain, and prevention and early detection of complications. The convalescent phase is a transition period from the time of hospital discharge to full recovery. The trend toward earlier postoperative discharge after major surgery has shifted the venue of this period.

2.1 The Immediate Postoperative Period

The primary causes of early complications and death following major surgery are acute pulmonary, cardiovascular, and fluid derangements. The postanesthesia care unit (PACU) is staffed by specially trained personnel and provided with equipment for early detection and treatment of these problems. All patients should be monitored in this specialized unit initially following major procedures unless they are transported directly to an intensive care unit. In the PACU, the anesthesiology service generally exercises primary responsibility for cardiopulmonary function. The surgeon is responsible for the operative site and all other aspects of the care not directly related to the effects of anesthesia. The patient can be discharged from the recovery room when cardiovascular, pulmonary, and neurologic functions have returned to baseline, which usually occurs 1–3 hours following operation. Patients who require continuing ventilatory or circulatory support or who have other conditions that require frequent monitoring are transferred to an intensive care unit.

2.1.1 Monitoring

(1) Vital signs

Blood pressure, pulse, and respiration should be recorded frequently until stable and then regularly until the patient is discharged from the recovery room. Continuous electrocardiographic monitoring is indicated for most patients in the PACU. Any major changes in vital signs should be communicated to the anesthesiologist and attending surgeon immediately.

(2) Central venous pressure

Central venous pressure should be recorded periodically in the early postoperative period if the operation has entailed large blood losses or fluid shifts, and invasive monitoring is available.

(3) Fluid balance

The anesthetic record includes all fluid administered as well as blood loss and urine output during the operation. This record should be continued in the postoperative period and should also include fluid losses from drains and stomas. This aids in assessing hydration and helps to guide intravenous fluid replacement.

(4) Other types of monitoring

Depending on the nature of the operation and the patient's preexisting conditions, other types of monitoring may be necessary.

2.1.2　Administration of fluid and electrolytes

Orders for postoperative intravenous fluids should be based on maintenance needs, operative losses, and the replacement of gastrointestinal losses from drains, fistulas, or stomas.

(1) Drainage tubes

Details such as type and pressure of suction, irrigation fluid and frequency, skin exit site care and support during ambulation or showering should be specified. Surgeon should examine drains frequently, since the character or quantity of drain output may herald the development of postoperative complications such as bleeding or fistulas. Careful positioning and reinforcement of anchors can prevent the dreaded early loss of key placement of nasogastric tubes, chest tubes, and drains.

(2) Position in bed and mobilization

The postoperative orders should describe any required special positioning of the patient. Unless doing so is contraindicated, the patient should be turned from side to side every 30 minutes until conscious and then hourly for the first 8–12 hours to minimize atelectasis. Early ambulation is encouraged to reduce venous stasis; the upright position helps to increase diaphragmatic excursion.

2.2　The Intermediate Postoperative Period

The intermediate phase begins with complete recovery from anesthesia and lasts for the rest of the hospital stay. During this time, the patient recovers most basic functions and becomes self-sufficient and ready to continue convalescence at home. Transfer from the PACU/SICU to a less monitored setting usually occurs at the start of this period.

2.2.1　Postoperative pain

Severe pain is a common sequela of intrathoracic, intra–abdominal, and major bone or joint procedures. About 60% of such patients perceive their pain to be severe, 25% moderate, and 15% mild.

The factors responsible for these differences include duration of operation, degree of operative trauma, type of incision, and magnitude of intraoperative retraction. Gentle handling of tissues, expedient operations, and good muscle relaxation help lessen the severity of postoperative pain. Objective measures of pain remain elusive.

The physiology of postoperative pain involves transmission of pain impulses via splanchnic (not vagal) afferent fibers to the central nervous system, where they initiate spinal, brain stem, and cortical reflexes. Spinal responses result from stimulation of neurons in the anterior horn, resulting in skeletal muscle spasm, vasospasm, and gastrointestinal ileus. Brain stem responses to pain include alterations in ventilation, blood pressure, and endocrine function. Cortical responses include voluntary movements and psychologic changes, such as fear and apprehension. These emotional responses facilitate nociceptive spinal transmission, lower the threshold for pain perception, and perpetuate the pain experience.

Postoperative pain serves no useful purpose and may cause alterations in pulmonary, circulatory, gastrointestinal, and skeletal muscle function that contribute to postoperative complications. Pain following thoracic and upper abdominal operations, for example, causes voluntary and involuntary splinting of thoracic and abdominal muscles and the diaphragm. The patient may be reluctant to breathe deeply, promoting atelectasis. The limitation in motion due to pain predisposes to venous stasis, thrombosis, and embolism. Release of catecholamines and other stress hormones by postoperative pain causes vasospasm and hypertension, which may in turn lead to complications such as stroke, myocardial infarction, and bleeding. Prevention of postoperative pain is thus important for reasons other than the pain itself. Effective pain control may improve the outcome of major operations.

2.2.1.1　Communication

Close attention to the patient's needs, frequent reassurance, and genuine concern help to minimize postoperative pain. Spending a few minutes with the patient every day in frank discussions of progress and any complications does more to relieve pain than many physicians realize.

2.2.1.2　Parenteral opioids

Opioids are the mainstay of therapy for postoperative pain. Their analgesic effect is via two mechanisms：①A direct effect on opioid receptors. ②Stimulation of a descending brain stem system that contributes to pain inhibition. Morphine is the most widely used opioid for treatment of postoperative pain. Morphine may be administered intravenously, either intermittently or continuously.

2.2.1.3　Nonopioid parenteral analgesics

Nonsteroidal anti-inflammatory drug (NSAID) with potent analgesic and moderate anti-inflammatory activities is available in injectable form suitable for postoperative use, such as Ketorolac tromethamine.

2.2.1.4　Oral analgesics

Within several days following most abdominal surgical procedures, the severity of pain decreases and oral analgesics suffice for control.

For most patients, a combination of acetaminophen with codeine or propoxyphene suffices.

2.2.1.5　Patient-controlled analgesia

Patient-controlled analgesia (PCA) puts the frequency of analgesic administration under the patient's control but within safe limits. A device containing a timing unit, a pump, and the analgesic medication is connected to an intravenous line. By pressing a button, the patient delivers a predetermined dose of analgesic (usually morphine, 1–3 mg). This method appears to improve pain control and even reduces the total dose of opioid given in a 24-hour period.

2.2.1.6　Continuous epidural analgesia

Topicalmorphine does not depress proprioceptive pathways in the dorsal horn, but it does affect nociceptive pathways by interacting with opioid receptors. Therefore, epidural opioids produce intense, prolonged segmental analgesia with relatively less respiratory depression or sympathetic, motor, or other sensory disturbances. Patients managed in this way are more alert and have better gastrointestinal function.

2.2.1.7　Intercostal block

Intercostal block may be used to decrease pain following thoracic and abdominal operations. Since the block does not include the visceral afferent nerve fibers, it does not relieve pain completely, but it does eliminate muscle spasm induced by cutaneous pain and helps to restore respiratory function.

2.2.1.8　Direct Infiltration

Direct administration of a combination of short-and long-acting local anesthetics can help significantly in management of postoperative pain in a variety of settings. Optimally, wound infiltration or local nerve block should occur following the induction of intravenous anesthesia and prior to skin incision but may still be beneficial a er incision.

(1) Postoperative care of the gastrointestinal tract

Following laparotomy, gastrointestinal peristalsis temporarily decreases. Peristalsis returns in the small intestine within 24 hours, but gastric peristalsis may return more slowly. Function returns in the right colon by 48 hours and in the left colon by 72 hours.

Nasogastric intubation is probably useful after esophageal and gastric resections and should always be used in patients with marked ileus or a very low level of consciousness (to avoid aspiration) and in patients who manifest acute gastric distention or vomiting postoperatively. The nasogastric tube should be connected to low intermittent suction and assessed frequently to ensure patency. The tube should be left in place for 2–3 days or until there is evidence that normal peristalsis has returned (e. g. , return of appetite, audible peristalsis, or passage of flatus).

Once the nasogastric tube has been withdrawn, fasting is usually continued for another 24 hours, and the patient is then started on a liquid diet. Opioids may interfere with gastric motility and should be limited if possible for patients who have slow gastric emptying beyond the first postoperative week.

Gastrostomy and jejunostomy tubes should be connected to low intermittent suction or dependent drainage for the first 24 hours after surgery. Enteral nutrition through a jejunostomy feeding tube may be started on the second postoperative day even if motility is not entirely normal. Gastrostomy or jejunostomy tubes should not be removed before the third postoperative week once firm adhesions have developed between the viscera and the parietal peritoneum.

After most operations in areas other than the peritoneal cavity, the patient may be allowed to resume a regular diet as soon as the effects of anesthesia have completely resolved.

(2) Care of the wound

Within hours after a wound is closed, the wound space fills with an inflammatory exudate. Epidermal cells at the edges of the wound begin to divide and migrate across the wound surface. By 48 hours after closure, deeper structures are completely sealed off from the external environment. Sterile dressings applied in the operating room provide protection during this

period. Removal of the dressing and handling of the wound during the first 24 hours should be done with aseptic technique.

Dressings over closed wounds should be removed by the third or fourth postoperative day. If the wound is dry, dressings need not be reapplied; this simplifies periodic inspection. Dressings should be removed earlier if they are wet or placed in a contaminated setting, because soaked dressings increase bacterial contamination of the wound. Dressings should also be removed if the patient has new manifestations of infection (such as fever or increasing wound pain). The wound should then be inspected and the adjacent area gently compressed. Any drainage from the wound should be examined by culture and Gram-stained smear.

Generally, skin sutures or skin staples may be removed by the fifth postoperative day and replaced by tapes. Sutures should be left in longer (e. g. , for 2 weeks) for incisions that cross creases (e. g. , groin, popliteal area) , for incisions closed under tension, for some incisions in the extremities (eg, the hand), and for incisions of any kind in debilitated patients. Sutures should be removed if suture tracts show signs of infection. If the incision is healing normally, the patient may be allowed to shower or bathe by the seventh postoperative day (and often sooner, depending on the incision).

Wounds are traditionally classified according to whether the wound inoculum of bacteria is likely to be large enough to overwhelm local and systemic host defense mechanisms and produce an infection (Table 8-2-1). In the years before prophylactic antibiotics, as well as during the early phases of their use, there was a very clear relation between the classification of the operation (which is related to the probability of a significant inoculum) and the rate of wound infection. This relation is now less dominant than it once was.

Table 8-2-1   National research council classification of operative wound

Classification	Performance
Clean (class I)	Nontraumatic No inflammation encountered No break in technique Respiratory, alimentary, or genitourinary tract not entered
Clean-contaminated (class II)	Gastrointestinal or respiratory tract entered without significant spillage Appendectomy Oropharynx entered Vagina entered Genitourinary tract entered in absence of infected urine Biliary tract entered in absence of infected bile Minor break in technique
Contaminated (class III)	Major break in technique Gross spillage from gastrointestinal tract Traumatic wound, fresh Entrance of genitourinary or biliary tracts in presence of infected urine or bile
Dirty and infected (class IV)	Acute bacterial inflammation encountered, without pus Transection of "clean" tissue for the purpose of surgical access to a collection of pus Traumatic wound with retained devitalized tissue, foreign bodies, fecal contamination, or delayed treatment, or all of these; or from dirty source

(3) Management of drains

Drains are used either to prevent or to treat an unwanted accumulation of fluid such as pus, blood, or serum. Drains are also used to evacuate air from the pleural cavity so that the lungs can re-expand. When used prophylactically, drains are usually placed in a sterile location. Strict precautions must be taken to prevent bacteria from entering the body through the drainage tract in these situations. The external portion of the drain must be handled with aseptic technique, and the drain must be removed as soon as it is no longer useful. When drains have been placed in an infected area, there is a smaller risk of retrograde infection of the peritoneal cavity, since the infected area is usually walled off. Drains should usually be brought out through a separate incision, because drains through the operative wound increase the risk of wound infection. Closed drains connected to suction devices are preferable to open drains (such as Penrose) that predispose to wound contamination. The quantity and quality of drainage should be recorded and contamination minimized. When drains are no longer needed, they may be withdrawn entirely at one time if there has been little or no drainage or may be progressively withdrawn over a period of a few days.

2.3   The Convalescent Phase

Determination and planning for discharge should start even before the operation and should be modified accordingly. Plans should be made early for home assistance in the activities of daily living and in assisting recovery from surgery including education on the care of ostomies, new tubes/drains, intravenous or intramuscular medications.

Chapter 3

Management of Postoperative Complications

Complications occur after operations and surgeons must be versed in anticipating, recognizing, and managing them. The spectrum of these complications ranges from the relatively minor, such as a small postoperative seroma, to the catastrophic, such as postoperative myocardial infarction or anastomotic leak. The management of these complications also spans a spectrum from nonoperative strategies to those requiring an emergent return to the operating room.

When considering postoperative complications, it is helpful to categorize them in a system-based method that has additional usefulness in clinical research.

3.1 Mechanical Complications

Mechanical complications are defined as those that occur as a direct result of technical failure from a procedure or operation. These complications include postoperative hematoma and hemoperitoneum, seroma, wound dehiscence, anastomotic leak, and those related to lines, drains, and retained foreign bodies.

3.1.1 Bleeding

Bleeding is the most common cause of shock in the first 24 hours after abdominal surgery. Postoperative bleeding—a rapidly evolving, life-threatening complication—is usually the result of a technical problem with hemostasis, but coagulation disorders may play a role. Causes of coagulopathy, such as dilution of hemostatic factors after massive blood loss and resuscitation, mismatched transfusion, or administration of heparin, should also be considered. In these cases, bleeding tends to be more generalized, occurring in the wound, venipuncture sites, etc.

Hemoperitoneum usually becomes apparent within 24 hours after the operation. It manifests as intravascular hypovolemia: tachycardia, hypotension, decreased urine output, and peripheral vasoconstriction. If bleeding continues, abdominal girth may increase and intra-abdominal hypertension or abdominal compartment syndrome may ensue. Changes in the hematocrit are usually not obvious for 4-6 hours and are of limited diagnostic help in patients who sustain rapid blood loss.

The differential diagnosis of immediate postoperative circulatory collapse also includes pulmonary embolism, cardiac dysrhythmias, pneumothorax, myocardial infarction, and severe allergic reactions. Infusions to expand the intravascular volume should be started as soon as other diseases have been ruled out. If hypotension or other signs of hypovolemia persist, one usually must reoperate promptly. At operation, bleeding should be stopped, clots evacuated, and the peritoneal cavity rinsed with saline solution.

3.1.2 Hematoma

Wound hematoma, a collection of blood and clot in the wound, is a common wound complication and is usually caused by inadequate hemostasis. The risk is much higher in patients who have been systemically anticoagulated and in those with preexisting coagulopathies. Vigorous coughing or marked arterial hypertension immediately after surgery may contribute to the formation of a wound hematoma.

Hematoma produces elevation and discoloration of the wound edges, discomfort, and swelling. Blood sometimes leaks between skin sutures. Neck hematoma following operation on the thyroid, parathyroid, or carotid artery are particularly dangerous, because it may expand rapidly and compromise the airway. Small hematomas may resorb, but they increase the incidence of wound infection. Treatment in most cases consists of evacuation of the clot under sterile conditions, ligation of bleeding vessels, and reclosure of the wound.

3.1.3 Seroma

A seroma is a fluid collection in the wound other than pus or blood. Seromas often follow operations that involve elevation of skin flaps and transection of numerous lymphatic channels (e. g. , mastectomy, operations in the groin). Seromas delay healing and increase the risk of wound infection. Those located under skin flaps can usually be evacuated by needle aspiration if necessary. Compression dressings can then occlude lymphatic leaks and limit reaccumulation. Small seromas that recur may be treated by repeated evacuation. Seromas of the groin, which are common after vascular operations, are best left to resorb without aspiration, since the risks of introducing a needle (infection, disruption of vascular structures, etc.) are greater than the risk associated with the seroma itself. If seromas persist or if they leak through the wound—the wound should be explored in the operating room and the draining sites oversewn. Open wounds with persistent lymph leaks can be treated with wound vacuum devices.

3.1.4 Wound dehiscence

Wound dehiscence is partial or total disruption of any or all layers of the operative wound. Rupture of all layers of the abdominal wall and extrusion of abdominal viscera is evisceration. Wound dehiscence occurs in 1% –3% of abdominal surgical procedures. Systemic and local factors contribute to the development of this complication.

3.1.5 Systemic tisk factors

Dehiscence after laparotomy affects about 5% of patients older than 60 years. It is more common in patients with diabetes mellitus, uremia, immunosuppression, jaundice, sepsis, hypoalbuminemia, cancer, obesity, and in those receiving corticosteroids.

3.1.6 Local risk factors

The three most important local factors predisposing to wound dehiscence are inadequate closure, increased intra-abdominal pressure, and deficient wound healing.

3.1.6.1 Closure

This is the single most important factor. The fascial layers give strength to a closure, and when fascia disrupts, the wound separates. Accurate approximation of anatomic layers is essential for adequate wound closure. Most wounds that dehisce do so because the sutures tear through the fascia. Prevention of this problem includes performing a neat incision, avoiding devitalization of the fascial edges by careful handling of tissues during the operation, placing and tying sutures correctly, and selecting the proper suture material. Sutures must be placed 2-3 cm from the wound edge and about 1 cm apart. Wound complications are decreased by obliteration of dead space. Stomas and drains should be brought out through separate incisions to reduce the rate of wound infection and disruption.

3.1.6.2　Intra-abdominal pressure

After most intra-abdominal operations, some degree of ileus exists, which may increase pressure by causing distention of the bowel. High abdominal pressure can also occur in patients with chronic obstructive pulmonary disease who use their abdominal muscles as accessory muscles of respiration. In addition, coughing produces sudden increases in intra-abdominal pressure. Other factors contributing to increased abdominal pressure are postoperative bowel obstruction, obesity, and cirrhosis with ascites formation. Extra precautions are necessary to avoid dehiscence in such patients.

3.1.6.3　Poor wound healing

Infection is an associated factor in more than half of wounds that rupture. The presence of drains, seromas, and wound hematomas also delays healing.

3.1.7　Diagnosis and management

Although wound dehiscence may occur at any time following wound closure, it is most commonly observed between the fifth and eighth postoperative days, when the strength of the wound is at a minimum. Wound dehiscence may occasionally be the first manifestation of intra-abdominal sepsis. The earliest sign of dehiscence is often discharge of serosanguineous fluid from the wound or, in some cases, sudden evisceration. The patient may describe a popping sensation associated with severe coughing or retching.

Patients with dehiscence of a laparotomy wound and evisceration should be returned to bed and the wound covered with moist towels. With the patient under general anesthesia, any exposed bowel or omentum should be rinsed with lactated Ringer solution containing antibiotics and then returned to the abdomen. After mechanical cleansing and copious irrigation of the wound, the previous sutures should be removed and the wound reclosed using additional measures to prevent recurrent dehiscence, such as full-thickness retention sutures of number 22 wire or heavy nylon. Evisceration carries a 10% mortality rate due both to contributing factors (e. g. , sepsis and cancer) and to resulting local infection.

Wound dehiscence without evisceration is best managed by prompt elective reclosure of the incision. If a partial disruption is stable and the patient is a poor operative risk, treatment may be delayed and the resulting incisional hernia accepted. It is important in these patients that skin stitches, if present, not be removed before the end of the second postoperative week and that the abdomen be wrapped with a binder or corset to limit further enlargement of the fascial defect or sudden disruption of the covering skin.

In patients at high risk for wound dehiscence, placement of retention stitches at the initial operation should be considered. Although these do not prevent dehiscence, they may prevent evisceration and the morbidity and mortality that are associated with it.

3.2   Pulmonary Complications

Respiratory complications are the most common single cause of morbidity after major surgical procedures and the second most common cause of postoperative deaths in patients older than 60 years. Patients undergoing chest and upper abdominal operations are particularly prone to pulmonary complications. Special hazards are posed by preexisting chronic obstructive pulmonary disease (chronic bronchitis, emphysema, asthma, pulmonary fibrosis). Elderly patients are at much higher risk because they have decreased compliance, increased closing and residual volumes, and increased dead space, all of which predispose to atelectasis.

3.2.1   Atelectasis

Atelectasis, the most common pulmonary complication, affects 25% of patients who have abdominal surgery. It is more common in patients who are elderly or overweight and in those who smoke or have symptoms of respiratory disease. It appears most frequently in the first 48 hours after operation and is responsible for over 90% of febrile episodes during that period. In most cases, the course is self-limited and recovery uneventful.

Atelectasis is usually manifested by fever (pathogenesis unknown), tachypnea, and tachycardia. Physical examination may show elevation of the diaphragm, scattered rales, and decreased breath sounds, but it is often normal. Postoperative atelectasis can be largely prevented by early mobilization, frequent changes in position, encouragement to cough, and use of an incentive spirometer. Preoperative teaching of respiratory exercises and postoperative execution of these exercises prevent atelectasis in patients without preexisting lung disease.

Treatment consists of clearing the airway by chest percussion, coughing, or nasotracheal suction. Bronchodilators and mucolytic agents given by nebulizer may help in patients with severe chronic obstructive pulmonary disease. Atelectasis from obstruction of a major airway may require intrabronchial suction through an endoscope.

3.2.2   Postoperative pneumonia

Pneumonia is the most common pulmonary complication among patients who die after surgery. It is directly responsible for death—or is a contributory factor—in more than half of these patients. Patients with peritoneal infection and those requiring prolonged ventilatory support are at highest risk for developing postoperative pneumonia. Atelectasis, aspiration, and copious secretions are important predisposing factors.

More than half of the pulmonary infections that follow surgery are caused by gram-negative bacilli. They are frequently polymicrobial and usually acquired by aspiration of oropharyngeal secretions. Occasionally, infecting bacteria reach the lung by inhalation—for example, from respirators. Pseudomonas aeruginosa and Klebsiella can survive in the moist reservoirs of these machines, and these pathogens have been the source of epidemic infections in intensive care units.

The clinical manifestations of postoperative pneumonia are fever, tachypnea, increased secretions, and physical changes suggestive of pulmonary consolidation. A chest X-ray usually shows localized parenchymal consolidation.

Maintaining the airway clear of secretions is of paramount concern in the prevention of postoperative pneumonia. Respiratory exercises, deep breathing, and coughing help prevent atelectasis, which is a precursor of pneumonia. The prophylactic use of antibiotics does not decrease the incidence of gram-negative colonization of the oropharynx or that of pneumonia.

Treatment consists of measures to aid the clearing of secretions and administration of antibiotics. Sputum obtained directly from the trachea, usually by endotracheal suctioning, is required for specific identification of the infecting organism

3.2.3　Pulmonary embolism

Pulmonary embolism (PE) is a blockage of anartery in the lungs by a substance that has moved from elsewhere in the body through the bloodstream (embolism). PE may result from a blood clot, air, fat, or amniotic fluid. The risk of blood clots is increased by cancer, prolonged bed rest, smoking, stroke, certain genetic conditions, estrogen-based medication, pregnancy, obesity, and after some types of surgery.

Symptoms of a PE may include shortness of breath, chest pain particularly upon breathing in, and coughing up blood. Symptoms of a blood clot in the leg may also be present such as a red, warm, swollen, and painful leg. Signs of a PE include low blood oxygen levels, rapid breathing, rapid heart rate, and sometimes a mild fever. Severe cases can lead to passing out, abnormally low blood pressure, and sudden death.

Pulmonary embolism can be diagnosed by echocardiography, ventilation/perfusion scan, and formal angiography; however, helical CT angiography is the most commonly utilized technique.

Once symptoms develop, supportive treatment should be provided until respiratory insufficiency and central nervous system manifestations subside. Respiratory insufficiency is treated with positive end-expiratory pressure ventilation and diuretics. The prognosis is related to the severity of the pulmonary insufficiency.

3.2.3.1　Venous thromboembolism

Postoperative patients should be carefully monitored for lower extremity swelling, hypoxia, or new-onset pleuritic chest pain, as these may be harbingers of the syndrome. Risk factors include those that are nonmodifiable (thrombophilia, prior VTE, congestive heart failure, chronic lung disease, paralytic stroke, malignancy, spinal cord injury, obesity, age > 40, varicosities) and modifiable (type of surgery: hip, lower extremity, major general surgery, mechanical ventilation, major trauma, central venous lines, chemotherapy, hormone replacement therapy, pregnancy, immobility).

Prevention of VTE is much more effective than management of this complication. The CHEST guidelines are a useful adjunct to stratifying risk and assigning appropriate preventive therapy. This usually requires heparin therapy with regular or low-molecular-weight heparin, sequential compression stockings, and early ambulation. Inferior vena cava filters may be considered as a preventive method in patients who have contraindications to anticoagulation or have progression of disease despite adequate anticoagulation.

Diagnosis of deep vein thrombosis may be performed in a cost-effective manner by utilizing duplex ultrasonography. CT, MRI, or traditional venography.

The goals of treatment of VTE remain stabilization of clot, revasculature of a ected vessels, and prevention of long-term complications. The majority of these patients respond to anticoagulation with intravenous heparin or higher doses of subcutaneous low-molecular-weight heparin and, subsequent, conversion to oral therapy with warfarin. In patients who have hemodynamic instability due to a pulmonary embolus, consideration to system thrombolysis, suction embolectomy, or a Trendelenburg procedure should be given.

3.2.3.2　Postoperative fever

Fever occurs in about 40% of patients after major surgery. In most patients the temperature elevation resolves without specific treatment. However, postoperative fever may herald a serious infection, and it is therefore important to evaluate the patient clinically. Features often associated with an infectious origin of the fever include preoperative trauma, ASA class above 2, fever onset after the second postoperative day, an initial temperature elevation above 38. 6 ℃, a postoperative white blood cell count greater than 10 000/L, and a postoperative serum urea nitrogen of 15 mg/dL or greater. If three or more of the above are present, the likelihood of associated bacterial infection is nearly 100%.

When fever appears after the second postoperative day, atelectasis is a less likely explanation. The differential diagnosis of fever at this time includes catheter-related phlebitis, pneumonia, and urinary tract infection. A directed history and physical examination complemented by focused laboratory and radiologic studies usually determine the cause.

Patients without infection are rarely febrile a er the fi h postoperative day. Fever this late suggests wound infection or, less o en, anastomotic breakdown and intra-abdominal abscesses. A diagnostic workup directed to the detection of intra-abdominal sepsis is indicated in patients who have high temperatures (> 39 ℃) and wounds without evidence of infection 5 or more days postoperatively. CT scan of the abdomen and pelvis is the test of choice and should be performed early, before overt organ failure occurs.

Fever is rare a er the first week in patients who had a normal convalescence. Allergy to drugs, transfusion-related fever, septic pelvic vein thrombosis, and intra-abdominal abscesses should be considered.

3.2.3.3　Surgical site infection

The Center for Disease Control (CDC) classifies SSIs into three locations: superficial incisional; deep incisional; organ space.

The risk for developing an SSI has been estimated at 4% rate in clean wounds and 35% in grossly contaminated wounds.

Risk factors for SSI include systemic factors (diabetes, immunosuppression, obesity, smoking malnutrition, and previous radiation) and local factors (surgical wound classification and surgical techniques).

Prevention of SSI includes meticulous surgical techniques (skin preparation, maintaining sterility, judicious use of cautery, respecting dissection planes, approximating tissue neatly, etc.) and administration of appropriate preoperative antibiotics as determined by the type of operation being performed.

The diagnosis of SSI is primarily clinical. Common symptoms include pain, warmth, and erythema with drainage through the incision. Deep and organ space infections may be further diagnosed with radiographic imaging.

Treatment for an SSI emphasizes primary source control. Gaining such control may require an operative procedure such as an incision and drainage of the infectious source. For superficial infections, the treatment would simply include opening the incision, exploring the space, irrigating, debriding, and leaving the wound open with local wound care. Deep incisional and organ space infections may necessitate open operative drainage and debridement or percutaneous drainage procedures. Antibiotics by themselves do not usually address the underlying focus of infection.

3.3　Genitourinary Complications

3.3.1　Postoperative urinary retention

Inability to void postoperatively is common, especially after pelvic and perineal operations or operations conducted under spinal anesthesia. Factors responsible for postoperative urinary retention are interference with the neural mechanisms responsible for normal emptying of the bladder and overdistention of the urinary bladder. When its normal capacity of approximately 500 mL is exceeded, bladder contraction is inhibited. Prophylactic bladder catheterization should be considered whenever an operation is likely to last 3 hours or longer or when large volumes of intravenous fluids are anticipated. The catheter can be removed at the end of the operation if the patient is expected to be able to ambulate within a few hours.

The treatment of acute urinary retention is catheterization of the bladder. In the absence of factors that suggest the need for prolonged decompression, such as the presence of 1000 mL of urine or more, the catheter may be removed.

3.3.2 Urinary tract infection

Infection of the lower urinary tract is the most frequently acquired nosocomial infection. Preexisting contamination of the urinary tract, urinary retention, and instrumentation are the principal contributing factors.

Cystitis is manifested by dysuria and mild fever and pyelonephritis by high fever, flank tenderness, and occasionally ileus. Diagnosis is made by examination of the urine and confirmed by cultures. Prevention involves treating urinary tract contamination before surgery, prevention or prompt treatment of urinary retention, and careful instrumentation when needed. Treatment includes adequate hydration, proper drainage of the bladder, and specific antibiotics.

Part 9

Surgical Infection

Chapter 1

Introduction

Surgical infections occur because of a breakdown of the equilibrium that exists between organisms and the host. This may be due to a breach in a protective surface, changes in host resistance, or particular characteristics of the organism. The possible outcomes are resolution, abscess formation, extensive local spread with or without tissue death, and distant spread.

1.1 Host Defense Mechanisms

Areas of the body that are in contact with an external environment are protected by elaborate barrier mechanisms. Parts of these barriers are mechanical in nature, such as the keratinized layer of skin. Such physical barriers are augmented by powerful innate immune mechanisms (e. g. , the low pH and fatty acid content of normal skin inhibits bacterial growth). An additional factor is that all mucous membranes are protected by lymphocyte–mediated events that result in the secretion of immunoglobulin A (IgA) antibodies. In the gut, the rapid turnover of the mucosal cells along the crypto–villus axis has a protective function because enteropathogens must adhere to enterocytes in order to cause clinical problems.

Tissue injury stimulates a cascade of events that lead to the formation of granulation tissue and eventual healing. However, extensive tissue damage inhibits the inflammatory response (e. g. , the low oxygen tensions in poorly vascularized tissues impairs the oxidative killing of microbes by phagocytes). Damaged tissue also forms a nidus for bacterial growth. These factors explain the need to debride wounds in order to avoid infection.

The response of the body to microbes can be affected by immunodeficiencies of genetic origin (which are rare) or by acquired deficiencies (e. g. , protein–energy undernutrition; diseases such as diabetes, cancer and AIDS; or by the administration of immunosuppressive or cytotoxic drugs). Infections often arise in immunocompromised individuals with microbes that are not usually regarded as pathogens (e. g. , opportunistic infections caused by fungi).

1.2　The Organisms

The pathogenicity of microbes is determined by their capacity to adhere to and damage host cells, and then to produce and release a variety of enzymes and exotoxins. Staphylococcus has surface receptors that allow it to bind to host cells and extracellular matrix proteins, especially those covered by protein A molecules, which bind to the Fc portion of antibodies. Streptococcus and Haemophilus secrete proteases that degrade antibodies, and other enzymes such as haemolysins and kinases that assist in the spread of infection in the form of cellulitis or erysipelas. Escherichia coli carries K−antigen, which prevents the activation of complement via the alternate pathway.

Foreign bodies increase the pathogenicity of microbes by impairing local defense mechanisms. It is important to explore deep wounds adequately in order to remove foreign bodies and devitalized tissues. This is a critical issue because the use of antibiotics is no substitute for poor surgical technique. It should also be appreciated that although prosthetic materials are made of "inert materials" they are still foreign bodies, and it is difficult to control associated infections without removing the offending prosthesis. Examples of this range from infected central venous lines to infected vascular grafts and orthopedic implants.

Chapter 2

Superficial Suppurative Infections

2.1　Folliculitis

This is a superficial pustular eruption localized to the opening of the hair follicle, commonly caused by S. aureus infection. Predisposing factors include obesity, diabetes, moist humid climate, and tight or occlusive clothing. A small pustule with a hair emerging is the typical clinical finding. Healing usually occurs without scarring. Contact with mineral oils or tar products may produce a sterile folliculitis; a similar sterile folliculitis may occur beneath adhesive plasters or adhesive dressings. Differential diagnoses includes miliaria pustulosa (see above), inflammatory tinea, and moniliasis.

Therapy: Folliculitis is often self-limiting. Improvement in hygiene and the use of antibacterial scrubs such as 3% hexachlorophene or chlorhexidine gluconate may clear the infection; wearing of loose-fitting cotton clothing often helps. If the infection is persistent or extensive, treatment with dicloxacillin or erythromycin (each 250 mg four times daily for 7 days) is usually sufficient. Recurrence is common.

2.2　Abscess (furuncle, boil)

An abscess is a localized collection of pus within the skin associated with erythema, tenderness, and showing marked infiltration by polymorphonuclear leucocytes. An abscess that involves the hair follicle is termed a furuncle. Staphylococcus aureus is the most common causative organism; streptococci and Gram-negative organisms may also be present.

2.2.1　Epidemiology

Furuncles are uncommon in children, except in those with atopic dermatitis; the incidence increases at puberty, becoming common in adolescents and young adults. Men are more frequently affected than women. Most patients have intact immune systems. Local mechanical factors participate in the pattern of distribution of lesions.

2.2.2 Clinical appearance

The earliest lesion is a small, tender, inflammatory nodule in a follicular location. Pustulation occurs, followed by necrosis and discharge. Healing results in scar formation. Furuncles may be single or multiple. Common sites are the buttocks, anogenital area, face, neck, arms, wrists, and fingers. Cystic acne, hidradenitis suppurativa, and inflamed epidermal inclusion cysts are the lesions that most commonly need to be distinguished from furuncles.

2.2.3 Therapy

Since the course of furuncles is often self-limiting, therapy may not be necessary. Large lesions should be treated by incision and drainage. Antibiotic therapy, such as dicloxacillin 250–500 mg every 4 h for 7 days, is also warranted in this situation. Patients who show persistent recurrences may be nasal or perineal carriers of the causative organism.

2.3 Carbuncle

A carbuncle is a suppurative extension of several contiguous furuncles into the subcutaneous fat. The maintenance of fascial attachments to the skin results in the production of multilocular compartments, particularly in the nape of the neck, upper back, hips, and thighs. Men in middle to late life are most commonly affected; predisposing factors include malnutrition, diabetes, cardiac failure, prolonged steroid therapy, and generalized dermatoses. Staphylococcus aureus is the most common cause.

2.3.1 Clinical features

The initial lesion is a painful, dome-shaped nodule, which may increase in size over several days to 10 cm or more. After about 1 week, pus-draining follicular orifices are noted, followed by necrosis of skin and deep ulceration. Fever and malaise may precede or accompany the development of the lesion.

2.3.2 Treatment

A carbuncle should be treated with a penicillinase-resistant systemic antibiotic such as dicloxacillin (250–500 mg every 6 h), particularly if cellulitis is suspected. If the lesion is large, incision and drainage is indicated.

2.4 Impetigo

This superficial infection of the outer layers of the skin is characterized by the presence of honey-colored crusts. Previously, most cases were due to infection by streptococci; occasionally, mixed streptococcal-staphylococcal infection was seen. Now the majority of cases are caused by staphylococci alone; a few mixed infections are still seen. This condition is especially common in small children. The differential diagnosis includes contact dermatitis and infected atopic dermatitis.

Treatment: Traditionally, treatment required a 10-day course of oral antibiotics, either penicillin VK, 250 mg every 6 h (or the equivalent dose in small children), or erythromycin, 250 mg every 6 h. Topical treatment with mupirocin ointment (Bactroban) 3 times daily has recently been used successfully, with the addition of oral antibiotics if topical therapy fails. For extensively crusted areas, wet-dry saline soaks help debride and dry the area. Complications of impetigo are unusual, but rare cases of post-streptococcal glomerulonephritis have been reported.

Chapter 3

Acute Cellulitis

3.1 Pathogenesis

Cellulitis is a diffuse, spreading infection of the deeper layers of the skin and the subcutaneous tissues. By far the most common infective organisms are the β-hemolytic streptococci, e. g. , Strep. pyogenes (group A streptococcus). Staphylococcus aureus is also a major cause of cellulitis after the β-hemolytic streptococci. These bacteria produce enzymes that break down intercellular barriers and promote spread. Despite the fact that cellulitis is thought to be an infective process, bacteria can only be isolated by needle aspiration or biopsy in 30% of cases (technique may cause variations in results). This is probably due to the fact that the bacteria are being rapidly cleared and diluted by the inflammatory process. The release of the cytokines IL-1 and tumor necrosis factor from the Langerhans' cells in the skin increase the phagocytosis and clearance of the bacteria. The heat, redness, and swelling seen in cellulitis are probably due to the small number of residual bacteria and bacterial remnants triggering the inflammatory response and the release of the cytokines and other inflammatory mediators rather than the infection itself.

3.2 Clinical Features

A patient with cellulitis usually presents with an area of swelling (oedema), erythema, heat, and tenderness. Most commonly this occurs after minor trauma, such as a laceration or deep abrasion. It is also seen after any break in the skin, such as an area of dermatophyte infection. In many cases there is no obvious break. The red, thickened, oedematous area spreads and is clearly demarcated from the surrounding skin. The patient will have systemic features of inflammation, including malaise, fever, and leucocytosis. If severe, the patient may develop bacteraemia and hypotension.

If untreated, lymphangitis develops, with red streaking over the lymphatics draining the area and passing to the local lymph nodes, which also become inflamed (lymphadenitis). Blisters, local abscesses, and areas of local necrosis of the skin may develop in advanced, untreated cases. Cellulitis can predispose to the development of thrombophlebitis, especially in older people.

Predisposition to cellulitis occurs in a number of conditions, including the following. ①In patients with lymphoedema of either the upper or lower limb. The common causes of this would be lymphadenectomy, radiotherapy, or neoplastic involvement of the nodes concerned. This can also involve the vulva in the case of inguinal nodes or the breast and chest wall in axillary nodes. ②Chronic oedema due to venous stasis predisposes to cellulitis, but less frequently. ③Diabetic patients with peripheral neuropathy and ulcer formation in lower limbs are particularly prone to superficial cellulitis around an ulcer (as well as developing deep necrotizing infection). ④Postoperatively, where there may be cellulitis surrounding a surgical wound. ⑤Orbital cellulitis.

Occasionally, in severe cases of cellulitis, there may be concern that the patient could be suffering from necrotizing fasciitis or gas gangrene.

Erysipelas is uncommon, but when it does occur is more often seen in children and older adults. It is painful and has distinctive, elevated margins that are clearly demarcated from the surrounding skin. It sometimes has a peau d'orange appearance.

3.3　Management

Cellulitis, if recognized and treated early, will often respond to oral antimicrobials and rest in the community setting. Failure of response to these measures or in compromised patients will require intensive, intravenous antimicrobial therapy together with bed rest, elevation of the affected limb, and careful observation in the hospital setting. Any predisposing cause will require prompt and thorough treatment. In particular, fungal infection between the toes will require antifungal therapy. Wound infections may require drainage and patients with diabetic feet will require full and thorough investigation and management. Patients with leg oedema will require compression stockings.

Most initial therapy is empirical. In some absence of distinctive features, the most likely causative agent is either Strep. pyogenes or, to lesser extent, Staph. aureus, and an antimicrobial regimen should cover both of these bacteria; di(flu)cloxacillin 2 g intravenously (children 25-50 mg/kg up to 2 g) every 6 h. In mild cases, oral di(flu)cloxacillin can be used. Dicloxacillin has taken on popularity because flucloxacillin can cause severe hepatitis and cholestatic jaundice, which may be protracted. This reaction is more frequent in older patients and those who take the drug for prolonged periods. However, the intravenous administration of dicloxacillin has been associated with moderate to severe phlebitis, which may require discontinuation of treatment.

If the patient is hypersensitive to penicillin, a first-generation cephalosporin [e. g. , cephazolin (cefazolin), cephalexin, or cephalothin] can be used. However, if severe hypersensitivity to penicillin is reported, cross-reaction between b-lactams is possible and then an agent like clindamycin should be considered. Vancomycin can be used if the cellulitis is caused by, or suspected of being caused by, MRSA.

Patients with impaired immunity are susceptible to developing cellulitis from unusual bacteria including Serratia, Proteus, Strep. pneumoniae and Haemophilus influenzae type b, together with the yeast Cryptococcus neoformans.

Failure to respond to intensive antimicrobial therapy, the presence of immunosuppression or of areas of fluctuance indicate the need for needle aspiration to obtain cultures. If the infection and systemic effects are severe or there is any doubt, a full-thickness biopsy to exclude necrotizing fasciitis is indicated.

Diabetic pedal wound infections and orbital (pre-and postseptal) cellulitis require urgent surgical intervention together with potent, rapidly acting, broad-spectrum antimicrobial regimens.

Patients with recurrent episodes of cellulitis, especially if associated with lymphoedema, may require prophylactic antimicrobials.

If predisposing conditions such as oedema and fungal foot infections exist, they should be identified and treated concurrently or after the infection has settled (varicose veins/neuropathic ulcers).

Chapter 4

Acute Lymphangitis and Lymphadenitis

4.1 Acute Lymphangitis

Lymphangitis refers to inflammation of subcutaneous lymphatic channels, typically in an extremity, and can represent an acute bacterial infection or a more chronic, indolent process due to a fungal, mycobacterial, or parasitic pathogens.

4.1.1 Etiologic agents

S. pyogenes is the leading cause of acute lymphangitis. Less commonly, S. aureus or other streptococci can cause lymphangitis, as can Pasteurella species after cat or dog bite and Spirillum minor after a rat bite.

4.1.2 Clinical manifestations

Acute bacterial lymphangitis can accompany cellulitis or can occur in association with minor or inapparent skin infection. Lymphangitis is recognized from the rapid appearance of tender, red, linear streaks proceeding from the site of cutaneous (frequently minor) infection toward the regional lymph nodes. Tender lymphadenopathy typically is present, as are systemic symptoms such as fever, chills, and malaise. Most often infection manifests on the hands and upper extremities. Subcutaneous nodules varying from 2 to 20 mm in size appear indolently as the infection advances along the course of the lymphatic channel. These nodules are either small and freely mobile or adherent to the superficial skin. Larger nodules often exhibit overlying erythema, but rarely are painful. Nodules sometimes ulcerate, releasing serosanguineous fluid.

4.1.3 Differential diagnosis

Acute lymphangitis is a clinical diagnosis made in the febrile patient with tender, linear red streaking that extends proximally from a site of peripheral infection. Thrombophlebitis is the major differential diagnostic consideration, but this condition lacks the characteristic inciting lesion (unless it is associated with an intravascular cannula) and the tender regional lymphadenopathy associated with acute lymphangitis. The precise etiologic agent (usually S. pyogenes) can be identified with Gram stain and culture of a specimen from the cutaneous lesion or, not uncommonly, by culture of the blood. Acute lymphangitis develops in about

20% of patients with animal bites infected with Pasteurella canis (dogs) or P. multocida (cats). Finally, Spirillum minor infection should be considered in a child living in a crowded urban dwelling that is prone to rat infestation, because the superficial bite wound often completely heals during the 1−3−week incubation period before development of acute lymphangitis.

4.1.4 Therapy

Since S. pyogenes is the predominant cause of acute lymphangitis, penicillin is the preferred initial treatment. Children with mild disease can be treated with oral penicillin V (50 mg/kg per day). Patients with S. pyogenes disease and concurrent BSI should be treated with intravenous penicillin G, 100,000 − 400,000 U/kg per day), depending upon illness severity; resistance to penicillin has never been documented. Penicillin also is the drug of choice for Pasteurella lymphangitis and S. minor rat−bite fever. Those with prominent systemic symptoms and unknown or possible bacteremia should receive intravenous therapy with an antibiotic that also provides adequate coverage for S. aureus.

4.2 Lymphadenitis

Lymphadenitis is the inflammation of lymph nodes. It is often a complication of bacterial infections, although it can also be caused by viruses or other disease agents. Lymphadenitis may be either generalized, involving a number of lymph nodes, or limited to a few nodes in the area of a localized infection. Lymphadenitis is sometimes accompanied by lymphangitis, which is the inflammation of the lymphatic vessels that connect the lymph nodes.

4.2.1 Description

The lymphatic system is a network of vessels (channels), nodes (glands), and organs. It is part of the immune system, which protects against and fights infections, inflammation, and cancers. The lymphatic system also participates in the transport of fluids, fats, proteins, and other substances throughout the body. The lymph nodes are small structures that filter the lymph fluid and contain many white blood cells to fight infections. Lymphadenitis is marked by swollen lymph nodes that develop when the glands are overwhelmed by bacteria, virus, fungi, or other organisms. The nodes may be tender and hard or soft and "rubbery" if an abscess has formed. The skin over an inflamed node may be red and hot. The location of the affected nodes is usually associated with the site of an underlying infection, inflammation, or tumor. In most cases, the infectious organisms are Streptococci or Staphylococci. If the lymphatic vessels are also infected, in a condition referred to as lymphangitis, there will be red streaks extending from the wound in the direction of the lymph nodes, throbbing pain, and high fever and/or chills. The child will generally feel ill, with loss of appetite, headache, and muscle aches.

The extensive network of lymphatic vessels throughout the body and their relation to the lymph nodes helps to explain why bacterial infection of the nodes can spread rapidly to or from other parts of the body. Lymphadenitis in children often occurs in the neck area because these lymph nodes are close to the ears and throat, which are frequent locations of bacterial infections in children.

Lymphadenitis is also referred to as lymph node infection, lymph gland infection, or localized lymphadenopathy.

4.2.2　Causes and symptoms

Streptococcal and staphylococcal bacteria are the most common causes of lymphadenitis, although viruses, protozoa, rickettsiae, fungi, and the tuberculosis bacillus can also infect the lymph nodes. Diseases or disorders that involve lymph nodes in specific areas of the body include rabbit fever (tularemia) , cat-scratch disease, lymphogranuloma venereum, chancroid, genital herpes, infected acne, dental abscesses, and bubonic plague. Lymphadenitis can also occur in conjunction with cellulitis, which is a deep, widespread tissue infection that develops from a cut or sore.

The early symptoms of lymphadenitis are swelling of the nodes caused by a build-up of tissue fluid and an increased number of white blood cells resulting from the body's response to the infection. Further developments include fever with chills, loss of appetite, heavy perspiration, a rapid pulse, and general weakness.

4.2.3　Diagnosis

4.2.3.1　Physical examination

The diagnosis of lymphadenitis is usually based on a combination of the child's medical history, external symptoms, and laboratory cultures. The doctor will press (palpate) the affected lymph nodes to see if they are sore or tender, and search for an entry point for the infection, like a scratch or bite. Swollen nodes without soreness are sometimes caused by cat-scratch disease, which is an uncommon illness. If the lymphadenitis is severe or persistent, the doctor may need to rule out mumps, HIV, tumors in the neck region, and congenital cysts that resemble swollen lymph nodes.

4.2.3.2　Laboratory tests

The most significant tests are a white blood cell count (WBC) and a blood culture to identify the organism. A high proportion of immature white blood cells indicates a bacterial infection. Blood cultures may be positive, most often for a species of staphylococcus or streptococcus. In some cases, a biopsy of the lymph node is also needed to look for unusual infection or lymphoma.

4.2.4　Treatment

4.2.4.1　Medications

The medications given for lymphadenitis vary according to the bacterium or virus that causes it. For bacterial infections, the child will be treated with antibiotics, usually a penicillin, clindamycin, a cephalosporin, or erythromycin.

4.2.4.2　Supportive care

Supportive care of lymphadenitis includes resting the affected area and applying hot moist compresses to reduce inflammation and pain.

4.2.4.3　Surgery

Cellulitis associated with lymphadenitis should not be treated surgically because of the risk of spreading the infection. Pus is drained only if there is an. In some cases, biopsy of an inflamed lymph node is necessary if no diagnosis has been made and no response to treatment has occurred.

Inflammation of lymph nodes due to other diseases requires treatment of the underlying causes.

Chapter 5

Tetanus

This is caused by a spore-forming obligate anaerobe, C. tetani, found in the feces of humans and animals, and capable of prolonged survival in soil. Two exotoxins are produced: tetanospasmin, a neurotoxin, and tetanolysin, a hemolysin. Dead muscle and clotted blood provide an ideal culture medium for the germination of tetanus spores, and compound fractures with devitalization of muscle are very susceptible to such infection, as are small puncture wounds harboring a clot deep in the tissues. Locally produced tetanolysin contributes to optimal growth conditions through its lecithinase, gelatinase, esterase, and lipase activities. Tetanospasmin, the neurotoxin responsible for the clinical features of the disease, does not act peripherally or locally but is carried to, and acts on, the central nervous system. In order to neutralize blood-borne toxin, antitoxin must be present before tetanospasmin becomes fixed by nerve cells. Antitoxin given when symptoms are apparent only limits further intoxication of nerve cells and can not reverse developing symptoms.

5.1　Clinical Manifestations

There is considerable variability in the progression of the disease from its onset. There may be a prodromal period of headache, stiff jaw muscles, restlessness, yawning, risus sardonicus, and wound pain, typically beginning 1-2 weeks after trauma but occasionally as early as 1 day or as late as 2 months after injury. The active stage follows in 12-24 h, with trismus, facial distortion, opisthotonos, pain, clonic spasms, and seizures. Acute asphyxia is a major hazard; it may result from either spasm of the respiratory muscles or aspiration. The shorter the incubation period, the poorer the prognosis.

5.2　Therapy

Human immune globulin, 3000 units intramuscularly, should be given immediately to neutralize circulating toxins. An additional 1000 units are injected into and immediately proximal to the wound, followed by wide debridement. 500 units of intramuscular immune globulin may subsequently be given daily. If symptoms persist for longer than 2 weeks, the large initial doses of immune globulin may be repeated. An airway must be established; tracheostomy will be needed in every patient with more than prodromal symptoms and should be performed before the situation becomes urgent. Respirator support and oxygenation may be needed. Muscle spasms may be controlled with intravenous midazolam or diazepam, or with intramuscular meprobamate or chlorpromazine. If spasms persist, curare or another muscle blocker should be given. Additional sedation is usually not needed if muscle relaxant therapy has been adequate, but is best achieved with intramuscular barbiturates if required. The patient should be placed in a quiet room, with environmental stimulation kept at a minimum to avoid triggering seizures.

Intravenous thiopental (pentothal) may be needed to control seizures. High doses of penicillin G (5–10 million units) will establish a sufficient antibacterial tissue concentration. With appropriate early care, 75% of patients survive with no neurologic impairment.

5.3　Principles for Tetanus Prophylaxis

Tetanus is absolutely preventable by prior active immunization. Effective active immunization (not in association with a fresh wound) is accomplished by the injection of 0.5 mL fluid or adsorbed toxoid, repeated after 2 and 20 months.

Immediate meticulous surgical care of the fresh wound is of prime importance. Removal of devitalized tissue, blood clots, and foreign bodies, obliteration of dead space, and prevention of tissue ischemia in the wound are the objectives of initial treatment. If the wound is grossly contaminated, penicillin should be administered. Wounds seen late or grossly contaminated should be left unsutured after debridement, protected by a sterile dressing for 3–5 days, and closed by delayed primary sutures if the tissues appear clean and healthy. Active and passive immunization should be accomplished with 0.5 mL tetanus toxoid and tetanus immune globulin, 250–1000 units. Patients not previously immunized should receive injections of 0.5 mL fluid or adsorbed toxoid, repeated after 2, 6, and 20 months.

Part 10

Burns and Cold Injury

Chapter 1

Burns and other Thermal Injuries

A burn is an injury to the skin or other organic tissue primarily caused by heat, electricity, or contact with chemicals, or due to radiation. Thermal injury, the most common kind of burn, occur when skin or other tissues are destroyed by hot liquids (scalds), hot solids or flames.

1.1 Structure and Function of the Skin

1.1.1 Structure of the skin

Skin is the largest organ of the body and consists of three layers, that is the epidermis, the dermis (corium) and subcutaneous tissue (Figure 10-1-1).

The outermost cells of the epidermis are dead cornified cells that act as a tough protective barrier against the environment. Cell division is limited to the basal cell layer of the epidermis, it is necessary during the process of the reepithelialization. The second, thicker layer, the dermis (0.06-0.12 mm), is composed chiefly of fibrous connective tissue. The dermis contains the blood vessels and nerves to the skin and the epithelial appendages with specialized function. The blood vessels and nerves in the skin run throughout the dermis but do not enter the epidermis. Since the nerve endings that mediate pain are found only in the dermis, partial thickness injuries may be extremely painful, whereas full thickness burns are usually painless. Hair follicles and sweat glands originate in the dermis. These cutaneous appendages are lined with epidermis cells, which are important factors in reepithelialization of deep second-degree burns. The third layer of skin is subcutaneous tissue, which is composed primarily of areolar and fatty connective tissue. It contains skin appendages, glands, and hair follicles. Hair follicles extend in deep narrow pits or pockets that traverse the dermis to varying depths and usually extend into the subcutaneous tissue. Each hair follicle consists of a shaft that is projects above the surface and a root that is embedded within the skin.

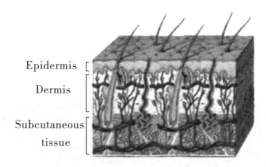

Figure 10-1-1   **Structure of skin**

1.1.2   Function of the skin

The main functions of the skin are as the following:

· Skin, especially the dermis, offers special protective functions.

· Prevents loss of body fluid by evaporation and loss of excess body heat.

· Maintains body temperature by controlling the amount of water evaporated.

· Excretes small amounts of electrolytes and metabolic products.

· Produces some materials (e. g. , vitamin D).

· Mediates various sensations.

1.2   Pathophysiology of Burn

All kinds of burn factors cause traumatic inflammation and let the vasoactive mediators release which lead to a transient increase in microvascular permeability at the injured area. Then a rapid loss of intravascular fluid and protein occurs through the injured capillaries. The blisters form at the injured site and much more body fluid is evaporated from the wound. If it is a moderate or severe burn, large quantities of body fluid loss bring about effective circulating blood volume (ECBV) deficiency or even hypovolemic shock. Swelling will appear at the burn areas and even nonburned tissues because of exudation and hypoproteinemia. This process is greatest in the first 6-8 hours postburn, with capillary integrity returning toward normal by 36-48 hours.

1.3   Metabolic Response to Burns and Metabolic Support

The initial metabolic response appears to be activated by proinflammatory cytokines and in turn oxidants. The secretion of catecholamine, cortisol, glucagons, renin angiotensin, antidiuretic hormone and aldosterone is also increased. Early in the response, energy is supplied by the breakdown of stored glycogen and by the process of anaerobic glycolysis.

A profound hypermetabolism occurs in the post burn period, characterized by an increase in metabolic rate that approaches doubling of the basal rate in severe burns. The degree of response is proportionate to the degree of injury, with a plateau occurring when the burn involves about 70% of total body surface. The initiating and perpetuating factors are the inflammation mediators, especially the cytokines and endotoxin. Added environmental stresses, such as pain, cooling, and sepsis, increase the obligatory hypermetabolism.

During the first week postburn, the metabolic rate and oxygen consumption rise progressively from the normal level present during resuscitation and remain elevating until the wound is covered. The specific pathophysiologic mechanism remains undefined, but increased and persistent catecholamine secretion and excessive evaporative heat loss from the burn wound are major factors, as is increased circulating endotoxin from wound.

The evaporative water loss from the wound may reach 300 mL/($m^2 \cdot$ h), normal is about 15 mL/cm^2 $\cdot$ h). This produces a heat loss of about 580 kcal/L of water evaporated. Covering the burn with an impermeable membrane, such as skin substitute, reduces the hypermetabolism.

Similarly, placing the burn patient in a warm environment, where convection and radiant loss of heat are minimized, also modestly reduces the metabolic rate. Placing the burn patient in an unwarmed environment (room temperature at or below 27 ℃) accentuates heat loss and markedly increases the hypermetabolic state. The persistently elevated circulating levels of catecholamines stimulate an exaggerated degree of gluconeogenesis and protein breakdown. Protein catabolism, glucose intolerance, and marked total body weight loss result.

Aggressive nutritional support along with rapid wound closure and control of pain, stress, and sepsis are the only means available to decrease the hypermetabolic state. The use of selective antiinflammatory agents may be of some benefit in the future.

1.4   Clinical Stages of Burn

Based on the pathophysiology of burns, the clinical process undergoes the following three stages.

(1) The shock stage

It starts from the injury, and completely ends at a week. The main problems are hypovolemia and shock. The volume loss is greatest in the first 6−8 hours postbum. Prevention and correction the hypovolemia are the main measure in this stage.

(2) The infection stage

The stage begins with 2−3 days postburn and ends at the burn wound completely covered. The main treatment during the stage is to prevent infection and promote the wound healing.

(3) The rehabilitation stage

Most of the moderate and major burned patients need to do functional exercise and repair the residual wounds. This process starts from closure of the burn wound and may last several years.

1.5   Determination of Severity of Burn

The severity and death rate of burn patients are mainly related to the size (body surface area, BSA) and depth of the burn.

1.5.1   Size of burns

There are two methods to calculate the percentage of the burned area.

· The palm method: The whole surface area of the burned patient palm represents 1% total body surface area (TBSA). This method is convenient to determine the minor burn.

· Rule of nines: In rule of nines, TBSA of a person is divided into several 9%. The advantages of this model are reasonably accurate, relatively easy to use and remember.

1.5.1.1 Adult

A Chinese Adult: The head: 9×1% (face, scalp, neck 3 % respectively); The upper extremities: 9×2% (two hands 5 %, two forearms 6 %, and two upper arms 7 %); The trunk: 9×3% (anterior and posterior trunk 13% each, the genitalia 1%); The lower extremities: (9×5 +1)% (The buttocks 5%, two feet 7%, two legs 13%, two thighs 21%).

A Westerner Adult: The head: 9×1% (face, scalp, neck 3 % respectively); The upper extremities: 9×2%; The trunk: anterior and posterior trunk 18% each, the genitalia 1%; Each lower extremity 18%.

1.5.1.2 Children

Comparing children with adults, the surface area of the head in children is relative larger, and the area of the lower extremities is relative smaller. So calculating the surface area of the head and lower extremities in children should be changed as follow. The head: 9 + (12−age)%; The lower extremities: 41 − (12−age)%.

1.5.2 Depth of burns

A skin thermal injury is determined based on the layer affected, the temperature, and duration of exposure. Determining the depth of burn is essential for evaluating the severity of the burn and planning for wound care. The general classification for depth of burns is first−, second−, and third−degree. The features of different degree burns are as follows:

1.5.2.1 First−degree burn

First−degree burn involves only the epidermis and is characterized by erythema, pain, and a lack of blisters. The most common causes of this degree burn are overexposure to sunlight and brief scalding. Healing occurs rapidly. In 5−10 days, the damaged epithelium peels off in small scales, leaving no residual scarring.

1.5.2.2 Second−degree burn

Second−degree burn or partial thickness burn destroys the entire epidermis and varying depths of the dermis. The systemic severity of the burn and the quality of subsequent healing are directly related to the amount of undamaged dermis.

The superficial second−degree burn is characterized by blister, pain and a moist, red basal surface. Complications are rare from the superficial second−degree burns, which usually heal with minimal scarring in 10−14 days unless they become infected.

The deep second−degree burns have blister and a mottled−red appearance or a layer of whitish nonviable dermis firmly adherent to the remaining viable tissue. Deep dermal burns heal over a period of 25 − 35 days with a fragile epithelial covering that arises from the residual uninjured epithelium of the deep dermal sweat glands and hair follicles. However, a superimposed bacterial infection can seriously interfere with healing and may convert into a full thickness injury. Severe hypertrophic scarring occurs when such an injury heals.

1.5.2.3 Third−degree burn

If the injury reaches the subcutaneous tissue, it is considered a full thickness or third−degree burn. All epithelial elements of skin are destructed completely leaving no potential for reepithelialization. Third−degree burn is characterized by a dry, painless, dark and leathery appearance, or may appear mottled, or waxy white surface. The destroyed skin will separate as a slough (eschar). If the diameter of this degree burn is larger than 2.5-3.0 cm, skin grafting is generally needed before healing occurs.

Burns can extend into subcutaneous tissue, underlying muscle, or bony tissue. These burns are sometimes classified as fourth-degree or char burns.

Generally the first-degree burn and the superficial second-degree burn are called the superficial burn. The deep burn involves the deep second-degree burn and third-degree burn.

1.5.3   Burn severity categorization

The burn severity categorization by the Chinese Burn Association (CBA) are listed as the following.

(1) Mild degree burns: TBSA of second-degree burn< 9%.

(2) Moderate degree burns : TBSA of second-degree burn 10% -29% or TBSA of third-degree burn <10%.

(3) Severe degree burns : TBSA of burn 30% -49%; or TBSA of third-degree burn 10% -19%; TBSA of burn <30%, but with one of the following conditions: ①severe general condition or be in shock; ②moderate or severe inhalation injury; ③burn injury complicated by other major trauma.

(4) Major degree burns: TBSA of burn >50%; or TBSA of third-degree burn>20%.

1.6   Burn Management

1.6.1   First aid of burn

Burn care should begin at the site of injury and continue through prehospital care. Basic guidance on first aid for burns is provided below.

· Extinguish flames by allowing the patient to roll on the ground, or by applying a blanket, or by using water or other fire-extinguishing liquids.

· Remove charred clothing when appropriate.

· Cold therapy: Minor superficial burns can be cooled with running tap water or immersed in cold water as early as possible for 20-30 minutes to relieve pain and limit tissue damage. But do not apply ice water or apply ice directly to the burn wound because it deepens the injury.

· In chemical burns, remove or dilute the chemical agent by irrigating with large volumes of water.

· Do not apply paste, oil, or any other foreign materials on the burn wound as they might interfere with determination of the burn depth and become infected.

· Perform a rapid primary survey and immediately correct any problems found.

· Concurrently with airway and circulatory management, make an effort to stop the burning process.

· Wrap the patient in a clean cloth or sheet and transport to the nearest appropriate facility for medical care.

1.6.2   Fluid resuscitation

All patients with a moderate and major burn injury must receive fluid resuscitation. It is critical within the first 24 hours. The amount of fluid resuscitation can be determined from the percentage of the BSA involved. But only the area covered by second-degree burns and third-degree is taken into consideration, as the first-degree burns do not cause hemodynamically significant fluid shift to warrant fluid replacement.

1.6.2.1   Determination the volume of intravenous infusion

The following formulas are commonly used in determination the volume of fluid required for adults.

Alarge-bore intravenous catheter should be inserted into a large peripheral vein, not into the central lines, because of increasing risk of infection.

(1)The combination formula of crystalloids and colloids

This formula is developed and widely applied in China. Fluid for first 24 hours (mL)= % TBSA burned ×body weight (kg)×(1.0 mL crystalloids +0.5 mL colloids)+2000 mL(water). Lactated Ringer's solution is commonly used of crystalloids. The first choice of colloids is fresh plasma, other alternatives include frozen fresh plasma, plasma substitute:e. g. ,low molecular dextran, and even whole blood. Here water often means 5%-10% glucose solution. Half of the total volume is infused in the first 8 hours, the other half solution is delivered in the following 16 hours.

(2)The Parkland formula

The Parkland formula, a widely used formula in other countries, is a pure crystalloid resuscitation formula. The Parkland formula for calculating fluid needs for burn victims in the first 24 hours is as follows: Fluid requirement (mL)= (4 mL of crystalloid)× (% TBSA burned)× body weight (kg).

The first half of lactated Ringer's solution is delivered in the first 8 hours, and the remaining half is delivered in the remaining 16 hours. It has been demonstrated that patients can be adequately resuscitated with less fluid and, in turn, less edema if under monitoring serum sodium, a hypertonic salt solution is used instead of lactated Ringer's solution.

The Parkland formulas emphasize only crystalloids is infused during the early stage. Plasma proteins are not infused until after the initial plasma leak in nonburned tissues begins to decrease. This usually occurs 4-8 hours postburn.

1.6.2.2　Monitoring of fluid resuscitation

The volume of fluid calculated on above formulas is only theoretical result. The calculated volume is rarely equal to the required one. So we have to monitor the patients to adjust the infusion rate. The common items to be evidenced adequate resuscitation are as follows:

(1)Basic items

· Pulse: ≤120 beats/min.

· Blood pressure: ≥ 90/60 mmHg.

· Mental status:conscious or arousable, reflecting perfusion of the brain.

· Urine output:reflecting the blood flow of kidneys and other critical organs.

· Children younger than 2 years:1 mL/(lb · h).

· Older children:0.5 mL/(lb · h).

· Adults: ≥ 30-40 mL/h.

· Peripheral circulation:temperature and color, which reflect capillary refill of extremities.

(2)Special items

· CVP(central venous pressure) :5 cmH$_2$O.

· PAWP (pulmonary arterial wedge pressure):6-12 mmHg.

· Blood gas.

1.6.2.3　Management during postresuscitation period

(1)Intravenous fluid

The amount of fluid infused after the second 24 hours depends chiefly on the evaporative loss, sometime it includes the evaporation from the endotracheal intubation or the tracheostomy and the amount related to fever, etc. The fluid consists of glucose in water or hypotonic salt solution to replace evaporative losses and of plasma proteins to maintain adequate circulating volume. The amount of evaporative loss from the wound will be (mL/h):(25×% TBSA burned)×body surface(m^2)

(2)Nutritional support

It should begin as early as possible in the postburn period to maximize wound healing and minimize immune deficiency. Patients with moderate burns may be able to meet nutritional needs by voluntary oral intake. Patients with large bums invariably require calorie and protein supplementation by parenteral and enteral nutrition route.

(3)Antibiotics

Tetanus toxoid,0. 5 mL,should be administered to patients with any significant burn injury. Antibiotics does not be recommended to administrate prophylactically,especial the broad-spectrum antibiotics.

1.6.3   Burn wound management

The burn wound of moderate and large burns patients can't be debrided until intravenous fluids have been started and the vital signs are stabilized. The goals of burn wound care are preventing and /or controlling infection;preserving as much tissue as possible and preventing destruction of remaining viable epithelium;preparing a wound for the earliest possible closure either by primary healing or by grafting. Aggressive and thorough wound care helps to promote rapid healing in deep partial-thickness wound,to protect and promote good granulation tissue until grafting.

1.6.3.1   Circumferential eschar

Circumferential burns of an extremity or of the trunk pose special problems. Swelling beneath the unyielding eschar may act as a tourniquet to blood and lymph flows,and the distal extremity may become swollen and tense. More extensive swelling may compromise the arterial supply. Constriction involving the chest or abdomen may severely restrict ventilation. Escharotomy or excision of the eschar may be required before arterial ischemia develops or ventilation be influenced. The procedure can usually be performed in the patient's room and anesthetics are rarely required.

1.6.3.2   Topical antibacterial agents

All topical antibiotics retard wound healing to some degree and therefore should be used only on deep second-or third-degree burns or wounds with a high risk of infection. Topical agents have definitely advanced the care of burn patients. Although burn wound sepsis is still a major problem,the death rate has been reduced,particularly in burns of less than 50% of body surface area.

Silver sulfadiazine (SD-Ag)is now the most widely used topical antibacterial agent and is moderately effective in penetrating the burn eschar. SD-Ag can be applied directly to the wound or spread on coarse mesh gauze and secured to the wound. The drug prevents invasive burn wound sepsis and reduces mortality. It is particularly effective in burns of 30% -60% of the TBSA,although considerably less protection from infection is observed when the burn covers 60% or more of the TBSA. In any event,wounds are not sterilized by the topical agents,but there is a substantial reduction in bacterial counts in the wound. Mafenide, silver nitrate,povidone iodine,and gentamicin ointments are also used.

Topical antibiotics decrease microbial growth and reduce invasive infection. Prophylactic systemic antibiotics are not recommended because they do not prevent wound sepsis. Systemic antibiotics may be indicated when cellulitis is evident in surrounding unburned tissue.

1.6.3.3   Temporary skin substitutes

For the second-degree burn or the clean excised wound,skin substitutes are another alternative to topical agents and particularly effective. After the initial cleansing and removal blisters,these agents are immediate applied to prevents fluid loss, protects against infection, and stops pain. The resultant healing is associated with minimal scarring.

For this purpose, human skin (homograft) works better but is difficult to obtain. Split-thickness porcine (heterograft) are commercially available and have gained popularity as a biologic dressing that can be applied to clean partial-thickness wounds and to cover primarily excised areas when grafting must be delayed or when auto-grafts are not available. Other alternatives include a number of synthetic skin substitutes such as Biobrane, a thin plastic membrane that reduces water evaporative loss.

1.6.3.4 The operational process of burn wound care

(1) Cleansing

The wound is first gently washed with a mild detergent, sterile normal saline or distilled water, and then made antisepsis by application of mild, chemical antimicrobial agents, such as germicide.

(2) Treatment of burn blisters

The small blister is allowed absorption by itself. A large blister is ruptured with a surgical scissors and forced the blister fluid out, or drained the blister fluid with an injection syringe. After that the blister is retained in place intact. But for the blister of the deep second-degree burn, it is suggested to remove the blister with scissors to prevent infection.

(3) Management of the burn wound

There are two methods to care burn wounds, the closed and exposure technique.

1) The closed technique

The closed technique is suitable to partial-thickness burns of extremities and trunk. The advantages of this method are increasing the rate of reepithelialization and less heat loss. While the disadvantage is the risk of potential increase in bacterial growth, especially the deep second-degree burn.

After wound cleansing and dealing with the blisters, the burn wound is covered with a layer of vaseline gauze or antibiotic ointment, then bandaged with thick, dry and sterile cotton dressings. Fingers and toes should be wrapped individually, with fluffed gauze separating the digits.

For the clean burn wounds, especially superficial scald burns, change dressings every 1-2 days is suitable. If there are infection or excessive amounts of exudates on the wound. Twice-daily dressing changes are indicated.

Occlusive dressings is an alternate method of managing burn wounds and can be applied to a superficial partial-thickness burn that is clean and less than 24 hours post injury. These products such as Biobrane and TransCyte maintain a moist wound environment that enhances healing and eliminates the need for dressing changes. Currently, several different types of commercial occlusive dressings are available.

Superficial burns generally do not require the use of topical antibiotics. Occlusive dressings to minimize exposure to air increase the rate of reepithelialization and decrease pain. If there is no infection, burns will heal spontaneously.

2) The exposure technique

The indication of the exposure technique involves the deep second-or third-degree burns, contaminated wounds or wounds with a high risk of infection and the burned areas that is difficult to be closed, e. g. , face, perineum. Inhibiting the bacterial growth, remaining a wound visible and readily accessible are advantages of exposure method. But increasing pain and heat loss is the disadvantages.

After cleansing and debridement of the third-degree burns wound or some of the deep second-burns wounds with a high risk of infection, topical antibacterial agents, such as Silver sulfadiazine, are applied directly to the wound. And then the patients are placed in a clean, warm, dry environment.

Dry sterile mesh is applied to all areas that tend to remain moist with excessive exudate. The mesh is allowed to adhere for 2-5 minutes and then gently pulled from the wound, removing much of the exudative material. This procedure can be repeated until the area is clean and dry.

Sometimes layers of destroyed skin form a crust in the partial thickness burn. The crust protects underlying tissue from contamination. Healing proceeds beneath it.

The surgeon and patient must be aware that burn wound infection is a continual threat that can cause a partial-thickness burn to be converted to a full-thickness burn. Threat of hypertrophic scar formation, as well as pigmentary skin changes, also should be concerned. Remind patient to use a sun-blocking agent over the healed wounds for at least 6 months after injury to prevent the development of permanent pigmentary changes caused by sun exposure.

1.6.3.5　Debridement and grafting

Debridement is to remove away devitalized or contaminated tissue. The goal is to debride all necrotic tissue and to remove exudate and secretion on the wound so as to promote reepithelialization or formation of healthy granulation tissue. Five categories of debridement are surgical, mechanical, infection, natural enzymatic, and commercially prepared enzymatic.

Surgical management of burn wounds has now become much more aggressive, even beginning within the first several days postburn rather than after eschar has sloughed. Surgical debridement is often used to prepare the wound for skin grafting. Excision of eschar (escharectomy) should be carried down to fascia. Excision to viable tissue, referred to as tangential excision, is advantageous because it provides a vascular base for grafting while preserving remaining viable tissue, especially dermis. Blood loss is substantial in view of the vascularity of the dermis.

The standard management for full-thickness burns is burn wound excision and grafting. The mortality of patients with massive burns is reduced by early escharectomy and tangential excision of the entire wound, followed by skin closure with an autograft from unburned areas of the patient or an allograft, xenograft, or artificial skin. Allograft and xenograft may be usedas biological dressings to temporarily cover denuded areas, particularly in massive burns with insufficient donor sites, to help control infection, prevent serum loss, decrease pain, stimulate formation of epidermis and promote growth of granulation tissue. Permanent skin substitutes composed of both dermis and epidermis have been designed ın order to maintain coverage and improve skin function. But the efficacy of skin substitutes remains uncertain. Donor sites for autograft require 1-2 weeks to heal.

1.7　Prevention and Treatment of Burn Systemic Infection

Infection remains a critical problem in burns, though the mortality has been reduced by modern therapy with topical antibacterial agents. Systemic infections of burns involve bacteremia, septicemia and burn wound sepsis or septic syndrome. They usually occur in the first week after burn, minority in 2-3 weeks postburn. Burn wound sepsis is defined as bacteria growing in the burn wound containing 10^5 bacteria per gram of eschar and involving adjacent normal tissues.

Many of the burn wounds are relatively free of bacteria during the first 24 hours. From 3 days postburn, bacterial colonization increases on the surface of wound, and proliferation occurs into the depths of the hair follicles. The colonizing cells spread from the base of the hair follicles and, by the 4-5 days postburn, extensive involvement of the wound develops. Bacteria in large numbers permeate burn wound and invasion occurs.

Another source of infection is the external contamination of wounds. A concerted effort should also be made to avoid cross contamination between patients.

1.7.1　Clinical findings and diagnosis of burn systemic infection

- Temperature: hyperpyrexia with chill or falling below normal.
- The wound: purulence may be present, or wound surface may appear dry and pale.
- The white count: leukocytosis or may fall.
- Bacterial quantitative culture of the subeschar tissue: usually $> 10^5/g$.
- Pathological test of the subescher tissue: invasive activity of bacteria.
- Blood culture and antibiotic sensitivity testing: blood culture (+).

1.7.2　Treatment of burn systemic infection

(1) Prevention and treatment shock

For the patients with moderate and severe degree burns, if the hypovolemic shock is corrected effectively and easily, the systemic infection comes later and moderately. Otherwise the infection will be violently and earlier.

(2) Care the burn wound correctly

Management of the burn wound to prevent and control burn systemic infection involve effective, timely debridement and removing exudates; promotion formation of fresh granulation tissue; closure the burn wound with skin grafting as early as possible.

(3) Application of topical antibacterial agents and specific systemic antibiotics

Topical antibacterial agents such as SD-Ag should be applied on the wounds with a high risk of infection from the early stage to prevent and control the infection. Systemic antibiotics are generally only given for treatment of bacteremia or sepsis. Once the invasive infection is identified, specific antibiotics should be administered.

(4) Enhancement of the patient's conditions

- Providing nutrition with high calories, high proteins and high vitamins.
- Correcting water electrolyte and acid-base imbalance, and hypoproteinemia, anemia, etc.

1.8　Inhalation Injury

Today the major cause of death after burns is respiratory tract injury or complication in the respiratory tract. The problems include inhalation injury, bacterial pneumonia, pulmonary edema, pulmonary embolism, and posttraumatic pulmonary insufficiency.

Inhalational injury refers to airway and pulmonary problems resulting from thermal injury. Upper airway damage and edema is due to direct heat exposure, which usually does not affect the larynx. Lower airway injury can result from inhalation of a particulate (≤ 5 microns) and chemical damage from incomplete combustion products carried by smoke.

Direct burns to the upper airway are associated with burns of the face, lips, and nasal hairs and necrosis or swelling of the pharyngeal mucosa. Acute edema of the upper tract may cause airway obstruction and asphyxiation without lung damage. Inhalation injury causes severe mucosal edema followed soon by sloughing of the mucosa. The edema fluid enters the airway and, when mixed with the pus in the lumen, may form cast and plugs in the smaller bronchioles. Acute bronchiolitis and bronchopneumonia commonly develop within a few days.

Signs of inhalational injury include stridor, voice change, brassy cough, carbonaceous sputum or carbon particles in the oropharynx, etc. Flame face burns or burns in enclosed spaces are clues to inhalational injury. When inhalation injury is suspected, early endoscopic examination of the airway with fiberoptic bronchoscopy is helpful in determining the area of injury.

Unfortunately, the clinical manifestations of inhalation injury may be subtle and frequently do not appear in the first 24 hours. The severity of the injury can not be accurately quantified by bronchoscopy—it can only be shown that an injury is present. While waiting for evidence of pulmonary injury from an X-ray or a change in blood gas, upper airway edema may preclude intubation, forcing the need for a surgical airway.

Treatment is primarily supportive. The first priority is to assess the patient's airway, breathing and circulation. Others include mechanical ventilation (when indicated), and antibiotics. All patients who initially have evidence of smoke inhalation should receive humidified oxygen in high concentrations.

Laryngeal edema must be anticipated in patients with airway burns. If there is any concern about the patency of the airway, endotracheal intubation is essential and should be performed well in all doubtful cases before manifestation of airway obstruction appears. Because delayed intubation will be difficult to achieve in cases associated with pharyngeal edema or upper airway injury, and an emergency tracheostomy may become necessary later under difficult circumstances. The endotracheal tube should be large enough to allow removal of thick copious secretions during subsequent care.

When endotracheal intubation is used without mechanical ventilation (e. g. , for upper airway obstruction), mist and continuous positive pressure ventilatory assistance should be included. Tracheostomy is indicated in the first several days for patients who are expected to require ventilator support for a few weeks or more. But tracheostomy performed through burned tissue is associated with a prohibitively high complication rate and should only be done if endotracheal intubation is impossible.

Management of inhalation injury should also include frequent evaluation of the lungs throughout the hospital course.

Chapter 2

Electrical Injuries and Chemical Injuries

2.1　Electrical Injuries

There are three kinds of electrical injuries: electrical shock, electrical current injury, and electrothermal burns from arcing current. Occasionally, all three will be present in the same victim.

Arc burns are serious thermal injuries to the skin because the electrical arc has a temperature of about 2500 ℃. Treatment is the same as any other thermal injuries.

In electrical current injury, the severity of injury depends on the voltage and on the resistance provided by various parts of the body. Once current has entered the body, its pathway depends on the resistances it encounters in the various organs. The following are listed in descending order of the resistance: bone, fat, tendon, skin, muscle, blood, and nerve. If the current passes through the heart or the brain stem, death may be immediate from ventricular fibrillation or apnea. Current passing through muscles may cause spasms severe enough to produce long bone fracture or dislocations.

The type of current is also related to the severity of injury. The usual 60 cycle alternating current that causes most injuries in the home is particularly severe. Alternating current causes tetanic contractions, and the patient may become "locked" to the contact. Cardiac arrest is common from contact with house current.

Electrical current injuries are frequently more serious than they appear on the surface, resulting in deep tissue damage. Focal burns occur at the points of entrance and exit through the skin. The entry and exit wounds are usually a depressed gray or yellow area of full thickness destruction surrounded by a sharply defined zone of hyperemia. Thrombosis frequently occurs in vessels deep in an extremity, causing more widely tissue necrosis than the evidence at the initial examination. The greatest muscle injury is usually closest to the bone, where the highest heat of resistance is generated.

Electrical burns can result in rhabdomyolysis and develop compartment syndromes, cardiac arrest and myoglobinuria, which can lead to acute renal failure.

A rapid drop in hematocrit sometimes follows sudden destruction of red blood cells by the electrical energy. Bleeding into deep tissues may occur as a result of disruption of blood vessels. In some cases, thrombosed vessels disintegrate later and cause massive interstitial hemorrhage.

The treatment of electrical injuries depends on the extent of deep muscle and nerve destruction more than any other factors. Management of electrical burns should include paying close attention to the airway and breathing, establishing an IV line in an uninvolved extremity, monitoring the patient with an electrocardiogram and placing an indwelling catheter.

If the patient's urine is dark, it should be assumed that hemochromogens are in the urine. There is no need to wait for lab confirmation before instituting therapy for myoglobinuria. The urine output must be kept 2–3 times of normal with intravenous fluids. And alkalinization of the urine and osmotic diuretics may be indicated.

In general, the treatment of electrical injuries is complex at every step, and after initial resuscitation these patients should be referred to specialized centers.

The lesion should be debrided to underlying healthy tissue. This dead and devitalized tissue must also be excised. A second debridement is usually indicated 24–48 hours after the injury, because the necrosis is found to be more extensive than originally thought. The strategy of obtaining skin covering for these burns can tax ingenuity, because of the extent and depth of the wounds. Microvascular flaps are now used routinely to replace large tissue losses.

2.2　Chemical Injuries

The chemical burn a kind of injury caused by corrosive substances such as a strong acid or base, sulfuric acid (H_2SO_4), hydrochloric acid (HCl), nitric acid, sodium hydroxide (NaOH), etc. Effects depend on the substance. Chemical burns may occur through direct contact on body surfaces, including skin and eyes, via inhalation, and/or by ingestion.

Chemical burns may be extremely painful, and diffuse into tissue and damage structures under skin without immediately apparent damage to skin surface. Hydrofluoric acid, for instance, leaches into the bloodstream and reacts with calcium and magnesium, and the resulting salts can cause cardiac arrest. The degree of the chemical injury is influenced by the concentration and amount of agent and duration of exposure. Chemical burns follow standard burn classification and may cause extensive tissue damage.

Symptoms of a chemical burn include itching, bleaching or darkening of skin, burning sensations, trouble breathing, coughing blood and/or tissue necrosis.

The chemicals should be immediately removed by irrigation with water or brushing it away if it is dry powder. Alkali burns require longer irrigation with water than other chemical burns. The therapeutic principle of the wound is similar to the thermal injuries.

Chapter 3

Frostbite

Frostbite is the medical condition in which localized damage is caused to skin and other tissues due to freezing. Frostbite is most likely to happen in body parts farthest from the heart and those with large exposed areas. The first stage of frostbite is sometimes called frostnip. Two related injuries, trench foot and pernio which are belongs to non-freezing cold injury (NFCI), involve prolonged exposure to wet, cold conditions above freezing. Trench foot is damage to nerves and blood vessels, and is reversible if treated early. Pernio are inflammation of the skin, which can appears as various types of ulcers and blisters.

Frostbite effects can be magnified by moisture or wind. With wind chills approaching the single digits and below zero, it is possible to develop frostnip with progression to frostbite in exposed areas in as little as 20-30 minutes, especially in those patients with peripheral vascular disease, a history of smoking or diabetes.

3.1　Mechanism

Cooling of the body causes vasoconstriction. Frostnip is similar to frostbite, but without ice crystal formation in the skin. In frostbite, the resulting cellular dehydration coupled with ischemia due to vasoconstriction and increased blood viscosity is the mechanisms of tissue injury. Temperatures below -4 ℃ are required to form ice crystals between the cells, which in turn causes damage at the cellular level. Ice crystals can directly damage cell membranes and small blood vessels at the site of injury. Skin and muscle are considerably more susceptible to freezing damage than tendons and bones, which explain why the patient may still be able to move severely frostbitten digits. The risk of frostbite is increased by generalized hypothermia, which produces peripheral vasoconstriction as part of the mechanism for preservation of core body temperature. Scar tissue forms when fibroblasts replace the dead cells.

3.2　Clinical Findings

3.2.1　Frostnip

As the initial stage of frostbite, frostnip can cause skin redness, irritation, and a transient blanching and numbness of exposed parts. It often appears on the tips of fingers, ears, nose, chin, or cheeks. The damage of frostnip is not permanent but if no immediately be detected and be managed by rewarming through contact with warm parts of the body or warm air, frostnip may progress to frostbite.

3.2.2   Frostbite

The initial symptom of frostbitten part is typically numbness. This may be followed by clumsiness with a white or bluish appearance. With superficial frostbite, only the skin and subcutaneous tissues are frozen, so the tissues beneath are still compressible with pressure. Deep frostbite involves freezing of underlying issues, which imparts a wooden consistency to the extremity.

Complications may include hypothermia or compartment syndrome. Hypothermia is life-threatening should be treated first.

3.3   Diagnosis

Diagnosis is based on medical history and symptoms. Historically, frostbite has been classified by degrees according to skin and sensation changes, similar to burn classifications. However, the degrees do not correspond to the amount of long term damage. A simplification of this system of classification is superficial (1st and 2nd degree) or deep injury (3rd and 4th degree). Bone scans, MRI or CT angiography can be done to assess the extent of injury.

3.4   Treatment

Frostnipe should be managed by rewarming through contact with warm parts of the body or warm air. Whitening of the skin and numbness of these parts reverse quickly after rewarming.

The first priority in people with frostbite should be to assess for hypothermia and other life-threatening complications of cold exposure. Before treating frostbite, the core temperature should be raised above 35 ℃. Oral or intravenous (IV) fluids should be given. Other considerations for standard hospital management include as following.

3.4.1   Rewarming

If the area is still partially or fully frozen, it should be rewarmed in the hospital with a warm bath with povidone iodine or chlorhexidine antiseptic. Active rewarming seeks to warm the injured tissue as quickly as possible without burning. The faster tissue is thawed, the less tissue damage occurs. The recommendatory temperature for rewarming is 37–39 ℃. Warming takes 15 minutes to 1 hour. Rewarming can be very painful, so pain management is important. NSAIDs or opioids are recommended during the painful rewarming process.

After rewarming, the frostbitten area becomes mottled blue or purple, painful and tender. Rubbing or applying snow to the affected part is not recommended because it can increase tissue damage.

3.4.2   Medications

Aspirin and ibuprofen can be given to prevent clotting and inflammation. Blood vessel dilating medications such as iloprost may prevent blood vessel blockage. This treatment might be appropriate in grades 2–4 frostbite, when people get treatment within 48 hours. In addition to vasodilators, sympatholytic drugs can be used to counteract the detrimental peripheral vasoconstriction that occurs during frostbite. For severe injuries thrombolytics may be used.

People with potential for large amputations and who present within 24 hours of injury can be given TPA with heparin. These medications should be withheld if there are any contraindications.

Tetanus toxoid should be administered according to local guidelines. Uncomplicated frostbite wounds are not known to encourage tetanus. If there is trauma, skin infection or severe injury, antibiotics should also be administered.

3.4.3　Wound care

Swelling or blistering may occur following treatment. The blisters can be drained by needle aspiration, unless they are bloody (hemorrhagic). Then the wound is covered by protective dressings or bandages.

3.4.4　Surgery

Various types of surgery might be indicated in frostbite injury, depending on the type and extent of damage. Debridement or amputation of necrotic tissue is usually delayed for a few months to allow determination of the extent of injury unless there is gangrene or systemic infection. If symptoms of compartment syndrome develop, fasciotomy can be done to attempt to preserve blood flow.

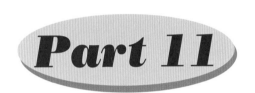

Part 11

Tumors

Tumor is very complicated and oncology is about the science of tumor. Clinical oncology will play an important role in this era.

Some basic concept in oncology:

Tumor: Tumor originally refered to any mass or swelling. The present meaning is generally synonymous with neoplasm (a new pathologic growth tissue). A neoplasm may be characterized as benign or malignant depending upon histologic and gross clinical features. From the molecular level, tumor is a kind of disorder of gene.

Malignant tumor: Usually show imperfect differentiation and structure atypical of tissue of origin, an infiltrative growth pattern not contained by a true capsule, frequent and abnormal mitotic figures. Growth rarely ceases, although the rate of growth may be irregular, and many malignant tumors have a propensity for metastasis.

Usually show imperfect differentiation and structure atypical compere with tissue of origin, an infiltrative growth pattern and not contained by a true capsule, frequent and abnormal mitotic. Growth of malignant tumors rarely stop although the rate of growth may be irregular. Many malignant tumors have a propensity for metastasis.

Benign tumor: Usually lack these features above mentioned, but occasionally it may be fatal as a result of impaction of other structures and impairment of function. For exmple, adenoma, papilloma, fibroma and so on.

Sarcoma and carcinoma: Neoplasms are classified according to their tissue of origin. Those from mesenchyma tissue (muscle, bone, fat, vessels, or lymphoid or connective tissue) are called sarcomas. Malignant tumors from epithelial origin are called carcinomas. According to their histologic appearance, as adenocarinoma, squamous, transitional, or undifferentiated carcinoma.

Epidemiology of tumor: Epidemiology of tumor research the distribution of tumor among population, including to the distributions of region, time, sex, age and so on. Its purpose is to identify the various factors which correlated with tumorigenesis, and in order to take effivtive measure to prevent tumorigenisis.

Molecular epidemiology research tumorigenesis is at the gene and protein level. It is a hot spot of tumor epidemiology.

Chapter 1

Etiology

The factors that result in tumor are very complicated. Up to now, though there are so many researches which want to interpret the causes of tumor, it is now impossible to really elucidate the etiopathology.

Some causes which are related with tumor are as follows:

(1)Chemical carcinogenesis: For example, waste gas, smoking and lung carcinoma. The cause of epithelial cancers (e. g., lung, esophageal, head and neck, gastric, pancreatic, and colon cancers)involves exposureto chemical carcinogens, high fat diet, smoking, alcohol, etc.

(2)Physical factors: For example, X-rays, cosmic ray, ultraviolet ray and skin cancer. Ionizing radiation disrupts chromosomes. Genes are broken apart in the malignancy. Encoded protein are also destructed.

(3)Biological factors: Mould may result in esophagus cancer. HP (is a kind of bacteria) and stomach cancer. EB(Epstein-Barr) virus and nasopharynx cancer. HBV(Hepatitis B virus) and liver cancer.

(4)Genetic factors: This is a hot spot of research now. For example, BRCA1, BRCA2 and breast cancer. In general, there are genetic characteristics in 5% tumor patients.

Chapter 2

Pathology of Tumor

Pathology of tumor has great prognostic value, enables prediction of probable biologic behavior. It is the only certain method of diagnosis and classification at this time.

Some basic concept:

(1) Precancerous lesions

There are certain states or conditions that predispose to the subsequent of tumor, particularly cancer. Such precancerous states are important from the clinical viewpoint because by recognition and treatment of them it may be possible to prevent subsquent cancer from arising, even though one does not understand the exact cause of the cancer. The few terms mentioned here will give an idea as to the scope of changes that have been suggested: ①Achlorhydria often precedes the development of cancer of the stomach. ②Cirrhosis precedes most liver cancer.

(2) Anaplasia

Anaplasia is a term implying a change in a cell or tissue from a more to a less highly differentiated form. A synonym is "dedifferentiation", implying that the cells or tissue have become more primitive, even embryonic. The term is used primarily to describe cancers and infrequently for nonneoplastic cellular proliferations.

(3) Carcinoma in situ

Carcinoma is located in mucosa.

(4) Atypical hyperplasia, or dysplasia

Dysplasia is a change affecting the size, shape, and orientationalrelationship of adult types of cell, primarily epithelial cells. Such cells exhibit pleomorphism that is vary in size and shape, posses larger hyperchrommatic nuclei and exhibit an increase in their nucleus cytoplasm ratio (Table 11-1-1).

Table 11-1-1　General morphologic features

Benign	Malignant
circumscribed	no capsule
noninvasive	invasive
no direct destruction tissue	destroys tissue
nuclear uniformity	nuclear pliomorphism

Continue to Table 11-1-1

Benign	Malignant
normal nuclear chromatin content; ploidy	increased nuclear chromatin; often polyploid or aneuploid
nucleocytoplasmic ratio near normal	nucleocytoplasmic high ratio
nucleoli normal	nucleoli prominent
structure simulates normal	structure parodies normal
cytoplasm less basophilic	cytoplasm more basophilic
cells polarized (put in order)	cells disoriented

Chapter 3

Diagnosis of Tumor

3.1 History

Mass is the most usual symptom. Bleeding is also an usual symptom, and it may result in anemia. Pain is a kind of symptom of the advanced tumor, in general, it is a chronic pain, not acute pain. Tumor itself is not pain, if only when tumor infiltrates the capsule of organ or nerves, the pain is likely to be emerged. Fever is a systematic symptom. Fatigue is a commonly stated or implied complaint that brings the patients to the oncologist's attention. Weight loss is an useful working definition for involuntary (weight loss is the loss of 5% of usual body weight over the previous 6 months, document by medical records). Unexplained significant involuntary weight loss is frequently a clue that has serious diseases.

A cancer produces symptoms largely because the primary tumor mass or its metastasis interfere with normal organ functions. For example, nausea and vomiting, diarrhea, superior vena cava syndrome. It may also produce remote effects on other organ not directly involved with the neoplasm. These remote effects are termed paraneoplastic syndrome. They occur in about 10% of patients with cancer, and occasionally they represent the first sign of the disease. The endocrine effects are understood best, since many cancers produce hormones or substances that mimic the physiologic effects hormones.

3.2 Physical Examination

It is analogous to physician's physical examination. The important point is mass's size, shape, border, hardened degree, activity and lymphatic node conditions.

3.3 Laboratory Examination

It includes serum assessment(CEA, PSA, AFP), etc. Occult blood in the stool is for gastric and colon and rectum cancer.

3.4   Special Examination

For example, aspiration of breast mass, needle biopsy, mammography, ultrasonography for breast cancer. Bone scan for bone metastasis. Upper gastrointestinal (GI) X-rays and upper GI endoscopy will evaluate gastric carcinoma. Ultrasound, CT, MRI for liver cancer. Barium contrast radiography is for colon and rectum cancer.

3.5   Pathological Examination

It is the only certain method of diagnosis and classification for carcinoma and sarcoma at this time. Histologic grading can also determine the degree of anaplasia of tumor cell, varying from grade I (very well differentiated) to the grade IV (undifferentiated).

Some Concept in Diagnosis:

(1) Staging of tumor

Staging of cancer is based upon the extent of its spread and has been degree of local extension at the primary site, N refers to the clinical findings in regional nodes, and M to the presence of distant metastasis. For example, in breast cancer T1 denotes <2 cm in diameter, N0 denotes no metastasis in axillary lymph nodes, and M1 means the appearance of distant metastasis.

An accurate delineation of the stage and the extent of disease is an important initial step in consideration of the most appropriate treatment for the patient.

(2) Tumor marker

Maybe demonstrated chemically by immunoassay or in tissue by immunohistochemically methods. Consist of protein, peptide hormone, and enzymatic moieties that are found in tumor cells, as well as released into circulation. In addition, intracellular filaments and surface elements may identify certain types of cells. For example, cytokeratin and membrane antigen: CEA, AFP, PSA, etc. It is helpful in diagnosis and follow up.

Chapter 4

Treatment of Tumor

4.1 Surgical Treatment

Surgical excision is the most effective means of removing the primary lesion of most neoplasms and achieves a higher rate of primary control than any other form of therapy. Resection of incurable but symptomatic tumors or bypass of unresectable tumors that obstruct the intestinal tract or bile ducts may provide worthwhile palliation. In a number of highly malignant tumors, where wide excision is impossible or would cause major deformity, excision with narrow margins combined with radiation and chemotherapy has been successfully employed.

Oncology surgery is different from general surgery. Oncology surgeon must have much knowledge about tumor. Except for the no bacteria principle, the no tumor principle is very important. For example: ①no touch isolation technique. ②en-bloc dissection of all tissue. ③early control of the venous supply to prevent tumor cell from embolization during manipulation of the tumor.

The mode of treatment chosen should ideally: ①prevent the development of the distant metastatic disease in those patients whose tumors have not yet seeded the lymphatics or the blood stream. ②prevent local recurrence of tumor. There are several methods of operation:

Radical operation: It is an offering hope of curing cancer of tumor. The results of such therapy, however, are profoundly affected by the growth rate of the cancer cells and the degree of host resistance. Neither of these factors can, at present, be identified or measured. Some standard radical operations include radical mastectomy, total gastrectomy, proximal or distant subtotal gastrectomy, colostomy, etc.

Palliative operation: The survival rate of palliative cases was generally poor. Relief of pyloric obstruction bypass, arrest of persistent bleeding.

Prophylactic operation: Prophylactic mastectomy for breast that are predisposed to cancer is in controversy. Ulcerative colitis may operate total removal of colonand rectum.

New techniques of oncology surgery: For example, sentinel lymphatic node biopsy is a kind of new technique for early breast cancer in order to remain patient's axillary.

4.2 Radiation Therapy

Radiation therapy deals with the treatment of disease using ionizing radiation. Since most diseases treated by radiation therapy are malignant tumors, radiation therapy actually a branch of oncology. Radiation therapy is the treatment of the choice for the control of cancer in many sites. In other situations it used in conjunction with surgery or chemotherapy. It is used for the relief of symptoms resulting from cancer.

(1) Radiation sources

The radiations commonly used in radiotherapy include X−rays, gamma rays, electrons and beta rays. These rays may be able to destroy protein or synthesize DNA, so as to result in tumor cell death.

(2) Preoperative radiation therapy

By killing the majority of cancer cell prior to resection, radiation therapy reduce the possibility of seeding or dissemination of viable cancer cells during surgery.

(3) Postoperative radiation therapy

When the surgical margins are close or positive, or when the risk of local recurrence is great because of extensive tumor invasion, postoperative radiation therapy is usually indicated.

(4) Intraoperative radiation therapy

It is a new radiotherapy modalities. It involves the administration of radiotherapy to microscopic or gross residual disease during an operation procedures. It can be delivered a large single dose. Normal tissue must be excluded from the radiation field.

(5) Three dimensional conformed radiotherapy

It involves the use of computerized imaging techniques and three dimensional computerized treatment planning system.

4.3 Chemotherapy

4.3.1 Scientific basis (selective toxicity)

①The qualitative approach: The chemotherapy drug have the selective toxicity against replicating tumor cells but which at the same time spare replicating host tissue. Such an ideal drug has not yet been found. ②The quantitative kinetic approach: According to quantitative difference in the proliferative kinetics of normal and neoplastic cell growth, chemotherapy is to be achieved.

4.3.2 Goal of chemotherapy

Curative chemotherapy is used for the tumors such as many Wilm's tumor, some testicular carcinomas in young men. Palliative chemotherapy may afford significant palliation and prolongation of life, e. g. , advanced breast cancer, ovarian cancer.

4.3.3 New adjuvant chemotherapy

New adjuvant chemotherapy is achieved before operation. Its purpose is to reduce tumor bulk and to kill micrometastasis.

Side effects:Nausea and vomiting is the most frequent toxicities. Bone marrow is restrained.

Combination chemotherapy blocks multiple biosynthetic pathways and are given in an attempt to exert a synergistic effect on the tumor. The drugs of a combination are selected to avoid overlapping toxicity. This approach has been of greatest value where no single agent is highly effective. For example, CMF, CAF, CAP, ELF. (C:cyclophosphamide, M:methotrexate, A:doxorubicin, F:fluorouracil, P:cisplatin.)

4.4 Immunotherapy

Better understanding of cellular and humoral immune mechanisms in the past decade has led to a different approach to cancer treatment. Terms for these new therapies include the following:

Antibodies in cancer treatment:Monoclonal antibodies that selectively react with human tumor associated antigens have now been used for tumor immunotherapy (e. g. ,Herceptin).

Nonspecific immunotherapy:In an effort to augment the endogenous host defenses,a number of agents have tested as nonspecific immunotherapy (e. g. ,bacilli calmette guerin).

Cytokines:Tumor necrosis factor (TNF) ,Interferon (INF) ,Interleukin (IL) and so on.

Adoptive immunotherapy:Circulating lymphocytes harvested from the patient were stimulated by IL-2 to proliferate in culture,and these autologous lymphokine-activated killer (LAK) cells were returned to the patients.

Active specific immunotherapy:Augmentation of antitumor immunity through the use of autologous tumor cell vaccines or immunization of the cancer patient with purified cellular components shared by many tumors has yet to produce worthwhile result. Current far efforts are directed at finding tumor antigens that are more immunogenic. A novel approach so far confined to animal studies is to transfect tumor cells with various cytokines before vaccination. The cytokine secreting cell are more likely to trigger an immune response toward otherwise weakly immunogenic tumor cells.

4.5 Pain Palliation in Cancer

Malignant disease may cause pain by obstruction of a hollow viscus,by destruction of the supporting architecture of weight bearing bones,by infiltration of nerve roots or plexusesby tumor. Pain may be controlled by decreasing tumor bulk by radiation,surgery,and chemotherapy. However,these measures are only temporarily or partially effective,and nonspecific symptomatic treatment of pain is required. WHO has indicated a principle that guide treatment of pain (see the detail at https://www. nccn. org/).

4.6 Other Therapy

(1) Interventional oncology:Take Seldinger technique (digital subtractive angiography, DSA) , and take advantage of needle,guide wire,catheter and introducer to inject drugs into tumor.

(2)Laser therapy and other local treatment methods.

(3)Traditional Chinese medicine therapy:This is a very useful therapy that had been used for 2000 years or so. At present,Chinese including you should research it.

Part 12

Organ Transplantation

Chapter 1

Summary

1.1 Overview

The concept of tissue replacement, or transplantation, is a medical technique of implant an organ or tissue from an individual to another part of his body or to another individual, so as to, it can be kept beyond the useful life of the organ or tissue. According to the different transplant, it can be divided into cell transplantation, tissue transplantation and organ transplantation. The individual that provides transplant is called donor, while the individual receiving the transplant is called recipient.

1.2 Brief History of Transplantation

The development of modern human transplantation is one of the most outstanding achievements in western medicine in the 20th century. In 1818, the first successful blood transfusion by an obstetrician, James Blundell, was the first cell transplantation. In 1905, Dr. Eduard Zirm successfully completed the first corneal transplantation in the world. The next year a kidney transplantation was attempted in France. During World War II, allogenic skin was transplanted to the wound of burn patient. Unfortunately, it failed because of rejection. In 1945, Owen reported the immune tolerance induced by allogeneic antigens. In 1953, Medawar made a further study of allogenic skin transplantation in mice and verified Owen's observation. It is revealed that when immune cells are in development stage, they can be induced artificially to tolerance to non-self-antigens. It laid the foundation for modern transplantation biology. In 1954, Murray et al. performed a successful kidney transplantation between genetically identical twins, indicating that organ transplantation entered the stage of clinical application. In 1960s, the first generation of immunosuppressive drugs (azathioprine, prednisone and anti-lymphocyte serum) and the improvement of organ preservation technique and vascular anastomosis technique have made a steady development of organ transplantation. After that, spleen transplantation (Woodruff, 1966), primary liver transplantation (Starzl, 1963), lung transplantation (Hardy, 1963), pancreas transplantation (Kelly, 1966), heart transplantation (Barnard, 1967), heart-lung transplantation (Cooley, 1968), and small intestine transplantation (Detterling, 1968) were carried out. Especially in the late 1970s and early 1980s, the advent of cyclosporine, a new immunosuppressive agent, improved the survival rate and the efficacy of organ transplantation. In recent years, due to the large increase of transplant cases, the shortage of donor is very prominent. Therefore, relatives as living donors, as well as patients with cardiac and brain death as deceased donors partially alleviated the shortage of human organs and tissues. In 1905, the world's first renal xenotransplantation was carried out. In the 1960s and 1980s, 8 cases of renal xenotransplantation, 3 cases of liver xenotransplantation and 2 heart xenotransplantation were reported, and the xenografts are from orangutans, monkeys and baboons. But severe rejection is still an insuperable obstacle to xenotransplantation. In the 21st century, the research and application of clinical transplantation have been brought to a climax again. Cell transplantation, such as bone marrow transplantation and islet transplantation have achieved remarkable results. Solid organ transplantation such as kidney, liver, pancreas, heart transplantation and multi-organ transplantation has become an effective way to treat end-stage diseases. In the last few years, there has been a breakthrough in regenerative medicine. Alexander Seifalian's laboratory inUniversity of London UK has developed a variety of human organs, such as noses, ears, tracheas and arteries. And in July 2011, they participated in the world's first artificial trachea transplantation successfully.

1.3   Classification

According to the individual, it can be divided into auto-transplantation and allo-transplantation. According to different implantation sites, it can be divided into orthotopic transplantation and heterotopic transplantation. According to the gene relationship between donor and recipient, grafts can be classified into autograft, isograft, allograft and xenograft. An auto graft is transplanted from one site of the body to another in the same individual. An isograft is transferred between genetically identical individuals, and no rejection will occur after transplantation. An allograft is transplanted between genetically dissimilar individuals of the same species, and rejection may occur after transplantation. A xenograft is tissue that is transferred between different species, and severe rejection will occur after transplantation. According to whether the donor survives, it can be divided into deceased donor transplantation and living donor transplantation. The former transplant comes from the donor of cardiac and brain death, and the latter transplant comes from natural persons who voluntarily donate their organs according to law.

Cell transplantation refers to the technique of transferring amount of living cells with a certain function into the recipient's blood vessel, body cavity, tissue or organ. The main indication is to replenish the cells that decreased or function reduced in vivo. Bone marrow transplantation and hematopoietic stem cell transplantation can be used for the treatment of hereditary immunodeficiency diseases, severe thalassemia, severe aplastic anemia, all kinds of hematologic malignancy including leukemia. In addition, islet cell transplantation for the treatment of diabetes mellitus, splenocyte transplantation for severe hemophilia, testicular Leydig cell transplantation for male sexual dysfunction (male hypoandrogenisim) and so on.

Tissue transplantation refers to transplant a kind of tissue such as cornea, skin, fascia, tendon, cartilage, bone, vessel, or the whole combination of several tissues such as cutaneous-muscular flap. Generally, autograft or allograft transplantation is usually used to repair the defect of some tissue. Living transplantation is mainly auto-transplantation. Autologous flap, muscle, nerve, bone and omentum majus transplantation can be performed through microsurgical techniques for blood vessels and/or nerves anastomosis. It is most commonly used for repairing wound skin defect with autologous skin transplantation.

Organ transplantation mainly refers to the transplantation of the whole or part of the solid organ and the reconstruction of the vascular and other functional pipeline structures, such as kidney, liver, heart, pancreas, lung, small intestine, spleen transplantation, and heart – lung, liver – kidney, pancreas – kidney, abdominal multiple organ transplantation.

Chapter 2

The Mechanism of Transplantation

2.1　Transplantation Immunology

At present, clinical transplantation is mostly allograft, and rejection is the biggest obstacle to successful transplantation. Rejection is an immunologic attempt to destroy foreign tissue after transplantation, with features of adaptive immune response, such as specificity and memorability, including T-cell-mediated cellular immune response and antibody mediated humoral immune response.

2.2　Transplantation Antigen

Transplantation antigen is antigen from donor transplant and can cause immune response, including major histocompatibility complex molecules (MHC), minor histocompatibility antigens (mH antigens) and endothelial glycoproteins (such as blood group antigens).

Histocompatibility refers to the degree of acceptance between recipient and transplant tissue or organ in different individuals. MHC molecules is the strongest antigen for transplantation, located on the short arm of the sixth chromosome in human. The MHC molecules are found by serological methods in white blood cells, so they are also called human leucocyte antigen (HLA). HLA is divided into three types of molecules, in which Class I and Class II HLA molecules are related to transplantation. Class I antigens are cataloged as HLA-A, B, or C. These antigens are expressed on almost all the surfaces of the nucleated cells. Class II antigens are cataloged as HLA-DR, DQ, or DP. These antigens are present on the surfaces of antigen presenting cells (APC), such as dendritic cells, macrophages, B-cells and other cells with antigen presenting function. The main reason for acute rejection is the MHC difference between donor and recipient because of the polymorphism of MHC.

mH antigens may cause weak rejection, including gender-related antigens (such as H-Y antigens), mH antigens expressed in non-Y chromosome chained leukemia cells or normal cell and so on. The peptide fragments formed by degradation of mH antigens have the same antigenic determinant with allografts, and can be recognized by T-cells in restriction.

ABO blood group antigens can also be expressed in vascular endothelium. When not meet the requirements of transfusion, ABO antigens can bind to the preformed antibodies in recipient, activating complements and coagulation response and then endothelial necrosis with vascular thrombosis occurs, leading to hyperacute rejection.

2.3　Recognization and Immune Response of Antigen

Recognition of transplantation antigen is divided into direct recognition and indirect recognition. Direct recognition refers to the antigen presenting cells from the donor migrate to the secondary lymphoid tissues (lymph nodes and spleen) via the blood. The MHC molecules or antigen peptide-MHC molecule complexes are presented directly to the recipient lymphocytes to be identified and responded. Indirect identification means that the detached cells or antigens of the donor graft are absorbed, processed by the antigen presenting cells in recipient. They are activated by T-cells in the form of antigen peptide-Class II MHC molecule complexes. Th-cells can secrete cytokines to promote proliferation for themselves after activated. At the same time, they can also activate CD8 positive cytotoxic T-cells and B-cells. Cytotoxic T-cells can damage the target cells of transplanted organs by secreting perforin and granzyme. B-cells can be converted into plasma cells, secreting antibodies, damaging the graft by humoral immunity or antibody-mediated cellular immune response. The immunoglobulin antibodies expressed on each B-cell surface are antigen-specific. IgD and IgM antibodies were expressed in the stationary phase B-cells. With the stimulation of antigens and cytokines, the antibody phenotype has changed. IgM and IgG are expressed in endogenous intravascular immune responses. IgM was expressed firstly, and then IgG gradually increased with the consumption of IgM. The ability of primed B-cells to increase the affinity of antibodies is called somatic hypermutation. Preformed antibodies such as ABO blood group antibodies and anti-MHC antibodies can activate complements and coagulation reactions, leading to vascular endothelial injury and intravascular coagulation. It is generally believed that direct recognition plays an important role in early acute rejection, and indirect recognition as the synergy. But in the late of acute rejection or chronic rejection, indirect recognition is more important.

2.4　Mechanism and Classification of Rejection

After organ transplantation, there are two different types of rejection due to different directions of immune response: one is host versus graft reaction (HVGR), the other is graft versus host reaction (GVHR). So-called rejection in clinic often means HVGR. According to the mechanism, rejection can be classified into T-cell-mediated rejection and antibody mediated rejection. According to the histological manifestations, it can be further classified into acute/chronic T-cell-mediated rejection and acute/chronic antibodies mediated rejection. For types of clinically identified rejection occur. The forms of allograft rejection are classified according to the time of occurrence and the immune mechanism involved: hyperacute rejection, accelerated acute rejection, acute rejection and chronic rejection.

Hyperacute rejection (HAR) is associated with preformed antibodies in the recipients directed toward either ABO blood group or HLA antigens. It occurs minutes to several hours after graft implantation. Preformed antibodies quickly bind to the graft endothelial cells, activating complements and coagulation response. Then histolysis and endothelial necrosis with vascular thrombosis occurs. It can be seen that the graft swelling, color darkening and blood flow decreasing. And the graft becomes soft and nonelastic, and then loses its function rapidly. The pathological features are extensive acute arteritis with thrombosis. It can be observed that obvious edema, hemorrhage and necrosis of the organ parenchyma. Thrombus is formed in capillaries and small blood vessels. Polymorphonuclear granulocyte infiltration and fibrous necrosis can be seen at the wall of the vessels. Once HAR occurs, the only way is to remove the graft and prepare for re-transplantation. It can be prevented by preoperative ABO blood group matching, lymphocyte toxicity test and anti-HLA antibody test.

Accelerated acute rejection is also called vascular rejection. It is usually caused by the low concentration of preformed antibodies against the graft in recipient, which is a typical humoral immune response, similar to hyperacute rejection. Damages are usually caused by antigen-mediated cytotoxicity and antibody-dependent cell-mediated cytotoxicity. It usually occurs 3-5 days after transplantation, which can result in transplant dysfunction rapidly, decline or failure of the graft function. The main pathological features are small vascular inflammation and fibrous necrosis of the vessels wall, as well as hemorrhage or infarction of the organ parenchyma. It is difficult to reverse accelerated acute rejection by immunosuppressive agents.

Acute rejection (AR) is the most common type of rejection in clinic. Both cellular immunity and humoral immunity play an important role in it. It was believed that the acute rejection occurred mainly within 3 months after transplantation. But due to the application of strong immunosuppressive agents, it did not have a definite time concept, and could be seen at any time after transplantation. There is no characteristic clinical manifestation when rejection is lightly, and it should be differentiated from primary graft dysfunction and toxic side effects of immunosuppressive agents. At present, no reliable biochemical or immunological indicators are available for early diagnosis, and the final diagnosis is still based on pathological examination. Its pathological features are obvious infiltration of inflammatory cells, including lymphocytes, monocytes and plasma cells, sometimes neutrophils and eosinophils can be observed as well. Once diagnosed, it should be treated as early as possible. High dose of corticosteroids or adjustment of immunosuppressive agents are usually effective.

Chronic rejection (CR) is a common cause of transplant dysfunction. Some have been found after biopsy for several months after transplantation. The mechanism of chronic rejection is remained unclear. Immune factors are treated as the main reason, such as recurrent acute rejection and chronic rejection promoted by various non-immune factors. Eventually, the transplant loses its function. The clinical manifestation is the decline of the function of the transplant. The main pathological features are that the transplant artery intima is thickened by repeated immune injury and repair, leading to vasculopathy in graft, which finally results in widespread graft ischemia, fibrosis even loss of function. At present, immunosuppressive agents is not effective in chronic rejection, which is one of the biggest obstacles in organ transplantation.

Graft versus host reaction (GVHR) is caused by the specific lymphocytes in the graft recognizing the host antigen, leading to a transplantation failure. It can induce graft versus host disease (GVHD) and cause multiple organ dysfunction syndrome (MODS) and death of the recipient.

2.5 Prevention and Treatment of Rejection

Cross match includes the following four aspects: ①Donor's ABO blood group should match with recipient. ②HLA cross-matching; HLA-A, B and DR loci are associated with transplantation. It is better to choose HLA cross-matching donors. It is generally believed that HLA-DR locus has the greatest long-term significance for kidney and heart transplantation recipients and graft survival, followed by HLA−B locus. The influence of HLA−A is small, and remains unclear on liver transplantation. ③Panel reactive antibody (PRA) test is used to detect the preformed HLA antibodies. More than 10% is regarded as positive. Transplantation, pregnancy and blood transfusion may cause sensitization of therecipient. ④Lymphocyte toxicity test: The potential donor's lymphocytes serve as antigen, plus recipient's serum, under the action of complement, then antigen antibody reaction occurs. Cross−matching test positive (>10%) is a contraindication for organ transplantation, especially for kidney transplantation and heart transplantation.

Immunosuppressive drug therapy is usually used in transplantation. Clinical treatment of acute rejection can be divided into basic treatment and resuscitation. Basic treatment is to apply immunosuppressive agents to prevent rejection effectively. The dosage of immunosuppressive agents in early postoperative period is higher because of immune response occurring just after graft implanted, and this period is called induction stage. Subsequently, it can be reduced gradually to prevent the occurrence of acute rejection, which is called maintenance stage. Generally, immunosuppressive agents should be taken for whole life. When acute rejection occurs, it is necessary to increase the dosage of immunosuppressive agents or adjust the combination to reverse the rejection, which is called rescue therapy. Clinical immunosuppressive agents include immuno−induction drugs and immuno−maintenance drugs.

(1) Immuno−induction drugs can be classified as follows:

1) Lymphocyte inhibitors are immunoglobulins including polyclonal antibodies and monoclonal antibodies. Polyclonal antibodies are extracted from serum and can directly produce cytotoxic effects on lymphocytes and dissolve them, such as antilymphocyte globulin (ALG) and antithymocyte globulin (ATG). It is mainly used in immuno−induction stage and corticosteroid−resistant rejection.

2) Monoclonal antibody: ①Anti−CD3 mAb is mainly OKT3, a kind of mouse anti human CD3 molecules antibody on the surface of lymphocyte, and it can inhibit the activity of T−cells and the expression of various cytokines. It can be used for immuno−induction and corticosteroid−resistant rejection. ②Anti−IL−2R mAb such as basiliximabt and daclizumab can combine with Tac site on IL−2R selectively, mainly used for immuno−induction. ③Anti−CD20 mAb (rituximab): CD20 is a transmembrane protein expressed on the surface of mature B−cells and pre−B−cells, and not expressed in the progenitor B−cells and mature plasma cells. CD20 plays an important regulatory role in cell cycle and differentiation. Fab fragments from rituximab can bind to CD20 antigens on the surface of B−cells, leading to the dissolution of B−cells. Initially, it was mainly used for lymphatic proliferative diseases after organ transplantation. Now rituximab is used in combination with immunosuppressive agents, plasma exchange and high dose intravenous immunoglobulin, to inhibit autoantibodies mediated immune response in recipients. It is also used to prevent rejection for kidney transplantation, which is incompatible with blood type.

3) Intravenous immunoglobulin (IVIG) is made from the plasma of the blood bank, containing all antibodies of normal population. It can be used for ABO incompatible and cross−matching positive recipients.

(2) Immuno−maintenance drugs can be classified as follows:

1) Corticosteroids include hydrocortisone sodium succinate, methylprednisolone sodium succinate, prednisone, prednisolone and dexamethasone. They have strong inhibitory effects on mononuclear macrophages, neutrophils, T−cells and B−cells. Corticosteroids are not only used in combination with anti−proliferation drugs and/or calcineurin inhibitors for basic treatment, but also the first choice for acute rejection. However, they can cause several side effects so that small doses are often used and low doses are used for maintenance.

2) Anti−proliferation drugs: Azathioprine (Aza) can inhibit nucleic acid synthesis, also can inhibit

T-cells proliferation significantly. The main side effects of azathioprine are liver and kidney toxicity and bone marrow depression. Mycophenolate mofetil (MMF) can inhibit the proliferation of lymphocytes and inhibit the generation of antibodies. The main side effect of mycophenolate mofetil is gastrointestinal side effect, and bone marrow depression is weak contrasted with azathioprine. Mycophenolate mofetil is often used for maintenance therapy. Leflunomide (a kind of pyrimidine antimetabolites) and its ramification and other inhibitors such as cyclophosphamide (CTX) are rarely used in clinic because of their toxic side effects.

3) T-cell-mediated immunosuppressive agents: ①Calcineurin inhibitors are the most essential drugs for immuno-maintenance, including cyclosporine A (CsA) and tacrolimus (TAC, FK506). CsA can be combined with Cyclophilin (CyP) in the cytoplasm of T-cells, and then tightly bound to calcineurin-calmodulin complex, which further inhibits the activation of calcium dependent phosphorylation and transcriptional regulatory factor NF-AT. It inhibits the expression of cytokines necessary for the activation of T-cells such as IL-2, and then inhibits the activation and proliferation of T-cells. TAC can bind to the FK binding protein in the cytoplasm, and then inhibit the activation and proliferation of T-cells similar to CsA. ②mTOR (target of rapamycin) inhibitors, such as rapamycin and everolimus, which can influence the downstream of the IL-2R signal transduction pathway. The immunosuppressive effect of mTOR inhibitors is to keep the cell cycle in G1 and S phase. mTOR inhibitors can be used combined with calcineurin inhibitors.

4) Lymphocyte isolator: The main mechanism of fingolimod (FTY720) is to inhibit the outflow of lymphocytes in peripheral lymphoid organs, and it can strengthen the connection of endothelial cells.

The ideal immunosuppressive therapy requires that the graft not be rejected, and has the least effects on the immune system. The basic principle of immunosuppressive agents is the combination of drugs, to increase curative effects and decrease toxic and side effects. Now the most used therapeutic regimen is a calcineurin inhibitor (CsA or FK506) combined with corticosteroid and proliferation inhibitor (Aza or MMF). And it can be modified to four or two drugs combination according to the condition. Generally, immunosuppressive agents should be taken for whole life. However, a small number of patients can maintain very few doses or completely stop using immunosuppressive agents after a long period, and achieve "clinical tolerance" or "almost tolerable" state.

2.6 Transplantation Tolerance

Transplantation tolerance refers to that the recipient immune system does not reject the graft without any immunosuppressive agents, and maintains the immune response to other antigens, thus the graft can survive for a long time. According to the mechanism, transplantation tolerance can be divided into central immune tolerance and peripheral immune tolerance. Central immune tolerance is refers to the tolerance produced by T-cells and B-cells from central organs. Peripheral immune tolerance is the same but lymphocytes are from peripheral lymphoid organs. In the process of differentiation and maturation, T-cells or B-cells have encountered self-antigens or exogenous antigens ever and generated tolerance for them. Induction of immune tolerance is an ideal strategy to solve clinical rejection and avoid toxic side effects of immunosuppressive agents. The methods to induction include injection of antigens in thymus, blocking costimulatory molecules, induction of mixed chimera, elimination of T-cells, regulating T-cell pathway, etc. Although the above methods have some effects in animal experiments, it is still difficult to produce reliable immune tolerance in clinic.

Chapter 3

Organ and Tissue Donation

3.1　Donor Management

Organs and tissues for transplantation come from either deceased donors or living donors. Deceased donors are the major source of graft tissues in China. In countries with no relevant legislation, or in countries with legislation but there are also religious and cultural influences, family donors are the only source of organs. Patients with brain death or cardiac death can be potential donors. Because of the shortage of organs, it is widely accepted by the medical community that living relatives have been donors for kidney and liver.

It is best to choose the organs from the young donors. With the accumulation of transplantation experience, and the shortage of organs, donors' age is no longer strictly limited. Donors for lung andpancreas should be younger than 55 years old. For heart, kidney and liver, it should be no more than 60,65 and 70 years old. Organs from people older than 70 are rarely used for transplantation. In theory, the volume of organs for transplantation (especially liver)should match those of the recipient.

The following conditions are contraindicated as donors for organ transplantation: Patients with systemic infections and positive blood cultures or not be cured completely, patients with human immunodeficiency virus (HIV)infections or patients with malignant tumors (except primary malignant tumors of the brain). Organs should be treated cautiously from patients with HBV or HCV infections, drug addiction or medical histories of related organs. But a kidney with a history of HCV infection can be used for a recipient with HCV infection.

It is of great significance to screen the donor and recipient by immunology requirements, in order to reduce the rejection after allograft transplantation. To prevent excessive and even fatal rejection, the following examinations should be done before transplantation:

(1)ABO typing: ABO antigens are expressed not only on the red blood cells, but also on the blood vessel endothelium. Thus, allograft transplantation usually requires the same blood type or meets the requirements of blood transfusion. Even if ABO blood type does not meet the requirements of transfusion, successful cases of liver transplantation have been reported.

(2)Lymphocyte cross - matching is a necessary examination before transplantation. The potential donor's lymphocytes serve as the target cells for the patient's serum. If a kidney transplantation is to be performed, the result must be negative or less than 10%. If a recipient had ever received blood transfusion, pregnancy or allogeneic transplantation, probably there are antilymphocyte antibodies in his serum, and he may be sensitive to human leukocyte antigen (HLA). In this condition, the lymphocyte toxicity test can be positive, and hyperacute rejection may occur after transplantation. A more sensitive technique is the flow cytometry crossmatching. But it is still controversial because it may exclude the donor that could have been transplanted successfully.

(3) HLA matching: International standard requires detection of Class I antigens within HLA–A and HLA–B loci and Class II antigens within HLA–DR locus from donor and recipient. A large number of studies show that 6 loci of HLA are closely related to the survival rate of kidney transplantation and bone marrow transplantation. The mismatch between HLA–A, B and DR affects the effect of organ transplantation. But with new immunosuppressive drugs used in clinic, this difference is decreasing gradually. Other HLA loci are not important in the transplantation of solid organs.

3.2   Organ Preservation

The method of excision and preservation depends on different organs and donor types. The process of acquiring organs mainly involves incision and exploration, in situ perfusion, organ excision, organ preservation and transportation. Organs can be acquired in one corpse such as heart, lung, kidney, liver, pancreas, cornea, so as to transplant them into several recipients.

After blocking the blood supply and excising, organ tends to lose its activity in a short time at 35–37 ℃. In order to ensure the function and the survival rate after organ transplantation, it is important to shorten warm and cold ischemic time, storage at low temperature, avoid cell swelling and damage. Warm ischemic time is the interval from blocking the blood supply to flushing in situ with a cold solution. This period does most harm to organ and should be less than 10 minutes. Cold ischemia time is the interval from cold perfusion to opening blood supply in recipient, including preservation of the organ. Too long cold ischemia time has bad effects on the function recovery and long–term survival of the transplanted organs. In addition, the mechanical damage and destruction to the donor organs should be avoided to ensure the quality of the graft. The most critical step in the preservation of solid organs is rapid organ cool perfusion to flush blood out as much as possible at 0–4 ℃. Usually, perfusion pressure is at 60–100 cmH$_2$O. The total perfusion volume of liver is 2–3 L, and 200–500 mL for kidney or pancreas. After perfusion, organs should be preserved in the perfusion liquid at 2–4 ℃ until transplantation.

UW (the University of Wisconsin solution), HTK (histidinetryptophan–keto glutarate) and Hartmann are the most commonly used in clinic as organ perfusion andpreservation liquid. The cationic concentration of UW solution is similar to that of intracellular fluid. Hartmann solution is composed of Ringer lactate solution and albumin, similar to extracellular fluid. HTK solution is non – intracellular and non – extracellular like. Hartmann solution is used for organ excision and cold perfusion. UW and HTK solutions are used to preserve organs. In theory, kidney or pancreas can be preserved in UW solution for 72 hours, and liver for 20–24 hours. However, clinical organ preservation is often limited as follows: heart for 5 hours, kidney for 40–50 hours, pancreas for 10–20 hours and liver for 12–15 hours.

Chapter 4

Organ Transplantation

Organ transplantation is now the preferred treatment modality for a variety of different types of organ failure, such as kidney, liver, heart, pancreas, lung, intestine, spleen, adrenal gland, parathyroid gland, testis and ovary. Besides, heart-lung, liver-intestine, heart-liver, pancreas-kidney transplantation and abdominal multiple organ transplantation have been performed already. With the increasing of the transplantation effect, a large number of long-term survivors have returned to normal life and work.

4.1 Kidney Transplantation

Renal transplantation is regarded as the most effective treatment in all kinds of organ transplantation. Long-term survivors are satisfied with their work, life, psychology and mental state. The effect of living donor kidney transplantation is better than that of deceased donor kidney. The 1-year graft survival rate for a genetically identical twin is more than 95%. The recipient mortality in the first year is less than 3%. At present, the 3-year graft survival rates for zero mismatch of HLA-DR and HLA-B, zero mismatch of HLA-DR, one mismatch of HLA-DR and two mismatch of HLA-DR are 83%, 83%, 80% and 77%. The 10-year graft survival rates for zero mismatch, one to two mismatch, three to four mismatch, five to six mismatch in all HLA loci are 63%, 58%, 52% and 47%. The statistics show that the earlier the patients with renal failure received dialysis, the higher the survival rate was. And the longer the dialysis time, the higher the proportion of delayed function recovery of transplanted kidneys. Therefore, kidney transplantation should be done as soon as possible.

The indication of kidney transplantation is all kinds of end-stage renal disease, including chronic glomerulonephritis (70%), chronic pyelonephritis, polycystic kidney, diabetic nephropathy, interstitial nephritis and autoimmune nephropathy, etc.

The surgical technique of renal transplantation is established. The transplant kidney is placed in the iliac fossa through an oblique lower abdominal incision, and the kidney will lie in an extraperitoneal position. An end-to-side anastomosis is performed between renal vein and iliac vein; an end-to-side anastomosis is then performed between the renal artery and the external iliac artery. An alternative technique is to connect the renal artery end-to-end to the internal iliac artery. Ureter is brought into the bladder through a submucosal tunnel and sutured to the mucosa of the bladder from the inside of the bladder, to prevent urine counterflow (Figure 12-4-1).

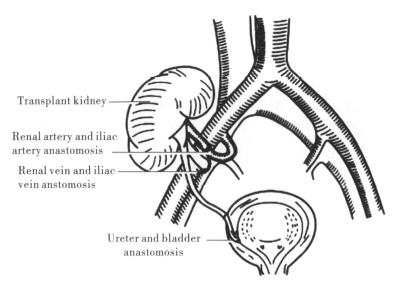

Figure 12-4-1　Technique of renal transplantation

4.2　Liver Transplantation

Liver transplantation has been explored and studied for more than half a century. The current 1-year survival rate is nearly 90% , and 3-year survivalrate is almost 80%. The longest survival time is nearly 40 years. The survival rate of children with liver transplantation is better than that of adults. It is frequently reported the normal pregnancy of adult female.

In principle, the indication of liver transplantation is progressive, irreversible and fatal end-stage liver disease, and there are no other effective treatments. It is also suitable for patients with liver malignant or benign lesions and are expected to survive less than a year. Benign lesions include viral or alcoholic cirrhosis decompensations, acute liver failure, congenital biliary atresia, hepatolenticular degeneration, etc. Malignant lesions include primary hepatocellular carcinoma. The 5-year survival rate of recipients with hepatocellular carcinoma is close to that of benign lesions. Currently, the international standard for liver transplantation includes Milan standard and Hangzhou standard. Milan standard requires that the diameter of a single tumor is no more than 5 cm, or the tumor number is less than three and the maximum diameter is no more than 3 cm. No major vascular invasion, lymph node or extrahepatic metastasis are also required.

Classic techniques of liver transplantation include orthotopic liver transplantation, piggyback liver transplantation and ameliorated piggyback liver transplantation. In orthotopic liver transplantation, the host liver is removed with the vena cava and the donor organ placed in an orthotopic position. The piggyback liver transplantation allows the liver to be dissected off the vena cava without division of vena cava. The donor hepatic vein is sewn to the recipient vena cava. The advantage of the piggyback liver transplantation is that when the anastomosis of vena cava and the portal vein is performed, the blood flow of the inferior vena cava can be retained completely or partially to maintain the stability of recipient's circulation (Figure 12-4-2). Ameliorated piggyback liver transplantation is to open the donor inferior vena cava and three recipient hepatic veins, expand them to the same shape of triangle, and then sew them together. In this way, it is conducive to the smooth outflow tract. Split-liver transplantation is to split a liver from deceased donor into two parts and transplant them into two recipients. Living-relate liver transplantation is to get a part of liver (left or right half of liver) from relatives and transplant it into recipient. The premise is to make sure that there is as little harm to the donor as possible, and the recipient can achieve a similar effect to normal liver transplantation. Besides, there are reduced-size liver transplantation, heterotopic and auxiliary liver transplantation, etc. But they are performed limitedly in clinic.

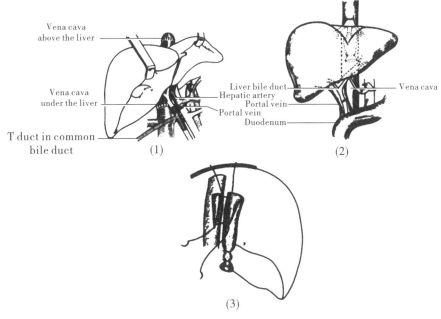

Figure 12-4-2   Technique of liver transplantation

(1) Orthotopic liver transplantation; (2) Piggyback liver transplantation; (3) Ameliorated piggy-back liver transplantation.

4.3   Pancreas Transplantation

There are three types in clinical practice: simultaneous pancreas-kidney transplantation (SPK), pancreas-after-kidney transplantation (PAK) and pancreas transplantation alone (PTA). The 1-year survival rate and the 1-year graft survival rate were different, SPK is 95% and 84%, PAK is 94% and 76%, and PTA is 94% and 76%.

Pancreas transplantation is an effective treatment for type 1 diabetes. It is expected to improve and even partially reverse the complications of cardiovascular disease and peripheral vascular disease caused by diabetic nephropathy or diabetes. In clinical practice, pancreas transplantation or SPK is only performed for patients with end-stage diabetes, especially with uremia, because it may cause some undesirable side effects after transplantation. Pancreas transplantation may also be considered for a few patients with type 2 diabetes and difficult to control blood glucose or complications occur obviously, as well as those who received total pancreatectomy for any reasons (trauma or tumor).

Bladder or enteric drainage may be performed for the exocrine secretions in pancreas transplantation. The donor duodenal C-loop is used to drain the donor pancreatic exocrine secretions. Duodenal stump is sutured to bladder in bladder drainage [Figure 12-4-3 (1)]. The main disadvantage is that a large amount of pancreatic juice is lost with urine, resulting in chronic metabolic acidosis which is difficult to correct, and It is easy to cause the long-term complications of chemical cystitis, chronic urethral infection and urethrostenosis.

In enteric drainage, the pancreas is transplanted into the abdominal cavity, and duodenal stump is sutured to small bowel [Figure 12-4-3 (2)]. Enteric drainage is more likely to physiology state, without the disadvantage of pancreatic juice excreted by urinary tract. In recent years, enteric drainage is more than 80%. There are two kinds of internal secretions drainage in pancreas transplantation, which are through systemic (external and internal iliac vein) and portal (inferior mesenteric vein and splenic vein) vein reflux. Physiologically, insulin reach to portal vein first. Systemic vein reflux is different from this so it can lead to hyperinsulinemia. And the advantage of the portal vein reflux is that it avoids hyperinsulinemia. It is good to insulin utilization that insulin gets to liver directly. In addition, because the venous blood of the transplanted pancreas is returned to the liver, antigens or antigen-antibody complexes can be treated in the liver. It helps to reduce the incidence of rejection and improve the metabolism and composition of lipoprotein. It is considered that the enteric drainage with portal vein reflux is the ideal operation for kidney-pancreas co-transplantation.

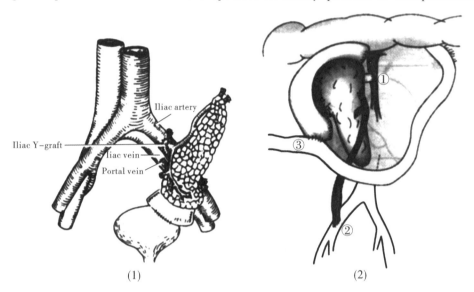

① Anastomosis between pancreatic vein and superior mesenteric vein; ② Anastomosis between pancreatic artery and Iliac artery; ③ Anastomosis between duodenal stump and small bowel.

Figure 12-4-3 Technique of pancreas transplantation

(1) Bladder drainage for exocrine secretions and venous drainage for insulin; (2) Enteric drainage for exocrine secretions and portal drainage for insulin.

4.4 Small Bowel Transplantation

Because of the special physiology features of small intestine, the incidence of rejection was high after transplantation, and serious infections are easily to occur. Moreover, intestinal function recovers slowly and GVHD often happens. It is reported that 1-year and 5-year survival rates after small intestinal transplantation have been more than 70% and 50%. At the same time, 91% and 75% can be reached in Starzl Transplantation Institute. The 1-year and 5-year survival rates of functional grafts are 86% and 61%. The prime indication for small intestinal transplantation is short-gut syndrome and those who can not adapt total parenteral nutrition (TPN). The syndrome is the result of many intestinal disorders, and patients eventually undergo extensive resection of the small bowel. If the recipient is only short-gut syndrome, it is feasible to transplant small intestine. If liver failure is complicated, liver-small intestine co-transplantation is suitable. A few patients require the co-transplantation of whole digestive tract (includes liver, stomach, pancreas, duodenum, small intestine, even a part of colon).

4.5   Lung Transplantation

Statistics data shows that 1–year survival rate of recipients with lung transplantation is 70% –90% , and 5–year survival rate is 40% –50% . The mainly reasons that affect thesurvival rate include early postoperative infection, primary graft failure and postoperative long–term bronchiolitis obliterans. The indication for lung transplantation is end–stage pulmonary disease not suitable for other medical or surgical therapy, such as emphysema, pulmonary fibrosis, cystic fibrosis, bronchiectasis. Only about 40% of the patients waiting for lung transplantation can receive a transplant because of the strict lung requirements for donors. The techniques of lung transplantation include single lung transplantation and dual lung transplantation (sequential or whole lung transplantation).

4.6   Heart Transplantation

The survival rates of 1, 5, 10–year after heart transplantation are 80% , 64% and 45% . It is coronary atherosclerosis caused by chronic rejection has bad influence on long–term survival after heart transplantation. The indication for heart transplantation is end–stage cardiac disease not amenable to other medical or surgical therapy, such as dilated myocardiopathy, coronary heart disease and valvular disease, or congenital complex cardiac malformation not suitable for surgical correction. In addition, heart–lung transplantation is suited for primary pulmonary hypertension, Eisenmann's syndrome, or severe myocardiopathy, ischemic heart disease, rheumatic heart disease together with irreversible pulmonary lesions or pulmonary vascular lesions. The techniques of orthotopic heart transplantation includes standard HT, total HT, and bi–venacava HT (Figure 12–4–4). At present, bi–venacava HT is more common abroad.

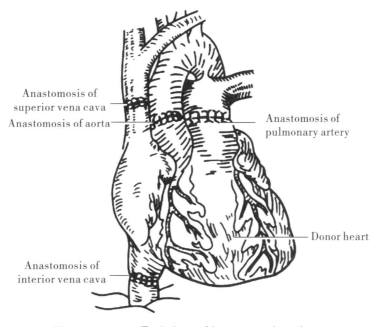

Figure 12–4–4   Technique of heart transplantation

Part 13

Pain Therapy

Chapter 1

Introduction and Definition

The subject of pain is a new branch emerging from medical field, In the past, doctors solved the painful problems just use "pain killers". Our knowledge of pain remains inadequate. It was not treated as a independent subject. During the last decades, there has been a tremendous surge of interest in the subject, "pain" was really begin to study specially, National and International societies (International Association for the Study of pain, IASP) have been formed, a journal is devoted exclusively to the subject, a textbook of pain was published, be a guideline on how to tackle the subject and how to practice, "pain clinics" and various pain control center have opened every where. It is obviously brought a widely research in this field, especially the study of pain control measures have made tremendous strides, SGB has extensively used in "pain clinics" for many disease. The study of pituitary gland destruction is an extremely useful method of reliving the persistent pain associated with malignancy. SCS has been applied for controlling pain much success. All of above have opened vistas undreamt of the study and treatment of pain emerges as a subject in it's own right.

1986. Mount castle Wrote simply:

Pain is that sensory experience evoked by stimuli that injury. The taxonomy committee of the IASP chaired by Mercy defined pain as "An unpleasant sensory and emotional experience" associated with actual or potential tissue damage, or described in term of such damage. They added crucial notes to this sentence: Pain is always subjective. Each individual learns the application of the word through experience related to injury in early life. It is unquestionably a sensation in a part of the body but it is also always unpleasant and therefore also an emotional experience.

Chapter 2

Classification

The subject of pan is a frontier science. Pain relief problems' are involving many other Medical branches. The range of treatment is extraordinarily extensive. We can say so：any formidable pain is the indication of the study of pain. Up to now，the simply classification of painful diseases is as follow：

(1) Chronic headache

· Migraine.

· Giant cell arthritis.

· Neurasthenia.

· Endocrines.

· Occipital neuralgia.

· Headache origin from cervicodynia.

· Atypical headache，etc.

(2) Neuralgia and peripheral neuropathy

· Sciatica.

· Trigeminal neuralgia.

· Radiculitis.

· Intercostal neuralgia.

· Neuralgia after herpes zoster.

· Post-amputation pain.

· Injury of rachial plexus.

· Injury of spinal nerve.

· Glosssopharyngeal neuralgia，etc.

(3) Acute and chronic soft tissue damage

· Fibromyositis.

· Bursitis.

· Ligament us sprains.

· Muscle spasm.

· Chronic strains.

· Disorders of joints and periarticular structure，etc.

(4) Degenerative disease

· Degenerative disease range from cervical segment to lumbosacral.

region.

· Intervertebral disk herniation.

· Osteoporosis, and so on.

(5) Joint pain

· Osteoarthritis (degenerative arthritis) rheum arthritis, rheumatoid arthritisl, etc.

(6) Viceral pain

labour pain, etc.

(7) Painful peripheral vascular disorders

Raynaud's disease, RD, Gangrene, etc.

(8) Malignant pain

The so called later periods cancerous pain.

Chapter 3

The Basic Therapeutics

(1) Drugs

Non-steroidal anti-inflammatory analgesic drugs.

"Three steps therpy" for cancerous pain:

· Non-narcotic analgesics

representative drug: Aspirin

· Weak, morpine-type

representative drug: codeine

· Strong morphine-type

representative drug: morphine

(2) Local and nerve block.

(3) Epidural therapeutics.

(4) Stellate gangline block.

(5) Pituitary destruction.

(6) Endocranial injection of morphine.

(7) Stimulation.

Transcutaneous and implanted nerve stimulation.

Acupuncture and related forms of folk medicine.

Spinal cord stimulation.

Brain stimulation.

(8) Physiotherapy.

Ultrasound.

Short wave.

Microwave.

Super lizer.

Superficial heat and cold in the treatment of pain.

(9) Biofeadack.

(10) Psychotherapy.

Hypnosis.

Behaviour therapy.

(11) Massage.

(12) Operative therapy and minimally invasive surgery.

(13) Injection of collagenase treat LDH.

(14) Destruction of spinal nerve with the injection of alcohol or other.

Destructive drugs.

(15) Neural regulation therapy.

(16) Spine intervention.

Percutaneous laser disc decompression.

Radiofrequency ablation nucleoplasty.

Chemical dissolving technique of pulposus of intervertebral disc.

Minimally invasive endoscopic technique.

Chapter 4

Clinical Application of Local and Nerve Block

4.1　Basis for Use

Local and regional analgesia, achieved by injecting a local anaesthetic into tissue or in proximity of certain parts of the peripheral nerve system, to relieve pain has been used for nearly a century. For many years these various techniques were used in an empirical and often haphazard fashion resulting not infrequently in failures and at times complications. Fortunately, during the past quarter–century a number of factors have helped to clarify their proper role as diagnostic and therapeutic tools in managing patients with acute and chronic pain. The purpose of this chapter is to present a brief discussion of the basis for use and side–effects and complications of local analgesia and regional nerve blocks.

The basis for the efficacy and utility of local analgesia and somatic nerve blocks in patients with acute or chronic pain is interruption of nociceptive fibres, eliminate the local inflammation, nutrition of the damaged nerve and tissue. In addition, blockade may interrupt the afferent fibres of abnormal reflex mechanisms which contribute to the pathophysiology of some pain syndromes. Moreover, block of sympathetic fibres may be used to eliminate sympathetic hyperactivity which often contributes to the pathophysiology of certain painsyndromes. On the other hand, in certain conditions it may be useful to block somatomotor nerve to relieve muscle spasm. By producing one or more of these effects, some disease can be cured, in certain conditions, the pain relief outlasts by days and weeks and monthes. For cancerous pain, if the related sensory merve was blocked with acolhol or other destructive drugs, the pain relief may outlasts very long periods even keep company with the patients of the later periods of his or her life.

In different parts of the boby, nerve block have different effects, for example:

Intercostal nerve block is to relieve sevevre pain that follws thoracotomy, fracture of ribs, slipped costovertebral joints, except eliminates muscle spasm and interrupts abnormal reflex phenomena that are initiated by nociceptive input. A number of studies have shown the superiority of intercostals nerve block over narcotics in managing thoracodynia, the PEF, FVC, FEV_1, PaO_2 which are usually reduced by 50% or more, but are markedly improved after intercostal block.

4.2   Side-effects and Complicatios

Different parts of the boby have different complications, to avoid repetition with each procedure, the following complications will be briefly considered:

(1)Systematic toxic reactions.

(2)Very high or total spinal anaesthesia.

(3)Pneumothorax.

(4)Neurological complications.

4.3   Preventative Measures

(1)Using the lowest concentration and volume of local anaesthetic that assures good results.

(2)Use of epinephrine 1 : 200 000 in the solution to retard the rate of LA absorption.

(3)Repeated aspiration to ascertain that the needle point is not in a blood vessel or other important structures prior to each injection.

(4)Prior to injecting large amounts, inject 3 mL of solution as a test dose.

Treatment of mild reactions includes encouragement of the patient and administration of oxygen. Convulsion must be treat immediately so that the patient dose not suffer asphyxia because as long as the patient is not ventilating adequately. Sometimes intravenous injection of 40-80 mg of succinylcholine is necessary. If any difficulty is encountered in keeping the airway patent, tracheal intubation is promptly carried out. In addition, 5-10 mg diazepam(valium) or 50-100 mg of thiopental sodium should be given i. v. To control seizure activity of the cerebral cortex, and additional increments of these drugs given as needed. Severe reactions require support of the circulation with fluids and vasopressors and artificial Ventilation.

Other treatment of side-effects will be discuss in related measures.

Chapter 5

Local Block

Infiltration or topical applications of local anesthetics are frequently used techniques in the treatment of pain. Simplicity, facility and apparent innocuousness make the method of choice among many doctors. By producing physicochemical interruption of nervous pathways almost at the very source of the nociceptive process, it effectively relieves the pain and othersymptoms of many disorders including myofascial pain syndromes, sprains and strains, tendonitis, epicondylitis, periarthritis, severe muscle spasm and some simple fractures.

5.1 Techniques

One of the most productive clinical applied of local block therapy is in the management of myofascial pain syndromes with trigger points. Trigger points can be found in virtually every muscle of the body, in tendons and in ligaments. The injection of the trigger point is accomplished with a 25 or 22-gauge; 5 cm needle Usually 5-10 mL of a dilute solution is sufficiency, e. g. , 0. 25% bupivacaine or 0. 5% lidocaine with other drugs is necessary for lxal anaesthetic (LA). As the point of needle nears or actually touches the trigger point the patient experiences exaggeration of local and referred pain and tenderness and this is further aggravated during the injection. A fan-like approach is made by inserting the needle at different angles until the most sensitive region is contacted. Since many patients have more than one trigger point, it is essential to block all of them to obtain optimal results. Some clinicians have found saline injections almost as effective as the injection of the local anesthetics.

The relief of pain, tenderness, and muscle spasm persists for several hours and sometimes for days and weeks or even months, especially if the condition is treated early. In acute cases one or two treatments are sometimes sufficient, whereas in chronic cases a series of treatments is usually necessary. Injections are repeated every second, third, or fourth day, depending on the severity and acuteness of the conditions. After the trigger points have been injected. Adjunctive therapy including physical therapy, massage, application office or spraying of coolant should be used.

5.2   Indications

Infiltration of dilute solution of LA into the muscle is effective in relieving very severe pain of muscle spasm caused by trauma. This technique is also effective in relieving severe lower back pain (lumbago) due to sudden lumbosacral muscle strain or caused by poor posture or deformity of the spine. Pain due to disorders of joints and periarticalar structures: simple joint sprains may be effectively treated with infiltration of the most sensitive areas followed by a pressure with elastoplast. Immediate resumption of active motion, made possible by complete pain relief, enhances the circulation of the part, reduces the edema, helps drainage of hemotoma and consequently results in more rapid healing, the procedure is repeated as frequently as necessary until the pain and edema subside. This method must not be used for fractures and structural instability due to severe ligamentous tears. Acute bursitis is another important indication for infiltration of local anaesthetics and long-lasting steroids. Usually 10-15 mL of dilute solution of a long-acting agent such as 0.25% bupivacaine with 40 mg of methylprednisolone or other long-acing steroids. Pain relief occurs in 10-15 minutes and is likely to last 4-8 hours, after which pain returns and is often more intense. Therefore, the patient should be given systemic analgesics to manage the post-block pain. Frequently several injections are necessary. Subacromial, subscapular, prepatellar bursitis are best known with this proledure. If the effusion of the joints is pronounced, frequent aspiration of the bursa is indicated. Tendonitis is another very painful condition for which local block is effecive in relieving the associated pain, e. g. , lateral humeral epicondilitis (tennis elbow), medial humeral epicondilitis (golfers elbow), supraspinous tendonitis. Ligamentous strains is another indication for LA infiltration therapy. This condition may affect ligaments of any major joint, including the lumbosacral, sacroiliac, coccydynia, interspinous and lateral or medial patellar ligaments. Intra-articular injection of LA alone or in combination of steroids is also indicated in patients with severe pain or chronic arthritis involving major joints in the limbs or spine or the temporomandibular joint. Other painfull disorders including painful scars, neuroma with post-amputation pain in the stump or phantom limb, can be usefully treated and relieved.

Chapter 6

Nerve Block

6.1　Cervical Paravertebral Nerve Block

6.1.1　Technique

The lateral approach is the most frequently used technique of blocking the cervical spinal nerve. For example, to block the 8 th nerve. Note that the patient's head is turned to the opposide side and a small pillow is placed under the portion of thoracic spine and neck in older to make the transverse processes of cervical vertebrae more prominent. The tips of the transverse processes may be palpated. After preparation, a skin weal is made over the transverse process of the cervical and a 5 cm 22-gauge needle is inserted to contact the processes at a depth of 2-2.5 cm, and then the needle is slightly caudad to near the cervical nerve, fixing the needle and with extreme caring aspiration, no fluid, no blood, the injection can be made.

6.1.2　Indications

Paravertebral block of the cervical nerves can be as a diagnostic procedure to identify the specific nerve segment in pationts with segmental neuralgia due to intervertebral disc, root-sleeve fibrosis or osteophytes. Since these patients already have a mechanical neuropathy extreme care must be exercised to aoid further damage to the nerve with the needle point, It is also may be used to relieve cancer pain and severe pain due to musculoskeletal pathology.

6.1.3　Complications

These include accidental injection into the subarachnoid, with consequent total spinal anaesthesia, or injection into the vertebral artery which promptly brings bolus of drug to the brain with consequent transient paralysis of vital centers and often unconsciousness. Both of these complications must be treated promptly with artifical ventilation and support of the circulation until the local anaesthesia drug is redistributed and biotransformed. Side offects which may occur include concomitant block of the cervical sympathetic chain, the superior and recurrent laryngeal nerve and perhaps even the trunk of the vagus. All of these can be avoid by using proper techniques and small volumes of solutions.

6.2   Occipital Nerve Block

Block of the greater and smaller occipital nerve may be used as a diagnostic or therapeutic measure in managing patients with occipital headache, neuralgia and other painful condition in the posterior portion of the head.

Technique

The greater occipital nerve is usually blocked just above the superior nuchal line 2.5-3 cm lateral to the external occipital protuberance. At the point, we can palpate the occipital artery, the needle is introduced perpendicular to the scalp just medial to the artery. It is advanced until paraesthesia along the course of the nerve is obtained where upon 2-3 mL of solution is injected. The smaller occipital nerve is just beside the greater nerve and is often involved in the block.

Side-effects is none, other than accidental intra-arterial injection, which is usually of no consequence because of the small volume of the drug.

6.3   Brachial Plexus Block

Block of the brachial plexus may be used as a diagnostic or therapeutic measure in patients with causalgia and other sympathetic dystrophy, phantom limb pain and other types of peripheral neuralgia. It is also useful in providing temporary relief of severe acute pain that followed trauma or operation, or in patients with severe pain consequent to an embolus, in such circumstances, prolonged sympathetic block and analgesia enhance the survival of the limb and concomitantly provides pain relief.

6.3.1 · Technique

Although many techniques to block the brachial plexus have been describe, the most commonly used are the supraclavicular, interscalenus and axillary approaches.

Supraclavicular brachial plexus block: First, identify the two ends of clavicle and palpate the subclavian artery. Then sterilize the skin, towels are placed along the inferior and posterior edge of the triangle of the neck and the skin wheal is formed about 1 cm above the midpoint of the clavicle and just posterior to the palpable artery. A 22-gauge 5 cm needle is inserted in a caudad and slightly dorsad and mesiad direction until paraesthesia is elicited, whereupon the needle is arrested, aspiration in two places is carried out and if negative, 3-4 mL of solution is injected. The needle is then carefully advanced until the upper surface of the first rib just posterior to the artery is contacted, after injecting 2-3 cm on the rib, the remainder of the solution is injected as the needle is withdrawn between the first rib and superficial fascia.

The interscalenus brachial plexus block: The interscalennus groove is identified and a line is drawn extending laterally from the cricoid cartilage to intersect the groove which is just over the transverse process of C6. After formation of a skin wheal and with the second and third fingers of the left hand palpating the groove, a 22-gauge 3 cm needle is inserted in the direction almost perpendicular to the skin being directed into the sulcus of C6 transverse process. The needle is advanced slowly for 1.5-2.0 cm until paraesthesia is elicited indicating contact with the nerve. The needle need not be inserted more than 1.5-2.0 cm. since the fascia of the anterior and middle scalene muscle provide a relatively closed space within which the brachial plexus and subclavian artery are located, the injection of 15–20 mL of local anaesthetic solution will diffuse up and down and laterally to block the roots of the brachial plexus and often those of the cervical plexus.

Axillary block of the brachial plexus: With the patient supine, the arm abducted to 90 ℃ and externally rotated, the axillary artery is palpated and traced as far as possible toward the axilla. After appropriate preparation on the skin, a skin wheal is formed over the artery and a 25–gauge 3 cm needle is inserted perpendicular to the skin and directed laterally to a point just anterior to the artery. By using a short bevel needle, one can feel it penetrating the sheath within which the axillary artery and the three major nerves of the plexus lie. Injection of 15–20 mL of solution is necessary.

6.3.2 Compliations

The most serious complication of supraclavicular brachial plexus block is pneumothorax, which is reported to occur in between 0.5% and 6%, but in the hands of the skilled operator, it occurs in less than 1% of the blocks. Other complications with large volumes of drug include ipsilateral block of the phrenic nerve, which cause no symptomatology except in patients with severe lung disease, and /or block of the cervicothoracic sympathetic chain with consequent Horner's syndrome. Accidental intravenous injection with consequent systemic toxicity can occur if repeated aspiration tests are not used. As already mentioned. Transient or prolnged nerve dysfunction due to trauma by the needle–point is rare. The possible complication of interscalene block is accidental epidural or subarachnoid injection or injection into the vertebral artery, all of which can be obviated with proper technique. Phrenic nerve block occurs more frequently with this technique than with the supraclavicular approach. Possible complications of axillary block include accidental intravenous injection with systemic reaction, haematoma or nerve damage if poor techniques are used.

6.4 Suprascapular Nerve Block

Block of the suprascapular nerve, a branch of the brachial plexus and the major senory nerve supply to thc shoulder point, is useful for the management of severe pain due to bursitis, periarthritis or arthritis.

Suprascapular nerve block is accomplished at the suprascapular notch. Although in most instances this block is relatively simple, occasionally it is difficult to contact the nerve and the solution is injected within the muscle mass, resulting in failure. Side–effects include pneumothorax, bleeding and damage of suprascapular nerve.

6.5 Block of Thoracic Spinal Nerve

Paravertebral block of the thoracic spinal nerve is useful procedure in managing painful disorders involving the thoracic spine, the thoracic cage and the abdominal wall, e. g. , it is useful for the relief of severe pain of rib fracture, acute or chronic neuralgia of herpes zoster, acute of post–thoracotomy pain, segmental neuralgia due to osteoporosis or osteophyetes, and cancer pain in the related region.

6.5.1 Technique

Patient lie on health side, a skin wheal is formed 1.5 cm lateral to the tip of the spinous process of the vertebrae, A 22–gauge 10 cm needle with a short bevel is inserted through the skin wheal perpendicular to the skin and advanced until the lateral edge of the lamina is contacted, the needle is then withdrawn until its point is in the subcutaneous tissue, the skin moved laterally about 0. 5cm and the needle then readvanced until it slips just lateral to the lateral edge of the lamina and its point engages the anterior costotransverse ligament, and there is some resistance. By exerting slightly pressure on the plunger of the syringe and advancing the needle very slowly, a lack of resistance is felt as soon as the bevel of the needle passes through the ligament and is in the paravertebral region in the immediate vicinity of the nerve, with repeated aspiration, if negative, the solution can be injected.

6.5.2   Complications

Possible complication with the paralaminar technique include accidental subarachnoid, intravenous injection and pneumothorax. All of these can be obviated by using patience, caution and skill in carrying out the procedures.

6.6   Intercostal Nerve Block

Intercostal nerve block is one of the most useful procedures for relief of a severe acute post−traumatic, postoperative or postinfectious pain in the thoracic or abdominal wall. It is highly effective in relieving severe pain from fracture of one or more ribs or fracture of the sternum or dislocation of the costochondral junction. Slipped rib cartilage, contusion chest pain, pleurisy and neuralgia from herpes zoster.

6.6.1   Technique

The intercostal nerves may be bocked at any point along their course, but there are three basic puncturing points in common use, the posterior (angulus costae), lateral (posterior axillary line), and anterior (midclavicular line). The method of them is same, but the posterior block is the best site of block. After choose the point, with the second finger of the left hand placed over the intercostal space and pushes the skin cephalad slightly so that the lower edge of the rib above can be palpated and at the same time immobilize the skin over the rib. This finger also protects the intercostal space and thus decrease the risk of passing the needle too far into the lung. A 25−gauge short bevel needle 1−2 cm in length (depending on the thickness of the subcutaneous tissues) is inserted perpendicular the skin and advanced until the lowermost part of the rib is contacted. The skin is moved caudad with the left index fingle to allow the needle to slip below the lower border of the rib. It is then advanced (about 0. 5 cm) until the paraesthesia was elicited, with the needle held steady in left hand an attempt at aspiration is made and, if negative, 3−4 mL of solution is injected.

6.6.2   Complications

The most important complication of intercostals block is pneumothorax. Because the absorption of local anaesthetic from the intercostals space is faster and greater than after injection in other sites, systemic toxic reactions may occur after the injection of large therapeutic doses. This problem can be obviated or at least minimized by adding epinephrine to the solution to retard absorption, and by using optimal concentrations and reasonable volumes of the drug.

6.7　Lumber Paravertebral Block

Lumber paravertebral block is very useful method to manage the painful conditions including lumbago, neuralgia from nerve root and other related vertebral pathology. The technique is similar to the thoracic nerves. Complications of lumber paravertebral block are similar to those of thoracic block, except pneumothorax. If without caution, nerve damage by the needle may occur.

6.8　Sciatic Nerve Block

Since the sciatic nerve contains the majority of the sensory and sympathetic fibres for the lower extremity, sciatic nerve block may be used to control severe acute or chronic pain associated with leg and foot. Complications are rare and are limited to accidental intravenous injection or transient nerve dysfunction due to trauma during the procedure.

Technique

The patient lies in Sims position. Drawing a line extending from the upper portion of the greater trochanter to the posterior superior iliac spine is bisected and a perpendicular line is drawn from the point of bisection in an inferior and medial direction for a distance of 3 cm. This is the site of the puncture. After formation of the skin weal a 10 cm 22-gauge needle is introduced in a direction perpendicular to the skin and advanced until paraesthesia is obtained or bone is coatacted. If paraesthesia is not obtained, the skin weal is moved 0.5 cm cephalad and the needle reintroduced until paraesthesia is elicited or bone contacted and 15-20 mL solution is injected.

6.9　Femoral Nerve Block

Block of the femoral nerve is used to manage the neuralgia and other severe pain in the anterior thigh, or it can be used concomitantly with sciatic block to effect sympathetic interruption of the entire lower limb.

Technique

After preparation of the skin and anaesthetic weal is made 1 cm external and lateral to the femoral artery and a 22-gauge 5 cm needle is introduced perpendicular to the skin and advanced until paraesthesia is elicited in the distribution to the cutaneous branches of the femoral nerve. Injection of 8-10 mL of solution in the region of the nerve usually is effective in blocking it.

6.10　Lateral Femoral Cutaneous Nerve Block

It is used to manage the severe pain in the anterolateral aspect of the thigh and in managing neuralgia paraesthesia. The technique; After identifying the anterior superior iliac spine and inguinale ligament, the skin is sterilized and a skin weal is made 1.5 cm medial to the spine immediately below the inguinal ligament. Then a 5 cm 22-gauge needle is introduced through the skin weal in a diection perpendicular to the skin and slowly advanced until paraesthesia is obtained and the Injection of 5 mL of solution suffices.

6.11　Obturator Nerve Block

This method may be used in the management of adductor muscle spasm and severe intractable pain in the hips due to osteoarthritis.

Although this procedure is rarely used, the technique is discussed for the sake of completeness. With the patient lying supine and thighs separated, the pubic tubercle of the affected side is palpated and the skin weal raised 1 cm lateral and inferior to it. A 22-gauge 8 cm needle is introduced through the weal in a direction perpendicular to the skin and slowly advanced until the upper part of the inferior ramus of the pubis is contacted. A needle recorder is placed 2.5 cm from the skin and the point of the needle is redirected in a lateral and slightly superior and posterior direction so that the shaft is parallel with the superior ramus of the pubis and the point of needle directed laterally and slight superiorly. The needle is then slowly advanced while its point is kept in constant contact with the inferomedian surface of the superior ramus of the pubis until the recorder is flush with the skin or contact with the bone is lost, since the paraesthesia is rather difficult to elicit, we just request the point of needle near the nerve. 10 mL of solution is injected after negative aspiration.

6.12　Block of Cranial Nerve

6.12.1　Trigeminal nerve block

Trigeminal nerve block is used to manage the trigeminal neuralgia and other painful conditions in the face and the anterior 2/3 of the head. The common complications is the laceration of vessels caused by needles with hooks or repeated haphazard insertions and adjacent nerve involving.

6.12.2　Technique

We just discuss the common using method: the block of pterygopalatine fossa. The point of entrance into the skin just below the midpoint of the zygomatic arch. After preparation 10 cm 22-gauge needle is inserted in a direction perpendicular to the skin and advanced slowly until the needle point contact with the lateral pterygoid plate. To carry out maxillary nerve block, the needle is withdrawn until is point is in the subcutaneous region and then reinserted so that it will pass slightly anterior and superior, and advanced until its point enters the pterygopalatine fossa and concacts the maxillary nerve therein. In carrying out mandibular nerve block, Needle is withdrawn and reinserted in a direction slightly posterior, It is advanced until its point contacts the mandibular nerve just below the foramen oval. After contacting each nerve and eliciting paraesthesia, 2 - 3 mL of solution is injected. Injection of large amounts of solution may involve the gasserian-ganglia.

6.13   Epidural Analgesia

The spinal epidural nerve block has been extensively used to manage many painful problems and malignant pain. The puncture is same with the puncture of epidural anaesthesia. The injected solution is basically same with the solution in nerve block.

Chapter 7

Stellate Ganglion Block

The sympathetic supply to the head, neck and arm can be interrupt at the stellate ganglion.

7.1 Regional Anatomy

The sympathetic chains originating from the upper thoracic segments extend through the neck as far as the base of the skull. The cervical chain no white rami and usually only three ganglia, a superior, middle and lower. The lower ganglion is usually fused with the first thoracic ganglion to form the stellate ganglion. It usually lies over the neck of the first rib and just anterior to the transverse process of seventh cervical vertebra. Gray rami leave the stellate ganglion to provide the sympathetic supply to the arm via the brachial plexus. Postganglionic fibers are also distributed to the subclavian artery and the vertebral artery and their branches. Anterior to the sympathetic chain lies the carotid sheath and medially the pharynx with the recurrent laryngeal nerve between them. Inferior to the stellate ganglion lies the dome of the pleura. Many of the complications of stellate ganglion block are related to its proximity to important anatomical structure.

7.2 Technique

Moore(1945) has described 16 possible approaches to the cervical sympathetic chain. These are variations of anterior lateral and posterior approaches. The anterior approache is most commonly used and the objective is to place a needle in the correct plane well above the pleura, and upper thoracic sympathetic chains. Smith(1951) described such an approach but more recently Lofstron(1969) and Carron & Litmiller (1975) have described an anterior paratracheal approach at C6 and this is the very popular method used by pain clinicians.

The patient lies supine with the head slightly raised and extend on a flat pillow. A finger between the sternomastoid and the trachea feels for the most prominent transverse process which should be the sixth, at or slightly above the level of the cricoid cartilage, palpation may be facilitated by a slight opening of the patient's mouth. A skin weal is made at this point. The essential maneuver in this technique is using the middle and index fingers of the operator's left hand to compress groove between the sternomastoid and trachea and to gently hook the carotid sheath and its contents laterally. This has the effect of making the anterior tubercle of C6 almost subcutaneous so that it can be reached with a 2. 5 cm 20-gauge needle attached to a 10 mL syringe. If the palpating fingers of the left hand are separated slightly they can straddle the transverse process of C6 and the needle can be inserted at right angles to the skin to contact the anterior aspect of the transverse process. It should be possible to dance the needle lightly on the bone and demonstrate the sensation to an observe. If the bone is not contacted the needle may have passed between the transverse process and could penetrate the vertebral artery or a dural sleeve. It is vitally important not to inject local anaesthetic unless the operator is confident of being anterior to the transverse process. When the needle rests securely on the transverse process the palpating fingers can be moved to hold the hub of the needle after which the needle should be withdrawn 2-3 mm and fixed with the left hand. After careful aspiration the injection is made with the right hand and the needle withdraw.

Signs of success is Horner's syndrome. it can be observed on the injectede side.

(1)Ptosis: droping of eyelid.

(2)Moistening and suffusion of the conjunctiva.

(3)Enophthalmos.

(4)Miosis: constriction of the pupil.

(5)The nose may become blocked on the injected Side.

(6)The face become flushed and dry.

If Horner's syndrome could not be observed after injection, the blocked should be failure and the effect may be not good.

7. 3   Indications

Stellate ganglion blockade has been used for a wide variety of conditions. The two main indications have been vascular insufficiency and pain. Acute vascular occlusion lead to spasm and pain which may be relieved by stellate ganglion block and the method has been used to treat arterial spasm following embolectomy and at onc time was used in the early treatment of cerebrovascular occlusions. Sudden deafness may respond to sympathetic block by relief of arterial spasm. And remissions are occasionally produced in Meniere's-disease. The accidental intra-arterial injection of drags such as thiopentone leads to intense spasm which may be relieved by sympathetic block. The commonest vascular disorder to be treated by the method has been Raynaud's disease and severe cases showing gangrene of the finger tips have respond well to alternate daily blocks. Causalgia, reflex sympathetic dystrophy and Sudeck's atrophy are the major painful indications for cervical sympathetic block. Many various chronic headache are respond very well to SGB, also which is a very useful method for treating cervicodynia. But a number of other painful peripheral states may benefit, particularly when the pain is accompanied by hyperpathia. These conditions include post-herpetic neuralgia, post-amputation pain, painful scars, pain due to carcinoma and Paget's disense. In some cases of pain due to lesions of the central nervous system. It is unusual for pain relief to be permanent after a single stallate ganglion block, repeated blocks need 5-8 times as normal.

7.4   Complications

Incorrectly performed stellate ganglion block can produce some alarming complications. If the injection is made too low the pleura may be penetrated, if the needle insertion produces coughing it should be withdrawn and a chest X−ray should be carried out subsequently. Injection of local anesthetic drugs into the vertebral artery may lead to dizziness, convulsions and unconsciousness. Injection into the dura will produce high spinal anaesthesia and possible respiratory arrest and circulatory collapse. Inject too medially may puncture the pharynx and produce an unpleasant sensation in about 10% of cases with resulting hoarseness for several hours, so that the block should be carried out one side at a time and opposing side blockade should be carried out alternate days. It is possible the bilateral blockade could result in bilateral recurrent laryngeal palsy can cause respiratory obstruction. The brachial plexus may also be affected resulting in temporary loss of sensation in arm. Hematoma are not uncommon in such a vascular region but minimized by the use of fine needles. With careful attention to asepsis infection is uncommon but osteitis and mediastinitis have been reported.

Part 14

Intracranial Hypertension

Raised intracranial pressure is quite common in neurosurgical and neurological clinical practices, which is the fundamental knowledge in learning neurosurgical disease. In this chapter, you will learn how intracranial pressure is generated and regulated normally and abnormally. Patients with intracranial hypertension (IHT) usually possess some common manifestations. You can also learn the symptoms and signs of IHT and differential diagnoses. Meanwhile, the most serious complications of IHT, i. e. , cerebral herniations, will also be introduced. We will focus two kinds of most common herniations, including transtentorial herniation and foraminal impaction. Finally, you will learn some treatment principles for patient with IHT.

Chapter 1

Pathophysiology

Contents in the cranial cavity include brain, blood and CSF, each of which occupies volume and generate its own pressure. All the pressures together form intracranial pressure (ICP). Although each of these can change in volume, neither brain nor CSF does more rapidly or flexible than intracranial blood volume. Fluctuations of blood volume in patients suffered from more slowly developed space-occupying lesions may aggravate or mitigate the effects on ICP.

1.1　Cerebral Blood Flow (CBF)/Cerebral Blood Volume (CBV)

Changes in blood volume could result from physiological (changes in posture, coughing, sports, and stooling) or pathological (breath inadequacy, respiratory obstruction, uncontrolled hypertension) reasons. These changes also come from clinical interventions, mechanical and pharmacological reasons.

Blood flow is dependent on blood pressure and the vascular resistance, of which the relationship is shown as below.

$$\text{Blood flow} = \frac{\text{Blood pressure}}{\text{Vascular resistance}}$$

Within the cranial cavity, the ICP must be taken into account. Thus, CBF could be expressed as below.

$$\text{CBF} = \frac{\text{CPP}}{\text{CVR}} = \frac{\text{MAP}-\text{ICP}}{\text{CVR}}$$

Where, CBF is cerebral blood flow, CPP is cerebral perfusion pressure, CVR is cerebral vascular resistance, MAP is mean arterial pressure, and ICP is intracranial pressure.

Cerebral blood flow is defined as the blood supply to the brain in a given time, which is usually represented by the blood volume (mL) passed through 100 g of brain per minute. In an adult, CBF is typically 750 mL per minute or 15% of the cardiac output. This equates to 50-55 mL of blood per 100 g of brain tissue per minute (Figure 14-1-1).

In normal condition, cerebral blood flow is coupled to the energy requirement of brain tissue. CBF is regulated by various mechanisms, which effects on the cerebral vessels mainly and finally maintains sufficient cerebral blood flow to meet the metabolic demands. Energy requirement differs in different parts of the brain. In the white matter, CBF is 20 mL/100 g · min, whereas in the gray matter flow is as high as 100 mL/100 g · min.

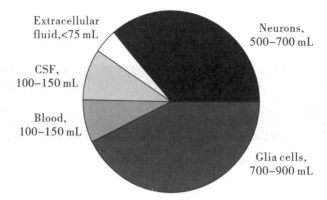

Figure 14-1-1　Pie chart of intracranial contents (by volume)

1.2　Factors Affecting the Cerebral Vasculature

Cerebral arterioleis sensitive to chemical factors. Changes of extracellular pH or accumulation of metabolic by-products directly affect the cerebral vascular contraction and dilation. Any change of arterial partial pressure of CO_2 ($PaCO_2$) has direct effect on cerebral vessels. Chemical signal change of $PaCO_2$ will be captured by the chemical sensors in carotid body and transmitted to the central followed by cerebral vascular automatic regulation.

When $PaCO_2$ rises from 40 to 80 mmHg, there is a doubling of the CBF, and the increased intracranial blood volume causes ICP to rise. Changes in blood gases are usually due to respiratory inadequacy. Hypoventilation may be caused by respiratory depression from drugs or from other cerebral condition. For example, respiratory obstruction could be caused by aspiration of vomit, swallowing the tongue, and glottis closure during seizure. Any respiratory obstruction will cause additional rise in ICP by passive venous engorgement. As intracranial venous sinuses contact with the superior vena cava indirectly and there are no venous valves in the sinuses, any changes in central venous pressure will be transferred to the intracranial cavity. Patients with conscious disorders are vulnerable to these events, whether their condition is traumatic or not. Seizures, some sedatives or analgesics also inhibit respiratory and aggravate the situation. Alone or in combination, these factors participate the crisis in patients whose compensatory capacity for temporary rises of intracranial blood volume has been already impaired.

1.2.1　Cerebral vascular automatic regulation

When ICP<35 mmHg and CPP>40-50 mmHg, CBF is regulated by chemical factors mainly, especially $PaCO_2$. The arterial partial pressure of CO_2 will effect on the sensors in carotid body and initial cerebral vascular automatic regulation, which is regulated by negative feedback. Cerebral perfusion pressure change results in cerebral vascular caliber change. Any change in blood vessel diameter results in considerable variation in cerebral blood volume, and in turn, this directly affects intracranial pressure.

When $PaCO_2$ rises, cerebral vessels dilate and CBF increases, which will make ICP go up. Negatively, the increased ICP will reduce $PaCO_2$ through accelerating respiratory frequency and increasing depth of respiration to expirate extra CO_2 in blood. Once $PaCO_2$ decreased, cerebral vessels contract and CBF decreases followed by ICP goes down. Generally, any changes of 2 mmHg of $PaCO_2$ will introduce 10% changes in CBF.

Cerebral vascular automatic regulation is a compensatory mechanism that permits fluctuation in the cerebral perfusion pressure within certain ranges without significantly altering cerebral blood flow.

A drop in CPP produces vasodilatation to maintain CBF, which is probably due to the direct "myogenic" effect on the vascular smooth muscles. On the contrary, a rise in the CPP causes vasoconstriction, which is also to maintain CBF.

1.2.2   Autonomic nervous system regulation

Neurogenic influences appear to have little direct effect on the cerebral vessels, but they may alter the ranges of pressure change over which cerebral vascular automatic regulation acts.

Cerebral vascular automatic regulation fails when the CPP falls below 40 mmHg or rises above 160 mmHg. At these extremes, CBF is more directly related to the perfusion pressure. In damaged brain (e. g. , cerebral injury and subarachnoid hemorrhage), cerebral vascular automatic regulation is impaired. A drop in CPP is more likely to reduce CBF and cause ischemia. Conversely, a high cerebral perfusion pressure may increase CBF, break down the blood-brain barrier and produce cerebral edema as in hypertensive encephalopathy.

When ICP>35 mmHg and CPP<40-50 mmHg, cerebral vascular automatic regulation is out of work. Instead autonomic nervous system takes the place to regulate CBF, where Cushing reaction presents. Cushing reaction (or Cushing reflex, Cushing effect) refers to a kind of physiological nervous system response to extreme high ICP that results in Cushing's triad of increased blood pressure, irregular/decreased breathing, and a reduction of the heart rate. Cushing reaction is the compensation of maintaining proper CPP at the moment of raised intracranial pressure. During Cushing reaction, heart rate decreases. However, cardiac output (CO) gets increased. Meanwhile, mean blood pressure (MAP) rises. Thus, both the increased CO and MAP facilitate increased CPP to maintain necessary CBF.

1.3   CSF Volume and Circulation

CSF is mainly secreted from the choroid plexuses or choroid tissue in the ventricles. On average, CSF is produced about 500 mL per day. It flows through the ventricular system and enters the subarachnoid space via the foramens of Magendie and Luschka of the fourth ventricle.

CSF is secreted from the choroid plexuses in the two lateral ventricles. It passes through the foramen of Monro (interventricular foramen) and goes into the third ventricle. Together with the CSF secreted by the choroid tissue on the roof of third ventricle, it flows through the aqueduct of Sylvius (cerebral aqueduct) and travels into the fourth ventricle, of which choroid plexus also secret CSF and mix with the previous CSF. Finally, it escapes into cistema magna through the median foramen of Magendie and the lateral foramens of Luschka (Figure 14-1-2). Some fluid then passes into the spinal subarachnoid space but most probably passes up through the cistema ambiens, a narrow space between the midbrain and the edge of the tentorial notch (Figure 14-1-3) to enter the subarachnoid space over the surface of the cerebral hemispheres, followed by absorption into the sagital sinus via arachnoidal granulations. Some CSF is produced and absorbed all along this route, but most originates in the lateral ventricle and is absorbed by the sagittal sinus. 15% -

20% of CSF volume is formed this way.

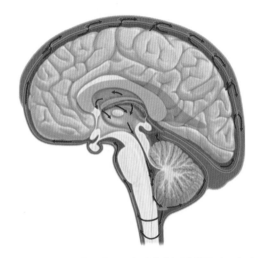

Figure 14-1-2   Cerebrospinal fluid (CSF) circulation

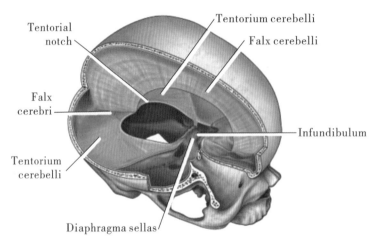

Figure 14-1-3   Tentorial notch

In normal conditions, CSF flows freely through the subarachnoid space and is absorbed into the venous system through the arachnoidal granulations. When ventricular pathways are obstructed, CSF may likewise be absorbed via retrograde flow into the extracellular fluid, which is so-called transependymal absorbtion. This may be visible on CT scan as a low-density area around the ventricles. If the CSF flow is obstructed at any place on the way, hydrocephalus with the associated rise in intracranial pressure develops, as a result of continued CSF production. Blockage leads to dilatation of any cavity above the obstruction, affecting one or both lateral ventricles if the foramen of Monro is blocked. When the aqueduct is involved, the third ventricle also dilates. So does the fourth ventricle if its outlet is obstructed. Patients with obstructive hydrocephalus can develop very high intracranial pressures that may persist over long periods, although the pressure probably fluctuates. It is such patients who commonly develop secondary changes in the skull related to raised pressure.

1.4 Brain Volume

Brain edema is a term often loosely used anywhere of swelling of the brain. Whereas, "brain edema" should be used restricting to water increasing in brain, which normally comprises 70% of white matter and 80% of gray matter which is more cellular.

There are two types of brain edema to be distinguished, which are vasogenic edema and cytotoxic edema. Vasogenic edema is characterized by the increase in extracellular fluid, largely due to impaired permeability of the endothelium of brain capillaries. This is the type of edema that is commonly associated with tumor, abscess, contusion, and hemorrhage. It is often focal and may contribute to brain shift and herniation thereafter. Cytotoxic edema is associated with macrophages, glia cells or neurons, which is due to the accumulation of intracellular water and sodium. The most common reason is hypoxia, particularly due to cardiac arrest. Therefore, this effect is usually widespread throughout the brain.

Focal infarcts initially cause cytotoxic edema but this often progress to vasogenic edema. With ischemic damage, cell metabolism fails, intracellular Na^+ and Ca^{2+} increase, and the cells swell, i. e. , cytotoxic edema, followed by capillary damage and vasogenic edema thereafter.

1.5 The Space–occupying Lesion

The accumulation of additional intracranial matter, which might be neoplasm, blood clot, pus, and abscess, must occupy spaces in the cranial cavity and eventually raise intracranial pressure. Initially it causes intracranial contents redistribution, some of which are displaced into the spinal canal. This is the stage of compensation before ICP rising.

Eventually this can no longer sustain the situation. The extent of the effects produced depends mostly on the size of the lesion, but somewhat on the speed of development and on the extent to which the pathological process destroys the brain, rather than expanding it with pathological tissue. Blood flow mapping studies indicate that expanding mass lesions compress the surrounding brain and reduce perfusion of tissue around the lesion, which induces an ischemic lesion which may worsen brain edema or swelling.

1.6 Volume/Pressure Relationships

The main factor influencing the effect of alteration of the volume of intracranial contents on ICP is the elasticity or stiffness of the brain, which partially depends on the extent to which normal compensatory processes have been exhausted. By decreasing the capacitance of intracranial vessels, the intracranial blood volume is decreased. Then CSF is displaced from the intracranial cavity into the expanded spinal canal, and brain then takes up the subarachnoid space vacated by CSF. Brain shift may also develop with the formation of herniation and the related distinctive clinical effects. Once these compensatory mechanisms are exhausted, the quite a little additional increase in volume, such as due to temporary cerebral vasodilatation, can produce a remarkable rise in ICP and initial a clinical crisis. This is because that the additional volume causes much greater effect on pressure when reserve compensation is no longer available (Figure 14–1–4).

However, intracranial elasticity is not only dependent on the existing volume of intracranial contents, but also their proportional disposition. Some other factors, which are under clinical control sometimes, have been found to affect elasticity rather than ICP directly (Table 14-1-1).

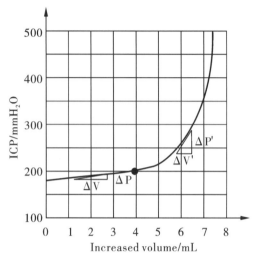

Figure 14-1-4   The relationship between intracranial pressure and increased intracranial volume

Table 14-1-1   Factors affecting elasticity of the brain

Increased elasticity (more softness of the brain)	Decreased elasticity (more stiffness of the brain)
Hypercapnia (any degree)	Hypocapnia (any degree)
Hypoxia (PaO$_2$<50 mmHg)	Hyperoxia (PaO$_2$ ranges 100-150 mmHg)
Rapid eye movement (REM) sleep	Hypothermia
Volatile anesthetic agents	Barbiturates
Nitrous oxide (NO)	Neurological analgesia
	Increased intra-thoracic pressure
	Increased intra-abdominal pressure

1.7   Interrelationships

Many factors affect intracranial pressure and these should not be considered isolated. Interrelationships are complex and feedback pathways may merely serve to cause the brain damage.

Chapter 2

Clinical Features

Patients diagnosed as space-occupying lesions usually complain of suffering from the classical triad of headaches, vomiting, and papilloedema, with most of the remainder having at least two of the complaints. Many also present mental disorder, which varies differently including personality change, dementia, drowsiness, and coma.

None of these features is peculiar to raised pressure. Indeed with the exception of papilloedema these are many common causes of each of them alone. It is their occurrence together which raise the suspicion of raised ICP. However, evidence for a causal relationship between high pressure and the classical symptoms is incomplete and there is no consistent correlation between the pressure and the severity of the symptoms. These features are conventionally ascribed to raised ICP, and are commonly referred to as the general symptoms and signs of intracranial tumor, in contract to localizing features.

Clinical features due to raised ICP include the following:

(1) Headache: worse in the mornings, aggravated by stooping and bending.

(2) Vomiting: occurs with an acute rise in ICP.

(3) Papilloedema: occurs in a proportion of patients with raised ICP.

2.1　Headache

2.1.1　Mechanism of production

Many structures in the cranial cavity are insensitive to pain. Indeed neurosurgeons used to operate almost exclusively under local anesthesia, knowing that the bony skull and the brain itself could be handled painlessly. Distension or traction of the arteries of the scalp and at the base of the brain, or the venous sinuses and their tributaries, gives rise to ill-localized pain. More localized pain results from stretching or distortion of certain areas of the dura mater and of the trunks of the cranial nerves V, IX, and X. Headache also origins from spasm of the large muscles at the base of the skull, and this may occur alone or as an added reflex activity when one of the other painful mechanisms is in play. Whatever the origin is, the final common path for pain is limited to the trigeminal, glossopharyngeal and vagus nerves, together with the posterior roots of the first three cervical segments.

2.1.2　Characteristics of pressure headache

The patient commonly wakes with rising headache dispersing within an hour. It may disappear for days or even weeks. Sometimes after months of regular morning, headache there may be a complete remission, although the pressure is unrelieved. Pressured headache is frequently not very intense, which is often being described as pulsing, throbbing, or bursting. Headache usually aggravates by coughing, sneezing, stooping or exertion, and gets relieved by simple analgesics or by staying in bed for a few days.

The distribution of the headache seldom gives any useful clue to the site of the lesion. It is because not only that the headache often felt at a situation remote from its origin, but also that the site of origin may be away from the lesion. Most pressured headaches are felt bilaterally in frontal or occipital regions. However, headache that is initially or exclusively occipital, radiating down the neck, is common with a mass in the posterior fossa. Tumors in the cerebellopontine angle area often cause persistent aches in the area.

Severe obstructive hydrocephalus may produce a syndrome of intense episodic headache associated with acute rises of pressure, which may be induced by neck or head movements. These so-called hydrocephalic attacks are alarming. Patients may cry out with pain, consciousness may be clouded, pulse and respiration become irregular and followed by sudden death occasionally. This attack warns of extremely dangerous high pressure, which requires emergency prompt intervention immediately.

2.1.3　Other causes of headache

(1) Hypertension. Although there may be a specific vascular component to hypertensive headache, it is largely due to raised ICP. Occurring in the morning, and sometimes accompanied by vomiting, it is frequently more severe than headaches due to tumor. Episodes of hypertensive encephalopathy can closely resemble hydrocephalic attacks. The relief of hypertensive headache, when the blood pressure is lowered by drugs, is not a reliable diagnostic test. The similar improvement can be observed in patients with tumor during the lowering of intracranial pressure secondary to a drop in arterial pressure. The remarkable efficacy of splanchnicectomy in relieving hypertensive headache, even when the blood pressure was not greatly altered, has never been satisfactorily explained.

(2) Migraine. The severe episodic headache usually begins in adolescents, tending to run in families. Sometimes it is accompanied by focal neurological disorders such as visual disorders (fortification spectra, hemianopia, or blindness), paraesthesia or weakness on one side of the limbs, dysphasia, and numbness around the lips bilaterally. The headache is often a hemicrania, altering from side to side in different attacks, and lasting for several hours to a day or so. It seldom returns within a fortnight but more commonly attacks recur monthly or even sporadically over years. Some patients recognize specific precipitating factors such as menstruation, the weekend or emotional stress. Vomiting is common and alarming prostration can occur. Ergot preparations, if given at the onset, may abort an attack.

(3) Anxiety states and neurosis. Headache is one of the most common psychosomatic symptoms, when it tends to have certain characteristics. Unremitting over weeks, months or years, even without an hour's relief, it is often said to be worse anytime, but never better. The sensation is reported of pressing, burning, or "like a tight hand round the head". It is usually uninfluenced by analgesics.

(4) Ear, nose and throat (ENT), eye, and dental diseases. Sinusitis, glaucoma, and toothache all give rise to pain in the trigeminal distribution, but there is often radiation or referral to the head. Secondary muscle spasms can cause headache, which are frequently occurred with cervical spondylosis.

(5) Meningism. Irritation of meninges on the skull base, whether by subarachnoid hemorrhage or by

pus from meningitis, gives rise to severe pain in the head and neck associated often with restlessness and noisiness.

(6) Temporal arteritis. The elderly patients who suffer this condition complain less of headache than of localized pain or tenderness in the scalp, and the affected artery may be palpated. The pain can be very severe and unremitting until the artery is divided surgically or prednisolone is given. Some patients may suffer from visual symptoms like sudden blindness and visual field impairment.

(7) Lumbar puncture(low-pressure-headache state). Traction and distortion of structures at the base of brain, similar to that which occurs with raised pressure, causes the head—that may follow drainage of CSF by lumbar puncture. This often appears to be aggravated by sitting up, and relieved by a high fluid intake and take supine position. Low CSF pressure be one factor but headache is very variable after lumbar puncture, because some patients denying any discomfort whatever.

2.2 Vomiting

This may be a sign of increased intracranial pressure but also occurs as a focal manifestation of lesions in the fourth ventricle. Such lesions almost always bring raised pressure due to CSF circulation obstruction and it is not easy to determine which mechanism is dominant.

Vomiting due to increased intracranial pressure usually occurs before breakfast, frequently with the complaint of morning headache. Although it is referred to as projectile, this is seldom a striking feature. Certainly it can occur without much nausea or omen. Children with tumors vomit more frequently than adults and often without any complaint of headache. This may be related to the posterior fossa tumors in children, which produce both raised ICP and local pressure on the medulla. 5/6 of the patients with infra-tentorial tumors have vomiting compared with less than half of the patients with supra-tentorial tumors.

Vomiting due to a local lesion in the fourth ventricle is uncommon and more likely to appear long before headache. It may occur daily for many months before signs of pressure or neurological disorder leading to the correct diagnosis.

The two most common causes of morning vomiting are pregnancy and migraine. The latter is usually recognized by the episodic nature of the attacks and other features such as hemicrania and visual disorders.

2.3 Papilloedema

The optic nerve is an extension of the brain, covered with meninges, and communicates with subarachnoid space in the cranial cavity. Intracranial tension is thereby transmitted to the site where the effects in the cranial cavity may be directly observed through the eye fundus. There are two factors limiting the reliability of such observations, i. e. , the time needed for papilloedema developing and the possibility that the subarachnoid extension to the optic disk is blocked pathologically. Although large blot or splash hemorrhages can occur at the time of a severe subarachnoid hemorrhage, it probably takes some days of abnormally high ICP before papilloedema is evident.

2.3.1 Mechanism of production

Papilloedema is probably due to obstruction of axoplasmic flow resulting swelling of the nerve head.

Unilateral disc swelling may result from an orbital lesion affecting the optic nerve, or from generalized pressure when there is anatomical or pathological blockage of the subarachnoid space around the other optic nerve. A tumor may cause ipsilateral optic atrophy by direct compression and papilloedema on the contralateral by the mass effect (the Foster–Kennedy syndrome).

Papilloedema seldom develops in infants, except following sagital sinus thrombosis. Because the skull bones can separate from each other and the sutures widen. The tension of fontanel is the best guide to ICP in infants. The elderly also have rare papilloedema as a sign of intracranial tumor because the large subarachnoid spaces and dilated ventricles leave more space for the expanding lesion.

2.3.2 Appearance

The swelling of the nerve head may be measured in diopter by comparing the lenses required to bring to the disc to focus and the peripheral retina get into focus. This maneuver requires experience, and even skilled observers often get conflicted conclusions about the degree of swelling. A qualitative assessment based on a number of factors is more useful.

The earliest change is filling of the depression in the nerve head, from which the vessels emerge and where the nerve fibers are seen end–on normally form a stippled patch (cribral lamina). Then the medial half of the disc becomes pink and its edge becomes indistinct, until no normal disc remains visible and the vessels climb out over the heaped–up pink swelling. The veins appear engorged at an early stage and later flame–shaped hemorrhages may develop alongside the vessels usually. In more severe degrees, small circular "blob" hemorrhages and exudates appear.

Papilloedema eventually subsides either because of the fading natural resolution of the responsible process or following surgical relief of pressure. Depending on the severity and duration of the swelling, the disc and the nerve may be restored to normal appearance and full function, or consecutive optic atrophy may develop.

Once started, atrophy often progresses, even though the pressure has been relieved. The patient may be left blind, with a pale disc that is permanently blurred at the edges. Patients with severe papilloedema should be put into the urgency treatment for the sake of avoiding this sequel, even when there appears to be no immediate danger from herniation.

2.3.3 Symptoms

Most patients are unaware of papilloedema and are astonished by the seriousness with other complaints are taken after their fundi have been examined. A lot of brain tumors are firstly detected by ophthalmologists who examine the fundi before prescriptions. The visual fields show blind spot enlargement followed by peripheral field constriction. Children under 9 years old seem curiously reluctant to complain of deteriorating vision, and may present blindness before other features of raised pressure become obvious.

Intermittent loss of vision is more common than consecutive deterioration. Episodes termed as amblyopic attack, which could be complained as obscurations of vision or amaurosis fugax, consist of brief periods of partial or complete blindness, usually lasting less than one minute, occurring many times per day, often occurred repeatedly for several months. There may be complete black out of vision, only blurring, and graying with loss of color perception. Episodes are sometimes precipitated by sudden rising from the horizontal or sitting position and stooping. Postural alterations in local blood supply probably account for these weeks or months of headache. This symptom is often misinterpreted as a form of epilepsy, vertigo, dizziness, or fainting. It is important to recognize because it indicates that sight is in peril and relief of pressure is needed urgently.

Differential diagnoses for bilateral fundi changes include arterial hypertension, pseudo-papilloedema, and prolonged carbon dioxide retention in advanced emphysema. Unilateral fundus changes are mostly due to retrobulbar neuritis, which is usually induced by demyelinating diseases. Visual acuity is affected early and severely, due to a paracentral scotoma impairing central vision. The globe is often painful to move and tender on palpation. The marked swelling of the disc may be indistinguishable from papilloedema, but hemorrhages and exudates are rare. Occasionally the other eye is affected. A less common cause is orbital tumor, which is usually associated with proptosis, failure of vision, and eye movement limitation sometimes.

Thrombosis of the central retinal veinhappens suddenly at the beginning, which also presents with vision loss, as if that in retrobulbar neuritis. But the fundus changes are quite different. Hemorrhages spread widely to the peripheral retina, which is edema with severe engorgement of veins. Cavernous sinus thrombosis and carotid cavernous fistula may manifest similar but less acute and dramatic appearance.

Chapter 3

Effects of Brain Shift

With pressure rising, the brain itself moves sooner or later. How it makes moving depends on the pressure differences between adjacent subdivided compartments separated by dura mater and its special structures, which is driven by expanding lesion. The brain shifts from high-pressure compartment to low-pressure compartment and enters into the larger subarachnoid spaces, the cisterna ambiens, and cisterna magna. In this process, CSF is also redistributed.

Sometimes even though brain shifts, there is no obvious related symptom and sign. Neurological dysfunction could be observed only if the brain shifts greatly enough. Neurological examinations can indicate whether the primary mass is more likely above or below the tentorium, which also warn that the brain is dangerously compressed.

The tentorium is the specific structures of dura mater, which divides the posterior fossa from the supratentorial compartment. This division is complete but for the hiatus which is passed through by the midbrain and filled with the narrow cisterna ambiens. Masses above the tentorium push the midbrain and part of the cerebral hemisphere downward through the tentorial hiatus, the only exit from this compartment. Posterior fossa tumors drive the cerebellar tonsils and medulla oblongata through the foramen magnum. These comprise the two most important brain shifts. Either puts a vital part of the brain in jeopardy.

The word "cone" was first applied to herniation of the cerebellum through the foramen magnum to form a cone-shaped plug of tissue. The verb "to cone" is in common usage among neurosurgeons and neurologists to describe the development of clinical syndromes associated with transtentorial herniation or foraminal impaction.

3.1   Transtentorial Herniation (tentorial or temporal cone)

3.1.1   Pathology

The medial part of the temporal lobe (the uncus and hippocampus) is packed down into the cisterna ambiens forming a hernia (Figure 14-3-1). There are some results induced by the herniation. Midbrain is compressed from ipsilateral to contralateral. The thrust push downwards through the hiatus, the midbrain suffers stresses parallel or perpendicular to its longitudinal axis, i. e. , shearing force and stretching force. Conscious could be impaired, which is resulted from the involvement of reticular formation of brain stem. The third cranial nerve and posterior cerebral artery, which are being fixed above normally, are stretched during herniation. The ipsilateral nerve may also be compressed against the firm petroclinoid ligament as well as being pushed downward by the temporal herniation. Posterior cerebral artery occlusion may result in hemorrhagic infarction of the occipital lobe. The pituitary stalk may be stretched across the dorsum sellae, leading to diabetes insipidus.

Not only the neurons and tracts of the brainstem are distorted, but also the deep vessels are involved. It frequently results in local hemorrhages, which is most likely due to tearing of stretched arterioles and capillaries. Hemorrhage is most striking after acute compression, in which condition it usually does not have time to produce typical tentorial herniation. Whereas, gross herniation and midbrain distortion can occur without any hemorrhage when compression develops slowly.

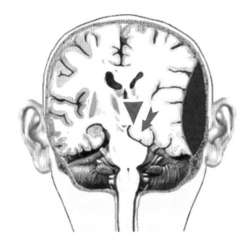

Figure 14-3-1 The formation of tentorial herniation

3.1.2 Clinical manifestation

3.1.2.1 Acute tentorial cone

This critical condition is most often encountered in patients who suffered cerebral hemorrhage, massive infarction followed by edema, necrotizing encephalitis, rapid accumulating traumatic hematoma, and progressing malignant tumors above the tentorium.

Deterioration of conscious level is usually the first evidence of acute coning. At first there may be noworse than somnolence. But soon confusion occurs and there is progression down the coma scale.

The third cranial nerve palsy on the side of the compression is most readily detected by pupil dilatation with loss of both direct and indirect light reflexes. Other third nerve functions are difficult to test in patients with conscious disorder. But in the quite a few who will cooperate, ptosis and eyeball movement restriction (especially upward) may be discovered. Relief of the compression frequently reverses the oculomotor palsy immediately, but it may recover only gradually over days or weeks. If the condition is not relieved the opposite pupil follows the course of the first one. Meanwhile, the recovery is rare once the condition has advanced to the stage of bilaterally fixed and dilated pupils.

Other causes may account for unilateral dilated pupil, including atropine drops, posterior communicating artery aneurysm, and certain recent head injury, in which optic nerve was damaged and the afferent path for the light reflex was impaired, while the pupil will constrict normally when light is shined in the opposite eye (indirect reaction). Bilaterally fixed dilated pupils occur during epileptic seizures and this possibility must be considered when papillary change and coma develop very suddenly. If it is due to epilepsy, the pupils will usually recover within minutes.

Extension posturing of the limbs, which is called decerebrate rigidity previously, results from loss of cortical inhibition. The increased extension tone in the limbs is often associated with neck retraction. The hip joints and knee joints are extended extremely with strong plantar flexion, while the arms are hyper-pronated with the fists clenched and the elbows extended extremely. This posture is often aggravated during the hyperpnoeic phase of periodic respiration or this abnormal tonus may be presented only when painful stimuli are applied. Only the stimulated limb may become decerebrate, and sometimes the response may be generalized.

Autonomic abnormalities include slowing of the pulse and a rising blood pressure. The latter response to rising ICP helps to maintain adequate blood flow to the brain, especially medulla oblongata. If the blood pressure is elevated when the patient first presents, the diagnosis of pre-existing hypertension with cerebral vascular accident must be considered. Respiration may be slow and is periodic-slow and shallow for a few breaths and then more rapid and deep, which is also termed as Cheyne-Stokes breathing.

3.1.2.2   Chronic tentorial cone

Any slowly growing supratentorial mass canraise intracranial pressure even to chronic tentorial cone. But the most striking example is recognized as chronic bilateral subdural hematoma.

Loss of conjugate upward gaze with bilateral ptosis is probably the result of compression of the dorsal midbrain. Ptosis is easily neglected when the patient is in bed. But the wrinkled forehead and surprising look (due to over action of frontalis) with the eyes only partly opened imply some clues and are the characteristics of ptosis. If cooperation is poor, the eyes may be induced to turn up reflexive by touching the cornea, and a diminution in upward movement can be detected. Both ptosis and loss of upward movement are sometimes more marked on one side than the other. A tumor in the pineal region may be suspected. But dilated pupil reacting is only dull to light, which is common in pineal tumors, but rarely a feature of a chronic cone.

The fluctuating conscious level is a striking feature, which is probably due to impairment of function in the midbrain reticular formation. The patient who is somnolence and almost inaccessible may appear normally alert only a few hours later, and this cycle may be repeated many times without any obvious precipitating factors.

Ipsilateral hemiplegia, which could be induced by supratentorial mass or chronic subdural hematoma, is due to compression of contralateral corticospinal tract of the cerebral peduncle against the contralateral tentorium notch, terming the Kenohan-Woltman notch phenomenon.

Homonymous hemianopia, from posterior cerebral artery compression, is not often detected clinically.

Occasionally a mass in the posterior fossa causes upward displacement of the upper part of the vermis through the tentorial hiatus. This upward transtentorial herniation may compress the dorsal midbrain, which is encouraged to lower the supratentorial pressure by external lateral ventricle drainage rather than lower the infratentorial pressure by decompression craniotomy of the posterior fossa.

3.2   Foraminal Impaction (cerebellar or tonsillar cone)

3.2.1   Pathology

Normally the tonsils just reach the level of the foramen. When pressure in the posterior fossa reaches critical level, the cerebellar tonsils will crowd into the foramen magnum, followed by medulla oblongata being pushed forward and compressed against the anterior bony margin. In this case, the tonsils are often found as low as axis (second cervical vertebra) of the spine.

3.2.2   Clinical manifestation

A foraminal conemay lead to apnea with little or no warning due to acute compression, or it may develop as the terminal stage of a neglected tentorial cone.

Abnormal neck posture behaves several forms. A child may have a tilted head when he walks because of vestibular imbalance or the sixth nerve weakness, the reason of which is that the head position is adapted to avoid diplopia. However, this tilted head is seldom noticed by the patient or the relatives.

Stiff neck, due to irritation of the dura mater around the foramen magnum by the tightly packed structures, may raise the signs of meningitis. Tingling in the arms on extension of the neck is due to compression on the cervical spinal cord by the prolapsed plug in the foramen magnum. Some patients may be "black-out" if they flex the neck too far. This movement reduces volume of cervical canal and raises pressure through complete blockage of CSF circulation and causing pressure directly impacted on the medulla oblongata. Thus, opisthotonos occurs, which is the extreme opposite posture of flexion.

Abnormalities of respiratory rate and rhythm are quite danger signs in posterior fossa compression. A slow rate, even 9 breaths a minute, may be continued with complete regularity for days but this is uncommon. Periodic breathing is common. In the classical form (Cheyne–Stokes breathing) it consists of a crescendo of breaths of increasing depth and frequency followed by a period of total apnea of up to a minute or so, probably until the accumulating carbon dioxide reaches a high enough level to stimulate the failing respiratory center. Any irregularity of respiration should raise suspicion of a foraminal cone, which is probably the final stage of cerebral compression of whatever origin. When foraminal cone happens induced by the mass is in the posterior fossa, however, apnea is frequently quite sudden, without impaired consciousness or any other warning signs.

Chapter 4

Differential Diagnoses

Intracranial space–occupying lesions may present with clinical evidence of increased pressure and focal neurological disorders. The differential diagnosis varies with the type of presentation, and any evidence of brain shift.

4.1　Increased Intracranial Pressure with Focal Features

This combination leaves little doubt that the patient issuffering from an intracranial mass. Tumor may be distinguished in most instances from abscess to hematoma by the preceding histories. However, neither sudden onset nor spontaneous remission excludes tumor. Moreover, the patients with tumor may have raised blood pressure either from preexisting hypertension or as a reaction to raised ICP.

4.2　Focal Features Alone

This opens a wider field of differential diagnosis. Confusion most often arises with cerebrovascular disease, cerebral atrophy, and demyelinating disorders. However, careful histories collection is invaluable in differentiation from brain tumor. The steady progressive development of dysfunction that is confined to a single, even if extensive, area of the brain is suggestive of tumor. Nearly all patients developing persist or progress focal neurological signs should be investigated as to confirm brain tumor, unless there are definite indications of cerebrovascular diseases or demyelization diseases, of which the present features are different from the previous disturbance episodes of functional area.

4.3　Raised Pressure Alone

This is a more frequent and a more pressing situation. Likely causes include midline masses blocking CSF flow and causing obstructive hydrocephalus, silent and slowly growing supratentorial masses (usually non primary frontal or temporal), and chronic bilateral subdural hematoma. Progressive loss of vision from papilloedema occurs with relatively few headaches in patients with benign meningioma or neurofibroma. Mental disorder happens even in patients without any suspicious of organic disease, which may be referred to psychiatric consultation thereafter.

A number of patients with raised pressure alone appear having no local lesion after investigation, and are diagnosed as suffering from the unexplained but not uncommon conditions known as pseudotumor cerebri, otitic hydrocephalus, serous meningitis, and benign intracranial hypertension. It is most common in adolescents, especially in women, and may be associated with pregnancy and obesity, sometimes with infections, especially of the ear. Headaches, seldom of great severity, are followed by diplopia due to sixth nerve weakness from raised ICP. There is severe papilloedema. In some cases, obscuration of vision progresses to blindness due to consecutive atrophy. With all these evidences of severe raised ICP, the patients hardly stay full healthy.

The natural history is towards resolution but it may be many months before papilloedema subsiding completely. Treatment is usually applied with steroids and the diet to reduce weight, if required. Lumbar puncture, which was sometimes done repeatedly as an aid to recovery previously, shows that the pressure fluctuates widely day to day. A further curious feature is the abnormal low CSF protein (100–200 mg/L). Some patients require a lumbo–peritoneal shunt. But subtemporal decompression craniotomy is rarely required as an attempt to save sight.

The association between otitis media and the leading term "otitic hydrocephalus" is explained in theory that it was due to thrombosis spreading from the lateral to the sagital sinus with impaired CSF absorption. This explains the symptoms in a proportion of the patients. But in majority the pathogenesis remains unexplained. The ventricles are never dilated. Accurate measurement shows a reduction in ventricular size, giving the impression that they are being squeezed by the swollen brain.

There are other causes of raised pressure other than brain tumor. Arterial hypertension, polycythaemia, and chronic emphysema are more common. Each must be quite severe before it affects ICP, and therefore is obvious if general physical examination is conducted, as which should be done in every suspected brain tumor case.

Emphatically, patients with suspected raised intracranial pressure require a CT scan immediately.

Chapter 5

Treatment of Intracranial Hypertension

In some patients, despite the above measures, cerebral swelling may produce a marked increase in intracranial pressure. This may follow removal of a tumor or hematoma, and may complicate a diffuse head injury. Artificial methods of lowing intracranial pressure may prevent brain damage and death from brain shift, although the uses in some instances are still controversial. Treatment of raised intracranial pressure (in the absence of any identifiable cause, e. g. , hematoma or rising $PaCO_2$) is a controversial topic in head injury management. Some believe that active reduction of an elevated ICP significantly reduces management mortality and morbidity. Others feel that if brain damage is severe enough to cause a rise of ICP, the artificially reducing the ICP to normal levels does not alter the extent of the damage, even improve outcome. In adults, more and more evidences suggest that active ICP reduction benefit mortality or morbidity improvement. In children, even though the pathogenesis of raised ICP may differ, some studies suggest that cerebral vasodilatation with a subsequent increase in cerebral blood volume is a major factor, rather than an increase in brain water content (cerebral edema). Thus, treatment of raised ICP may well benefit.

Treatment may be instituted when the mean ICP is over 30 mmHg. This may be reduced by hyperventilation (reducing the $PaCO_2$), repeated mannitol infusion, and CSF drainage, etc. These artificial methods to ICP reduction are maintained until the level falls spontaneously back to normal ranges. In many patients, this treatment fails to produce a sustained effect and the ICP returns to previous levels or continues to rise unabated until death ensues. Some clinicians still use barbiturate therapy when the ICP fails to respond to other measures, but its value remains unproven. When a rising intracranial pressure is caused by an expanding mass, or is accompanied by respiratory problems, the mass must be removed and blood gas restored to normal by ventilation, if necessary.

5.1 Hypertonic Solutions

Hypertonic solutions, given intravenously, take into effect depending osmotic dehydration of the brain, which results into blood volume increasing and inducing diuresis. Reduction of ICP is evident within about 15 minutes of rapid infusion and the effect lasts for 4–6 hours. A saturated solution of mannitol (20%) is most commonly used, but this must be kept in a warm cupboard to prevent crystallization. The full dose is 250 mL given over 20 minutes, but smaller amounts may be effective. Usually the unit dosage ranges 0. 25–

1 g/kg (1.25–5 mL/kg). It reduces ICP by establishing an osmotic gradient between the plasma and brain tissue. Mannitol is also used every 6–hour within 24–48 hours period in the attempt to reduce raised ICP. However, repeated infusions lead to equilibration and high intracellular osmotic pressure, which will counteract further treatment. In addition, repeated dose may precipitate lethal rises in arterial blood pressure and acute tubular necrosis. Its usage is therefore best restricted for emergency situations. Frusemide may itself be effective. If given 30 minutes before mannitol, it will largely prevent the rise in blood pressure which is normally observed as the result of an increase in blood volume. In the operation room mannitol may be given as a routine after induction of anesthesia, so that its maximal effect peaks by the time that the bone flap is turned over. However, in most situations properly conducted anesthesia with good positioning on the table and controlled respiration will give sufficient slack brain. But disadvantages may result, in which brain shrinkage may tear bridging veins or avulse olfactory nerves, causing permanent anosmia.

5.2　Steroids

There is no doubt that steroids play an important role in treating patients with intracranial tumor and surrounding edema, in which cell membranes are stabilized. But it is not certain that their beneficial effect in tumor management is due to the result of reducing ICP. Steroids appear to be of no value in the treatment of traumatic or ischemic damage. Experimental evidences suggest that they may help if administered before the damage occurs. But apparently this is seldom of practical value.

Corticosteroids are less rapid in action but their effects can be never–the–less dramatic in patients with intracranial tumors. Although side effects tend to develop with prolonged using, patients with inoperable tumors may tolerate a low maintenance dose of 2 mg/day of dexamethasone and maintain a sustained improvement over months. But they will only to develop symptoms again as soon as this drug is withdrawn. In acute situations a dose of 4 mg four times a day is given, followed by to be reduced to 2 mg three times a day after 3 days and eventually down to 2 mg/day. Although sometimes it is employed as a routine postoperative method to prevent edema and brain swelling, steroids are probably not useful in the treatment of spontaneous or aneurysmal intracranial hematoma. They have no place in the treatment of head injury. To date several controlled trials as well as other studies have failed to show any better results in craniocerebral traumatic injured patients treated with steroids, even in mega dosage.

5.3　Hyperventilation

Hyperventilation, by inducing cerebral vasoconstriction secondary to hypocapnia, reduces ICP within minutes. If the patient is anesthetized and hyperventilation brings $PaCO_2$ down to 25 mmHg, the resultant vasoconstriction and reduction in cerebral blood flow lowers intracranial pressure. However, further drop in $PaCO_2$ risks ischemic damage due to severe vasoconstriction. Meanwhile, many patients adapt to the new $PaCO_2$ level, and after several hours the ICP gradually rises to previous levels again.

5.4   Barbiturate Therapy

Some doctors have advocated barbiturate therapy in the treatment of raised ICP following brain damage. Barbiturates reduce cerebral metabolism, thereby reducing metabolic requirements and activities of neurons. They also block free radical production. A fall in energy requirements may protect ischemic areas and subsequent vasoconstriction may reduce cerebral blood flow and intracranial pressure. Although some experimental studies have shown encouraging results, clinical trials have yet to show convincing benefit.

5.5   CSF Withdrawing

Removal of some CSF from the ventricle will immediately reduce the ICP. However, within minutes, the pressure rises and further CSF withdrawal will be required. In practice, this method is of limited value, since CSF outflow to the lumber theca results in a diminished intracranial CSF volume and the lateral ventricles are often collapsed. Continuous CSF drainage may make most advantage of this method. A ventricular catheter is inserted through a burr hole temporarily relieves pressure. CSF drains to a sterile transfusion bag. The height of the loop of tubing should be fixed at about 150 mm above the head. A patient who is critically ill with high pressure may be operated in better condition after 24–72 hours of continuous drainage. However, the risk of infection increases as the drainage period prolongs. Another danger of CSF drainage is upward herniation of the cerebellum through the tentorial hiatus.

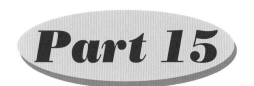

Part 15

Craniocerebral Trauma

Chapter 1

Scalp Injuries

Scalp consists of several distinct types of layers: ①The hairy skin. ②The subcutaneous fat and connective tissue layer. ③The galea or aponeurosis (a thin fibrous layer to which the flat epicranial muscles are attached). ④The thin layer of loose connective tissue and finally. ⑤The periosteum of the skull.

The scalp is susceptible to all types of injury, particularly laceration as it is readily crushed and split against the underlying bone. Such lacerations are often linear due to the convexity of the underlying skull. The scalp often swells markedly due to edema (water−logged tissues) or hematoma formation (raised swelling) due to bruising above or below the galeal layer. Dense hair may mask scalp injuries.

Types of Scalp Injuries:

(1) Laceration and hematoma: Apply direct pressure to control bleeding. Under sterile condition, inspect the wound for debris and palpate for fracture.

(2) Subgaleal hematoma: The galea is the aponeurotic part of the pericranial muscle overlying the periosteum, separated from it by loose alveolar tissue. The subgaleal hematoma presents as a localized or diffuse fluctuant swelling, usually in in−ants due to bloody fluid accumulation in the potential space between the galea and periosteum. A clinically significant hemorrhage may occur in infants and young children, which resolves and this lesion does not trans−illuminate.

(3) Subgaleal hygroma: This is an uncommon scalp accumulation of cerebrospinal fluid due to laceration of dura and arachnoid membrane by skull fracture. Clinically the condition resembles subgaleal hematoma except for the fact that hygroma trans−illuminate and is associated with skull fracture.

Chapter 2

Skull Fractures

2.1 Anatomy of Fracture

The causative forces and fracture pattern, type, extent, and position are important in assessing the sustained injury. The skull is thickened at the glabellas, external occipital protuberance, mastoid processes, and external angular process and is joined by 3 arches on either side. The skull vault is composed of cancellous bone (diploe) sandwiched between 2 tablets, the lamina externa (1. 5 mm), and the lamina interna (0. 5 mm). The diploe does not form where the skull is covered with muscles, leaving the vault thin and prone to fracture.

The skull is prone to fracture at certain anatomic sites that include the thin squamous temporal and parietal bones over the temples and the sphenoid sinus, the foramen magnum, the petrous temporal ridge, and the inner parts of the sphenoid wings at the skull base. The middle cranial fossa is the weakest, with thin bones and multiple foramina. Other places prone to fracture include the cribriform plate and the roof of orbits in the anterior cranial fossa and the areas between the mastoid and dural sinuses in the posterior cranial fossa.

2.2 History of the Skull Fracture

Skull fracture is described in Edwin Smith's papyrus, the oldest known surgical paper (Atta, 1999). The papyrus describes a conservative and expectant approach to skull trauma, With better results compared to a more aggressive and less favorable approach described in Hippocratic medicine (Prioreschhi, 1993).

Charles Bell first described occipital condylar fracture in 1817 based on an autopsy finding (Bell, 1817). The same fracture was described for the first time as an X-ray finding in 1962 (Ahlgren, 1962) and by computed tomography (CT) in 1983 (Peeters, 1983).

2.3　Classification

Fractures of the skull can be classified as linear or depressed. Linear fractures are either vault fractures or skull base fractures. Vault fractures and depressed fractures can be either closed or open (clean or dirty/contaminated).

2.4　Linear Skull Fracture

Linear fracture results from low–energy blunt trauma over a wide surface area of the skull. It runs through the entire thickness of the bone sand, by itself, is of little significance except when it runs through a vascular channel, venous sinus groove, or a suture. In these situations, it may cause epidural hematoma, venous sinus thrombosis and occlusion, and sutural diastases, respectively. Differences between sutures and fractures are summarized in Table 15–2–1.

Table 15–2–1　Differences between skull fractures and sutures

Fractures	Sutures
Greater than 3 mm in width	Less than 2 mm in width
Wisest at the center and narrow at the ends	Same width throughout
Runs through both the outer and the inner lamina of bone, hence appears darker	Lighter on x–rays compared to fracture lines
Usually over temporoparietal area	At specific anatomic sites
Usually runs in a straight line	Does not run in a straight line
Angular turns	Curvaceous

2.5　Basilar Skull Fracture

In essence, a basilar fracture is a linear fracture at the base of the skull. It usually is as sociated with a dural tear and is found at specific points on the skull base.

2.6　Temporal Fracture

The three subtypes of temporal fractures are longitudinal, transverse, and mixed (Wennmo, 1993).

Longitudinal fracture(Figure 15–2–1) occurs in the temporoparietal region and involves the squamous portion of the temporal bone, the superior wall of the external auditory canal, and the tegmen tympani. These fractures may run either anterior or posterior to the cochlea and labyrinthine capsule, ending in the middle cranial fossa near the foramen spinosum or in the mastoid air cells, respectively. Longitudinal fracture is the most common of the three subtypes (70% –90%).

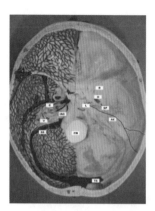

Figure 15-2-1   Internal aspect of the skull base that represents, in black and blue colors, the pathway of the longitudinal temporal bone fracture lines

Transverse fractures (Figure 15-2-2) begin at the foramen magnum and extend through the cochlea and labyrinth, ending in the middle cranial fossa (5%-30%).

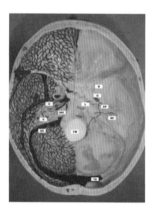

Figure 15-2-2   Internal aspect of the skull base that represents, in black and red colors, the pathways of the transverse temporal bone fracture lines

Mixed fractures have elements of both longitudinal and transverse fractures.

2.7   Occipital Condylar Fracture

Occipital condylar fracture results from a high-energy blunt trauma with axial compression lateral bending, or rotational injury to the alar ligament. These fractures are subdivided into three types based on the morphology and mechanism of injury (Anderson, 1988). An alternative classification divided theses fractures into stable and displaced, i. e. , with and without ligamentous injury (Tuli, 1997).

Type I fracture is secondary to axial compression resulting in comminution of the occipital condyle. This is a stable injury.

Type II fracture results from a direct blow, and despite being a more extensive basioccipital fracture, type II fracture is classified as stable because of the preserved alar ligament and tectorial membrane.

Type III fracture is an avulsion injury as a result of forced rotation and lateral bending. This is potentially an unstable fracture.

2.8   Depressed Skull Fracture

Depressed skull fractures (Figure 15-2-3) result from a high-energy direct blow to a small surface area of the skull with a blunt object such as a baseball bat. Comminution of fragments starts from the point of maximum impact and spreads centrifugally. Most of the depressed fractures are over the frontoparietal region because the bone is thin and the specific location is prone to an assailants attack. A free piece of bone should be depressed greater than the adjacent inner table of the skull to be of clinical significance and requiring elevation.

A depressed fracture may be open or closed. Open fractures, by definition, have either a skin laceration over the fracture or the fracture runs through the paranasal sinuses and the middle ear structures, resulting in communication between the external environment and the cranial cavity. Open fractures may be clean or contaminated/dirty.

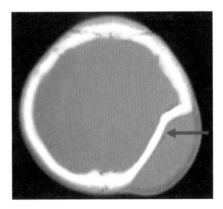

Figure 15-2-3   Depressed skull fractures

2.9   Frequency

Simple linear fracture is by far the most common type of fracture, especially in children younger than 5 years. Temporal bone fractures represent 15%-48% of all skull fractures. Basilar skull fractures represent 19%-21% of all skull fractures. Depressed fractures are frontoparietal (75%), temporal(10%), occipital (5%), and other (10%). Most of the depressed fractures are open fractures (75%-90%).

2.10   Etiology

In newborns, "ping-pong" depressed fractures are secondary to the baby's head impinging against the mother's sacral promontory during uterine contractions(Ingram,1950). The use of forceps also may cause injury to the skull, but this is rare skull fractures in infants originate from neglect, fall, or abuse. Most of the fractures seen in children are a result of falls and bicycle accidents. In adults, fractures typically occur from motor vehicle accidents or violence

2.11 Clinical

2.11.1 Linear skull fracture

Most patients with linear skull fractures are asymptomatic and present without loss of consciousness. Swelling occurs at the site of impact, and the skin may or may not be breached.

2.11.2 Basilar skull fracture

Patients with fractures of the petrous temporal bone present with CSF otorrhea and bruising over the mastoids, i. e. , Battle sign. Presentation with anterior cranial fossa fractures is with CSF rhinorrhea and bruising around the eyes, i. e. , "raccoon eyes". Loss of consciousness and Glasgow coma score may vary depending on an associated intracranial pathology.

Longitudinal temporal bone fractures result in ossicular chain disruption and conductive deafness of greater than 30 dB that lasts longer than 6–7 weeks. Temporary deafness that resolves in less than 3 weeks is due to hemotympanum and mucosal edema in the middle ear a. Facial palsy, nystagmus, and facial numbness are secondary to involvement of the Ⅶ, Ⅵ, and Ⅴ cranial nerves, respectively. Transverse temporal bone fractures involve the Ⅷ cranial nerve and the labyrinth, resulting in nystagmus, ataxia, and permanent neural hearing.

Occipital condylar fracture is a very rare and serious injury (Legros, 1999). Most of the patients with occipital condylar fracture, especially with type Ⅱ, are in a coma and have other associated cervical spinal injuries. These patients also may present with other lower cranial nerve injuries and hemiplegia or quadriplegia Vernet syndrome or jugular foramen syndrome is involvement of the Ⅸ, Ⅹ, and Ⅺ cranial nerves with the fracture. Patients present with difficulty in phonation and aspiration and ipsilateral motor; paralysis of the vocal cord, soft palate (curtain sign), superior pharyngeal constrictor; sternocleidomastoid, and trapezius.

Collet–Sicard syndrome is occipital condylar fracture with Ⅸ Ⅹ, Ⅺ and Ⅻ cranial nerve involvement (Collet, 1917 ; Sicard, 1917; Rebattu, 1925).

2.11.3 Depressed skull fracture

Approximately 25% of patients with depressed skull fracture do not report loss of consciousness, and another 25% loose consciousness for less than an hour. The presentation may vary depending on other associated intracranial injuries such as epidural hematoma, dural tears, and seizures.

2.12 Lab Studies

In addition to a complete neurological examination, baseline laboratory analyses, and tetanus toxoid (where appropriate, as in open skull fractures), the diagnostic workup for fractures is radiological.

2.13   Imaging Studies

(1) Radiographs

In 1987, the skull X−ray referral criteria panel decided that skull films are suboptimal in detecting basilar skull fractures. Hence, other than a fracture at the vertex that might be missed by CT scan and picked up by a plain film, skull X−ray is of no benefit when a CT scan is performed.

(2) CT scan

CT scan is the criterion standard modality for aiding in the diagnosis of skull fractures. Thinly sliced bone windows of up to 1−1. 5 mm thick, with sagittal reconstruction, are useful in assessing injuries. Helical CT scan is helpful in occipital condylar fractures, but 3−dimensional reconstruction usually is not necessary.

(3) MRI

MRI or magnetic resonance angiography is of ancillary value for suspected ligamentous and vascular injuries. Bony injuries are far better visualized using CT scan.

2.14   Other Tests

Bleeding from the ear or nose in cases of suspected CSF leak, when dabbed on a tissue paper, will show a clear ring of wet tissue beyond the blood stain, called a "halo" or "ring" sign. CSF also can be detected by analyzing the glucose level and by measuring tau−transferrin.

2.15   Treatment

2.15.1   Medical therapy

Adults with simple linear fractures who are neurologically intact do not require any intervention and may even be discharged home safely and asked to return if symptomatic. Infants with simple linear fractures should be admitted for overnight observation regardless of neurological status. Neurologically intact patients with linear basilar fractures also are treated conservatively, without antibiotics. Temporal bone fractures are managed conservatively, at least initially, because tympanic membrane rupture usually heals on its own.

Simple depressed fractures in neurologically intact infants are treated expectantly. These depressed fractures heal well and smooth out with time, without elevation. Seizure medications are recommended if the chance of developing seizures is higher than 20%. Open fractures, if contaminated, may require antibiotics in addition to tetanus toxoid. Sulfisoxazole is a common recommendation.

Type II and III occipital condylar fractures are treated conservatively with neck stabilization achieved in a hard (Philadelphia) collar or halo traction.

2.15.2   Surgical therapy

The role of surgery is limited in the management of skull fractures. Infants and children with open depressed fractures require surgical intervention. Most surgeons prefer to elevate depressed skull fractures if the depressed segment is more than 5 mm below the inner table of adjacent bone. Indications for immediate elevation are gross contamination, dural tear with pneumocephalus, and an underlying hematoma. Another indication for early surgical intervention is an unstable occipital condylar fracture (type Ⅲ) that requires atlantoaxial arthrodesis.

Delayed surgical intervention is required in ossicular in－congruencies resulting from a longitudinal skull base fracture of the temporal bone. Ossiculoplasty may be needed if hearing loss persists for longer than 3 months or if the tympanic membrane has not healed on its own. Another indication is persistent CSF leak after a skull base fracture. This requires precise detection of the site of leak before any surgical intervention is instituted.

2.15.3　Preoperative details

Blind probing of skull wounds should be avoided. Patients are prepared for surgery, and exploration is performed in the operating suite under direct vision to prevent loose pieces of bone from damaging the underlying brain. Patients with open contaminated wounds are treated with tetanus toxoid and broad－spectrum antibiotics, especially in a delayed presentation.

2.15.4　Intra－operative details

To maintain intracranial pressure, mannitol (1 g/kg) may be given at the beginning, and the PaO_2 should be kept at 30－35 mmHg during the surgery. Patients should be secured firmly to the table, allowing Trendelenburg or reverse Trendelenburg positioning if required. A lazy "S" or a horseshoe－shaped incision is made over the depression. A bicoronal incision is preferred for forehead depressions.

Bony fragments are elevated, and the dura is inspected for any tears. If a dural tearis found, it should be repaired. Special attention is given to homeostasis to prevent postoperative epidural collection. Bony fragments are soaked in antibiotic/isotonic sodium chloride solution and are reassembled. Larger pieces may be wired together. Alternatively, titanium mesh also may be used to cover the defect. Methyl methacrylate can be used instead of the bone pieces J but this should be avoided in children.

Depressed fracture over a venous sinus poses a unique situation requiring special attention. The decision to operate is based on the neurological status of the patient, the exact location of the sinus involved, and the degree of venous flow compromise. A preoperative angiogram with venous flow phase or magnetic resonance angiography is recommended whenever a depressed fracture is thought to be over a venous sinus. Useful data regarding the position and extent of occlusion and transverse sinus dominance is obtained that can affect decisions regarding surgery.

A neurologically stable patient with a closed depressed fracture over a venous sinus should be observed. A patient with an open depressed fracture over a patent venous sinus who is neurologically stable should undergo skin debridement without elevation of the fracture, but if the patient is neurologically unstable, urgent elevation of the depressed fragment is required. On the other hand, if the patient is neurologically stable and the sinus is thrombosed, it can be assumed that ligation of the sinus will be tolerated.

Usually, the anterior one third of the superior sagittal sinus can be ligated without any consequences; however, tears in the posterior two thirds need repair, either primarily or with a galea or pericranium patch. Alternatively, a piece of muscle or gelfoam may be sutured over the sinus.

2.15.5　Postoperative details

Other than the usual immediate postoperative care, the risk of intracranial hematoma and venous sinus thrombosis should be kept in mind in contaminated depressed fractures.

2.16　Follow-up care

Adults with simple linear fractures of the vault, without any loss of consciousness at the time of initial presentation and with no other complications, do not require long-term follow-up. On the other hand, infants with similar fractures with dural tears need to be monitored more closely because of the possibility of the skull fracture expanding.

Patients with contaminated open depressed skull fractures treated surgically should be monitored with repeat CT scans a few times over the next 2-3 months to check for abscess formation. Follow-up also is dictated by the complications associated with skull fractures, for example, seizures, infections, and removal of bone pieces at the time of initial debridement.

2.17　Complications

Failure to recognize skull fracture has more consequences than the complications resulting from treatment. The chance of a concomitant cervical spine injury is 15%, and this should be kept in mind when assessing a patient with skull fracture.

2.17.1　Linear skull fracture

In infants and children, a simple linear fracture, if associated with a dural tear, can lead to subepicranial hygroma or a growing skull fracture (leptomeningeal cyst). This may take up to 6 months to develop, resulting from the brain pulsating against a dural defect that is larger than the bone defect. Repair of such a defect is performed using a split-thickness bone graft. A fracture line crossing over a vascular groove, such as the middle meningeal artery, may form an epidural hematoma (Epstein, 1961). Similarly, a fracture line that crosses over a suture may cause sutural diastases.

2.17.2　Basilar skull fracture

The risk of infection is not high, even without routine antibiotics, especially with CSF rhinorrhea. Facial palsy and ossicular chain disruption associated with basilar fractures are discussed. However, notably, facial palsy that starts with a 2- to 3-day delay is secondary to neuropraxia of the VII cranial nerve and is responsive to steroids, with a good prognosis. A complete and sudden onset of facial palsy at the time of fracture usually is secondary to nerve transection, with a poor prognosis.

Other cranial nerves also may be involved in basilar fractures. Fracture of the tip of the petrous temporal bone may involve the gasserian ganglion. An isolated VI cranial nerve injury is not a direct result of fracture, but it may be affected secondarily because of tension on the nerve. Lower cranial nerves (IX, X, XI, and XII) may be involved in occipital condylar fractures, as described earlier in Vernet and Collet-Sicard syndromes (vide supra). Sphenoid bone fracture may affect the III, IV, and VI cranial nerves and also may disrupt the internal carotid artery and potentially result in pseudo-aneurysm formation and caroticocavemous fistula (if it involves venous structures).

2.17.3 Depressed skull fracture

In addition to the risk of infection in contaminated depressed skull fractures, a risk of developing seizures also exists. The overall risk of seizures in low, but it is higher if the patient loses consciousness for longer than 2 hours, if an associated dural tear is present, and if the seizures start in the first week of injury.

Chapter 3

Primary Cerebral Injury

Primary brain injury refers to brain injury that occurs immediately after violent action on the head, mainly including cerebral concussion, contusion and/or laceration, diffuse axonal injury and so on.

3.1 Concussion of the Brain

3.1.1 Definition and background

Concussion of the brain is the most common type of traumatic brain injury. Frequently defined as a head injury with a transient loss of brain function, concussion can cause a variety of physical, cognitive, and emotional symptoms. Treatment of concussion involves monitoring and rest. Symptoms usually go away entirely within 3 weeks, though they may persist, or complications may occur. Repeated concussions can cause cumulative brain damage such as dementia pugilistica or severe complications such as second−impact syndrome. Due to factors such as widely varying definitions and possible underreporting of concussion, the rate at which it occurs annually is not known; however it may be more than 6 per 1000 people. Common causes include sports injuries, bicycle accidents, car accidents, and falls; the latter two are the most frequent causes among adults. Concussion may be caused by a blow to the head, or by acceleration forces without a direct impact. The forces involved disrupt cellular processes in the brain for days or weeks. It is not known whether the concussed brain is structurally damaged the way it is in other types of brain injury or whether concussion mainly entails a loss of function with physiological but not structural changes. Cellular damage has reportedly been found in concussed brains, but it may have been due to artifacts from the studies.

3.1.2 Mechanism

The brain is surrounded by cerebrospinal fluid, one of the functions of which is to protect it from light trauma, but more severe impacts or the forces associated with rapid acceleration may not be absorbed by this cushion. Concussion may be caused by impact forces, in which the head strikes or is struck by something, or impulsive forces, in which the head moves without itself being subject to blunt trauma (for example, when the chest hits something and the head snaps forward).

3.1.3　Pathophysiology

Concussion involves diffuse (as opposed to focal) brain injury, meaning that the dysfunction occurs over a widespread area of the brain rather than in a particular spot. Concussion is thought to be a milder type of diffuse axonal injury because axons may be injured to a minor extent due to stretching. Animal studies in which primates were concussed have revealed damage to brain tissues such as small petechial hemorrhages and axonal injury. Axonal damage has been found in the brains of concussion sufferers who died from other causes, but inadequate blood flow to the brain due to other injuries may have contributed to the damage. Findings from a study of the brains of dead NFL athletes who received concussions suggest there is lasting damage to the brain after experiencing one; this damage can lead to a variety of other health issues.

3.1.4　Concussion grading systems

Three concussion grading systems are followed most widely: one was developed by Robert Cantu, one by the Colorado Medical Society, and a third by the American Academy of Neurology. Each divides concussion into three grades, as summarized in the following table(Table 15-3-1).

Table 15-3-1　Comparison of concussion grading scales

Classification	Crade I	Crade II	Crade III
Cantu guidelines	Post-traumatic amnesia < 30 min, no loss of consciousness	Loss of consciousness<5 min or amnesia lasting 30 min-24 h	Loss of consciousness > 5 min or amnesia >24 h
Colorado Medical Society guidelines	Confusion, no loss consciousness	Confusion, post-traumatic amnesia, no loss of consciousness	Any loss of consciousness
American Academy of Neurology guidelines	Confusion, symptoms last < 15 min, no loss of consciousness	Symptoms last >15 min, no loss of consciousness	Loss of consciousness(III a, coma lasts seconds, III b for minutes)

3.1.5　Signs and symptoms

Concussion can be associated with a variety of symptoms, which typically occur rapidly after the injury. Early symptoms usually subside within days or weeks. The number and type of symptoms a person suffers varies widely.

Headache is the most common mild traumatic brain injury (MTBI) symptom. Other symptoms include dizziness, vomiting, nausea, lack of motor coordination, difficulty balancing, or other problems with movement or sensation. Visual symptoms include light sensitivity, seeing bright lights, blurred vision, and double vision. Tinnitus, or a ringing in the ears, is also commonly reported. In one in about seventy concussions, concussive convulsions occur, but these are not actual post-traumatic seizures and are not predictive of post-traumatic epilepsy, which results from structural brain damage. Concussive convulsions are thought to result from temporary loss of brain function rather than from structural damage and are usually associated with a good outcome.

Cognitive symptoms include confusion, disorientation, and difficulty focusing attention. Loss of consciousness may occur but is not necessarily correlated with the severity of the concussion if it is brief. Post-traumatic amnesia, in which the person can not remember events leading up to the injury or after it, or both, is a hallmark of concussion. Confusion, another concussion hallmark, may be present immediately or may develop over several minutes. A patient may, for example, repeatedly ask the same questions, be slow to respond to questions or directions, have a vacant stare, or have slurred or incoherent speech. Other MTBI symptoms include changes in sleeping patterns and difficulty with reasoning, concentrating, and performing everyday activities.

Affective results of concussion include crankiness, loss of interest in favorite activities or items, tearfulness, and displays of emotion that are inappropriate to the situation. Common symptoms in concussed children include restlessness, lethargy, and irritability.

3.1.6　Diagnosis

Diagnosis of concussion of the brain is based on physical and neurological exams, duration of unconsciousness (usually less than 30 minutes) and post-traumatic amnesia (PTA; usually less than 24 hours), and the Glasgow coma scale (MTBI sufferer have scores of 13-15). Neuropsychological tests exist to measure cognitive function. The tests may be administered hours, days, or weeks after the injury, or at different times to determine whether there is a trend in the patient's condition. Athletes may be tested before a sports season begins to provide a baseline comparison in the event of an injury.

Most concussions can not be detected with MRI or CT scans. However, changes have been reported to show up on MRI and SPECT imaging in concussed people with normal CT scans, and post-concussion syndrome may be associated with abnormalities visible on SPECT and PET scans. Mild head injury may or may not produce abnormal EEG readings.

3.1.7　Treatment

Usually the symptoms of concussion of the brain go away without treatment, and no specific treatment exists. Traditionally, concussion sufferers are prescribed rest, including plenty of sleep at night plus rest during the day.

Medications may be prescribed to treat symptoms such as sleep problems and depression. Analgesics such as ibuprofen can be taken for the headaches that frequently occur after concussion, but paracetamol (acetaminophen) is preferred to minimize the risk for complications such as intracranial hemorrhage. Concussed individuals are advised not to drink alcohol or take drugs that have not been approved by a doctor, as they could impede healing.

Observation to monitor for worsening condition is an important part of treatment. Health care providers recommend that those suffering from concussion return for further medical care and evaluation 24-72 hours after the concussive event if the symptoms worsen. Repeated observation for the first 24 hours after concussion is recommended.

3.1.8　Prognosis

Concussion of the brain has a mortality rate of almost zero. The symptoms of most concussions resolve within weeks, but problems may persist. It is not common for problems to be permanent, and outcome is usually excellent. People over age 55 may take longer to heal from MTBI or may heal incompletely. Similarly, factors such as a previous head injury or a coexisting medical condition have been found to predict longer-lasting post-concussion symptoms. Other factors that may lengthen recovery time after MTBI include psychological problems such as substance abuse or clinical depression, poor health before the injury or addi-

tional injuries sustained during it, and life stress. Longer periods of amnesia or loss of consciousness immediately after the injury may indicate longer recovery times from residual symptoms. For unknown reasons,
having had one concussion significantly increases a person's risk of having another. Having previously sustained a sports concussion has been found to be a strong factor increasing the likelihood of a concussion in
the future. Other strong factors include participation in a contact sport and body mass size. The prognosis
may differ between concussed adults and children; little research has been done on concussion in the pediatric population, but concern exists that severe concussions could interfere with brain development in children.

3.2   Cerebral Contusion and Laceration

3.2.1   Definition and background

Cerebral contusion and laceration is a form of primary traumatic brain injury which is associated with
multiple micro-hemorrhages, small blood vessel leaks into brain tissue. Contusion occurs in 20% -30% of
severe head injuries. A cerebral laceration is a similar injury except that, according to their respective definitions, the pia-arachnoid membranes are torn over the site of injury in laceration and are not torn in contusion. The injury can cause a decline in mental function in the long term and in the emergency setting may
result in brain herniation, a life-threatening condition in which parts of the brain are squeezed past parts of
the skull. Thus treatment aims to prevent dangerous rises in intracranial pressure, the pressure within the
skull(Figure 15-3-1).

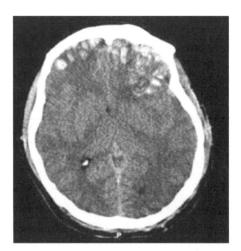

Figure 15-3-1   CT scan showing cerebral contusions, hemorrhage within the hemispheres, subdural
hematoma on the left, and skull fracture

3.2.2   Causes

Often caused by a blow to the head, contusions commonly occur in coup or contre coup injuries. In
coup injuries, the brain is injured directly under the area of impact, while in contrecoup injuries it is injured
on the side opposite the impact.

Contusion and laceration occur primarily in the cortical tissue, especially under the site of impact or in areas of the brain located near sharp ridges on the inside of the skull. The brain may be contused when it collides with bony protuberances on the inside surface of the skull. The protuberances are located on the inside of the skull under the frontal and temporal lobes and on the roof of the ocular orbit. Thus, the tips of the frontal and temporal lobes located near the bony ridges in the skull are areas where contusions frequently occur and are most severe. For this reason, attention, emotional and memory problems, which are associated with damage to frontal and temporal lobes, are much more common in head trauma survivors than are syndromes associated with damage to other areas of the brain.

3.2.3   Features

Contusion and laceration, which are frequently associated with edema, are especially likely to cause increases in intracranial pressure and concomitant crushing of delicate brain tissue. The distinction between contusion and intra-cerebral hemorrhage is blurry because both involve bleeding within the brain tissue; however, an arbitrary cutoff exists that the injury is a contusion if two thirds or less of the tissue involved is blood and a hemorrhage otherwise. The contusion and laceration may cause swelling of the surrounding brain tissue, which may be irritated by toxins released in the contusion. The swelling is worst at around 4-6 days after the injury. Extensive contusion associated with subdural hematoma is called burst lobe. Cases of a burst frontal or temporal lobe are associated with high mortality and morbidity.

3.2.4   Multiple petechial hemorrhages

Numerous small contusions from broken capillaries that occur in grey matter under the cortex are called multiple petechial hemorrhages or multifocal hemorrhagic contusion. Caused by shearing injuries at the time of impact, these contusions occur especially at the junction between grey and white matter and in the upper brain stem, basal ganglia, thalamus and areas near the third ventricle. The hemorrhages can occur as the result of brain herniation, which can cause arteries to tear and bleed. The types of diffuse brain injury, multiple petechial hemorrhages are not always visible using current imaging techniques like CT and MRI scans. This may be the case even if the injury is quite severe, though these may show up days after the injury. Hemorrhages may be larger than in normal contusions if the injury is quite severe. This type of injury has a poor prognosis if the patient is comatose, even with no apparent causes for the coma.

3.2.5   Signs and symptoms

The symptoms of the contusion and laceration (bruising on the brain) depend on the severity of the injury, ranging from minor to severe. Individuals may experience a headache; confusion; sleepiness; dizziness; loss of consciousness; nausea and vomiting; seizures; and difficulty with coordination and movement; lightheadedness; tinnitus; spinning sensations. They may also have difficulty with memory, vision, speech, hearing, managing emotions, and thinking. Signs depend on the contusion's location in the brain.

3.2.6   Treatment

Since cerebral swelling presents a danger to the patient, treatment of cerebral contusion aims to prevent swelling. Measures to avoid swelling include prevention of hypotension (low blood pressure), hyponatremia (insufficient sodium), and hypercapnia (increased carbon dioxide in the blood). Due to the danger of increased intracranial pressure, surgery may be necessary to reduce it. People with cerebral contusion may require intensive care and close monitoring.

3.2.7   Prognosis

A cerebral laceration with large amounts of blood apparent on a CT scan is an indicator of poor prognosis. The progression and course of complications do not appear to be affected by a cerebral laceration's location or a mass effect it causes.

3.3   Primary Brain Stem Injury

3.3.1   Definition and background

The incidence of brain stem injury (BSI) varied 8.8% –52% and TBSI might induce a serious impact on brain tissue as a form of diffuse axonal injury (DAI). Poor prognosis was a common feature following severe traumatic brain injury, and furthermore, it was more common in those with BSI. However, BSI is no more considered as powerful indicator to predict bad outcome. Many clinical case reports were publicized to elucidate the causal relationship between BSI and outcome by means of radiologic findings and anatomical studies, and now some aspects of its pathomechanism could be revealed. Therefore, we conducted this study to reappraise the correlationship among clinical variables, such as impact site on scalp and radiologic finding on Glasgow coma score (GCS) and Glasgow outcome score (GOS).

3.3.2   Features and causes

Nervous and/or vascular compression against the tentorial notch mostly occurs at its lateral portion due to the shortest distance to the brain stem and near the level of pontomesencephalic junction. These lesions are considered to result from the shearing mechanism in and around the brain stem very close to the tentorial edge. For example, an injury of lower brain stem could be caused by hyperextension of the cervical vertebrae or reciprocal actions of fracture of the clivus and the direct effect on the brain stem by acceleration or rotational forces. According to TBSI case reports to date, the frequent site of hemorrhage or contusion site is confined to dorsal side of midbrain, cranial nerves, whole brain stem, cerebellum, combined with upper cervical spinal injuries, clinically presenting as hemiparesis. In terms of cranial impact site, literature reviews addressed there is an association between occipital blows and primary cerebellar and brain stem lesions. But, another supportive review showed a preponderance of occipital impacts among the cases with primary brain stem lesions which were associated with cerebellar contusion, laceration, and hemorrhage. This clinical evidence was well verified in animal study using fluid percussion injury model under the hypothesis that the cerebellum is susceptible to selective Purkinje cell loss as well as white matter dysfunction. In addition to that, all impacts to the neck, although few in numbers, was known to give primary brain stem lesions.

3.3.3   Diagnosis

Before CT era, midbrain damage as a major DAI site, could be only and easily determined by autopsy, volumetric proton study, and/or evoked potential study. The prognosis of patient is dependent on the severity and site of head injury incurred. After CT era, due to its ability to demonstrate the nature, sites, and multiplicity of traumatic brain injury, CT is now the primary diagnostic method for head injury. It is also very useful to elucidate classical DAI and posterior fossa lesions based on direct and indirect signs which include focal hemorrhage, significant contrast enhancement, hemorrhagic contusion, and edema of brain stem, appearing as areas of high-, mixed-, and low-density on the scan. Indirect signs are obliteration of the pontine, cerebello-pontine angle, and perimesencephalic cisterns. Therefore, many cases of TBSI as an indirect evidence were reported where the hematoma were localized along tentorium, for which proposed supratentorial impact site as mostly occipital region, midbrain tegmentum, interpedunculo-ambient cisterns, cisterna magna, and cerebellum with or without supratentorial abnormalities. There were many DAI-compatible cases not detected even with CT whose clinical severity could not be evaluated in acute stage. Instead, MRI provides a more sophisticated display of brain stem with improved contrast resolution of structures not appreciated on CT. Therefore, acute stage MRI is used in place of CT or added to CT, because of some limitation of CT in detecting, localizing, and characterizing diffuse injury and posterior fossa lesions; for example, in differentiating between two patterns of TBSI such as ventral or dorsal location. Additionally, MRI is more helpful than CT in detecting non-hemorrhagic lesions, cortical contusions, diffuse axonal injury such as supratentorial injury in corpus callosum, and even in normal CT finding when neurological condition could not be explained. Nowadays, electrophysiological study could be added as a more powerful prognostic tool.

3.3.4 Treatment

Severe primary brain stem injury with a long duration of coma should be treated with tracheotomy, ventilator assisted breathing and mild hypothermia as soon as possible. For patients with mild brain stem injury, can be treated according to brain contusion, some patients can obtain good curative effect, and for the serious, its mortality is very high, so the treatment should be careful and careful, to have a long-term plan, and nursing work is particularly important, at the same time, pay close attention to the prevention and treatment of various complications.

3.3.5 Prognosis

From a prognostic model study for BSI, age, skull fracture and superimposed mass lesion are the most prognostic factors among the large number of variable tested, where age is the most reliable prognostic variable available at the time of admission. The gender of patient, previous history of hypertension, diabetes mellitus, or alcoholism may also influence the prognosis. In pediatric cases, the frequency and distribution of TBSI are similar to those of adults, but the skull fracture is associated with reduced death rate in the younger age group due to dissipated kinetic energy in fracturing the skull, and outcome did not correlate with significantly with morphological patterns of injury or the presence of extracranial injuries. Generally, poor prognosis is a common feature following severe traumatic brain injury, especially more common in those with BSI. However, many cases of TBSI following closed head injury were verified and have been increasingly reported with good outcome, especially in those with a single brain stem lesion. BSI is no more an absolute indicator of poor outcome, because the relationship between BSI and outcome is still unclear and the types of BSI are still poorly understood. Therefore, the understanding of anatomy and extent of BSI, as well as its relationship to supratentorial abnormalities is strongly recommended to estimate actual outcome. The first hypothesis is an anatomical variation in tentorial apertures and their relationship to adjacent structures such as midbrain, cerebellum, and oculomotor nerve which may influence the degree of brain stem distortion in case of acceleration-deceleration injuries. The second hypothesis is that BSI may occur alone or in association with other cranial injuries. Head injury carries a much graver prognosis when brain stem is involved. Since severe head injury is often characterized by injury to several sites, both intra-and extra-axial, there may be no clear-cut clinical evidence of a specific brain stem lesion. The most significant lesion may not be suspected until the patient fails to exhibit normal signs of recovery or it may be an unexpected autopsy findings.

Relating the location of the lesions and outcome, the death appeared to be closely linked to the phenomenon of bilateral pontine lesions, especially if bilateral upper pontine lesions are involved. The extent of supratentorial lesions had no bearing on survival in the absence of brain stem lesions.

3.4　Diffuse Axonal Injury

3.4.1　Definition and background

Diffuse axonal injury (DAI) is a brain injury in which scattered lesions in white matter tracts as well as gray matter occur over a widespread area. DAI is one of the most common and devastating types of traumatic brain injury and is a major cause of unconsciousness and persistent vegetative state after severe head trauma. It occurs in about half of all cases of severe head trauma and may be the primary damage that occurs in concussion. The outcome is frequently coma, with over 90% of patients with severe DAI never regaining consciousness. Those who do wake up often remain significantly impaired.

3.4.2　Causes

DAI is the result of traumatic shearing forces that occur when the head is rapidly accelerated or decelerated, as may occur in car accidents, falls, and assaults. Vehicle accidents are the most frequent cause of DAI; it can also occur as the result of child abuse such as in shaken baby syndrome.

Immediate disconnection of axons could be observed in severe brain injury, but the major damage of DAI is delayed secondary axon disconnections slowly developed over an extended time course. Tracts of axons, which appear white due to myelination, are referred to as white matter. Lesions in both grey and white matters are found in postmortem brains in CT and MRI exams.

Besides mechanical breaking of the axonal cytoskeleton, DAI pathology also includes secondary physiological changes such as interrupted axonal transport, progressive swellings and degeneration. Recent studies have linked these changes to twisting and misalignment of broken axon microtubules, as well as tau and APP deposition.

3.4.3　Features

Lesions typically exist in the white matter of brains injured by DAI; these lesions vary in size from 1 – 15 mm and are distributed in a characteristic way. DAI most commonly affects white matter in areas including the brain stem, the corpus callosum, and the cerebral hemispheres. The lobes of the brain most likely to be injured are the frontal and temporal lobes. Other common locations for DAI include the white matter in the cerebral cortex, the superior cerebral peduncles, basal ganglia, thalamus, and deep hemispheric nuclei. These areas may be more easily damaged because of the difference in density between them and the rest of the brain.

3.4.4　Diagnosis

DAI is difficult to detect since it does not show up well on CT scans or with other macroscopic imaging techniques, though it shows up microscopically. However, there are characteristics typical of DAI that may or may not show up on a CT scan. Diffuse injury has more microscopic injury than macroscopic injury and is difficult to detect with CT and MRI, but its presence can be inferred when small bleeds are visible in the corpus callosum or the cerebral cortex. MRI is more useful than CT for detecting characteristics of diffuse axonal injury in the subacute and chronic time frames. Newer studies such as diffusion tensor imaging are able to demonstrate the degree of white matter fiber tract injury even when the standard MRI is negative. Since axonal damage in DAI is largely a result of secondary biochemical cascades, it has a delayed onset, so a person with DAI who initially appears well may deteriorate later. Thus injury is frequently more severe than is realized, and medical professionals should suspect DAI in any patients whose CT scans appear normal but who have symptoms like unconsciousness.

MRI is more sensitive than CT scans, but MRI may also miss DAI, because it identifies the injury using signs of edema, which may not be present. DAI is classified into grades based on severity of the injury. In Grade I, widespread axonal damage is present but no focal abnormalities are seen. In Grade II, damage found in Grade I is present in addition to focal abnormalities, especially in the corpus callosum. Grade III damage encompasses both Grades I and II plus rostral brain stem injury and often tears in the tissue.

3.4.5 Treatment

DAI currently lacks a specific treatment beyond what is done for any type of head injury, including stabilizing the patient and trying to limit increases in intracranial pressure.

3.4.6 Prognosis

DAI is a serious but common type of traumatic brain injury. It can be fatal, but it is also possible to regain consciousness after a DAI. For those who recover, intensive rehabilitation will be needed.

Chapter 4

Intracranial Hemmorage

The process of hemorrhage results in the formation of a localized accumulation of blood, orhematoma. There are four types of intracranial hemmorage(ICH).

4.1　Epidural Hematoma

4.1.1　Background

Epidural hematoma (EDH) is a traumatic accumulation of blood between the inner table of the skull and the stripped-off dural membrane. The inciting event often is a focused blow to the head, such as that produced by a hammer or baseball bat. In 85%-95% of patients, this trauma results in an overlying fracture. Blood vessels in close proximity to the fracture are the sources of the hemorrhage. Because the underlying brain has usually been minimally injured, prognosis is excellent if treated aggressively. Outcome from surgical decompression and repair is related directly to patient's preoperative neuralgic condition.

4.1.2　Pathophysiology

70%-80% of EDHs are located in the temporoparietal region where skull fractures cross the path of the middle meningeal artery or its dural branches. Frontal and occipital EDHs each constitute about 10%, with the latter occasionally extending above and be low the tentorium. Association of hematoma and skull fracture is less common in young children because of calvarial plasticity.

EDHs are usually arterial in origin but result from venous bleeding in one third of patients. Occasionally, tom venous sinuses cause EDH, particularly in the parietal-occipital region or posterior fossa. These injuries tend to be smaller and associated with a more benign course. Usually, venous EDHs only form with a depressed skull fracture, which strips the dura from the bone and, thus, creates a space for blood to accumulate. In certain patients, especially those with delayed presentations, venous EDHs are treated nonsurgically.

Expanding high-volume EDHs can produce a midline shift and subfalcine herniation. Compressed cerebral tissue can impinge on the third cranial nerve, resulting in ipsilateral pupillary dilation and contra-lateral hemiparesis or extensor motor response.

EDHs are usually stable, attaining maximum size within minutes of injury; however, Borovich demonstrated progression of EDH in 9% of patients during the first 24 hours. Re−bleeding or continuous oozing presumably causes this progression. EDH occasionally runs a more chronic course and is detected only days after injury.

4.1.3   Frequency:In the US

EDH occurs in 1%−2% of all head trauma cases and in about 10% of patients who present with traumatic coma.

4.1.4   Mortality/Morbidity

Reported mortality rates range from 5% to 43%. Higher rates are associated with advanced age, intradural lesions, temporal location, increased hematoma volume, rapid clinical progression, pupillary abnormalities, increased intracranial pressure, lower GCS. Mortality rates are approximately 0% for patients not in coma preoperative−ly, 9% for obtunded patients, and 20% for patients in deep coma.

4.1.5   Age

Patients younger than 5 years and older than 55 years have an increased mortality rate. Patients, younger than 20 years account for 60% of EDH incidences. EDH is uncommon in elderly patients because the dura is strongly adhered to the inner table of the skull. In case series of EDH, fewer than 10% of patients are older than 50 years.

4.1.6   History

Fewer than 20% of patients demonstrate the classic presentation of a lucid interval. Following injury, the patient may be continually comatose, briefly comatose and recovered, or continually conscious. Severe headache, vomiting and seizure may occur. Patients with posterior fossa EDH may have a dramatic delayed deterioration. The patient can be conscious and talking and a minute later apneic, comatose, and minutes from death.

4.1.7   Physical

Cushing response consisting of the hypertension, bradycardia and bradypnea can indicate increased ICP. Level of consciousness may be decreased, with decreased or fluctuating GCS. Contusion, laceration, or bony step−off may be observed in the area of injury. Dilated, sluggish, or fixed pupil (s), bilateral or ipsilateral to injury, suggest increased ICP or herniation. Classic triad indicating transtentorial herniation consists of the coma, fixed and dilated pupils (s) and decerebration. Hemiplegia contra lateral to injury with herniation may be observed.

4.1.8   Causes

EDH results from traumatic head injury, usually with an associated skull fracture and arterial laceration.

4.1.9   Lab studies

Perform appropriate lab work for associated trauma. No specific tests are required. Coagulation abnormalities are a marker of severe head injury. Breakdown of the blood−brain barrier with exposed brain tissue is a potent cause of disseminated intravascular coagulation (DIC).

4.1.10 Imaging studies

The immediate CT scan is the procedure of choice for the diagnosis of epidural hematoma. Head CT scan shows location, volume, effect, and other potential intracranial injuries. EDH forms an extra axial, smoothly marginated, lenticular, or biconvex homogenous density. EDH rarely crosses the suture line because the dura is attached more firmly to the skull at sutures. Focal isodense or hypodense zones within EDH indicate active bleeding. Irregular hypodense swirling indicates active bleeding in the majority of patients. Air in acute EDH suggests fracture of sinuses or mastoid air cells. At surgery or autopsy, 20% of patients have blood in both epidural and subdural spaces.

4.1.11 Other tests

Cervical spine evaluation usually is necessary because of the risk of neck injury associated with EDH.

Procedures: Perform burr hole(s) if the patient is herniating, all other treatments prove insufficient and air or ground medical transport is prolonged. Burr-hole procedure includes the drill hole adjacent to, but not over the skull fracture or in the area located by CT scan. In the absence of CT scan, place a burr hole on the side of the dilated pupil, 2 finger widths anterior to tragus of ear and 3 finger widths above.

4.1.12 Treatment

(1) Pre-hospital care

Stabilize acute life-threatening conditions and initiate supportive therapy. Airway control and blood pressure support are the most important issues. Establish IV access, administer oxygen, and monitor. Administer IV crystalloids to maintain systolic blood pressure (SBP) greater than 90 mmHg. Intubationsf sedation, and neuromuscular blockade per protocol. Emergency Department Care

Establish IV access, administer oxygen, monitor, and administer IV crystalloids as necessary to keep SBP greater than 90 mmHg. Intubate using rapid sequence induction (RSI), which generally includes premedication with lidocaine, a cerebroprotective sedating agent (e. g. , etomidate), and neuromuscular blockade. Lidocaine may have limited effect in this situation, yet it carries virtually no risk. Intubate after a basic neurological examination to facilitate oxygenation, protect airway, and allow for hyperventilation as needed. Elevate head 30° after the spine is cleared, or use reverse Trendelenburg position to reduce ICP and increase venous drainage. Administer mannitol 0. 25 - 1 g/kg IV after consulting a neurosurgeon if SBP is greater than 90mm Hg with continued clinical signs of increased ICP. This reduces both ICP (by osmotically reducing brain edema) and blood viscosity, which increases cerebral blood flow and oxygen delivery. Hyperventilation to partial pressure of carbon dioxide (PCO_2) of about 30 mmHg treats incipient herniation or signs of increasing ICP; however, this is controversial. Be careful not to lower PCO_2 too far (<25 mmHg). Perform hyperventilation if clinical signs of increased ICP progress ; this procedure reduces ICP by hypocarbic vasoconstriction and reduces risks of hypoperfusion and death of injured cells. Phenytoin reduces the incidence of early posttraumatic seizures, although it does not affect late-onset seizures or the development of a persistent seizure disorder.

(2) Further inpatient care

Transfer to operating room (OR) for EDH evacuation and repair. Admit to neurosurgical ICU after surgery or directly for monitoring. This will likely include ICP, partial pressure oxygen (PO_2), or other intracranial monitoring devices. Repeat CT scan in the event of clinical deterioration.

（3）Deterrence/Prevention

Encourage use of seat belts and car seats. Advocate helmets for bicycling, skateboarding, snowboarding, rollerblading, and horse and motorcycle riding.

（4）Complications

Neurobehavioral changes such as post-concussive syndrome can last hours to months, vegetative state and death.

4.1.13　Prognosis

Mortality rates approximate 0% for patients not in coma preoperatively, 9% for obtunded patients, and 20% for patients in a deep coma before surgery. If treated early, prognosis usually is excellent, because the underlying brain injury generally is limited.

Right temporal epidural hematoma with midline shift（Figure 15-4-1）. Patient should be taken immediately to the operating room for neurosurgery. Brain CT scans of a 45 year-old man who slipped on a waxed floor（Figure 15-4-2）. Witnesses reported loss of consciousness followed by a lucid interval. CT scan indicates epidural hematoma.

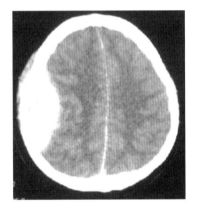

Figure 15-4-1　Right temporal epidural hematoma

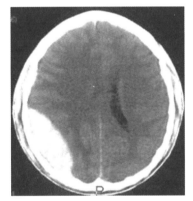

Figure 15-4-2　Acute epidural hematoma

4.2　Subdural Hematoma

4.2.1　Background

An acute subdural hematoma (SDH) is a rapidly clotting blood collection below the inner layer of the dura but external to the brain and arachnoid membrane. Two further stages, subacute and chronic, may develop with untreated acute SDH. Each type has distinctly different clinical, pathological, and imaging characteristics. Generally, the subacute phase begins 3-7 days after acute injury (Surgical literature favors 3 days; radiological, 7). The chronic phase begins 2-3 weeks after acute injury.

4.2.2　Pathophysiology

Typically, low-pressure venous bleeding of bridging veins (between the cortex and venous sinuses) dissects the arachnoid away from the dura and layers out along the cerebral convexity. Cerebral injury results from direct pressure, increased intracranial pressure, or associated intraparenchymal insults. In the subacute phase, the clotted blood liquefies. Occasionally, in the prone patient, the cellular elements layer, this can appear on CT imaging as a hematocrit-like effect. In the chronic phase, cellular elements have disintegrated, and a collection of serous fluid remains in the subdural space. In rare cases, calcification develops.

4.2.3　Frequency

In the US: Frequency is related directly to the incidence of blunt head trauma. An SDH is the most common type of intracranial mass lesion, occurring in about 1/3 of those with severe head injuries GCS score < 9).

4.2.4　Mortality/Morbidity

Acute SDH is associated with high mortality and morbidity rates. Simple SDH accounts for about half of all cases and implies that no parenchymal injury is present. Simple SDH is associated with a mortality rate of about 20%. Complicated SDH accounts for the remaining cases and implies that parenchymal injury (e. g. , contusion or laceration of a cerebral hemi-sphere)is present. Complicated SDH is associated with a mortality rate of about 50%.

4.2.5　Age

The majority of SDHs are associated with age factors related to the risk of blunt head trauma. Certain age factors are related to more unusual variants of this disease. SDH is more common in people older than 60 years. The elderly are predisposed to cerebral atrophy because they have less resilient bridging veins. Moreover, these veins can be damaged more easily in the elderly. Since the adhesions existing in the subdural space are absent at birth and develop with aging, bilateral SDHs are more common in infants. Interhemispheric SDHs often are associated with child abuse.

4.2.6　History

Suspect acute SDH whenever the patient has experienced a mechanism of moderately severe to severe blunt head trauma. Patients generally lose consciousness, but this is not an absolute. Chronic SDH is more difficult to anticipate, and about half of such cases offer no history of head trauma. Patient often present with progressive symptoms such as unexplained headache, personality changes, signs of increased ICP, or hemiparesis/plegia. Any degree or type of coagulopathy should heighten suspicion of SDH. Hemophiliacs can develop SDH with a seemingly trivial head trauma. An aggressive approach to diagnosis and immediate correction of the factor deficiency Io 100% activity is paramount. Alcoholics are prone to thrombocytopenia, prolonged bleeding times, and blunt head trauma. Maintain a high level of suspicion in this population. Promptly obtain a CT scan of the head when the degree of trauma is severe, focal neurological signs are noted, or intoxication does not resolve as anticipated. In alcoholics, more than any other cohort, acute or chronic SDHs can be due to the deadly combination of repetitive trauma and alcohol-associated coagulopathies. Patients on anticoagulants can develop SDH with minimal trauma and warrant a lowered threshold for obtaining a head CT scan.

4.2.7　Physical

Physical examination of patients with head trauma should emphasize assessment of neurological status using the GCS. Search for any focal neurological deficits or signs of increased ICP. Signs of external trauma alert the physician to the expected location of coup or counter-coup injuries on CT scan. Any abnormality of mental status that can not be explained completely by alcohol intoxication or the presence of another mind-altering substance should increate suspicion of SDH in the patient with blunt head trauma. Obtain an urgent CT scan. GCS score less than 15 after blunt head trauma ᵥ in a patient with no intoxicating substance use (or impaired mental status baseline), warrants consideration of an urgent CT scan. Presence of a focal neurological sign following blunt head trauma is ominous and requires an emergent explanation.

4.2.8　Lab studies

The laboratory studies include the complete blood count, coagulation profile, electrolytes, type and screen/cross.

4.2.9　Imaging studies

While MRI 19 superior for demonstrating the size of an acute SDH and its effect on the brain, non-contrast head CT scans are the primary means of making a diagnosis and suffice for immediate management purposes. Acute SDH typically appears on a non-contrast head CT scan as a hyperdense (white) crescentic mass along the inner table of the skull, most commonly over the cerebral convexity in the parietal region (Figure 15-4-3). The second most common area i, above the tentorium cerebelli. Small SDHs may blend in with the adjacent skull and may be appreciated only by adjusting the CT scan window width to between those generally used to view brain and bone. Some degree of midline shift should be present with moderate or large SDHs. Suspect a contralateral mass when midline shift is absent. If midline shift seems excessive, suspect underlying cerebral edema. SDHs are relatively uncommon in the posterior fossa since the cerebellum undergoes little movement, which is protective of its bridging cortical veins. SDHs that do occur in that location are usually a result of parenchymal cerebellar injury. Interhemispheric SDH causes the falx cerebri to appear thickened and irregular and often is associated with child abuse. In the sub-acute phase, the lesion becomes CT(with respect to the brain) and is more difficult to appreciate on a non-contrast head CT scan (Figure 15-4-4). For this reason, cither contrast-enhanced CT scan or MRI is widely recommended for imaging 48-72 hours head injury. On T_1-weighted MR images, sub-acute lesions are hyper-dense. On contrast-enhanced CT scans, cortical veins over the cerebral surface are opacified and help delineate the lesion. Sub-acute SDHs often become lens-shaped and can be confused with an epidural hematoma. In the chronic phase, the lesion becomes hypo-dense and is easy to appreciate on a non-contrast head CT scan.

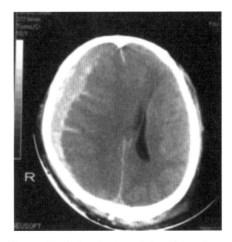

Figure 15-4-3　**Acute subdural hematoma**

Note the bright (white) image properties of the blood on this non-contrast cranial CT scan. Note also the midline shift.

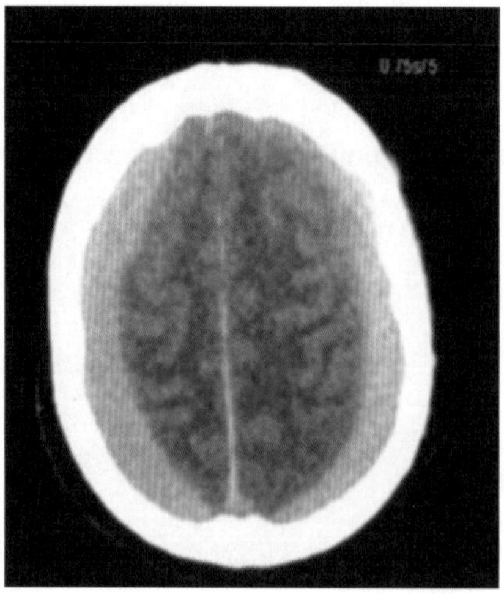

Figure 15-4-4　Subacute subdural hematoma

The crescent-shaped clot is less white than on CT scan of acute subdural hematoma.

4.2.10　Treatment

(1) Emergency department care

Consider endotracheal intubation when GCS score is less than 12 or other indications are present; this guarantees airway protection during the diagnostic workup. Obtain an immediate head CT scan in patients with head trauma who experienced clear loss of consciousness, are symptomatic, are disoriented/amnestic, or have any focal neurological signs. Burr holes are a temporizing option when rapid demise is associated with severe head trauma, especially if a herniation syndrome is clinically evident. Burr holes can guide surgical therapy when head CT imaging is unavailable. Generally, because the lesion represents clotted blood, the burr hole is not curative, and emergent craniotomy is necessary.

(2) Consultations

When a patient who experienced head trauma presents with a GCS score less than 12, consider immediate neurosurgical consultation while stabilizing and diagnostic maneuvers are in progress. Small, asymptomatic and acute SDHs may be managed by, observation, serial examinations and serial CT scanning. Patients with focal findings, neurological worsening, significant midline displacement (>5.0 mm), or increased intracranial or posterior fossa pressure require operative intervention. The usual treatment for acute SDH is craniotomy and evacuation. After making a large cranial flap, open the dura. Remove the clot with suction, cop forceps, and/or irrigation. Identify and control bleeding sites.

(3) Transfer

Detected SDHs require patient transfer to facilities offering neurosurgical evaluation and treatment. Transfer may be emergent, with appropriate stabilization measures taken and with appropriately skilled personnel accompanying the patient.

(4) Complications

Postoperative complications include elevated ICP, brain edema, new or recurrent bleeding, infection, and seizures. In chronic SDH the most common complications are recurrent hematoma (50%), infection (e. g. , subdural empyema, wound) and seizures (up to 10%).

(5) Prognosis

Definitive prognosis often is not possible at the time of emergency department evaluation. Ultimate prognosis is related to the amount of associated direct brain damage and the damage resulting from the mass effect of the SDH.

4.3   Subarachnoid Hemorrhage

4.3.1   Background

Subarachnoid hemorrhage (SAH) implies the presence of blood within the subarachnoid space from some pathologic process. The common medical useof the term SAH refers to the nontraumatic types of hemorrhages, usually from rupture of a berry aneurysm or arteriovenous malformation (AVM). The scope of this article is limited to these nontraumatic hemorrhages.

4.3.2   Frequency

In the US: Annual incidence of nontraumatic aneurysmal SAH is 6–25 per 100 000. More than 27 000 Americans suffer ruptured intracranial aneurysms each year. Annual incidence increases with age and probably is underestimated, because death is attributed to other reasons that are not confirmed by autopsies. Internationally: Varying incidences have been reported in other areas of the world (2–49 per 100 000).

4.3.3   Mortality/Morbidity

An estimated 10%–15% of patients die before reaching the hospital. Mortality rate reaches as high as 40% within the first week. About half die in the first 6 months. Mentality and morbidity rates increase with age and poorer overall health of the patient. Advances in the management of SAH have resulted in a relative reduction in mortality rate that exceeds 25%. However, more than 1/3 of survivors have major neurological deficits.

4.3.4   Sex

Incidence of aneurysmal SAH is higher in women than in men.

4.3.5   Age

Mean age of SAH is 50 years.

4.3.6   History

Patient experiences sudden onset of a severe headache. Prodromal (warning) headache (s) from minor blood leakage (referred to as sentinel headache) is reported in 30%–50% of aneurysmal SAHs. Sentinel headaches may occur a few hours to a few months before the rupture, with a reported median of 2 weeks prior to diagnosis of SAH. Minor leaks commonly do not demonstrate signs of elevated intracranial pressure or meningeal irritation. Minor leaks are not a feature of AVM. More than 25% of patients experience seizures close to the acute onset; the location of a seizure focus has no relationship to the location of the aneurysm, and/or vomiting may occur. Symptoms of meningeal irritation (e. g. , neck stiffness, low back pain, bilateral leg pain): These are seen in over 75% of SAH, hut many take several hours to develop. Photophobia and visual changes can occur. Loss of consciousness: About half of patients experience this at the time of bleeding onset.

4.3.7　Physical

Physical examination findings may be normal, or the clinician may find global or focal neurological abnormalities in more than 25% of patients. Syndromes of cranial nerve compression such as oculomotor nerve palsy (posterior communicating artery aneurysm) with or without ipsilateral mydriasis, abducens nerve palsy and monoocular vision loss (ophthalmic artery aneurysm compressing the ipsilateral optic nerve) maybe present. A motor deficit from middle cerebral artery aneurysms is seen in 15% of patients. No localizing signs in 40% of patients. Seizures and ophthalmologic signs such as subhyaloid retinal hemorrhage (small round hemorrhage, perhaps with visible meniscus, near the optic nerve head); other retinal hemorrhage are also observed. Papilledema is present. About half of patients have mild to moderate blood pressure (BP) elevation. BP may become labile as ICP increases. Fever is unusual at presentation but becomes common after the fourth day from blood breakdown in the subarachnoid space. Tachycardia may be present for several days after the occurrence of a hemorrhage. Grade SAH according to the following scheme:

Grade I: Mild headache with or without meningeal irritation.

Grade II: Severe headache and a nonfocal examination, with or without mydriasis.

Grade III: Mild alteration in neurological examination, including mental status.

Grade IV: Obviously depressed level of consciousness or focal deficit.

Grade V: Patient either posturing or comatose.

4.3.8　Causes

Primary SAH may result from rupture of the following types of pathologic entities (the first two are most common): ①Saccular aneurysm. ②AVM. ③Mycotic aneurysmal rupture. ④Angioma. ⑤Neoplasm. ⑥Cortical thrombosis.

SAH may reflect a secondary dissection of blood from an intraparenchymal hematoma (e. g, bleeding from hypertension or neoplasm). 2/3 of non-traumatic SAH are caused by rupture of saccular aneurysms. Congenital causes also may be responsible for SAH. Association of aneurysms with specific systemic diseases, including Ehlers-Danlos syndrome, Mar fan's syndrome, coarctation of the aorta, and polycystic kidney disease may also be present. Environmental factors associated with acquired vessel wall defects include age, hypertension, smoking, and arthrosclerosis.

4.3.9　Lab studies

The laboratory studies include complete blood count, prothrombin time, activated partial thromboplastin time, blood typing and screening, blood bank typing is indicated when SAH is identified or a severe bleed is suspected. Intra-operative transfusions may be required.

4.3.10　Imaging studies

The initial study of choice is an urgent CT scan without contrast (see Figure 15-4-5). Sensitivity decreases with time from onset and with older resolution scanners. CT scan is 90% sensitive within the first 24 hours, 80% sensitive at 3 days, and 50% sensitive at 1 week. CT also can detect intracerebral hemorrhage, mass effect, and hydrocephalus. A falsely negative CT scan can result from severe anemia or small-volume SAH. Distribution of SAH can provide information about the location of an aneurysm and prognosis. Intraparenchymal hemorrhage may occur with middle communicating artery and posterior communicating artery aneurysms. Interhemispheric and intraventricular hemorrhages may occur with anterior communicating artery aneurysms. Outcome is worse for patients with extensive clots in basal cisterns than for those with a thin diffuse hemorrhage. Cerebral angiography is performed once the SAH diagnosis is made. This study assesses the vascular anatomy, current bleeding site and presence of other aneurysm. This study helps plan operative options. Angiography findings are negative in 10% –20% of patients with SAHs. If negative, some advocate repeating angiography a few weeks later. Magnetic resonance imaging (MRI) is performed if no lesion is found on angiography. Its sensitivity in detecting blood is considered equal or inferior to that of CT scan. The higher cost, lower availability, and longer study time make it less optimal for detecting SAH. MRI mostly is used to identify possible AVMs that are not visible on angiography. MRI may miss small symptomatic lesions that have not yet ruptured. Magnetic resonance angiography (MRA) is less sensitive than angiography in detecting vascular lesions; however, many believe CT angiography and/or MRA one day will play a more central role.

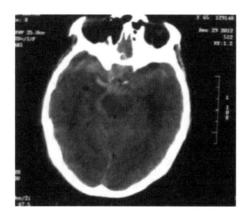

Figure 15 – 4 – 5　Brain CT scans showing subtle finding of blood at the circle of Willis consistent with acute subarachnoid hemorrhage

4.3.11　Other tests

Electrocardiogram (ECG): About 20% of SAH cases have myocardial ischemia from the increased circulation of catecholamines. Typical results are nonspecific ST – and T – wave changes, prolonged QRS segments, U waves, and increased QT intervals. ECG changes reflect myocardial ischemia or infarction and should be treated in the usual manner. Suspicion of SAH is a contraindication to thrombolytic and anticoagulant therapy.

4.3.12　Procedures

Lumbar puncture: Lumbar puncture (LP) is indicated if the patient has possible SAH and negative CT scan findings. Perform CT scan prior to LP to exclude any significant intracranial mass effect or obvious intracranial bleed. LP may be negative less than 2 hours after the bleed. LP is most sensitive at 12 hours after symptom onset. Red blood cells (RBCs) in the cerebrospinal fluid (CSF) remain consistently elevated in 2 sequential tubes or punctures in SAH, whereas the numbers of RBCs in technically traumatic punctures decrease over time. Xanthochromia (yellow – to – pink CSF supernatant) usually is seen by 12 hours after the onset of bleeding; ideally this is measured spectrographically, although many laboratories rely on visual inspection. LP findings can be positive in 5% −15% all SAH presentations that are not evident on the CT scan.

4.3.13 Prehospital care

Address the ABCs. Transport patients with altered level of consciousness or an abnormal neurological examination to the closest medical center with a CT scan and neurosurgical back−up. Ideally, avoid sedating these patients en route.

4.3.14 Emergency department care

In patients with a suspected grade Ⅰ or Ⅱ SAH, emergency department(ED) care essentially is limited to diagnosis and supportive therapy. Early identification of sentinel headaches is the key to reduced mortality and morbidity rates. Use sedation judiciously. Secure intravenous (IV) access during ED stay and closely monitor the patient's neurological status. In patients with a grade Ⅲ, Ⅳ, or V SAH (i. e. , altered neurological examination) , ED care is more extensive. Address the ABCs. Endotracheal intubation of obtunded patients protects from aspiration caused by depressed airway protective reflexes. Intubate to hyperventilate patients with signs of herniation. Thiopental and etomidate are the optimal induction agents in SAH during an intubation. Thiopental is short acting and has a barbiturate cytoprotective effect. It should be used only in hypertensive patients because of its propensity to drop systolic blood pressure (SBP) , which is the leading cause of secondary brain injury. In hypotensive and normotensive patients use etomidate. Use rapid sequence intubation if possible. In the process, to blunt ICP increase, ideally use sedation, defasciculation, short−acting neuromuscular blockade, and other agents with ICP−blunting properties (such as Ⅳ lidocaine). Avoid excessive or inadequate hyperventilation. Target the PCO_2 at 30−35 mmHg to reduce elevated ICP. Excessive hyperventilation may be harmful to areas of vasospasm. Avoid excessive sedation. It makes serial neurological exams more difficult and has been reported to increase ICP directly. Reliable neurological examinations before and after initial treatment are critically important to optimizing management and to deciding on the appropriate neurosurgical intervention. Use osmotic agents, such as mannitol, which reduces ICP 50% in 30 minutes, peaks after 90 minutes, and lasts 4 hours. Loop diuretics, such as furosemide, also decrease ICP without increasing serum osmolality. Ⅳ steroid therapy to control brain edema is controversial and debated. Monitor cardiac activity, oximetry, automated BP, and end−tidal carbon dioxide, when applicable. End−tidal carbon dioxide monitoring of intubated patients enables the clinician to avoid excessive or inadequate hyperventilation. Target the PCO_2 at 30−35 mmHg to reduce elevated ICP. Invasive arterial line monitoring is indicated when dealing with labile BP (common in high−grade SAH). Antihypertensive agents previously were advocated for an SBP greater than 160 mmHg or diastolic BP (DBP) greater than 90 mmHg. Current recommendation is to intervene judiciously for a mean blood pressure (MBP) that exceeds 130 mmHg. This is calculated using the formula: MBP = [(2×DBP) + SBP]/3. Consult critical care providers who will be involved in ongoing care of the patient, as individual practices vary. Use medications that can be titrated rapidly. Vasopressors may be indicated to keep SBP over 120 mmHg; this avoids CNS damage in the ischemic penumbra from the reactive vasospasm seen in SAH. Provide supplemental oxygen for all patients with CNS impairment. Elevate the head of the bed 30° to facilitate intracranial venous drainage. Administer IV crystalloid fluids to maintain volume. Do not over hydrate patients because of risks of hydrocephalus. Patients with SAH also may have hyponatremia from cerebral salt wasting. Consider antiemetics for nausea or vomiting. Sedate cautiously to avoid masking the neurological examination, which may jeopardize the reliability of the findings. However, avoid any increase in ICP due to excessive agitation from pain and discomfort. Prophylactic use of anticonvulsants does not acutely prevent seizures after SAH, but use anticonvulsants in patients who have had a seizure or if local practice dictates routine use. Begin with anticonvulsants that do not change the level of consciousness (i. e. , phenytoin first; barbiturates or benzodiazepines only to stop active seizures). Calcium channel blockers decrease the incidence and severity of cerebral vasospasm. Judicious use is essential because of the risk of detrimental primary or secondary hypotension. Short-acting medication is recommended; discuss this intervention with the neurosurgeon. Use of antifibrinolytics, such as epsilon aminocaproic acid, is controversial. They competitively inhibit plasminogen activation and have been reported to reduce the incidence of rebleeding. Other reports warn of their detrimental vasospastic effect and increased occurrence of hydrocephalus. Consult a neurosurgeon concerning their use. Emergent ventricular drain-age by the neurosurgeon may be necessary.

4.3.15   Consultations

Obtain emergent neurosurgical consultation for definitive treatment. Interventional radiology may be needed when surgical intervention is deemed necessary by the neurosurgical consultant (e. g. , a large clot causing a mass effect is present and needs to be evacuated emergently). Many centers opt for early angiography in all patients.

4.3.16   Further inpatient care

Admit to ICU for serial neurological examinations and for hemodynamic monitoring. Arrange for a darkened, quiet, private room to minimize stimuli that may lead to an elevation of ICP. Closely monitor BP and appropriately. Some centers favor volume expansion to treat vasospasm that develops days after the initial bleeding episode. Neurosurgical team should institute a workup and treatment plan. No clear difference exists in outcome with early (0–3 days) or late (11–14 days) surgical intervention; however, many centers favor early surgery in patients with grade Ⅰ or Ⅱ SAH. Emergent imaging and intervention may be necessary if mass effect or rebleeding develops.

4.3.17   Transfer

Patients with possible ruptured or leaking SAH should be transferred emergently to the closest center with CT scan and neurosurgical staff. Stabilize patients promptly for transfer in an advanced cardiac life support (ACLS) monitored unit. Address airway and the possible need for intubation or other emergent interventions, such as mannitol and hyperventilation, prior to transfer.

4.3.18   Complications

Hydrocephalus may develop within the first 24 hours because of obstruction of CSF out-flow in the ventricular system by clotted blood. Rebleeding of SAH occurs in 20% of patients in the first 2 weeks. Peak incidence of rebleeding occurs the day after SAH. This may be from lysis of the aneurysmal clot. Vasospasm from arterial smooth muscle contraction is symptomatic in 36% of patients. Neurological deficits from cerebral ischemia peak at days 4–12. Hypothalamic dysfunction causes excessive sympathetic stimulation, which may lead to myocardial ischemia or labile detrimental BF. Hyponatremia may result from cerebral salt wasting. Aspiration pneumonia and other complications of critical care may occur.

4.3.19   Prognosis

Cognitive deficits are present, even in many patients considered to have a good outcome. More than 1/3 of survivors have major neurological deficits. Factors that affect morbidity and mortality rates are severity of hemorrhage, degree of cerebral vasospasm, and occurrence of re-bleeding, location of bleeding, age and o-verall health of the patient presence of comorbid conditions and the hospital course (e. g. , infection, myo-cardial infection). Survival correlates with the grade of SAH upon presentation. Reported figures include a 70% survival rate for grade Ⅰ, 60% for grade Ⅱ, 50% for grade Ⅲ and 40% for grade Ⅳ, and 10% for grade Ⅴ.

4.4　Intracerebral Hemorrhage

Intracerebral hemorrhage involves bleeding in the brain caused by the rupture of an intracranial blood vessel.

4.4.1　Causes

Internal bleeding can occur in any part of the brain. Blood may accumulate in the brain tissues or in the space between the brain and the membranes covering the brain (subarachnoid space). The bleeding may be isolated to part of one cerebral hemisphere (lobar intracerebral hemorrhage) or it may occur in other brain structures, such as the thalamus, basal ganglia, pons, or cerebellum (deep intracerebral hemorrhage).

Intracerebral hemorrhage can be caused by trauma (brain injury) or abnormalities of the blood vessels (aneurysm or angioma). When it is not caused by one of these conditions, it is most commonly associated with high blood pressure (hypertensive intracerebral hemorrhage). In some cases, no cause can be found.

4.4.2　Clinical manifestations

4.4.2.1　Symptoms

Headache may occur when lying flat, may awaken patient from sleep, may increase with change in posi-tion and may increase with bending, straining or coughing. Nausea and vomiting may be present. Change in conscious level (sleepy, lethargic, somnolent, stupor) or coma may occur. Visual changes such as decreased vision, loss of all or part of vision, different size of pupils, uncontrollable eye movements and eyelid drooping may also be found. Decrease sensation, numbness, tingling and facial paralysis can be seen. The patient may have difficulty in speaking or understanding speech, difficulty in swallowing, difficulty in writing or reading and movement changes. Loss of coordination, loss of balance seizure and abnormal taste can be seen in some patients.

4.4.2.2　Signs

Neuromuscular examination may indicate increased intracranial pressure or focal neurological deficits (decreases in brain function). The specific pattern of symptoms and changes may indicate the location of the intracerebral hemorrhage. Eye examination may show optic nerve swelling caused by increased pressure in the brain, or there may be changes in the eye movement. Abnormal reflexes may be present, or there may be an abnormal extent of normal reflexes.

4.4.2.3　Lab studies

Tests to determine the amount and cause of bleeding may include the complete blood count, platelet count, bleeding time, prothrombin time or partial thromboplastin, liver function tests and kidney function tests.

4.4.2.4   Imaging studies

These may confirm the intracerebral hemorrhage. The location and amount of bleeding can be determined by these tests. Head CT scan (preferred if the bleeding is less than 48 hours). Head MRI or MRA. Angiography of the head (if symptoms allow enough time) can determine whether an aneurysm or arteriovenous malformation (abnormal collection of blood vessels) is present.

4.4.2.5   Treatment

Intracerebral hemorrhage is a sever condition requiring prompt medical attention even if symptoms are episode (occurring occasionally, and then disappearing). It may develop quickly into a life threatening situation.

Treatment goals include life saving interventions, supportive measures and control of symptoms. Treatment varies, depending on the specific location, extent and cause of the bleeding. Surgical removal of hematomas may be appropriate, especially if there is a hematoma in the cerebellum. Surgical repair of structures causing the bleed (repair of aneurysm, arteriovenous malformation) may be appropriate in some cases. Medicines used may include corticosteroids or diuretics to reduce swelling, anticonvulsants to control seizures, analgesics to control pain and others.

Blood, blood products, intravenous fluids, or medications may be appropriate to counteract bleeding and loss of blood volume.

4.4.2.6   Complications

The main complications include hemorrhagic stroke, permanent loss of any brain function, side effects of medications used to treat the disorder and complications of surgery.

4.4.2.7   Prognosis

The outcome varies highly. Death may occur rapidly despite prompt medical treatment. Recovery may occur completely or with a permanent loss of some brain functions. Medications, surgery or treatments for this condition can have severe side effects.

4.4.2.8   Glasggow coma scale

The GSC is a 3−15 point scale that reflects the level of arousal, as determined by using the patient's motor, verbal and eye responses. The severity of injury can then is stratified immediately, moderate and severs. Mild brain injury corresponds to a GCS score of 13−15, moderate corresponds to a score of 9−12, and sever injury corresponds to a score of 3−8. The GSC defines the severity of traumatic brain injury within 48 hours of injury.

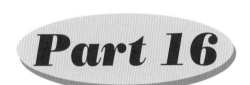

Part 16

Intracranial Neoplasms

Chapter 1

General Consideration

Intracranial neoplasms can be grouped into two broad categories: primary neoplasms, secondary or metastatic neoplasms. Primary tumors may arise from the brain itself (e. g. , gliomas), from its coverings(meninges, skull, and nerve sheaths)and its embryonal rest (dermoid, epidermoid and craniopharyngioma), or from other sites, such as the anterior(pituitary adenoma)or the pineal regions and gland. Primary CNS neoplasms are the sixth most common tumors in adults with an average incidence of 5–6 per 100 000. The most common central nervous system tumors occur in patients over 45 years old. In children, intracranial neoplasms are second in occurrence only to leukemias (Odom et al. ,1956). In adult, 70% of primary brain tumors arise above the tentorium cerebelli, the others 30% originate in the infratentorial compartment. In children, the incidence is the reverse. The most brain tumors eventually produce increased intracranial pressure, either by virtue of their bulk, by production of cerebral edema, or by obstruction of the flow of cerebrospinal fluid. For the purposes of this discussion, primary neoplasms are divided into glial (neuroeetoderal) and nonglial.

Chapter 2

Histological Classification

The development of a systematic taxomomy for primary brain neoplasma is an ongoing process which began in the late 19th century. In 1993, a significant revised version of these proceeding was published by the World Health Organization as Histologic typing of tumors of the central nervous system (WHO-1-4) (Klciliues 1993). Although these lesions may be histologically benign, the location of any particular neoplasm, i. e., ependmoma of the 4th ventricle or meningioma of the clivus, may render the lesion incurable.

Outline of primary CNS tumors and tumor-like masses

(1) Diffuse astrocytic and oligodendroglial tumours

Diffuse astrocytoma, IDH-mutant

Gemistocytic astrocytoma, IDH-mutant

Diffuse astrocytoma, IDH-wildtype

Diffuse astrocytoma, NOS

Anaplastic astrocytoma, IDH-mutant

Anaplastic astrocytoma, IDH-wildtype

Anaplastic astrocytoma, NOS

Glioblastoma, IDH-wildtype

Giant cell glioblastoma

Gliosarcoma

Epithelioid glioblastoma

Glioblastoma, IDH-mutant

Glioblastoma, NOS

Diffuse midline glioma, H3 K27M-mutant

Oligodendroglioma, IDH-mutant and 1p/19q-codeleted

Oligodendroglioma, NOS

Anaplastic oligodendroglioma, IDH-mutant and 1p/19q-codeleted

Anaplastic oligodendroglioma, NOS

Oligoastrocytoma, NOS

Anaplastic oligoastrocytoma, NOS

(2) Other astrocytic tumours

Pilocytic astrocytoma

Pilomyxoid astrocytoma

Subependymal giant cell astrocytoma

Pleomorphic xanthoastrocytoma

Anaplastic pleomorphic xanthoastrocytoma

(3) Ependymal tumours

Subependymoma

Myxopapillary ependymoma

Ependymoma

Papillary ependymoma

Clear cell ependymoma

Tanycytic ependymoma

Ependymoma, RELA fusion-positive

Anaplastic ependymoma

(4) Other gliomas

Chordoid glioma of the third ventricle

Angiocentric glioma

Astroblastoma

(5) Choroid plexus tumours

Choroid plexus papilloma

Atypical choroid plexus papilloma

Choroid plexus carcinoma

(6) Neuronal and mixed neuronal-glial tumours

Dysembryoplastic neuroepithelial tumour

Gangliocytoma

Ganglioglioma

Anaplastic ganglioglioma

Dysplastic cerebellar gangliocytoma (Lhermitte-Duclos disease)

Desmoplastic infantile astrocytoma and ganglioglioma

Papillary glioneuronal tumour

Rosette-forming glioneuronal tumour

Diffuse leptomeningeal glioneuronal tumour

Central neurocytoma

Extraventricular neurocytoma

Cerebellar liponeurocytoma

Paraganglioma

(7) Tumours of the pineal region

Pineocytoma

Pineal parenchymal tumour of intermediate differentiation

Pineoblastoma

Papillary tumour of the pineal region

(8) Embryonal tumours

Medulloblastoma

Medulloblastoma, NOS

Medulloblastomas, genetically defined

Medulloblastoma, WNT-activated

Medulloblastoma, SHH-activated and TP53-mutant

Medulloblastoma, SHH-activated and TP53-wildtype

Medulloblastoma, non-WNT/non-SHH

Medulloblastomas, histologically defined

Medulloblastoma, classic

Desmoplastic/nodular medulloblastoma

Medulloblastoma with extensive nodularity

Large cell / anaplastic medulloblastoma

Embryonal tumour with multilayered rosettes, C19MC-altered

Embryonal tumour with multilayered rosettes, NOS

Other CNS embryonal tumours

Medulloepithelioma

CNS neuroblastoma

CNS ganglioneuroblastoma

CNS embryonal tumour, NOS

Atypical teratoid/rhabdoid tumour

CNS embryonal tumour with rhabdoid features

(9)Tumours of the cranial and paraspinal nerves

Schwannoma

Cellular schwannoma

Plexiform schwannoma

Melanotic schwannoma

Neurofibroma

Atypical neurofibroma

Plexiform neurofibroma

Perineurioma

Hybrid nerve sheath tumours

Malignant peripheral nerve sheath tumour (MPNST)

MPNST with divergent differentiation

Epithelioid MPNST

MPNST with perineurial differentiation

(10)Meningiomas

Meningioma

Meningioma variants

Meningothelial meningioma

Fibrous meningioma

Transitional meningioma

Psammomatous meningioma

Angiomatous meningioma

Microcystic meningioma

Secretory meningioma

Lymphoplasmacyte–rich meningioma

Metaplastic meningioma

Chordoid meningioma

Clear cell meningioma

Atypical meningioma

Papillary meningioma

Rhabdoid meningioma

Anaplastic (malignant) meningioma

(11)Mesenchymal, non–meningothelial tumours

Solitary fibrous tumour / haemangiopericytoma

Haemangioblastoma

Haemangioma

Epithelioid haemangioendothelioma

Angiosarcoma

Kaposi sarcoma

Ewing sarcoma / peripheral primitive

neuroectodermal tumour

Lipoma

Angiolipoma

Hibernoma

Liposarcoma

Desmoid–type fibromatosis

Myofibroblastoma

Inflammatory myofibroblastic tumour

Benign fibrous histiocytoma

Fibrosarcoma

Undifferentiated pleomorphic sarcoma / malignant

fibrous histiocytoma

Leiomyoma

Leiomyosarcoma

Rhabdomyoma

Rhabdomyosarcoma

Chondroma

Chondrosarcoma

Osteoma

Osteochondroma

Osteosarcoma

(12) Melanocytic tumours

Meningeal melanocytosis

Meningeal melanomatosis

Meningeal melanocytoma

Meningeal melanoma

(13) Lymphomas

Diffuse large B-cell lymphoma of the CNS

Corticoid-mitigated lymphoma

Sentinel lesions

Immunodeficiency-associated CNS lymphomas

AIDS-related diffuse large B-cell lymphoma

EBV+ diffuse large B-cell lymphoma, NOS

Lymphomatoid granulomatosis

Intravascular large B-cell lymphoma

Miscellaneous rare lymphomas in the CNS

Low-grade B-cell lymphomas

T-cell and NK/T-cell lymphomas

Anaplastic large cell lymphoma (ALK+/ALK-)

MALT lymphoma of the dura

(14) Histiocytic tumours

Langerhans cell histiocytosis

Erdheim-Chester disease

Rosai-Dorfman disease

Juvenile xanthogranuloma

Histiocytic sarcoma

(15) Germ cell tumours

Germinoma

Embryonal carcinoma

Yolk sac tumour

Choriocarcinoma

Teratoma

Mature teratoma

Immature teratoma

Teratoma with malignant transformation

Mixed germ cell tumour

(16) Familial tumour syndromes

Neurofibromatosis type 1

Neurofibromatosis type 2

Schwannomatosis

Von Hippel-Lindau disease

Tuberous sclerosis

Li-Fraumeni syndrome

Cowden syndrome

Turcot syndrome

Mismatch repair cancer syndrome

Familial adenomatous polyposis

Naevoid basal cell carcinoma syndrome

Rhabdoid tumour predisposition syndrome

(17) Tumours of the sellar region

Craniopharyngioma

Adamantinomatous craniopharyngioma

Papillary craniopharyngioma

Granular cell tumour of the sellar region

Pituicytoma

Spindle cell oncocytoma

Chapter 3

Clinical Findings

Generally, intracranial lesions have a number of features that set the apart from neoplasms in other parts of the body. Intracranial structures are surrounded by tbe cranium, resulting in a vault which, in the mature person, does not expand. There is a very limited space for intracranial masses to enlarge before decompensation occurs. Likewise the cranium prohibits the identification of neoplasms by palpation, a common diagnostic practice for other parts of the body.

Signs and symptoms of intracranial neoplasms may be divided into those related to the generalized increase in intracranial pressure and those resulting from direct involvement of the cerebral structure with the neoplasm. Symptoms of generally increased pressure include headache, nausea, vomiting, papilledemam, 6th nerve palsies, and deterioration on the level of consciousness. Localized signs and symptoms include focal seizures, paresis, discrete sensory loss, lateralized ataxia, and dysfunction of cranial nerves other than the 6th. Localized signs and symptoms may appear after evidence of generalized increase in intracranial pressure, or may antedate the evidence of generalized increase in pressure depending upon the location and type of lesion. In children, before closure of the suture, progressive enlargement of the head and bulging of the anterior fontanelle are seen with increased in intracranial pressure.

3.1 Tumors of Neuroglial Cells

3.1.1 Astrocytomas

Astrocytomas make up 40% of gliomas and may occur in any part of the central nervous system. Symptoms and physical signs depend upon the site of the lesion. Lesions occurring in an optical nerve may produce unilateral blindness, which may become bilateral when the optical chiasm is involved. Lesions in the brain stem usually produce cranial nerve signs, early, followed by pyramidal tract signs and, ultimately, obstructive hydrocephalus. Hemispheric lesions cause lateralizing motor or sensory deficits and, frequently, seizures. Cerebellar astrocytomas are common in children and may be solid or comprised of a large cyst with a "mural nodule" of tumor in the cyst wall.

Treatment consists of excision where feasible, e. g. , cerebellar or some cerebral lesions. Cures be common on resection of cerebellar astrocytomas, rare when the lesions are located in the cerebral hemispheres.

Astrocytomas within the brain stem are difficult to resect. Those located within the visual pathways may be resected if they be confined to one optic nerve. Nonresectable lesions may be biopsied, if feasible, and irradiated(Figure 16-3-1).

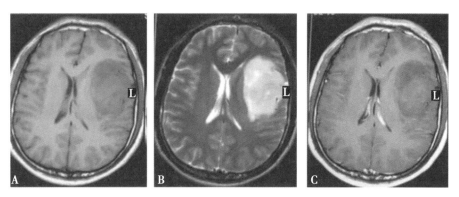

Figure 16-3-1   MRI T_1, T_2 and enhanced image of Astrocytomas

3.1.2   Oligodendrogliomas

Oligodendrogliomas are slowly growing lesions, usually occurring in the cerebral hemispheres. They occur much less frequently than astrocytomas or glioblastomas and are usually seen in young adults. Seizures are often the first indication, but the patients may later have other localizing symptoms and signs relating to the specific site of the lesion. Diagnostic studies and their findings are similar to those of astrocytomas of the cerebral hemispheres. The primary difference is that a much greater percentage of oligodendrogliomas has stippled calcification than other gliomas.

Treatment consists of resection followed by irradiation. As with glioblastomas, the objective of therapy is to decompress the brain and prolong life. Postoperative progression is often much more rapid than the long period of preoperative symptoms would imply. However, survival of a few years is not uncommon.

3.1.3   Ependymal tumors

Ependymomas occur throughout the central nervous system but are concentrated within the ventricular system. A high percentage of those occurring in infants and children are seen in the posterior fossa. Ependymomas often grow slowly, and rarely metastasize until they are attacked surgically. Obstructive hydrocephalus and signs of ataxia are associated with lesions of the posterior fossa. Supratentorial lesions produce signs localized to the site of the lesions.

Treatment is excision wherever possible. One must be satisfied with less than complete removal of those lesions attached to the floor of the 4th ventricle or other vital areas. Irradiation is used when resection is incomplete, which is quite frequent Figure 16-3-2.

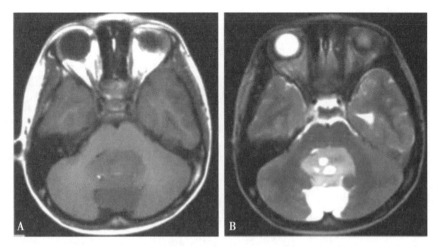

Figure 16-3-2   MRI T₁ and T₂ image of ependymomas

3.1.4   Medulloblastomas

Medulloblastomas are highly malignant tumors, usually seen in children, and usually originating in the 4th ventricle. Initial symptoms and signs result from the cerebellar involvement as well as from occlusion of the ventricular outflow. The fontanels may be full and the head enlacing if the fontanels and sutures are open at the time of onset. If the fontanels have closed, headache, nausea and vomiting, papilledema, 6th nerve palsies, and ataxia with or without nystagmus are usually present. Metastasis within the central nervous system is common, often along the spinal canal.

Treatment includes resection of as much tumor as possible without increasing the neurological deficit. Shunting should be performed when free communication is not easily obtained. Some authors recommend inclusion of a filter in shunts to avoid seeding of the neoplasm outside the central nervous system. The tumor is quite radiosensitive, 30% -40% of patients surviving 5 years. Prolongation of useful survival by chemotherapy is reported.

Metastasis may occur throughout the nervous system and irradiation of the entire neuroaxis is recommended. After surgery, metastasis may occur throughout the body(Figure 16-3-3).

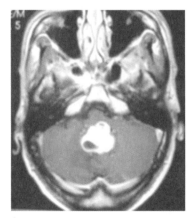

Figure 16-3-3   MRI enhanced image of medulloblastoma

3.1.5　Glioblastoma multiforme

Glioblastoma multiforme is the most common primary intracranial neoplasm and one of the most malignant. It can occur throughout the central nervous system, but most frequently affects predominately the cerebral hemispheres. It occurs during middle age. Symptoms and signs depend upon the location of the lesion, but are usually rapid in progression. They include evidence of generalized increased intracranial pressure, i. e. , lethargy and confusion plus localizing signs, i. e. , focal seizures, dysphasia, hemiparesis, or alteration of sensation.

Treatment is resection of all of the grossly apparent tumor. Resection is usually confined to the tumor in order not to increase neurological deficits. Cure is virtually never need. Postoperative irradiation is usually recommended but of questionable value. Chemotherapy is being attempted in a number of centers but its value is still not clear. The median postoperative survival without adjunctive forms of therapy 19 approximately 6 months.

3.2　Nonglial Tumors

3.2.1　Meningiomas

Meningiomas represent the largest group of bening intracranial tumors, accounting for roughly 15% of all intracranial masses. A rare lesion is malignant. They are thought to originate from the arachnoid villi, which are concentrated in the walls of venous sinuses but are also quite widely dispersed. Meningiomas preferentially occur along the superior sagittal sinus, under the sutures of the skull, along the lesser wing of the sphenoid, in the floor of the frontal fossa, on the clivus, in the cerebellopontine angles, along the lateral sinuses of the posterior fossa, on the rim of the foramen magnum and in the ventricles, in approximately that order of frequency. Overall, they are more common in females by a ratio of nearly 2 : 1. The duration of symptoms may be prolonged, offering a clue to the benign nature of the lesion. There are several histoiogical types, the most common being syncytial and transitional. The type appears to make little difference clinically. Symptoms and signs depend on the location. Lesions along the sagittal sinus may produce hemiparesis or paraparesis. Anteriorly placed lesions a long the sinus may be associated with behavioral changes and incontinence in addition to pyramidal tract signs. Lesions along the sphenoid wing may cause proptosis, unilateral visual impairment, and oculomotor impairment if they encroach on the superior orbital fissure. Severe pain may acompany involvement of the first division of the trigeminal nerve. Lesions in the floor of the frontal may produce headache and loss of smell. If they are situated in the region of the tuberculum sellae, they may embarrass the optic nerves on one or both sides.

Lesions of the clivus may produced pyramidal tract signs, oculomotor palsies, and loss of facial sensation. Lesions in the cerebellopontine angle may be indistinguishable clinically from acoustic neurinomas producing loss of hearing, impairment of facial sensation, and loss of motor activity in the muscles of facial expression. Ataxia may accompany lesions in these areas as well as lesions attached below the lateral sinus.

Lesions on the rim of the foramen magnum may produce pyramidal tract signs and weakness occurring in the upper extremities before it is apparent in the lower extremities. Lower cranial nerve palsies may also occur.

Treatment is total excision whenever possible. Resection may be difficult or impossible for those lesions originating around the brain stem and base of the skull, and it may be similarly unwise to attempt complete removal of lesions invading the sagittal sinus over its posterior two thirds because acute occlusion of this structure will produce severe neurological deficits(Figure 16-3-4).

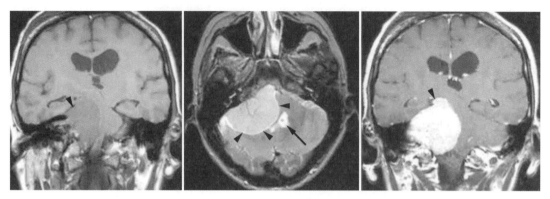

Figure 16-3-4   MRI T_1, T_2 and enhanced image of Meningiomas

3.2.2 Pituitary adenomas

Tumors of the pituitary usually originate in the adenohypophysis. By increase in size, tumors may produce symptoms of neurological deficits, or they can cause a hormonal imbalance resulting in excess or decrease of hormonal output. Both neurological deficits and excessive secretions of certain hormones represent indications for surgical correction. Deterioration of visual fields is usually the first neurological deficit caused by gradually expanding tumors of the pituitary. Bitemporal defects are common. Defects classically originate in the upper-outer quadrants, progress to the lower-outer quadrants, and then the lower-inner quadrants, finally producing complete blindness. These deficits result from involvement of the optic chiasm; they are often asymmetrical. Whether the deficits are consistently the result of direct pressure upon the optic pathways or the result of interruption of the vascular supply is not certain.

Tumors can enlarge so much that they cause total blindness, and impair hypothalamic function and even cause severe hydrocephalus by obstructing the flow of cecebrospinal fluid through the 3rd ventricle. Impairment of hypothalamic function can cause diabetes insipidus and stupor in addition to abnormalities in anterior pituitary function. Seizures may occur when tumors extend laterally into the region of the temporal lobe or anteriorally under the frontal lobe.

Hormonal indications for pituitaiy surgery include gigantism or acromegaly, Cushing's disease, Nelson's syndrome (increasing pigmentation of the skin following adrenalectomy for Cushing's disease), and syndromes associated with amenorrhea and galactorrhea. Very rarely, adenomas have been resected for excessive secretion of thyroid stimulating hormoneor gonadotrophins(Figure 16-3-5).

Treatment is surgical resection by the transfrontal approach if the lesion extends far above the clinoids, especially if the extrasellar extension is located anteriorly or laterally. The transsphenoidal approach is used if the lesion is confined to the sella and sphenoid-sinus or extends "moderately" above the sella in the midline. If resection is not considered complete, it should be followed by irradiation therapy.

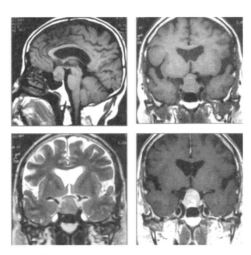

Figure 16-3-5   MRI T_1, T_2 and enhanced image of pituitary adenoma

3.2.3   Acoustic neurinomas

Acoustic neurinomas, also called schwannomas or neurilemonas, originate from the vestibular division of the 8th nerve in the internal auditory meatus. They are known to occur with increased frequency in patients with neurofibromatosis. They closely resemble neurofibromas pathologically. Symptoms usually begin with tinnitus or "ringing in the ear". There is progressive decrease in hearing. There may be headach lateralized to the involved side. As the lesion grows, it distorts structures in the cerebellopontine angle and may lead to loss of 5th nerve function and ataxia. Peripheral facial paralysis is usually a late sign. Distortion of the brain stem leads to a gradual obstruction of the aqueduct and 4th ventricle with papilledema and, subsequently, optic atrophy and blindness.

Treatment is excision, usually performed through the posterior fossa with microscope. This approach is mandatory for large lesions. Alternately, small tumors may be resected through the ear by the "translabyrinthine" approach, or through the middle fossa. Attempts should be made to preserve facial nerve function. If this is impossible, another cranial nerve (11th or 12th) may be anastomosed to its distal trunk at the base of the mastoid process(Figure 16-3-6).

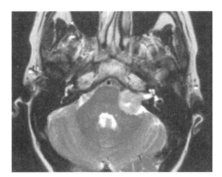

Figure 16-3-6   MRI T_2 image of acoustic neurinomas

3.2.4   Craniopharyngiomas

"Rathke's pouch tumors" or "suprasellar cysts" are thought to be remnants of Rathke's pouch, thus of developmental origin. Despite this embryological derivation, many are not manifested until the patient has reached adult life, and some craniopharyngiomas have been reported as incidental findings in autopsies of elderly individuals.

These lesions present with symptoms of hypothalamic or hypophyseal impairment, increased intracranial pressure, or visual field deficits. Visual deficits are usually bitemporal because of suprasellar masses pressing on the optic chiasm or tracts, although some lesions may compress an optic nerve and cause unilateral blindness.

Intracranial hypertension may result from compression of the 3rd ventricle, leading to obstructive hydrocephalus. Pituitary dysfunction will result in decreased output of adrenocorlicotrophic and thyroid stimulating hormones resulting in an electrolyte imbalance, decreased response to stress, and reduced blood pressure. The skin may be dry and pale, the hair fine. Decrease in gonadotrophins may result in loss of sexual development or loss of function. Some patients present with diabetes insipidus. The adiposogenital dystrophy syndrome of Frohlich, i. e. , obesity with infantile genitalia, is occasionally seen. Rarely, patients present in stupor from involvement of the hypothalamus and brain stem.

Treatment of craniopharyngiomas is surgical excisionif feasible. Extensive lesions or those densely adherent to the carotid arteries or hypothalamus may be impossible to completely remove. If there is a large cyst or multiple cysts, these may be drained. Irradiation therapy has been advocated and there seems to be little doubt that irradiation slows the progress of these lesions, although there is little evidence that many craniopharyngiomas are cured with radiotherapy(Figure 16-3-7).

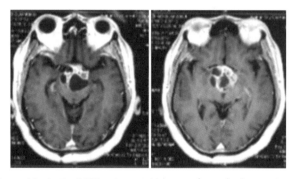

Figure 16-3-7   MRI enhanced image of craniopharyngiomas

3.2.5 Hemangioblastomas

Hemangioblastomas are benign tumors of capillaries involving the cerebellum. It is a fairly common primary tumor of the cerebellum seen in adults. The tumors of the cerebellum are frequently associated with similar lesions in the retinae (von Hippel-Lindau disease). Signs and symptoms are generalized increased CSF pressure and ataxia. Polycythemia may be an associated finding. Histologically, the tumors are identical with angioblastic meningiomas seen above the tentorium. Treatment is excision. Recurrence is a problem only when all the lesion is not removed.

Chapter 4

Diagnosis and Differential Diagnosis

A detailed history and neurological examination should be carried out on any patient who might have an intracranial neoplasm. A recent history of headaches, particularly when they occur predominantly early in the morning and are associated with nausea and projectile vomiting, focal seizures, deteriorating level of consciousness, lateralizing paresis or ataxia, or evidences of cranial nerve dysfunction of recent onset, should cause one to consider intracranial neoplasm in the differential diagnosis. Likewise, a history of hormonal dysfunction such as excessive growth, evidence of altered metabolism such as excessive weight gain or development of osteoporosis, hypertension and abdominal striae, or gonadal dysfunction in a young person should alert one to the possibility of a neoplasm in the region of the sella, as should the late onset of diabetes insipidus.

The neurological examination should include a discrete review of the cranial nerves. Particular attention should be paid to the ophthalmoscopic examination, where papilledema would suggest the presence of an intracranial expanding mass. Dysfunction of any of the cranial nerves evidences of lateralized paresis, sensory loss, nystagmus, ataxia, or depressed level of consciousness should lead one to consider further investigations.

Examintion may include an electroencephalogram, electronystagmography, audiometry, plain roentgenograms, isotopic brain scans, computer tomography and magnetic resonance imagine. CT and MRI are available in most intracranial neoplasms. When as-sessing either CT or MRI scans for neoplasm, the follow points should be ascertained: ①lesion location and extent-intraaxial versus extraaxial, supratentotial versus infratentorial, single versus multiple. ②tumor maiin or characterization-enhanced CT and MRI scans commonly demonstrate enhancement of the outer margin of more malignant tumors owing to the break-down in the blood-brain barrier and, to a lesser extent, the vascularity of the lesion itself. ③mass effect localized or generalized. Midline shift is indicated by displacement of the pineal gland, the ventricular system, or the falx. Effacement of the cortical sulci and CSF cisterns may occur as part of either a localized or a generalized process. ④the presence of edema at times, especially in lower grade tumors, it is difficult to separtate the tumor margin from edema ; steroid therapy may decrease the amount of edema. ⑤brain herniation of the brain may occur from one side to the other or from one fossa to another.

Differential diagnosis include brain abscess, vascular malformation, degeneration diseases, subdural hematoma and empyema, encephalitis, meningitis, congenital hydrocephalus. In children, unexplained seizures are usually the onset of idiopathic epilepsy but are often the first manifestation of brain tumors in adults.

Chapter 5

Treatment

The major objectives of treatment are as follow:

(1) Totally remove tumor when feasible, especial extra-axial tumor and cerebellar hemangioblastoma

(2) Subtotally remove tumor to relieve symptoms and prolong life when location, size, and vascularity preclude total extirpation.

(3) protection of brain from damage due to treatment.

Except cystic cerebellar astrocytomas, glial tumors are rarely curable by surgery alone. subtotal resection of glial tumor followed by postoperative radiation therapy consisting of 5000–6000 cGY delivered over 5–6 weeks affords temporary palliation. Chemotherapy has been used with increasing success for recurrent malignant gliomas and medulloblastomas and pineal germ cell tumors.

Part 17

Disease of the Neck

Chapter 1

Anatomy and Physiology

1.1　Summary

Thyroid gland is an endocrinal gland present in the neck secreting triiodothyronine (T_3) and thyroxine (T_4) hormones. It is richly vascular and highly functional. Effects of hormonal changes affect every part of the body such as central nervous system, cardiovascular system, gastrointestinal system and reproductive system. It is also the site of various diseases—a simple enlargement toxicity and malignant transformation.

1.2　Surgical Anatomy of Thyroid Gland

1.2.1　Development and anatomy

· It develops from median down growth(midline diverticulum) of a column of cells from the pharyngeal floor between first and second pharyngeal pouches.

· The decent is anterior to structures that from hyoid bone and larynx. (19.1)

· By 6 weeks of intrauterine life, the central column, which becomes the thyroglossal duct, gets reabsorbed.

· The duct bifurcates to form thyroid lobes.

· Pyramidal lobe is formed by a portion of the duct.

· Calcitonin producing parafollicular or C cells originate from the fourth branchial pouch.

· Thyroid gland is present in the neck, enclosed by pretracheal fascia which is a part of deep cervical fascia. It has a right and left lobe joined by the isthmus in front of 2nd, 3rd and 4th tracheal rings. It weighs 20–25 g. A projection from the isthmus usually on the left side is called pyramidal lobe. It is attached to the hyoid bone by a fibrous band or muscle fibers called levator glandulae thyroideae.

· Suspensory ligament of Berry: This pair of strong condenced connective tissue binds the glad firmly to each side of catil and upper trachead rings.

· Pretracheal fascia, which is part of deep cervical fascia splits to invest the gland. These structures (ligament of Berry and pretracheal fascia) are responsible for thyroid gland moving with deglutition.

1.2.2 Arterial supply(19.2)

· Superior thyroid artery, a branch of the external carotid artery, enters the upper pole of the gland. Divides into anterior and posterior branches and anastomoses with ascending branch of inferior thyroid artery. Since the upper pole is narrow, ligation is easy.

· Inferior thyroid artery is a branch of thyrocervical trunk gland and enters the posterior aspect of the gland. It supplies the gland by dividing into 4-5 branches which enter the gland at various levels(not truly lower pole).

· Inferior thyroid artery used to be ligated well away from the gland to avoid damage to RLN. However, ligation of these arteries on both sides will cause permanent hypoparathyroidism. Hence, the current practice is to identify and ligate the branches of inferior thyroid artery(3-4) separately.

· Thyroidea ima artery is a branch of either brachiocephalic trunk or direct branch of arch of aorta and enters the lower part of the isthmus in 2% to 3% of the cases.

1.2.3 Venous drainage

· Superior thyroid vein drains the upper pole and enters the internal jugular vein. The vein follows the artery.

· Middle thyroid vein is single, short and wide and drains into internal jugular vein.

· Inferior thyroid veins form a plexus which drain into innominate vein. They do not accompany the artery.

· Kocher's vein is rarely found(vein in between middle and inferior thyroid vein).

1.2.4 Nerves in relationship with thyroid gland

(1) Superior laryngeal nerve: The vagus nerve gives rise to superior laryngeal nerve, which separates from it at skull base and divides into two branches. The larger internal laryngeal nerve is sensory to the supraglottic larynx. The smaller external laryngeal nerve runs close to the superior thyroid vessels and supplies cricothyroid.

· This nerve is away from the vessels near the upper pole. Hence, during thyroidectomy, the upper pedicle should be ligated as close to the thyroid as possible.

(2) Recurrent laryngeal nerve (RLN) is a branch of vagus, hooks around ligamentum arteriosum on the left and subclavian artery on the right and runs in the tacheoesophageal groove near the posteromedial surface. Close to the gland. The nerve lies in between (anterior or posterior) branches of inferior thyroid artery (19.3 and 19.4).

· On the right side, it is 1 cm within the tracheoesophageal groove(key 19.1A B)

1.2.5 Lymphatic drainage of thyroid

· Subcapsular lymphatic plexus drains into pretracheal nodes (Delphic nodes means uncertain) and prelaryngeal nodes which ultimately drain into lower deep cervical nodes and mediastinal nodes. (19.5)

· The chief lymph nodes are middle and lower deep cervical lymph nodes(Level 3 and 4).

· Supraclavivular nodes and nodes in the posterior triangle can also be involved in malignancies of the thyroid gland, especially papillary carcinoma thyroid.

1.2.6   Histology(19.6)

- Microscopically, it is divided ito lobules.
- Each lobule has 20-40 follicles.
- Each follicle is lined by cuboidal epithelial cells.
- In the centre, colloid is present which is secreted from epithelial cells in response to calcitonin.
- Parafollicular cells are present in the interfollicular stroma.

1.3   Physiology

1.3.1   summary

Triiodothyronine and thyroxine are the hormones secreted by the thyroid gland. Dietary requirement of iodine per day is 100-200 μg or 0.1 mg. Sources of iodine are milk, dairy products and sea food.

1.3.2   Steps involved in the synthesis of these hormones

(1) Iodide trapping from the blood into the thyrocyte is the first step in the formation of T_3 and T_4.

- Thiocyanates and perchlorates block this step.

(2) Oxidation of iodide to inorganic iodine: This step needs the enzyme peroxidase.

- Drugs which block this stage (thioamides) are sulfonamide, PAS(para-amino-salicylic acid), carbimazole and propylthiouracil.

(3) Formation of iodotyrosines:

- Iodine + Tyrosine = MIT (monoiodotyrosine) and diiodotyrosine(DIT)
- This step is inhibited by thiourea group of drgs, i. e. , carbimazole.

(4) Coupling reactions

- Coupling of two molecules of DIT results in T_4 and one molecule of DIT and MIT reslts in T_3.
- This stage is blocked by carbimazole.

(5) Hydrolysis

- The hormones combine with globulin to form a colloidthyroglobulin. They are stored in the thyroid gland and releasd as required by process of hydrolysis.

T_3 is an important physiological hormone and is fast-acting (few hours). T_4 is a slow-acting hormone- and takes 4-14 days to act.

Chapter 2

Simple Goiter

2.1　Concept

Simple goiter is a thyroid gland goiter with normal thyroid function, thyroid enlargement due to inefficient thyroid tissue or iodine or related Enzyme deficiency and other causes that compensates for its inefficiency by enlarging, without obvious hyperthyroidism or hypothyroidism, called non-toxic goiter, which is characterized by falling ill in non-endemic goiter epidemic area, and is not associated with cancer and inflammation, the initial course of thyroid disease mostly manifested as diffuse swelling, later developed into multi-nodular swelling.

2.2　Etiology

Most patients with simple goiter have no obvious causes, the incidence of some patients may be related to the following factors:

(1) Iodine deficiency

Iodine is an essential element for the synthesis of thyroid hormones, under the situation of iodine deficiency, the body can not synthesize enough thyroid hormone, with pituitary TSH feedback stimulation, increased TSH promote thyroid hyperplasia, causing goiter. Our country is a country with serious iodine deficiency. The "universal salt iodization" policy promoted by the state is the most effective measure to prevent iodine deficiency.

(2) Enzyme deficiency

Congenital defects or acquired defects of some enzymes during thyroid hormone synthesis can lead to simple goiter, such as iodide transporter defect, peroxidase defect, dehalogenase defect, iodine tyrosine coupling enzyme defect, etc.

(3) Drug

Drugs such as iodide, fluoride, lithium salt, aminopyrine, aminoglutethimide, sulfonamides, phenylbutazone, amiodarone, sulfasalazine, methimazole, propylthiouracil and other drugs can cause simple goiter.

These drugs interfere with or inhibit all aspects of thyroid hormone synthesis through different mechanisms that ultimately affect thyroid hormone synthesis and feedback cause elevated TSH resulting in goiter.

(4) Smoking

Smoking can cause simple goiter, because the inhalation contains thiocyanate, which is a goiter-caused substance. Serum thyroglobulin levels of smokers are much more higher than non-smokers.

(5) Genetic factors

Brix (1999) studied more than 5000 identical twins of monozygotic and double-oviparous twins in endemic goiter areas and found that genetic susceptibility to simple goiter accounted for 82%, with 18% attributable to environmental factors, the result of this study is that sporadic goiter may be caused by genetic factors. So far it has been found that the genetic factors associated with sporadic goiter are 14q, multiple nodular goiter gene-1, 3q26, Xp22, thyroglobulin gene and so on. Epidemiological data show that familial aggregations take part in the cause of the goiter.

(6) Other illnesses

Cushing's disease, acromegaly and end-stage renal disease patients can lead to simple goiter.

2.3　Clinical Manifestations

2.3.1　Goiter or neck mass

Patients with the goiter often complain their necks become thicker or the tight collar. Thyroid is located in the anterior part of the neck and is easily found by patients or their families once swollen, and sometimes goiter can be extended down into the chest, which may be due to the thoracic negative pressure and tumor weight; occasionally goiter occurred in the vagina thyroid tissue.

The early course of the disease is diffuse goiter, check the body and we can see swollen thyroid surface smooth, soft, up and down with the swallowing activity, no tremor and vascular murmur, with the course of the disease, gradual thyroid nodular enlargement, generally not symmetry, multi-nodular nodules can be gathered together and manifested as the neck mass. Nodules vary in size, texture, location. Goiter generally causes no pain, patients can feel the pain if the nodules may be bleeding within. During the physical examination, if thyroid nodular activity found poor, malignant transformation should be wary of.

2.3.2　Compression symptoms

(1) Compression of the trachea

Mild tracheal pressure is usually asymptomatic, severe pressure can cause wheezing, breathing difficulties, coughing. Sternal-behind wheeze-induced wheezing and dyspnea often occur at night, and can occur with changes in position (such as patients with upper extremity lift).

(2) Compression of the esophagus

Lower esophageal position, the goiter generally is not easy to pressure, such as goiter growth and wrapped around the esophagus, can cause compression of esophagus or difficulty in swallowing.

(3) Compression of the recurrent laryngeal nerve

Simple goiter seldom compress the recurrent laryngeal nerve, unless combined with thyroid cancer, tumor infiltration unilateral recurrent laryngeal nerve can cause vocal cord paralysis, hoarseness, bilateral recurrent laryngeal nerve involvement can also cause breathing difficulties. Recurrent laryngeal nerve compression symptoms, to be highly alert that the goiter is malignant.

(4) Compression of blood vessels

Huge goiter, especially behind the sternum can compress the jugular vein, subclavian vein and even the superior vena cava, causing facial edema, superficial cervical vein and upper dilatation.

(5) Compression of phrenic nerve

Posterior thyroid goiter can compress the phrenic nerve, causing hiccups, diaphragmatic swelling. Phrenic nerve compression is less common.

(6) Compression of cervical sympathetic chain

Posterior thyroid goiter can compress the cervical sympathetic chain, causing Horners syndrome.

2.4   Detection

(1) Serum TSH, T_3, T_4 detection

Serum TSH, T_3, T_4 levels of patients with simple goiter are normal.

(2) Iodine 131 uptake rate

Iodine 131 uptake rate is normal or elevated.

(3) Serum TPOAb, TgAb

Generally negative, a few may be mildly elevated, may prompt the possibility of hypothyroidism greater in the future.

(4) Fine needle aspiration cytology

Hypoechoic nodules, calcified nodules diameter $\geqslant 1$ mm nodules, texture hard nodules or rapidly growing nodules should be taking fine needle aspiration cytology, fine needle aspiration cytology is the most effective method to the preoperative evaluation of benign and malignant thyroid nodules, the sensitivity of the cytology is $65\% - 98\%$, the specificity of which is $72\% - 100\%$.

(5) Neck X-ray examination

For longer course, obvious thyroid enlargement or respiratory obstruction or post-sternum goiter patients should be taken X-ray, in order to understand whether tracheal displacement, tracheal softening, and can determine the position and size of the post-sternum goiter.

(6) Neck ultrasound examination

Neck ultrasound is a convenient, reliable method of diagnosis of goiter. B-ultrasound can detect 2 - 4 mm small nodules, so B-ultrasound found the nodules which physical examination cannot touch the nodules, usually found in adult medical examination of the incidence of thyroid nodules was 4% to 7%, and B-ultrasound find 70% of the adults who have thyroid nodules.

(7) Nuclide imaging

Radionuclide imaging can evaluate thyroid morphology and thyroid nodule function. Thyroid volume of diffuse goiter can be seen increased, uniform distribution of radioactivity, nodular goiter got hot nodules or cold nodules.

(8) Neck CT and MRI

Neck CT or MRI does not provide more information and is more expensive than B-ultrasound but has a high diagnostic value for post-sternum goiter.

(9) Respiratory function test

Patients with large goiter or a post-sternum goiter should take a pulmonary function test to make a functional assessment of airway pressure.

2.5　Diagnosis

Residents of non-endemic goiter prevalence, diffuse thyroid enlargement or nodular enlargement, in the exclusion of hyperthyroidism, hypothyroidism, Hashimoto's goiter, acute thyroiditis, subacute thyroiditis, painless thyroiditis, thyroid cancer and other diseases can be diagnosed as simple goiter.

Diagnosis of non-toxic goiter must confirm thyroid function in normal conditions and serum T_3, T_4 levels were normal. Thyroid function is sometimes clinically difficult to assess because some patients with hyperthyroidism, especially the elderly, have mild or atypical clinical manifestations.

2.6　Differential Diagnosis

(1) Hashimoto goiter (chronic lymphocytic thyroiditis)

Manifested as bilateral or unilateral diffuse small nodular or massive mass, TPOAb, TgAb are positive, fine needle aspiration cytology can be diagnosed.

(2) Riedel thyroiditis (chronic fibroblastic thyroiditis)

Manifested as painless throat mass, hard texture, fixed, fine needle aspiration cytology is not meaningful, surgery and biopsy confirmed.

(3) Thyroid adenoma

Manifested as solitary thyroid mass, quality and tough, and hard to be identified with non-toxic goiter single nodules, ultrasound examination of the outer periphery of the capsule, fine needle aspiration cytology helps to identify.

(4) Thyroid cancer

Manifested as thyroid solitary or multiple lumps, hard, adjacent to lymph nodes, medullary carcinoma associated with elevated serum calcitonin levels, pathological examination confirmed.

2.7　Treatment

For the majority of simple goiter patients, whether diffuse or nodular, you can do without any special treatment.

2.7.1　Treatment indications

The following situations require treatment:

(1) There are local symptoms, from neck discomfort to severe oppression symptoms.

(2) Affect the appearance.

(3) Goiter progress faster.

(4) Posterior thyroid goiter.

(5) Nodular goiter can not rule out malignant.

(6) With thyroid dysfunction (including clinical hyperthyroidism).

2.7.2 Therapeutic principles

Simple goiter in patients with varying clinical manifestations, the difference is large, therefore, the treatment plan should be individualized. Because to simple goiter, thyroid function is normal and do not need treatment, unless there is oppression or even suspected tumor, then to take surgical treatment.

2.7.3 No treatment, clinical follow-up

Many simple goiter in patients with goiter growth slow, local asymptomatic, thyroid function is normal, may not be taken special treatment and just need clinical follow-up, regular physical examination, B-ultrasound. In addition, to regularly test serum TSH levels, and early detection of subclinical hyperthyroidism or hypothyroidism. If there is a clear cause of goiter factors, should be removed.

2.7.4 TSH inhibition treatment

Part of the pathogenesis of simple goiter are TSH stimulation related, to use exogenous thyroid hormone can inhibit the secretion of endogenous TSH so that to prevent the growth of goiter, TSH inhibition therapy has been widely used in the treatment of simple goiter.

Serum TSH levels should be detected before TSH inhibition treatment, if the serum TSH levels are normal, TSH inhibition treatment can be done, if the serum TSH <0.1 mU/L, suggesting subclinical hyperthyroidism, TSH suppression should not be treated. Serum TSH levels or thyroid uptake rates (RAIU) should be tested for TSH inhibition. Serum TSH <0.1 mU/L or RAIU <5% is generally considered as complete inhibition, above which partial inhibition is observed. It is generally believed that the serum TSH level can be suppressed to the lower limit of the normal range. The effectiveness of TSH suppressive therapy is a matter of debate, requiring treatment to reduce TSH below normal and noting that long-term suppression of TSH may cause heart and bone side effects.

2.7.5 Radioactive iodine 131 treatment

Radioiodine 131 has been widely used in the treatment of toxic goiter and has not been widely used in the treatment of non-toxic goiter. In recent years, the situation has changed, iodine 131 treatment of simple goiter has been paid more and more attention. In the past 10 years, many articles reported that the use of a one-time high-dose I treatment of simple goiter achieved good results, 80% -100% of patients thyroid volume can be reduced by 40% -60%.

2.7.6 Surgical treatment

Surgical treatment can quickly relieve the symptoms of local compression, therefore, surgical treatment of simple goiter has irreplaceable advantages.

2.7.7 Puncture aspiration or injection of anhydrous alcohol

For cystic nodules, aspiration or injection of anhydrous alcohol, can make a nodule reduced effectively.

Chapter 3

Hyperthyroidism

3.1 General Considerations

Hyperthyroidism is caused by the increased secretion of thyroid hormone (Graves' disease, Plummer's disease, amiodarone toxicity, TSH-secreting tumors) or by other disorders that increase thyroid hormone levels without increasing thyroid gland secretion (factitious hyperthyroidism, subacute thyroiditis). The most common type of thyrotoxicosis encountered in worldwide is Graves' disease; toxic nodular goiter is the second most common type of thyrotoxicosis.

Graves' disease accounts for 70% –80% of endogenous hyperthyroidism. The incidence of Graves' disease is five times higher in females than in males, with an annual incidence of up to 80 per 100 000 women, occurring generally during women's reproductive years, although it may occur at any age. Graves' disease is a syndrome that consists of hyperthyroidism, goiter, ophthalmopathy (orbitopathy), and occasionally a dermopathy referred to as pretibial or localized myxedema. Hyperthyroidism is the most common feature of Graves' disease, affecting nearly all patients, and is caused by autoantibodies to the TSHR (TSHR–Ab) that activate the receptor, thereby stimulating thyroid hormone synthesis and secretion as well as thyroid growth (causing a diffuse goiter).

3.2 Manifestations of Graves' Disease

The clinical presentation ranges from nosymptoms and a suppressed sensitive serum TSH level to overt or obvious clinical hyperthyroidism. The latter includes symptoms associated with increased adrenergic tone and resting energy expenditure and other hormonal effects. Features related to increased adrenergic tone include nervousness, tremor, increased frequency of defecation, palpitations, diaphoresis, irritability, insomnia, headaches, lid retraction and lid lag, muscle weakness, tachycardia, hyperreflexia, and widened pulse pressure. Those related to increased energy expenditure include heat intolerance, unintentional weight loss without anorexia, and warm, moist skin. In elderly subjects, the presentation may be subtle, with atrial fibrillation, weight loss, weakness, and depression. The patient on the verge of thyroid storm has accentuated symptoms and signs of thyrotoxicosis, with hyperpyrexia, tachycardia, cardiac failure, neuromuscular excitation, delirium, or jaundice(Table 17-3-1).

Table 17-3-1　Clinical manifestations of Graves' disease by system

System	Clinical finding
Central nervous system	Suppressed TSH; Anxiety decreased concentration and attention; Emotional lability; Rare Graves' encephalopathy
Constitutional	Weight loss; Fatigue; Nervousness; Dysthermia, usually heat intolerance; Increased oxygen consumption; Reduced fat mass
Ophthalmologic	Eyelid retraction; Edema to tissue around the eye; Constant stare; Dry eyes; Photophobia; Double vision; Infiltrative ophthalmopathy
Cardiac	Tachycardia; Increased contractility palpitations; Widened pulse pressure Increased risk of arrhythmias or heart failure if left untreated
Respiratory	Dyspnea air hunger
Gastrointestinal	Dysphagia; Direct compression from goiter; Myopathy causing pharyngeal or esophageal dysmotility; Hyperdefecation; Diarrhea; Increased appetite
Skin	Flushing; Sweating; Fragile or thinning hair; Onycholysis; Pretibial myxedema
Musculoskeleta	Proximal muscle weakness; Fatigability; Hand tremors; Increased bone turnover; Decreased bone density; Rare thyrotoxic periodic paralysis
Hematologic	Lymphadenopathy rare anemia or pancytopenia
Reproductive	Gynecomastia, erectile dysfunction; and decreased libido in men, oligomenorrhea and decreased fertility in women
Endocrine	Goiter; Increased secretion of T_3 and T_4; Dysregulation of calcium; Homeostasis

3.3　Laboratory Evaluation

Thyrotoxicosis caused by TNG or Graves' disease is usually characterized by a suppressed TSH level with either normal (subclinical) or elevated (overt) free thyroid hormone levels. Other serologic findings, such as antithyroid antibodies (antithyroid peroxidase and antithyroglobulin), that support the diagnosis of autoimmune thyroid disease may be detected in patients with Graves' disease. Serum TSHR-Ab is occasionally helpful in the diagnosis of Graves' disease.

Radioactive iodine uptake (RAIU) are useful tests to elucidate the cause of hyperthyroidism. In Graves' disease, because of diffuse thyroid involvement, the RAIU is always intense and increased.

3.4　Treatment

Once the diagnosis of Graves' disease is established, treatment must be tailored to each individual patient, based on both clinical manifestations of the disease and the personal preferences of the patient. If left untreated, thyrotoxicosis causes progressive and profound catabolic disturbances and cardiac damage. Death may occur in thyroid storm or because of heart failure or severe cachexia. Unfortunately, no treatment yet exists that is able to specifically target the underlying autoimmune condition, and treatment is aimed at correcting the endorgan thyroid dysfunction.

Maintenance of euthyroidism is the ultimate goal and can be achieved by one of three strategies: ①long-term course of antithyroid medication. ②radioactive iodine ablation (RAI). ③surgical thyroidectomy. Radioactive iodine and surgical thyroidectomy destroy the thyroid gland, and almost all patients end up with hypothyroidism that must be treated in the long term with levothyroxine. Treatment must be individualized and depends on the patient's age and general state of health, the size of the goiter, the underlying pathologic process, and the patient's ability to obtain follow-up care.

3.4.1 Antithyroid medications

Antithyroid medications are effective at quickly reducing the production and conversion of thyroid hormone. Remission occurs in 20%–30% of patients after a 12–18 months course of medication and 50%–60% after 5 years of treatment. Rates of remission are lower in men, smokers, those with large goiters, those with persistently elevated TRAb levels while on treatment, and those with high thyroid blood flow on Doppler ultrasound.

Propylthiouracil (PTU) used to be the favored antithyroid drug, but concerns about potentially fatal, fulminant, hepatic necrosis have limited its use today. For this reason, its use is now limited only to patients in the first trimester of pregnancy due to teratogenic effects of the alternative drug, methimazole. Methimazole and its precursor drug, carbimazole, work by inhibiting the enzyme thyroperoxidase, thus preventing the iodinization of thyroglobulin and decreasing the production of both T_3 and T_4. Methimazole also can cause hepatotoxicity, but this is usually cholestatic and not fulminant hepatocellular damage as seen in PTU therapy. A rare but serious side effect of both methimazole and PTU is agranulocytosis, which can lead to neutropenic fever and serious illness. Patients on either drug need baseline and periodic complete blood count and liver function tests. Methimazole can be effective when given once a day, but higher doses are sometimes needed to achieve euthyroid levels, and side effects increase in a dose-dependent manner.

Because antithyroid medication treatment provides the possibility of remission without the destruction or removal of the thyroid gland (unlike RAI and surgery), patients with a strong aversion to treatment that will render them permanently hypothyroid with a subsequent lifelong dependence on levothyroxine should consider this treatment option. Patients with serious comorbidities that would make surgery unacceptably high risk or patients who have had high previous radiation exposure making RAI higher risk should also consider this option. However, patients who are looking for a definitive and rapid treatment option may be frustrated by the low remission rate, the frequent blood draws for monitoring, and the potential—albeit rare—for serious side effects.

3.4.2 Radioactive iodine therapy

RAI therapy is established as an effective, relatively inexpensive, and safe treatment option for Graves' disease. The objective of RAI therapy is to destroy sufficient thyroid tissue to cure hyperthyroidism. The goal of treatment is to render the patient either euthyroid or hypothyroid, depending on the willingness of the physician to risk the possibility of persistent hyperthyroidism. Thyroid function is then assessed 6–8 weeks after RAI administration and possibly every month thereafter to monitor the development of hypothyroidism, especially during the first 6 months after RAI treatment. After the first year of treatment with radioiodine, the incidence of hypothyroidism increases about 3% per year. When hypothyroidism is detected by TSH elevations, levothyroxine treatment should be initiated to maintain the TSH level in the normal range.

RAI therapy is indicated for patients who are over 40 or are poor risks for surgery and for patients with recurrent hyperthyroidism. Hyperthyroid children and pregnancy women should not be treated with RAI therapy.

3.4.3 Surgery

Surgical treatment of Graves' disease indicated for the following: ①pregnant patients requiring high doses of an antithyroid drug or who are intolerant to antithyroid drugs. ②patients with a concomitant thyroid nodule that is malignant or suspicious for malignancy. ③failure of radioiodine therapy. ④massive thyroid enlargement with compressive symptoms. ⑤severe ophthalmopathy. ⑥patient preference. Patient preference is often related to the desire for the most rapid amelioration of symptoms, a reluctance to receive radioiodine because of having young children, a desire to become pregnant, and a fear of exposure to radiation. The advantages of surgical therapy are that patients experience immediate symptomatic improvement and, with subtotal thyroidectomy, the risk of recurrent hyperthyroidism is eliminated. It also allows for treatment of concomitant thyroid nodules and incidental thyroid carcinoma.

The disadvantage of surgical treatment of Graves' disease is the risk of complications from thyroidectomy, which include recurrent laryngeal nerve injury, hypoparathyroidism, neck hematoma, hypothyroidism and thyroid storm. Thyroid storm is a life-threatening condition that can be precipitated by surgery in a patient with poorly treated hyperthyroidism. It is characterized by severe manifestations of hyperthyroidism along with fever, nausea, vomiting, diarrhea, tachyarrhythmias, congestive heart failure, agitation, and delirium. The risk of thyroid storm can be eliminated by adequate preoperative preparation.

An antithyroid drug is used to normalize free T_4 and free T_3 levels prior to the operation. A beta-blocker is used for symptomatic treatment of adrenergic symptoms and tachycardia. Antithyroid drug is administered until the patient becomes euthyroid and is continued until the time of operation. 2-5 drops of potassium iodide solution or Lugol's iodine solution are then given for 10-15 days before surgery in conjunction with the antithyroid drug to reduces the rate of blood flow, thyroid vascularity, and intraoperative blood loss.

The surgical procedures most often performed for the treatment of Graves' disease are subtotal thyroidectomy with bilateral 2-4 gram thyroid remnants and a near-total thyroidectomy, with a remnant less than 1 gram, and a total thyroidectomy. Subtotal thyroidectomy is the preferred surgical option because of the relatively smaller risk of inducing complications and the limited access to postoperative thyroid hormone replacement medications(Table 17-3-2).

Table 17-3-2 Factors for providers and patient to consider for GD treatment options

	Antithyroid medications	Radioactive iodine	Thyroidectomy
Logistics	Daily medication	One time treatment, radiation precautions for 1-2 weeks after	Surgery
Benefits	Noninvasive; No radiation exposure	Permanent treatment option without surgical risk	Quickest, most predictable time course for cure
Speed of recovery	1 - 2 weeks after starting medications, but can take time to regulate dose	Hypothyroidism occurs anytime from 1 to 6 months after treatment	1 - 2 weeks from surgery, can start thyroid replacement immediately and avoid hypothyroid symptoms

Continue to Table 17-3-2

	Antithyroid medications	Radioactive iodine	Thyroidectomy
Drawbacks	Highest relapse rate	Variable time course: difficult to predict when to start thyroid replacement. Persistence of antibodies.	Most invasive, requires general anesthesia and surgical risk
Side effects	Rare fulminant liver failure, agranulocytosis, more common skin rash	Rare risk of secondary malignancy later in life can exacerbate eye disease	Hypoparathyroidism, damage to nerves controlling voice

Chapter 4

Hashimoto's Thyroiditis

Hashimoto's thyroiditis is not only the most common form of thyroiditis (inflammation of the thyroid gland) but also the most common thyroid disorder in America. The disease, which is also known as chronic lymphocytic thyroiditis or autoimmune thyroiditis, affects 14 million people in the United States alone.

4.1 Obstruction

Hashimoto's thyroiditis is named after the Japanese surgeon who discovered it in 1912. It is an autoimmune disorder, which means it occurs when immune cells attack healthy tissue instead of protecting it. In the case of Hashimoto's thyroiditis, immune cells mistakenly attack healthy thyroid tissue, causing inflammation of the thyroid. Autoimmune diseases affect women more than men, and women are 7 times more likely to have Hashimoto's thyroiditis.

When your thyroid gland comes under attack from malfunctioning immune cells, it impairs your thyroid's ability to make thyroid hormone. This can result in hypothyroidism.

Hashimoto's thyroiditis is the most common cause of hypothyroidism. If Hashimoto's thyroiditis attacks your thyroid to the point that the gland can no longer produce enough thyroid hormones for your body to function properly, then you will develop hypothyroidism.

But hypothyroidism isn't the only complication associated with Hashimoto's thyroiditis. In some people, the disorder causes the thyroid to become so inflamed and enlarged that a goiter develops.

For people who develop symptoms of Hashimoto's thyroiditis, such as hypothyroidism or goiter, thyroid hormone therapy is needed. You can read more about this treatment in our article about thyroid hormone replacement therapy.

It's possible to have Hashimoto's thyroiditis(inflammation of the thyroid gland for years without experiencing a single symptom. But there are hallmark signs and symptoms of this common disorder, and it's important that you know what they are. The sooner you recognize the symptoms, the sooner you can receive effective treatment.

If you have symptoms of Hashimoto's thyroiditis, they will be associated with the disorder's two primary complications—goiter and hypothyroidism.

（1）Hashimoto's thyroiditis signs and symptoms associated with goiter

When you have Hashimoto's thyroiditis, your immune cells mistakenly attack your healthy thyroid tissue. When this occurs, your thyroid can become inflamed and enlarged to the point that you develop a goiter.

The primary sign of a goiter is visible swelling in the front of your neck. At first, the bulge may be painless. But if left untreated, it can put pressure on your lower neck. In advanced stages, a goiter can interfere with proper breathing and swallowing.

（2）Hashimoto's thyroiditis signs and symptoms associated with hypothyroidism

Hashimoto's thyroiditis is the most common cause of hypothyroidism because it impairs the thyroid's ability to produce adequate amounts of thyroid hormone. Without enough thyroid hormone, your body cannot function properly. If you have hypothyroidism, you may experience fatigue, weight gain, increased sensitivity to cold, difficulty concentrating, dry skin, nails, and hair, constipation, drowsiness, muscle soreness, increased menstrual flow.

4.2　Causes of Hashimoto's Thyroiditis

Hashimoto's thyroiditis, or inflammation of the thyroid gland, is an autoimmune disorder. That means it is caused by a malfunction in your immune system. Instead of protecting your thyroid tissue, your immune cells attack it. These immune cells can cause hypothyroidism (underactive thyroid), a goiter(enlarged thyroid), or both. Eventually, the thyroiditis process can even destroy your entire thyroid, if left undetected or untreated.

In Hashimoto's thyroiditis, large amounts of damaged immune cells invade the thyroid. These immune cells are called lymphocytes; this is where Hashimoto's other name—chronic lymphocytic thyroiditis—is derived from.

When these lymphocytes enter the thyroid, they destroy the cells, tissue, and blood vessels within the gland. The process of destroying the thyroid gland is a slow one, which is why many people who have Hashimoto's thyroiditis go many years without any noticeable symptoms. You can read more about this in our article about the symptoms of Hashimoto's thyroiditis.

Because the thyroid is essentially coming under attack from invading cells, it isn't able to produce as much thyroid hormone as it normally would. Eventually, this causes hypothyroidism. And in extreme cases, the immune cells can cause the thyroid to become enlarged and inflamed to the point that it produces a visible mass in the neck—a goiter.

Doctors aren't entirely sure why the immune system, which is supposed to defend the body from harmful viruses and bacteria, sometimes turns against the body's healthy tissues. But what scientists do understand is that there are some factors that may make you more susceptible to this disease, and you can read about them in are article about risk factors for Hashimoto's thyroiditis.

4.3　Risk Factors of Hashimoto's Thyroiditis

Hashimoto's thyroiditis is an autoimmune disorder, so the main risk factor for developing this thyroid disorder is having a pre-existing autoimmune condition.

Autoimmune disorders occur when the body's immune cells attack healthy tissue instead of protecting it. In the case of Hashimoto's thyroiditis, immune cells attack the thyroid gland causing it to become inflamed and impairing its ability to produce enough thyroid hormone. You can read more about this in our article about what causes Hashimoto's thyroiditis.

If you have an autoimmune disorder, your immune system is malfunctioning in some way. That's why you are at a higher risk of developing Hashimoto's thyroiditis than someone who does not have an autoimmune disorder.

Below are examples of common autoimmune disorders: Addison's disease, rheumatoid arthritis, type 1 diabetes.

If you have an autoimmune disorder, that is a risk factor for developing Hashimoto's thyroiditis. That's why you should get checked for Hashimoto's thyroiditis every once in a while (your doctor will determine exactly how often you should get tested). That way, you will have the best chance of getting the disease detected early on. To learn more about the exams and tests you may need, read our article about diagnosing Hashimoto's thyroiditis.

4.4   Hashimoto's Thyroiditis Diagnosis

In addition to conducting a physical examination and taking your unique symptoms into account, your doctor will use one or more laboratory tests to diagnose Hashimoto's thyroiditis. This article will cover the three most common diagnostic tests that detect this common thyroid disorder: the thyroid–stimulating hormone test, anti–thyroid antibodies tests, and the free T_4 hormone test.

4.4.1   Thyroid–stimulating hormone test

A thyroid–stimulating hormone (TSH) test is a blood test that is one of the go–to tests for diagnosing hypothyroidism. Remember, Hashimoto's thyroiditis is the most common cause of hypothyroidism.

TSH is not produced by your thyroid—it's produced by your pituitary gland in your brain. When the pituitary detects even the slightest decrease in thyroid hormone production, it releases a greater amount of TSH to encourage the thyroid gland to make more hormones.

The goal of the TSH test is to determine whether your TSH levels are within the normal range. If they are higher than they should be, this may indicate Hashimoto's thyroiditis (and, in turn, hyperthxroidism). Remember, higher TSH levels mean that your brain thinks the thyroid is not producing enough hormones and needs stimulation (the "S" in TSH) to make more. TSH ranges are unique to each patient, and your doctor will determine your healthy TSH range.

You can read more about the TSH test in our article about hypothyroidism diagnosis.

4.4.2   Anti–thyroid Antibodies Tests

Anti–thyroid antibodies (ATA) tests, such as the microsomal antibody test (also known as thyroid peroxidase antibody test) and the anti–thyroglobulin antibody test, are commonly used to detect the presence of Hashimoto's thyroiditis.

Hashimoto's thyroiditis is an autoimmune disorder, and these types of disorders are caused by immune system malfunction. In other words, instead of protecting the body's healthy tissues, malfunctioning immune cells actually attack them.

When immune cells attack your thyroid gland, which is the case with Hashimoto's thyroiditis, antibodies are produced. Anti-thyroid antibodies tests detect the presence of these antibodies and measure their levels. This test is commonly used to confirm or exclude Hashimoto's thyroiditis as the reason for hypothyroidism.

4.4.3　Free T$_4$ Test

Thyroxine, or T$_4$, is the active thyroid hormone in the blood, and your doctor may measure the level of free T$_4$ in your bloodstream to help confirm a Hashimoto's thyroiditis diagnosis. Free T$_4$ is the portion of total T$_4$ thyroid hormone that is available to your tissues.

Typically, in Hashimoto's thyroiditis, the pituitary gland in the brain will make more TSH(your blood test for TSH comes back high) because it thinks the thyroid is not making enough thyroid hormone(your T$_4$ blood test may be below normal or on the low end of normal).

If your TSH test comes back normal, but your symptoms resemble those of hypothyroidism, a free T$_4$ test may help reveal any thyroid hormone problems. Low levels of free T$_4$ indicate some deficiency in thyroid hormone production, even if your TSH levels are normal.

There are numerous tests available today that your doctor may use to help diagnose Hashimoto's thyroiditis. If you notice any of the symptoms of Hashimoto's thyroiditis—or if you have risk factors associated with this thyroid disorder—don't hesitate to discuss testing options with your doctor.

4.5　Hashimoto's Thyroiditis Complications

Hashimoto's thyroiditis is a disorder characterized by inflammation of the thyroid gland. This condition can cause certain complications, including putting you at a higher risk for developing other autoimmune disorders and, to a lesser extent, thyroid lymphoma, a specific type of thyroid cancer.

4.5.1　Hashimoto's thyroiditis and other autoimmune disorders

Autoimmune disorders are caused by a malfunction in your immune system.

Hashimoto's thyroiditis is an autoimmune disorder, which is why the primary complication associated with Hashimoto's thyroiditis is that it increases your risk of developing other autoimmune disorders.

Hashimoto's thyroiditis increases your risk of developing a number of autoimmune disorders. Some examples include Addison's disease, Graves' disease, premature ovarian failure, type 1 diabetes, lupus erythematosus (a disorder that causes inflammation in a number of the body's systems, including the lungs and heart), pernicious anemia (a disorder that prevents the absorption of vitamin B$_{12}$), rheumatoid arthritis, thrombocytopenic purpura (a disorder that interferes with the blood's ability to clot), vitiligo (a disorder that produces white patches on the skin due to attacks on skin pigment cells).

4.5.2　Hashimoto's thyroiditis and thyroid lymphoma

It's a very rare complication, but Hashimoto's thyroiditis may increase your risk of developing a specific kind of thyroid cancer known as thyroid lymphoma. Thyroid lymphoma is highly treatable and curable when it's detected early on. That's why it's so important to pay attention to any thyroid nodules(or thyroid lumps) and get them examined by your doctor as soonas possible.

Because Hashimoto's thyroiditis can increase your risk for certain autoimmune disorders, you should talk to your doctor about what steps you should take to effectively manage these risks. Your doctor may recommend periodic tests to ensure that any associated complication is detected—and treated—as early as possible.

4.6   Preventing Hashimoto's Thyroiditis

Unfortunately, there is no known way to prevent Hashimoto's thyroiditis (or inflammation of the thyroid gland. But on the bright side, this disorder is very treatable. The sooner you get diagnosed, the sooner you can start receiving treatment.

Hashimoto's thyroiditis is an autoimmune disorder. In other words, it's caused by a malfunction of the immune system. It's still not fully understood why the immune system attacks the body's healthy tissues instead of protecting them, so preventing that mechanism isn't currently possible.

Since you can't prevent this disorder, it's that much more important to recognize the symptoms of Hashimoto's thyroiditis. If you understand the symptoms and visit your doctor as soon as possible after recognizing them, you'll have the best chance of preventing the disease's progression.

Like any disease, diagnosing Hashimoto's thyroiditis early is important because it gives you earlier access to treatment. Some of the most common symptoms of Hashimoto's thyroiditis— hypothyroidism and goiter—are highly responsive to treatment. You can read more about this in our article about thyroid hormone replacement therapy for Hashimoto's thyroiditis.

Though prevention isn't possible when it comes to Hashimoto's thyroiditis, keep in mind that this thyroid disorder is very treatable. If you are concerned about the presence of any possible symptoms, don't hesitate to discuss them with your doctor.

4.7   Hashimoto's Thyroiditis Facts and Tips

Hashimoto's thyroiditis affects 14 million people in the United States alone, making it not only the most common form of thyroiditis but also the most common thyroid disorder in America.

Hashimoto's thyroiditis is an autoimmune disorder. These types of disorders are caused by a malfunction in your immune system. Doctors aren't sure what causes autoimmune disorders to occur.

The main risk factor for developing Hashimoto's thyroiditis is having a pre-existing autoimmune condition, such as type 1 diabetes.

(1) Women are 7 times more likely to have Hashimoto's thyroiditis than men.

(2) Hypothyroidism and goiters are common symptoms associated with Hashimoto's thyroiditis.

(3) If you have Hashimoto's thyroiditis, you are at a higher risk of developing other autoimmune disorders and, to a lesser extent, a specific form of thyroid cancer.

(4) You can not prevent Hashimoto's thyroiditis. You can, however, prevent the progression of the disease by recognizing the symptoms of Hashimoto's thyroiditis early.

(5) Thyroid hormone replacement therapy is the only treatment available for Hashimoto's thyroiditis. Fortunately, it's highly effective at managing the condition.

Chapter 5

Tumor of Thyroid

5.1　Introduction

Thyroid cancer is the most common endocrine malignancy. In recent years, the incidence of thyroid cancer has increased significantly, which seriously threatens people's health. This chapter mainly introduces the etiology, diagnosis, case classification, treatment and prognosis of thyroid cancer, as well as the latest development of thyroid cancer diagnosis and treatment.

The increased detection of thyroid nodules of thyroid carcinoma in recent years has been attributed to the widespread use of high – resolution thyroid ultrasound (US) and fine – needle aspiration cytology (FNAC) under US guidance. Papillary throid cancer(PTC) is the most common histological type of differentiated thyroid cancer, and is characterized by early spread to regional lymphnodes and extracapsular invasion. However, PTC has a highly favourable prognosis, with a low incidence of distant metastasis and mortality. Other pathological types include follicular carcinoma, medullary carcinoma and undifferentiated carcinoma. The proportion was decreased, and the prognosis gradually decreased.

5.2　Epidemiology

The incidence rate of thyroid cancer rose rapidly in recent decades. However, the incidence rate of thyroid cancer also appears to have begun to stabilize in recent years, since changes in clinical practice guidelines were initiated in 2009. Papillary thyroid cancer accounts for 80% –90% of all thyroid malignancies, making it the most common type of thyroid malignancy.

5.3 Etiology

5.3.1 Gender and race-related risks

(1)Females are affected 2-3 times more often than males.

(2)People who are white or Asian are more likely to develop thyroid cancer.

5.3.2 Age and family-related risks

(1)Most cases of thyroid cancer affect people between the ages of 20 and 55.

(2)Multiple endocrine neoplasia, or multiple endocrine tumors (MEN2A and MEN2B)are tumors that affect glands of the endocrine system (e. g. ,thyroid,parathyroid,adrenal). MEN 2 tumors affecting the thyroid are medullary thyroid cancer. In rare cases,people have a family history of medullary thyroid cancer.

(3)According to the American Society of Clinical Oncology,anaplastic thyroid cancer is usually diagnosed adults older than 60.

(4)Although rare,medullary thyroid cancer may develop in infants 10 months and older and during adolescence if the child carries the RET proto-oncogene mutation.

5.3.3 DNA (deoxyribonucleic acid)makes up each person's biological blueprint

Genes are parts of the DNA that are inherited. An oncogene is a gene that has mutated and has the potential to cause cancer. Proto-oncogenes are genes that have mutated and can cause a cancer at the cellular level. There are different types of proto-oncogenes,such as RET.

5.3.4 Radiation exposure

Routine X-rays such as those performed during a dental examination or mammography do not cause thyroid cancer. The sources of radiation that may increase the risk for thyroid cancer include the following:

(1)Before 1950,low to moderate doses of X-ray therapy were used to treat adolescents with tonsillitis or acne.

(2)Radioactive fallout (e. g. ,Chernobyl)from atomic and nuclear disasters.

(3)Radiation therapy performed to treat Hodgkin lymphoma,such as the lymph nodes in the neck.

(4)If you have a family member with thyroid disease,even if non-cancerous,you should share that information with your doctor. Your doctor may run certain tests to evaluate your thyroid function and risk for developing thyroid cancer.

5.4 Pathological Classification

Cancers arise from cells that have undergone a change (malignant transformation)and begin to abnormally divide and multiply. Tumor growth may be slow or progress rapidly and invade or spread (metastasize)into other tissues. There are four types of thyroid cancer based on their cell of origin and their appearance and/or characteristics.

Thyroid cancer is generally first suspected by a lump or nodule in the thyroid gland. To make an accurate diagnosis of thyroid cancer, the thyroid cells will need to be closely examined. Since a cancer cell usually looks different than a normal cell, the type of thyroid cancer is determined by microscopic examination of the thyroid cells found in the nodule (neck lump) or growth. If surgery is recommended, the nodule(s) and/or mass is removed and examined by a pathologist to establish the diagnosis.

5.4.1　Papillary thyroid cancer

(1) Also termed papillary thyroid carcinoma.

(2) Is a differentiated thyroid cancer meaning the cells may resemble normal thyroid tissue.

(3) Most common type of thyroid cancer;70%–80% of all thyroid cancers are papillary thyroid cancer.

(4) Commonly diagnosed between the ages of 30 and 60, although it can occur at any age.

(5) Females are affected 3 times more often than males.

(6) Often more aggressive in elderly patients.

(7) May spread, but usually not beyond the neck.

(8) Papillary cells resemble finger-like projections.

(9) Tumor development can be related to radiation exposure, such as radiation treatments for acne or adenoid problems as a child.

5.4.2　Follicular thyroid cancer

(1) Also termed follicular thyroid carcinoma (FTC).

(2) Hürthle cell is a variant of FTC.

(3) It is a differentiated thyroid cancer meaning the cells may resemble normal thyroid tissue.

(4) Makes up 10%–15% of all thyroid cancers.

(5) More common in adults between the ages of 40 and 60.

(6) Females are affected 3 times more often than males.

(7) Cancer cells may invade blood vessels and travel to other body parts such as bone or lung tissues.

(8) Follicular cells are sphere-shaped.

(9) May be more aggressive in older patients.

5.4.3　Medullary thyroid cancer(MTC)

(1) Makes up 5%–10% of all thyroid cancers.

(2) More likely to run in families (familial medullary thyroid cancer, FMTC).

(3) Develops from the C Cells or parafolicullar cells that produce calcitonin (regulates calcium and phosphate blood levels and promotes bone growth).

(4) An elevated calcitonin level can indicate cancer.

(5) Often diagnosed between the ages of 40 and 50.

(6) Females and males are equally affected.

(7) Forms of medullary thyroid cancer include sporadic (not inherited), MEN 2A and MEN 2B (multiple endocrine neoplasia, genetic syndromes that involve other parts of the endocrine system), and familial (genetic, but not linked to other MEN-related endocrine tumors).

5.4.4　Anaplastic thyroid cancer

(1) This is an undifferentiated thyroid cancer meaning, under microscopic examination, the cancer cells

do not look like normal thyroid cells.

(2) Very rare—affects fewer than 2% of thyroid cancer patients.

(3) Usually occurs in patients older than 65 years.

(4) Females are slightly affected more often than males.

(5) Aggressive and invasive.

(6) Least responsive to treatment.

(7) Anaplastic (anaplasia) means the cells lose normal structure and organization.

5.5　Diagnosis

In order to accurately diagnose and treat thyroid cancer, we thoroughly reviews the patients' complete medical history, which may include information about family members who may have had a thyroid cancer, benign tumor, or multiple endocrine neoplasia.

During the physical exam, we palpates the patients' neck, which may require the patient to swallow and flex and bend your neck. We pay particular attention to the thyroid gland and surrounding tissues, such as the lymph nodes. The number, size, shape, and firmness of the nodule(s) are carefully examined. We correlates the physical findings with your medical history and reported symptoms, such as pain or hoarseness.

5.5.1　Family history as part of thyroid cancer diagnosis

If you have a family history of medullary thyroid cancer, the doctor will test your blood calcitonin and calcium levels. Calcitonin is a hormone important to calcium and phosphorus metabolism and bone growth. An elevated calcitonin level can indicate cancer.

5.5.2　Laboratory tests to diagnose thyroid cancer

Blood is drawn to test your thyroid gland function. Results from a thyroid-stimulating hormone test either confirms or rules out hypothyroidism (too low) or hyperthyroidism (too high) levels. If your thyroid gland does not function normally, a T_3 or Free T_3 and T_4 test is run to determine your thyroid hormone activity levels. It is important to remember that thyroid function tests are not indicators of thyroid cancer and most people with thyroid cancer have normal thyroid function.

5.5.3　Thyroid scan

A thyroid scan, or nuclear medicine scan, tests the gland's function. After a radioactive tracer is injected, a special camera captures images of the thyroid gland and measures the amount of dye the gland (nodules) absorbs.

Normal and abnormal test results are reported as functioning (normal), cold (underactive), or hot (overactive). Suspicious cold nodules can be further evaluated by a procedure called fine needle aspiration (needle biopsy). Hot nodules do not generally require biopsy.

5.5.4　Ultrasound guided biopsy fine needle aspiration

Fine needle aspiration (FNA) is one way of diagnosing thyroid cancer. A local anesthetic may be injected into/around the neck area. Using ultrasound to guide needle placement, your doctor takes several samples of the nodule or tumor. The samples are sent to pathology for microscopic evaluation.

Some fine needle aspiration biopsy results are indeterminate. This means it is not exactly known if the nodule or tumor is benign (noncancerous) or malignant (cancer). To help patients avoid unnecessary thyroid surgery, new molecular testing (gene expression classification) may be performed to help confirm an accurate diagnosis. Undergoing FNA can be a distressing time for patients.

5.5.5 Imaging studies

Results from imaging studies may assist your doctor in confirming your thyroid cancer diagnosis. Different types of imaging studies include X-ray, computed tomography scan, magnetic resonance imaging, and positron emission tomography (PET scan).

5.5.6 Laryngoscopy

Depending on your tumor's characteristics, and the close proximity of your thyroid gland to your voice box (larynx), your doctor may recommend laryngoscopy. A laryngoscope is a lighted and flexible tube with magnification used to examine your larynx.

5.5.7 Drawing conclusions

After your doctor has evaluated each piece of information about your health, including test results, he makes his diagnosis and outlines a treatment plan for your thyroid cancer.

5.6 Thyroid Tumor Staging

After thyroid cancer is diagnosed, it is staged. Staging is a tool your doctor uses to classify characteristics about your malignant thyroid tumor. Staging the tumor helps your doctor determine the best treatment for your thyroid cancer. The staging system was developed by the American Joint Committee on Cancer (AJCC) and is called the TNM System. The letter T stands for tumor, N for nodes and M means metastasis.

One or more of the following may help stage your thyroid cancer:

(1) Ultrasound examination.

(2) Pathology: biopsy obtained before or during surgery.

(3) Imaging: CT scan and/or MRI.

(4) Nuclear imaging: Full body scan may be performed using CT scan or PET scan and involves an intravenous injection of a radioactive substance. Thyroid cancer cells "take up" the radioactive tracer and can show if and where cancer has spread in other parts of your body.

TNM system basics:

T = size of the main tumor (there may be more than one tumor)

N = degree of spread to the local lymph nodes

M = indicates if the tumor has spread (metastasized) beyond the neck (e. g. , lungs)

"T" thyroid cancer categories:

TX = Tumor can not be evaluated

T0 = There is no primary tumor

T1 = Tumor size is 2 cm wide or smaller

T2 = Tumor size is 2-4 cm wide

T3 = Tumor size is greater than 4 cm or has started to grow outside the thyroid

T4a = The tumor (any size) has grown extensively beyond the thyroid gland into local neck tissues

T4b = Tumor has grown back toward the spine or into local large blood vessels

"N" thyroid cancer categories:

NX = Local lymph nodes cannot be evaluated

N0 = No spread to local lymph nodes

N1 = Tumor has spread to local lymph nodes

N1a = Tumor has spread to lymph nodes around the thyroid

N1b = Tumor has spread to lymph nodes in the sides of the neck or upper chest

"M" thyroid cancer categories

MX = Distant metastasis (i. e. , spread) can not be evaluated

M0 = No distant metastasis

M1 = Distant metastasis involves distant lymph nodes, internal organs, etcetera

5.7   Treatment

Different types of treatment are available for patients with thyroid cancer.

5.7.1   Surgery

Surgery is the most common treatment for thyroid cancer. One of the following procedures may be used:

Lobectomy: Removal of the lobe in which thyroid cancer is found. Lymph nodes near the cancer may also be removed and checked under a microscope for signs of cancer.

Near-total thyroidectomy: Removal of all but a very small part of the thyroid. Lymph nodes near the cancer may also be removed and checked under a microscope for signs of cancer.

Total thyroidectomy: Removal of the whole thyroid. Lymph nodes near the cancer may also be removed and checked under a microscope for signs of cancer.

Tracheostomy: Surgery to create an opening (stoma) into the windpipe to help you breathe. The opening itself may also be called a tracheostomy.

5.7.2   Radiation therapy, including radioactive iodine therapy

Radiation therapy is a cancer treatment that uses high-energy X-rays or other types of radiation to kill cancer cells or keep them from growing. There are two types of radiation therapy:

External radiation therapy uses a machine outside the body to send radiation toward the cancer. Sometimes the radiation is aimed directly at the tumor during surgery. This is called intraoperative radiation therapy.

Internal radiation therapy uses a radioactive substance sealed in needles, seeds, wires, or catheters that are placed directly into or near the cancer.

Radiation therapy may be given after surgery to kill any thyroid cancer cells that were not removed. Follicular and papillary thyroid cancers are sometimes treated with radioactive iodine (RAI) therapy. RAI is taken by mouth and collects in any remaining thyroid tissue, including thyroid cancer cells that have spread to other places in the body. Since only thyroid tissue takes up iodine, the RAI destroys thyroid tissue and thyroid cancer cells without harming other tissue. Before a full treatment dose of RAI is given, a small test-dose is given to see if the tumor takes up the iodine.

The way the radiation therapy is given depends on the type and stage of the cancer being treated. External radiation therapy and RAI therapy are used to treat thyroid cancer.

5.7.3　Thyroid hormone therapy

Hormone therapy is a cancer treatment that removes hormones or blocks their action and stops cancer cells from growing. Hormones are substances made by glands in the body and circulated in the bloodstream. In the treatment of thyroid cancer, drugs may be given to prevent the body from making TSH, a hormone that can increase the chance that thyroid cancer will grow or recur.

5.7.4　Targeted therapy

Tyrosine kinase inhibitor therapy is a type of targeted therapy that blocks signals needed for tumors to grow. Vandetanib and sorafenib are tyrosine kinase inhibitors that are used to treat certain types of thyroid cancer. New types of tyrosine kinase inhibitors are being studied to treat advanced thyroid cancer.

5.8　Thyroid Cancer Follow-up Care

After initial treatment for thyroid cancer, it is essential that the patients periodically follow-up to monitor the effectiveness of the medicine by checking TSH level.

Chapter 6

The Diagnosis and Treatment of Thyroid Nodules

Thyroid nodules are quite common diseases in endocrinology system. Presently, no known environmental factors have been identified to explain this increase in prevalence. Though often asymptomatic, thyroid nodules require evaluation primarily because of their risk of thyroid carcinoma and its potential dangers. Its clinical importance, is out of all proportion to its incidence, because cancers of the thyroid must be differentiated from the much more frequent benign adenomas and multinodular goiters. In the past 10 years, the incidence of thyroid cancer in the world is increasing rapidly year by year. It is increasing by 6% per year. The incidence of thyroid cancer in China has increased by nearly 5 times in 10 years. Therefore, how to correctly evaluate and handle thyroid nodules have important practical significance.

6.1 Diagnosis

6.1.1 History of nodules

Thyroid nodules grow slowly and may remain dormant for years. Factors that must be considered in reaching a decision for management include the history of the lesion, age, sex, and family history of the patient, physical characteristics of the gland, local symptoms, and laboratory evaluation. One clue to their origin is that they are 4 times more frequent in women than in men, but Male gender is believed to increase the risk a thyroid nodule>1 cm will prove cancerous. Nodules are less frequent in men, and a greater proportion are malignant. the family history may be helpful in the decision regarding surgery. Several features significantly increase the risk that a nodule >1 cm is cancerous. Perhaps most notable, thyroid exposure to ionizing radiation during childhood imparts significant risk.

An adenoma may first come to attention because the patient accidentally finds a lump in the neck or because a physician discovers it upon routine examination. Rarely, symptoms such as dysphagia, dysphonia, or stridor may develop, but it is unusual for these tumors to attain sufficient size to cause significant symptoms in the neck. Occasionally there is bleeding into the tumor, causing a sudden increase in size and local pain and tenderness.

6.1.2 Physical findings

The history of the neck lump itself is important. Recent onset, growth, hoarseness, pain, nodes in the supraclavicular fossae, symptoms of brachial plexus irritation, and local tenderness all suggest malignancy, but of course do not prove it. The usual cause of sudden swelling and tenderness in a nodule is hemorrhage into a benign lesion. Although the presence of a nodule for many years suggests a benign process, some cancers grow slowly.

6.1.3　Ultrasound examination

Ultrasound is part of the routine assessment of any patient with a suspected thyroid nodule. As part of the evaluation for any nodule suspected on physical examination, a thyroid ultrasound is required. Thyroid ultrasound allows for optimal radiologic visualization of the thyroid and associated nodules. For years, ultrasound has been the primary imaging tool for the thyroid nodules. It is cost effective, rapid in information accrual, and avoids radiation exposure. The principal goals and indications of thyroid ultrasonography: Assess thyroid nodularity and disease; Identify characteristics associated with malignancy; Monitor nodules, goiters, or lymph nodes in patients undergoing treatment or observation of thyroid disease. Ultrasound features associated with malignancy: Blurred or ill-defined margins; Absent or avascular halo; aspect ratio>1.

6.1.4　Fine needle nspiration

Thyroid nodules are typically discovered either by palpation or through an imaging study. A palpable thyroid nodule should undergo further evaluation to determine if an FNA is warranted. The aspiration is performed with thin needles (gauge ranging from 27 G to 20 G). the operator holds the sonographic probe with one hand and performs the aspiration with the other, typically with a syringe-holding pistol. Local anesthesia is not required in general. An FNA may also be carried out by simply moving the needle, without any connection to a suction device. In this technique, termed the cytopuncture technique, the cytologic material is extruded from the lesion by capillary action. The risk of complications is low even when the number of FNA passes. Once the needle is withdrawn from the lesion, the material is extruded onto glass slides and the smear is fixed with 95% ethyl alcohol for Papanicolaou staining. Or we can use Liquid-based cytology (LBC) techniques.

The core-needle biopsy (CNB) procedure involves the use of large-gauge needles (14-19 G). The advantages of this technique in combination with FNA include an increased amount of tissue, which may decrease the number of nondiagnostic samples and provides material for application of ancillary studies. The disadvantages of CNB include the increased possibility of complications, such as hemorrhage and local pain, and the difficulty in performing multiple samplings of the lesion.

In experienced hands, the diagnostic accuracy of thyroid FNA for technically satisfactory specimens is greater than 95%, with positive predictive values of 89% -98% and negative predictive values of 94% -99%.

6.1.5　Thyroid function tests

Serum thyrotropin (TSH) should also be assessed. A minority of patients will have a suppressed TSH below the reference range. If detected, this may suggest the possibility of afunctional (ortoxic) adenoma. The serum TG concentration may be elevated, as in all other goitrous conditions, and therefore is not a valuable tool in differential diagnosis. Calcitonin assay is indicated in the presence of a suggestive family history or of coincident features of the MEN-Ⅱ syndromes. Increasing concentrations of serum TSH appear to predict thyroid cancer risk in patients with thyroid nodules. Although MTC constitutes a small fraction of thyroid malignancies, and an even smaller proportion of thyroid nodules, several reports suggest that routine screening of nodular goiters by calcitonin assay is an appropriate approach.

6.1.6 Isotope scans

The scintiscan received much attention in the past as an aid in the differential diagnosis of thyroid lesions. The scan can provide evidence for a diagnosis in a multinodular goiter, in Hashimoto's thyroiditis, and rarely in thyroid cancer when functioning cervical metastases are seen. If the scan demonstrates a hyperfunctioning nodule suppressing the remainder of the gland, and the patient is thyrotoxic as demonstrated by an elevated serum FT_4 or FT_3 level, or suppressed sTSH, the chance of malignancy is very low. Tumors that accumulate RAI in a concentration equal to or greater than that of the surrounding normal thyroid tissue, but that do not produce thyrotoxicosis, are also typically benign Absence of ^{131}I (or ^{123}I) uptake is common and signals a nonfunctional, or "cold" nodule. This does not modify cancer risk. In contrast, radionuclide uptake into the discrete nodule signals autonomous functionality, or a "hot" nodule. When occurring, a toxic adenoma is confirmed, and the risk of malignancy is dramatically reduced. Though not indicated in the routine evaluation of euthyroid patients with nodularity, this radionuclide assessment can significantly modify cancer risk when performed in a hyperthyroid patient.

6.1.7 CT and MRI examination

Contrast enhanced CT or MRI imaging is commonly used in the head and neck in the evaluation of nodal metastases. They are not operator dependent, is done in a highly repeatable fashion.

CT is performed with 1.5 mm axial cuts. CT images are familiar to surgeons and can give detailed anatomic information. Additionally, CT is used as the test of choice for the evaluation of laryngeal or tracheal cartilage invasion in thyroid cancer. CT performs better than MRI in the determination of positive lymph nodes and has even been shown to have a higher sensitivity than PET-CT. MRI examination of multiple imaging and scanning range, higher resolution of soft tissue characteristics, can provide high quality images, can effectively display tumor to surrounding tissue invasion and lymph node metastasis. The characteristics of thyroid malignant tumor in MRI for T_1 weighted signal and normal thyroid tissue similar to or slightly lower, T_2 weighted images showed high signal, and follicular carcinoma on T_1 weighted and T_2 weighted images showed high signal. The tumor shape is irregular, inhomogeneous signal intensity and tumor envelope like low signal intensity is characteristic of MRI image for thyroid cancer.

6.1.8 Molecular diagnosis

Molecular diagnosis in clinical fields, such as lymphoma, lung cancer, breast cancer and gastrointestinal cancer, can assist the clinical diagnosis and prognosis evaluation, realize the individualized treatment and targeted therapy. This genes have been found in the cancer such as RET gene, ras gene, Bcl-2 gene, PAX8-PPAR γ1 fusion gene, BRAF gene, Trk gene; tumor suppressor gene such as p53 gene, PTEN gene, Rb gene. These genes play important roles in the pathogenesis of thyroid cancer, and they are closely related to the type and degree of tumor differentiation.

6.2 Treatment

All thyroid nodules should be treated once they are found complete diagnostic assessment, regardless of the presenting manifestation or size. This allows the selection of patients with nodules that are malignant or suspicious of malignancy and therefore eligible for surgery. In addition, surgical treatment may be needed for some benign nodules, either single or associated with multinodular goiter, when they are large or associated with signs and symptoms of compression, discomfort, or for cosmetic concerns. All other nodules can be followed without treatment. Many patients choose a more conservative approach, especially if older or suffering from other concurrent illness. Indeed, it may be reasonable to acknowledge that a low-risk thyroid carcinoma confined to the gland itself may pose less risk than the operative procedure itself, and with much less morbidity.

Thyroid surgical indications: ①Thyroid malignant tumor; ②Benign thyroid nodules compression of the trachea and esophagus, recurrent laryngeal nerve; ③Substernal goiter; ④Department of nuclear medicine, treatment of invalid or hyperthyroidism are taboo.

The extent of surgery of benign thyroid nodules: ①Bilateral lobectomy and multiple benign thyroid nodules, feasible or near total laryngectomy; ②Single, resection of benign thyroid nodules feasible lobe of thyroid function; ③Secondary hyperthyroidism, with total thyroidectomy or near total thyroidectomy. The main.

The scope of operation of differentiated thyroid carcinoma: 1 for low risk papillary thyroid carcinoma, can choose unilateral lobe with isthmus resection. The tumor diameter greater than 2 cm, the thyroid gland invasion, lateral neck or contralateral lymph node metastasis, there should be on the side of thyroid nodules underwent total thyroidectomy.

At least the ipsilateral central lymph node dissection, feasible therapeutic side cleaning lymph node of neck. Medullary thyroid carcinoma underwent total thyroidectomy for bilateral central clearing, and even to consider prophylactic lateral neck dissection in patients with central lymph nodes more.

Chapter 7

Primary Hyperparathyroidism

7.1 Definition

Primary hyperparathyroidism is usually caused by a tumor within the parathyroid gland. The symptoms of the condition relate to the elevated calcium levels, which can cause digestive symptoms, kidney stones, psychiatric abnormalities, and bone disease. Hyperparathyroidism, characterized by excess production of PTH, is a common cause of hypercalcemia and is usually the result of autonomously functioning adenomas or hyperplasia.

7.2 Located

The thyroid gland is located in the neck, anterior to the trachea, between the cricoid cartilage and the suprasternal notch. The thyroid (Greekthyreos, shield, plus eidos, form) consists of two lobes that are connected by an isthmus. It is normally 12 to 20 g in weight, highly vascular, and soft in consistency. Four parathyroid glands, which produce parathyroid hormone, are located in the posterior region of each pole of the thyroid. The recurrent laryngeal nerves traverse the lateral borders of the thyroid gland and must be identified during thyroid surgery to avoid vocal cord paralysis. Parathyroid glands (we all have four of them) are normally the size of a grain of rice. Occasionally they can be as large as a pea and still be normal. The four parathyroids are located behind the thyroid and are shown in this picture as the mustard yellow glands behind the pink thyroid gland. Normal parathyroid glands are the color of spicy yellow mustard(Figure 17-7-1).

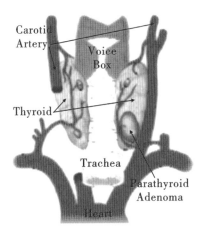

Figure 17-7-1   Schematic diagram of the location of the parathyroid glands(Dorsal view)

7.3   The Role of the Parathyroid Glands

The only purpose of the parathyroid glands is to regulate the calcium level in our bodies within a very narrow range so that the nervous and muscular systems can function properly. This is all they do. They measure the amount of calcium in the blood every minute of every day and if the calcium levels go down a little bit, the parathyroid glands recognize it and make parathyroid hormone (PTH) which goes to the bones and takes some calcium out (makes a withdrawal from the calcium vault) and puts it into the blood. When the calcium in the blood is high enough, then the parathyroids shut down and stop making PTH.

The single major disease of parathyroid glands is over-activity of one or more of the parathyroids which make too much parathyroid hormone causing a potentially serious calcium imbalance (too high calcium in the blood). This is called hyperparathyroidism and this is the disease that this entire web site is about.

7.4   Natural History and Incidence

Primary hyperparathyroidism is a generalized disorder of calcium, phosphate, and bone metabolism due to an increased secretion of PTH. The elevation of circulating hormone usually leads to hypercalcemia and hypophosphatemia. There is great variation in the manifestations. Patients may present with multiple signs and symptoms, including recurrent nephrolithiasis, peptic ulcers, mental changes, and, less frequently, extensive bone resorption. However, with greater awareness of the disease and wider use of multiphasic screening tests, including measurements of blood calcium, the diagnosis is frequently made in patients who have no symptoms and minimal, if any, signs of the disease other than hypercalcemia and elevated levels of PTH. The manifestations may be subtle, and the disease may have a benign course for many years or a lifetime. This milder form of the disease is usually termed asymptomatic hyperparathyroidism. Rarely, hyperparathyroidism develops or worsens abruptly and causes severe complications, such as marked dehydration and coma, so-called hypercalcemic parathyroid crisis. The annual incidence of the disease is calculated to be as high as 0.2% in patients>60 years old, with an estimated prevalence, including undiscovered asymptomatic patients, of ≥1%; some reports suggest the incidence may be declining, perhaps reflecting earlier overestimates. The disease has a peak incidence between the third and fifth decades but occurs in young children and in the elderly.

7.5   Etiology

7.5.1   Solitary adenomas

The cause of hyperparathyroidism is one or more hyperfunctioning glands. A single abnormal gland is the cause in>80% of patients; the abnormality in the gland is usually a benign neoplasm or adenoma and rarely a parathyroid carcinoma. Some surgeons and pathologists report that the enlargement of multiple glands is common; double adenomas are reported. In>15% of patients, all glands are hyperfunctioning; chief cell parathyroid hyperplasia is usually hereditary and frequently associated with other endocrine abnormalities.

7.5.2   Mul tiple endocrine neoplasia

Hereditary hyperparathyroidism can occur without other endocrine abnormalities but is usually part of a multiple endocrine neoplasia syndrome.

MEN 1 (Wermer's syndrome) consists of hyperparathyroidism and tumors of the pituitary and pancreas, often associated with gastric hypersecretion and peptic ulcer disease (Zollinger–Ellison syndrome). MEN 2A is characterized by pheochromocytoma and medullary carcinoma of the thyroid, as well as hyperparathyroidism; MEN 2B has additional associated features such as multiple neuromas but usually lacks hyperparathyroidism. Each of these MEN syndromes is transmitted in an apparent autosomal dominant manner, although, as noted below, the genetic basis does not always involve a dominant allele.

7.6   Pathology

Adenomas are most often located in the inferior parathyroid glands, but in 6%–10% of patients, parathyroid adenomas may be located in the thymus, the thyroid, the pericardium, or behind the esophagus. Adenomas are usually 0.5–5 g in weight but may be as heavy as 10–20 g (normal glands weigh 25 mg on average). Chief cells are predominant in both hyperplasia and adenoma. With chief cell hyperplasia, the enlargement may be so asymmetric that some involved glands appear grossly normal. If generalized hyperplasia is present, however, histologic examination reveals a uniform pattern of chief cells and disappearance of fat even in the absence of an increase in gland weight. Thus, microscopic examination of biopsy specimens of several glands is essential to interpret findings at surgery. Parathyroid carcinoma is usually not aggressive. Long–term survival without recurrence is common if at initial surgery the entire gland is removed without rupture of the capsule. Recurrent parathyroid carcinoma is usually slow–growing with local spread in the neck, and surgical correction of recurrent disease may be feasible. Occasionally, however, parathyroid carcinoma is more aggressive, with distant metastases (lung, liver, and bone) found at the time of initial operation. It may be difficult to appreciate initially that a primary tumor is carcinoma; increased numbers of mitotic figures and increased fibrosis of the gland stroma may precede invasion. The diagnosis of carcinoma is often made in retrospect. Hyperparathyroidism from a parathyroid carcinoma may be indistinguishable from other forms of primary hyperparathyroidism; a potential clue to the diagnosis, however, is provided by the degree of calcium elevation. Calcium values of 3.5–3.7 mmol/L (14–15 mg/dL) are frequent with carcinoma and may alert the surgeon to remove the abnormal gland with care to avoid capsular rupture.

7.7   Signs and Symptoms

Half or more of patients with hyperparathyroidism are asymptomatic. In series in which patients are followed without operation, as many as 80% are classified as without symptoms. Manifestations of hyperparathyroidism involve primarily the kidneys and the skeletal system. Kidney involvement, due either to deposition of calcium in the renal parenchyma or to recurrent nephrolithiasis, was present in 60%–70% of patients prior to 1970. With earlier detection, renal complications occur in <20% of patients in many large series. Renal stones are usually composed of either calcium oxalate or calcium phosphate. In occasional patients, repeated episodes of nephrolithiasis or the formation of large calculi may lead to urinary tract obstruction, infection, and loss of renal function. Nephrocalcinosis may also cause decreased renal function and phosphate retention.

The distinctive bone manifestation of hyperparathyroidism isosteitis fibrosa cystica, which occurred in 10%–25% of patients in series reported 50 years ago. Histologically, the pathognomonic features are an increase in the giant multinucleated osteoclasts in scalloped areas on the surface of the bone (Howship's lacunae) and a replacement of the normal cellular and marrow elements by fibrous tissue. X–ray changes include resorption of the phalangeal tufts and replacement of the usually sharp cortical outline of the bone in the digits by an irregular outline (subperiosteal resorption). In recent years, osteitis fibrosa cystica is very rare in primary hyperparathyroidism, probably due to the earlier detection of the disease.

With the use of multiple markers of bone turnover, such as formation indices (bone–specific alkaline phosphatase, osteocalcin, and type I procollagen peptides) and bone resorption indices (including hydroxypyridinium collagen cross–links and telopeptides of type I collagen), increased skeletal turnover is detected in essentially all patients with established hyperparathyroidism.

Computed tomography scan and dual–energy X–ray absorptiometry (DEXA) of the spine provide reproducible quantitative estimates (within a few percent) of spinal bone density. Similarly, bone density in the extremities can be quantified by densitometry of the hip or of the distal radius at a site chosen to be primarily cortical. Cortical bone density is reduced while cancellous bone density, especially in the spine, is relatively preserved. Serial studies in patients who choose to be followed without surgery have indicated that in the majority there is little further change over a number of years, consistent with laboratory data indicating relatively unchanged blood calcium and PTH levels. After an initial loss of bone mass in patients with mild asymptomatic hyperparathyroidism, a new equilibrium may be reached, with bone density and biochemical manifestations of the disease remaining relatively unchanged.

In symptomatic patients, dysfunctions of the CNS, peripheral nerve and muscle, gastrointestinal tract, and joints also occur. It has been reported that severe neuropsychiatric manifestations may be reversed by parathyroidectomy; it remains unclear, in the absence of controlled studies, whether this improvement has a defined cause–and–effect relationship. Generally, the fact that hyperparathyroidism is common in elderly patients, in whom there are often other problems, suggests the possibility that such coexisting problems as hypertension, renal deterioration, and depression may not be parathyroid–related and suggests caution inrecommending parathyroid surgery as a cure for these manifestations.

When present, neuromuscular manifestations may include proximal muscle weakness, easy fatigability, and atrophy of muscles and may be so striking as to suggest a primary neuromuscular disorder. The distinguishing feature is the complete regression of neuromuscular disease after surgical correction of the hyperparathyroidism.

Gastrointestinal manifestations are sometimes subtle and include vague abdominal complaints and disorders of the stomach and pancreas. Again, cause and effect are unclear. In MEN 1 patients with hyperparathyroidism, duodenal ulcer may be the result of associated pancreatic tumors that secrete excessive quantities of gastrin (Zollinger–Ellison syndrome). Pancreatitis has been reported in association with hyperparathyroidism, but the incidence and the mechanism are not established.

7.8 Diagnosis

The diagnosis is typically made by detecting an elevated immunoreactive PTH level in a patient with asymptomatic hypercalcemia (see "Differential Diagnosis: Special Tests," below). Serum phosphate is usually low but may be normal, especially if renal failure has developed.

Many tests based on renal responses to excess PTH (renal calcium and phosphate clearance; blood phosphate, chloride, magnesium; urinary or nephrogenous cyclic AMP) were used in earlier decades. These tests have low specificity for hyperparathyroidism and are therefore not cost–effective; they have been replaced by PTH immunoassays.

7.9 Treatment for Primary Hyperparathyroidism

7.9.1 Medical surveillance versus surgical treatment

The critical management question is whether the disease should be treated surgically. If severe hypercalcemia [3.7–4.5 mmol/L (15–18 mg/dL)] is present, surgery is mandatory as soon as the diagnosis can be confirmed by a PTH immunoassay. However, in most patients with hyperparathyroidism, hypercalcemia is mild and does not require urgent surgical or medical treatment.

The National Institutes of Health (NIH) held a consensus conference on management of asymptomatic hyperparathyroidism in 1990. Asymptomatic hyperparathyroidism was defined as documented (presumptive) hyperparathyroidism without signs or symptoms attributable to the disease. The consensus was that patients< 50 should undergo surgery, given the long surveillance that would be required. Other considerations that favored surgery included concern that consistent follow-up would be unlikely or that coexistent illness would complicate management. Patients >50 were deemed appropriate for medical monitoring if certain criteria were met, the patients wished to avoid surgery, or the guidelines for recommending surgery were not present. Careful evaluation of patients over the subsequent dozen years has both provided reassurance that in some patients medical monitoring rather than surgery is still prudent yet has promoted new questions about the natural history of the disease with or without surgery.

Data developed since the consensus conference indicated that a subgroup of patients had selective vertebral osteopenia out of proportion to bone loss at other sites and responded to surgery with striking restoration of bone mass (average>20%). In addition, as much as a 5% increase in bone mineral density in the spine and hip have been reported with alendronate use in asymptomatic hyperparathyroid patients. In light of this new information, the NIH convened a workshop on asymptomatic hyperparathyroidism in 2002, and an independent (non−NIH) panel offered a revised set of recommendations. The changes reflect both practical considerations (such as the difficulty in creatinine clearance measurements and therefore substituting calculations based on serum creatinine) and concerns regarding potential deleterious skeletal effects in untreated patients. Accordingly, indication for surgical intervention was lowered (i. e. , stricter serum calcium and bone density criteria). Asymptomatic patients should be monitored regularly. Surgical correction of hyperparathyroidism can always be undertaken when indicated, since the success rate is high (>90%), mortality is low, and morbidity is minimal. The goals of monitoring are early detection of worsening hypercalcemia, deteriorating bone or renal status, or other complications of hyperparathyroidism. No specific recommendations about medical therapy were made, but the promise of the newer agents was stressed, with the prediction that they would be used in clinical practice to increase bone mass in patients not electing surgery as further experience is gained. Neither panel recommended estrogen use in patients for whom surgery was not elected because there was insufficient cumulative experience with such therapy to balance theoretical risks (breast and endometrial cancer) versus benefits. Raloxifene (Evista) , the first of the SERMS, has been shown to have many of the bone−protective effects of estrogen in osteoporotic subjects yet at the same time lowers the incidence of breast cancer; preliminary use of this agent in a small series of hyperparathyroid patients led to increased bone density. Experience with calcimimetics, drugs that selectively stimulate the calcium sensor and suppress PTH secretion, indicates that these agents decrease calcium levels to normal and lower PTH levels by at least 50% for>1 year of continuous use.

7.9.2　Surgical treatment

7.9.2.1　Surgical removal

　　Surgical removal, or parathyroidectomy, is the only known cure for primary hyperparathyroidism and is currently the best treatment. In the hands of an experienced endocrine surgeon, success (cure) rates approach 95% −98%. Medications such as estrogen and bisphosphonates will not cure primary hyperparathyroidism but may decrease calcium or parathyroid hormone (PTH) levels and improve bone density. A new type of medication called calcimimetics (i. e. , Sensipar, Cinacalcet) may lower blood calcium levels and PTH levels, but they are not currently approved by the FDA for use in primary hyperparathyroidism and will not cure the disease. These medications have not been studied to determine whether or not they help decrease effects on other systems in the body or whether they improve the more subjective symptoms of primary hyperparathyroidism(depression, fatigue, muscle aches and pains, difficulty concentrating, memory problems, insomnia, constipation). The traditional technique for parathyroid surgery was bilateral neck exploration, in which the surgeon identifies all four of the parathyroid glands and determines which glands are diseased based on the size and appearance of the glands. This technique has been proven over time to be very safe and effective when performed by an experienced surgeon. However, since 80% −85% of patients with primary hyperparathyroidism have only one gland that is abnormal, many surgeons have shifted to doing a more limited and less invasive operation in patients thought to have a high likelihood of having a single abnormal gland. This more limited approach is often referred to as a focused parathyroidectomy. In a focused parathyroidectomy, the surgeon goes after and removes only the hyperactive gland that is identified on preoperative localizing tests. The term "minimally invasive parathyroid surgery" is often used to refer to focused parathyroidectomy, but really can be used for any parathyroid operation done through a very small incision. The length of the operation will vary depending on multiple factors including patient characteristics, whether a single gland is removed or if an exploration of both sides of the neck with removal of multiple glands is performed, and whether the operation is a first time surgery or a re-operation. Depending on the complexity of the surgery, the operation may last as little as 20 minutes or as long as several hours. There are many variations in how parathyroid surgery is performed based on surgeon preference. When deciding on a surgeon, it is important to remember that the type of technique used is far less important than the surgeon's personal experience and success rate. For example, whether the surgeon uses a radioguided technique or pre-operative imaging-based technique makes little difference when compared to the experience of the surgeon. Research has proven that the chance of being cured and of not having a complication after parathyroid surgery depends on the experience of the surgeon. In general, a surgeon should do more than 50 parathyroid operations a year to be considered an expert. Every surgeon has developed an approach based on their own experiences and resources that works well for them, so please discuss with your surgeon what approach they will use. Below is a description of some of the more commonly used techniques.

7.9.2.2　Bilateral Neck Exploration

Bilateral exploration was the traditional surgical approach to parathyroid surgery and may also be referred to as open parathyroidectomy, standard parathyroidectomy, four gland exploration, or conventional parathyroidectomy. This approach has proven over time to be highly successful with cure rates of 95% or greater when performed by an experienced surgeon. In order to be successful, the surgeon must identify all four parathyroid glands. In the past each parathyroid gland was biopsied to confirm that all glands were identified. However, due to the risk of injuring the blood supply to the parathyroid glands, biopsies of normal appearing glands is no longer recommended. Pre-operative localization and special intraoperative techniques (such as intraoperative parathyroid hormone, PTH-testing or radioguidance) are not required, but may be used to guide the surgeon. Traditionally a bilateral exploration was performed through a 5-7 inch incision. However, most surgeons are now able to do this operation through a much smaller 1.5-2 inch incision. The incision is usually located in the middle to lower portion of the neck and is curved to match the skin folds in your neck. The muscles are separated to expose the thyroid gland and the thyroid gland is retracted to expose the parathyroids. Temporary low calcium levels after surgery may occur in as many as 25% of patients. Low calcium levels after surgery can cause numbness and tingling in your lips, fingers, and toes. If this occurs it can usually be treated with calcium pills and the symptoms resolve within 15-30 minutes.

7.9.2.3　Focused parathyroidectomy

Focused exploration consists of "going after" a single abnormal gland and removing it. The surgeon will not plan on exploring the rest of the neck to find the other parathyroid glands. This technique may also be referred to as directed parathyroidectomy, minimally invasive parathyroidectomy or targeted parathyroidectomy. There are many different ways to perform a focused parathyroidectomy and these include image-guided, radioguided, and video-assisted techniques. Since the surgeon will not attempt to look at all four parathyroid glands in the operating room, it is crucial to perform pre-operative localizing tests. A patientmay be considered for focused parathyroidectomy if a pre-operative localization reveals a single abnormal gland (or two abnormal glands on the same side of the neck). Many surgeons will also use intraoperative PTH monitoring to confirm that there is no other hyperactive parathyroid tissue. Other adjuncts such as radio-guidance or video-assistance may also be used. Focused parathyroidectomy is typically performed through a smaller incision than the bilateral exploration, usually 1/2 or 1 1/4 inches long and can be performed through either a medial or lateral approach. For the medial approach the incision is typically 3/4 to 1 1/2 inches in size and is placed in the center of the neck. The muscles are separated along the midline and the thyroid is exposed and retracted medially. For the lateral approach, a 1/2 to 1 1/4 inch incision is made on the side of the neck over the muscle. The muscles are separated to expose the carotid artery and the edge of the thyroid gland. The thyroid is retracted medially and the carotid artery is retracted laterally to expose the space where the parathyroid glands lie. This approach works very well for glands that are located deep in the neck. In either method, once the abnormal gland is removed, many surgeons will use the intraoperative PTH test to confirm that all abnormal tissue has been removed. The cure rate of focused parathyroidectomy is 95% –98% and is the same as for bilateral neck exploration. There are several potential advantages of focused parathyroidectomy over a bilateral neck exploration including smaller incision size, improved cosmetic result, shorter operative time, creation of less scar tissue, and fewer problems with low calcium levels after surgery. The incidence of symptomatic low calcium levels has been shown to be reduced from 25% in a bilateral exploration to 7% or less with focused parathyroidectomy.

7.9.2.4   Radioguided parathyroidectomy

Radioguided parathyroidectomy is a type of focused parathyroidectomy and involves giving a small injection of Tc^{99m} sestamibi (the same agent used for the sestamibi scan, just a smaller dose) the morning of surgery. The surgeon then uses a handheld gamma probe (essentially a miniature Geiger counter) in the operating room to identify the hyperactive gland during surgery. The probe can also be used to help place the incision directly over the abnormal parathyroid gland as well as to lead the surgeon to it. The gamma probe is also used to confirm that the tissue that has been removed is indeed parathyroid tissue. The benefits of the intraoperative gamma probe have been debated. The greatest benefit appears to be in potentially reducing operative time when it is a reoperation, finding an ectopic parathyroid, and identifying the times the sestamibi scan incorrectly identifies a thyroid nodule as a parathyroid gland. The major downsides to using this technique include increased cost from the extra resources needed and additional radiation exposure. Although this technique can be useful, many surgeons feel that experience and a thorough knowledge of parathyroid anatomy make it unnecessary.

7.9.2.5   Video–assisted parathyroidectomy

Video–assisted parathyroidectomy is also known as minimally invasive video–assisted parathyroidectomy and endoscopic parathyroidectomy. Several techniques of video–assisted parathyroidectomy have been described using approaches from the middle of the neck or the side of the neck. The typical incision for this technique can be as small as 11/4 inches. The main benefit of the video–assisted technique is that it provides greater magnification and may allow the surgeon to do the operation through a smaller incision. The downsides to this procedure include a longer operating time, the need for additional equipment, and the fact that it can not reach certain areas of the neck. The safety and cure rate seem equal to other forms of focused parathyroidectomy.

7.9.2.6   Surgical options for four gland hyperplasia

Multiple abnormal parathyroid glands are found in 15% –20% of patients. Up to 10% of patients with primary hyperparathyroidism will have four hyperactive glands, a situation called four gland hyperplasia. If all four glands are abnormal then the treatment options are a subtotal parathyroidectomy (removal of 3 or 3 1/2 glands) or a total parathyroidectomy with autotransplantation (removal of all parathyroid tissue and placing a part of a parathyroid in the forearm or neck muscle). The autotransplanted parathyroid will grow a new blood supply and will typically start.

7.10   Secondary Hyperparathyroidism

In secondary hyperparathyroidism, a disease outside of the parathyroids causes all of the parathyroid glands to become enlarged and hyperactive. It is usually caused by kidney failure, a problem where the kidney is unable to clean the blood of phosphorus produced by the body and unable to make enough vitamin D (specifically calcitriol, the active form of vitamin D). The build-up of phosphorous leads to low levels of calcium in the blood, which in turn stimulates the parathyroid glands to increase PTH production which in turn causes them to grow. As the disease progresses, the parathyroid glands no longer respond normally to calcium and Vitamin D. During early secondary hyperparathyroidism, the blood calcium levels are normal or low, but the PTH level is high. As the disease gets worse, some of the treatments for the kidney disease (Vitamin D and calcium-containing phosphate binders) may eventually lead to abnormally high levels of calcium in the blood. High PTH levels can lead to weakening of the bones, calciphylaxis (when calcium forms clumps in the skin and leads to ulcers and potentially death of surrounding tissue), cardiovascular complications, abnormal fat and sugar metabolism, itching (pruritis), and low blood counts (anemia).

Chapter 8

Tuberculosis of Neck Lymph Nodes

Lymph node tuberculosis, occurring predominantly in the cervical region, is the most common manifestation of extrapulmonary tuberculosis. Tuberculous lymphadenitis is more common in females and younger age groups (highest among patients aged 30–40 years), which occurs when people with comprised immunity, in contrast to pulmonary tuberculosis, which is more common in males and in older age groups. However, tuberculous lymphadenitis can occur in adults and children at any time and at any age. Usually, mycobacterium tuberculosis invades through pave of tonsil and saprodontia. About 5% of CTBL is secondary to pulmonary and bronchial tuberculosis.

8.1 Clinical Manifestation

Cervical tuberculous lymphadenitis (CTBL) is the most common form of extrapulmonary tuberculosis, commonly is characterized by the multiple or single enlarged lymph nodes on one or both sides of the neck, which is/are typically located at the anterior or posterior edge of the sternocleidomastoid muscle. In the early stages of the disease, the affected lymph nodes are painless, harder and can be moved. When progressing, inflammation around the lymph nodes can occur enabling the involved lymph nodes to connect with the around tissue or skin. Furthermore, the affected lymph nodes can interconnect and form nodular masses that are not easily to be moved. In the late stages of the disease, lymph nodes undergo caseous necrosis and liquefaction forming the cold abscess that can lead to a long-lasting sinus or ulcer. Notably, different lymph nodes of the same patient can manifest as any features of different stage.

With respect to the systemic symptoms, a small number of patients can experience low fever, night sweats and inappetence.

8.2 Diagnose

CTBL is mainly diagnosed by analyzing tissue samples obtained by fine needle aspiration cytological analysis, and other techniques are available for diagnosing this disease, including analysis of tissue from excisional biopsy, isolation of mycobacteria in tissue cultures, molecular tests, and administration of the tuberculin skin test. Many authors have compared the utility of these techniques. Positivity for acid–fast bacilli (AFB) varies according to the technique used, with ranges of 0%–77.8% using Ziehl–Neelson (ZN) staining, 8%–80 % using tissue cultures, and 33.0%–94.6 % using polymerase chain reaction (PCR) analysis of tissues. Although the combination of FNA cytology, AFB smear, and culture may be sufficient to reach a reliable diagnosis of CTBL, culturing the bacilli remains the gold standard for diagnosis, and culturing may require 2–4 weeks to yield results. In contrast to culturing, PCR is a rapid and sensitive method that requires a small sample volume, and live bacilli are not required. In addition, although the sensitivity of PCR is the same as that of culturing, its specificity is 100%. However, the PCR technique can yield falsenegative results. Moreover, sometimes the possibility of tuberculosis is not suspected in the early stages of the diagnostic process.

According to the exposure history of mycobacterium tuberculosis, local signs especially the cold abscess, long–lasting sinus or ulcer, the diagnose of CTBL can be attained.

Differential diagnosis includes other infections, neoplasia, congenital conditions in the head and neck and rarely, drug reactions. Diagnosis should be made on the basis of histological evidence after lymph node biopsy. Diagnosis made on clinical grounds has poor specificity and will result in a great degree of over diagnosis.

8.3　Treatment

8.3.1　System treatment

Firstly, nutrition and rest are needed for patients. Secondly, patients should take isoniazid orally for 6–12 months. In addition, when patients with systemic symptoms or tuberculosis in other organs, ethambutol and rifampicin/amikacin should be added.

Most recent national and international treatment guidelines also recommend a 6 month therapy. The current meta–analysis supports these recommendations. Follow–up was at least 12 months after the end of treatment. In conclusion, it seems justified to administer medication for 6 months, including isoniazid, rifampicin and pyrazinamide, for tuberculous lymphadenitis.

8.3.2　Local treatment

(1) When lymph nodes are localized, enlargement and can be moved, surgical treatment can be considered and the protection of the accessory nerve should be noticed.

(2) When the cold abscess is not broken, puncture and suction treatment can be considered. The abscess puncturing via the normal skin are preferred. Suction and irrigation with 5% solution of isoniazid should be done thoroughly. Some mount of isoniazid can be left in the abscess cavity. This treatment needs to be done twice a week.

(3) When the sinus or ulcer without obvious secondary infection, curettage treatment can be considered. The wound should be drained and not sutured.

(4) When the sinus or ulcer obvious secondary infection, before the curettage treatment, section and drainage are needed in order to control the secondary infection.

Part 18

Disease of the Breast

Chapter 1

Anatomy and Physiology of the Breast

1.1　Anatomy of the Breast

1.1.1　Gross anatomy of the breast

Mammary gland secretion is a mammal characteristic. The breast extends laterally from the lateral edge of the sternum to the mid–axillary line and from the second rib superiorly to the sixth rib inferiorly. An axillary tail (of Spence)extends toward the axilla , or armpit. The human breast is plump and contains the mammary glands as well as an abundance of adipose tissue (the main determinant of size)and dense connective tissue. The mammary glands are located in the subcutaneous layer of the anterior and a portion of the lateral thoracic wall. Each breast contains 15 – 20 lobes (Figure 18 – 1 – 1)that each consist of many lobules. The nipples are located at the top of the breast where is a pigmented area. There is a horizontal fibrous septum and two vertical intervals that the course of the nerves and vessels to the nipple runs along. The horizontal fibrous septum originates at the pectoral fascia along the fifth rib , and the two vertical intervals contains the one along the sternum and the other at the lateral border of the pectoralis minor muscle. The breast is anterior to the deep pectoral fascia and is normally separated from it by the submammary space. The breast can mobility relative to the underlying musculature (the pectoralis major muscle , the serratus anterior muscle and the external oblique muscle)because of this space.

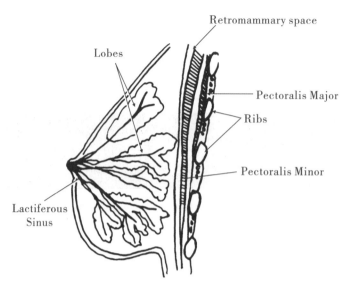

Figure 18-1-1 Sagittal section through the lactating breast

1.1.2 Nerve supply

The mammary gland is innervated by the somatic nerve. Innervation of the breast come from anterior and lateral cutaneous branches of intercostal nerves four through six, with the fourth nerve being the primary supply to the nipple. The lateral and anterior cutaneous branches of the second, third and sixth intercostal nerves, and the supraclavicular nerves (from C_3 and C_4), can also contribute to breast innervation. In many women, branches of the first and/or the seventh intercostal nerves also supply the breast. The areola and nipple are the most sensitive and are important for sexual arousal in many women because of the nipple's apical surface has abundant sensory nerve endings. In addition, the sympathetic fibers are distributed in the vascular, nipple, and the areola of the smooth muscle and mammary tissue with the lateral thoracic artery and the intercostal artery to the breast.

The sympathetic innervation does not cause a person's subjective sensation, but it controls the blood flow in the breast and the contraction of the smooth muscle under the skin. These nerves are mainly derived from the lateral anterior cutaneous branches of the second to seventh intercostal nerves, of which the branches of the fourth intercostal nerve are the most important. If this nerve is injured, the skin sensation of the nipple and the areola area will be diminished or disappearing. Nipple innervation is critical because the normal lactation needs the stimulation from infant suckling. Sympathetic fibers innervate the circular smooth muscle of the nipple (causing nipple erection), smooth muscle surrounding the lactiferous ducts and the arrector pili muscles.

1.1.3 Vascular supply

The arterial supply of the breasts mainly comes from the internal mammary artery and the axillary artery. The internal mammary artery is responsible for the internal blood supply of the breast, and the internal mammary veins are accompanied by the mammary artery, while the outside of the breast is supplied by the branches of the axillary artery (Figure 18-1-2).

The artery of the breast mainly comes from the lateral thoracic artery starts from the middle part of the axillary artery and goes along the lateral edge of the pectoralis major. In the female, the external mammary artery branch is supplied and the blood is supplied to the lateral side of the breast. The internal mammary artery, that is, the internal mammary artery, perforating through the second to fourth ribs, through the pectoralis major, and supply the blood to the inside of the breast. The lateral thoracic artery and the branch of the internal mammary artery and the corresponding intercostal artery have a rich anastomosis in the areola. The lateral thoracic artery is absent in a few patients. In a very few cases, the lateral thoracic artery is the only artery to supply blood to the nipple. For this case, excision of the lateral thoracic artery and excision of the lateral thoracic artery by 1/2 can cause ischemic necrosis of the nipple. The anterior branches of the third to fifth intercostal arteries were separated from the intercostal spaces and anastomosed to the branches of the lateral thoracic artery and the internal mammary artery, and the blood supply was given to the lower part of the breast.

The superficial vein of the breast is below the superficial fascia and can be displayed by infrared photography. Breast superficial vein divided into the transverse vein and the longitudinal vein. Go to the sternum, in the midline anastomosis in the parasternal across the chest, injected into the internal mammary vein, called transverse vein; to go into the neck and supraclavicular fossa, the lower part of the superficial vein, and finally into the anterior jugular vein, called longitudinal vein. Breast deep venous line can be divided into three ways: the internal mammary vein is a large vein in the breast, branch of the first, second, third intercostal space was the most obvious, the branch was injected into the ipsilateral innominate vein; the basilic vein and brachial vein confluence into axillary vein, all branches of the axillary vein receiving breast, axillary vein injection subclavian and innominate vein; breast vein injected directly into the intercostal vein, and then injected into the azygos vein. In breast cancer, the cancer cells can invade the lung through the superior vena cava through the above three pathways, and the lung metastasis occurs.

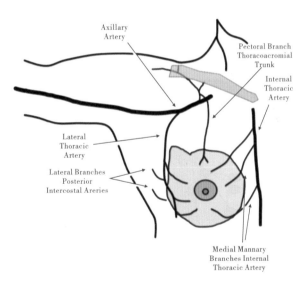

Figure 18-1-2　Vascular supply of the breast

Arterial blood is supplied by branches of the axillary artery (lateral thoracic and pectoral branch of the thoracoacromial trunk). Additional blood supply is from medial mammary branches of the internal thoracic (internal mammary) artery and from lateral branches of the posterior intercostal arteries. Venous drainage is via veins that parallel the arteries with the addition of a superficial plexus (not shown).

1.1.4　Lymphatic drainage

The lymphatic network of the breast is very rich, and the flow direction of the lymph is closely related to the spread of inflammation and the pathway of cancer cell metastasis, so it has important clinical significance. The lymphatic network of the breast can be divided into two groups, shallow and deep. The shallow group is located in the skin and subcutaneous. The deep group is located around the lobule of the breast and the wall of the mammary duct. The two groups are in extensive anastomosis. When breast cancer involves shallow lymphatic vessels, it can cause obstruction of lymphatic drainage, lymphedema and local skin punctuation, which is a "orange peel" change. It is an important basis for diagnosing breast cancer.

The main way of lymph drainage : ①Most of the lymph nodes on the lateral and upper part of the breast are drained into the axillary lymph nodes through the lateral border of the pectoralis major muscle, and then flow to the subclavian lymph nodes. This way drains 50% –75% lymph. ②The upper part of the mammary lymph can flow into the subclavian lymph node without the axillary passage through the lymphatic vessels through the pectoralis major, and then remittance to the supraclavicular lymph node. ③Part of the medial lymph of the breast, through the intercostal lymphatic vessels to the parastar lymph nodes, and then drainage to the supraclavicular lymph nodes. ④The bilateral breasts communicate with each other through a wide anastomosis of shallow lymphatic network, and the lymph of one side of the breast can flow to the opposite side. ⑤The deep lymph network of the breast can connect with the rectus abdominis sheath and the lymphatic vessels of the ligamentous ligaments of the liver, so that the lymph of the breast can be drained into the liver. ⑥The breast lymphatic sometimes directly injected into the inferior deep cervical lymph nodes(Figure 18-1-3).

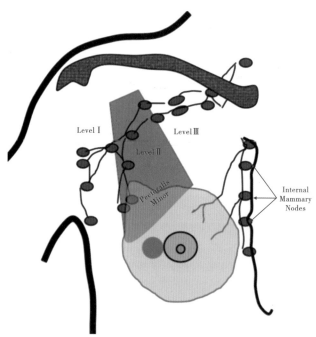

Figure 18-1-3　Lymphatic drainage of the breast

Most drainage is into the axillary nodes indicated as Level Ⅰ, Level Ⅱ, and Level Ⅲ, based on their relationship to the pectoralis minor muscle. Level I nodes are lateral to the muscle, Level Ⅱ are behind it, and Level Ⅲ are medial to it. Also, note the internal mammary nodes located just lateral to the edge of the sternum and deep to the thoracic wall musculature.

1.2 The Physiological Function of the Breast

1.2.1 Lactation

Breastfeeding is the most basic physiological function of the breast. Breast is a mammal's peculiar organ that breastfeeding offspring, and the development and maturity of the mammary glands are all prepared for mammalian activities. Under the stimulation of a large number of hormones after postpartum and the sucking of small babies, breasts begin to produce and discharge milk regularly for the growth and development of small infants.

1.2.2 Secondary sex characters

Breast is an important sign of female secondary sex characters. Generally speaking, the breast has developed at 2–3 years before menarche, that is to say, it has begun to grow at about 10 years old. It is the earliest secondary sex sign, and it is the sign of the onset of puberty.

1.2.3 Sexual activity

In sexual activity, breasts, as one of the sensitive areas of women, can produce a series of changes under the stimulation of touching and kissing. Such as nipple erection, breast fullness, is conducive to a harmonious sexual life, so as to enhance the feelings between husband and wife.

1.2.4 Endocrine hormones that affect the physiological function of the breasts

The hormonal control of human reproduction involves a hierarchy consisting of the hypothalamus, the anterior pituitary gland and the gonads: the hypothalamo–pituitary–gonadal (HPG) axis.

In the female, the main hormones involved are as follows: ①gonadotropin–releasing hormone (GnRH) from the hypothalamus. ②luteinizing hormone (LH) and follicle stimulating hormone (FSH) from the pituitary. ③ estrogen and progesterone, steroid hormones derived from cholesterol and made in the ovary (Figure 18–1–4). The levels of these hormones vary dramatically throughout each menstrual cycle, as well as during the various stages of a woman's lifetime.

1.2.4.1 Ovarian hormone

Estrogen: stimulating the growth of the milk tube (puberty) and the development of mammary lobule acinus and milk formation. Progestin: produces biological effects under the action of estrogen and acts on the mammary gland to promote its development. The proportion of the two is appropriate and the mammary gland develops normally.

1.2.4.2 Pituitary hormone

Prolactin: promote breast growth, development, start, maintain lactation. Gonadotropin: follicle stimulating hormone and luteinizing hormone (luteinizing hormone). Participate in the regulation of estrogen and progestin. Promoting thyroid hormone: promoting the secretion of thyroid, stimulating the whole body metabolism and indirectly promoting the growth and development of the breast. Growth hormone: the synergistic effect of thyroxine, which indirectly affects the development of the breast. Adrenocorticotropic hormone: promoting the secretion of estrogen and androgens, affecting the development of the breast.

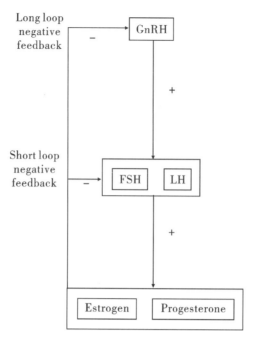

Figure 18-1-4   Endocrine feedback loops
in the hypothalamo-pituitary-gonadal axis

1.2.4.3   Changes in the breast during the menstrual cycle

Mainly for value-added breast before menstruation during the menstrual cycle, menstruation after involution, cycle, repeated. ①Hyperplastic period: 7-8 days after the end of menstruation. ②The secretory phase: proliferative phase to the end of menstruation. ③A period of decline: 7-8 days after the end of menstruation.

Chapter 2

Physical Examination of the Breast

Inspection should take palec in a good light. The bresats are first examined in the sitting or standing position.

2.1 Visual Inspection

Contour, symmetry, and skin changes are noted. The vascular pattern is observed and the condition of the areola and nipple recorded. The nipples are inspected and compared for the presence of retraction, nipple inversion, or excoriation of the superfcial epidermis. If carefully sought, dimpling of the skin or nipple retraction is a sensitive and specifc sign of underlying cancer.

2.2 Palpation

While the patient is still in the sitting position, the examiner supports the patient's arm and palpates each axilla to detect the presence of enlarged axillary lymph nodes. The supraclavicular and infraclavicular spaces are similarly palpated for enlarged nodes. Palpation of the breast is always done with the patient lying supine on a solid examining surface, with the arm stretched above the head. Palpation of the breast while the patient is sitting is often inaccurate because the overlapping breast tissue may feel like a mass or a mass may go undetected within the breast tissue. The breast is best examined with compression of the tissue toward the chest wall, with palpation of each quadrant and the tissue under the nipple−areolar complex.

Palpable masses are characterized according to their size, shape, consistency, and location and whether they are fxed to the skin or underlying musculature. Benign tumors, such as for adenomas and cysts, can be as firm as carcinoma; usually, these benign entities are distinct, well circumscribed, and movable. Carcinoma is typically firm but less circumscribed, and moving it produces a drag of adjacent tissue. Cysts and fbrocystic changes can be tender with palpation of the breast; however, tenderness is rarely a helpful diagnostic sign. Most palpable masses are self−discovered by patients during casual or intentional self−examination.

Patients with breast pain should also be examined with the woman lying on each side and the underlying chest wall palpated for areas of tenderness. Much of so called breast pain emanates from the underlying chest wall(Figure 18−2−1 to Figure 18−2−4).

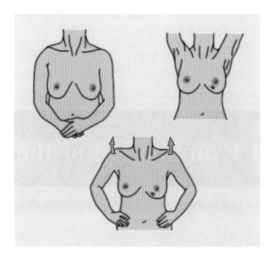

Figure 18-2-1 **Postions for breast inspection**

Skin dimpling in lower part of breast evident only when arms are elveated or pectoral muscles contracted.

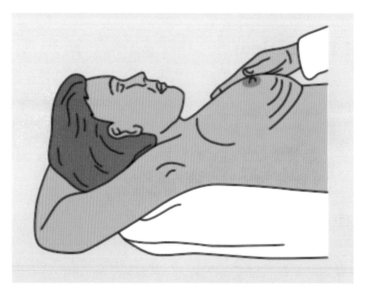

Figure 18-2-2 **Bresat palpation**

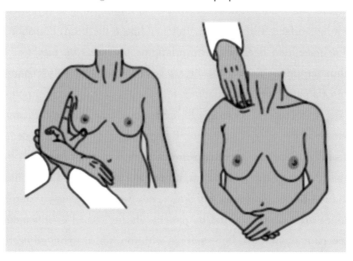

Figure 18-2-3 **Assessment of regional nodes**

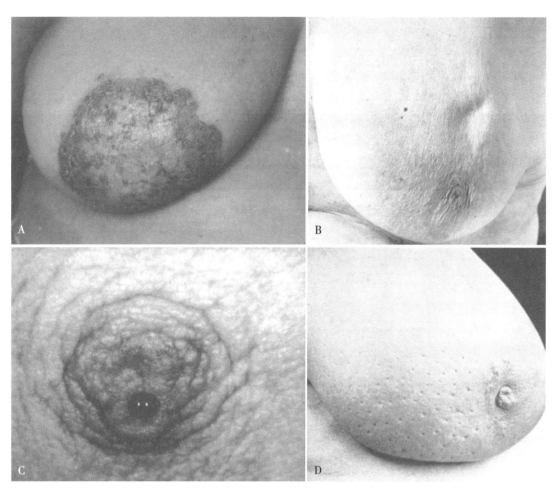

Figure 18-2-4   Common physical findings during breast examination

A , Paget's disease of the nipple. Malignant ductal cells invade the epidermis without traversing the basement membrane of the subareolar duct or epidermis. The disease appears as a psoriatic rash that begins on the nipple and spreads off onto the areola and into the skin of the breast. B , Skin dimpling. Traction on cooper's ligaments by a scirrhous tumor is distorting the surface of the breast and producing a dimple best seen with angled indirect lighting during abduction of the arms upward. C , Nipple discharge. Discharge from multiple ducts or bilateral discharge is a common finding in healthy breasts. In this case , the discharge is from a single duct orifice and may signify underlying disease in the discharging duct. In this patient , a papilloma was the source of her symptoms. D , Peau d'orange (skin of the orange) or edema of the skin of the breast. This finding may be caused by dependency of the breast , lymphatic blockage (from surgery or radiation) , or mastitis. The most feared cause is inflammatory carcinoma , in which malignant cells plug the dermal lymphatics—the pathologic hallmark of the disease.

Chapter 3

Special Examination of the Breast

Special examination of the breast are used to detect small, nonpalpable breast abnormalities, evaluate clinical fndings, and guide diagnostic procedures.

3.1 Mammography

Mammography requires compression of the breast between two plates and is uncomfortable. Two views—oblique and craniocaudal are usually obtained. With modern film screens a dose of less than 1.5 mGy is standard. Mammography allows detection of mass lesions, areas of parenchymal distortion, and microcalcifications. Breasts are relatively radiodense, so in younger women aged <35, mammography is of more limitde value and should not be performed in younger women unless there is suspicion on clinical examination or on cytology or core biopsy that the patient has a cancer. Mammographic sensitivity is limited by breast density, with as many as 10% –15% of clinically evident breast cancers having no associated mammographic abnormality. Digital mammography appears to be superior to traditional film-screen mammography for detecting cancer in younger women and those with dense breasts. All patient with breast cancer proved by cytology or biopsy, regardless of age, should undergo mammography before surgery for assessment of the extent of disease. The combination of a density with spiculated borders and distortion of surrounding breast architecture suggests a malignancy.

3.2 Ultrasonography

High frequency sound waves are beamed through the breast, and reflections are detected and turned into images. Cysts show up as transparent objects, and other benign lesions tend to have well demarcated edges whereas cancers usually have indistinct outlines. Blood flow to lesions can be imaged with colour flow than benign lesions, but the sensitivity and specificity of colour Doppler is insufficient to accurately differentiate benign from malignant lesions.

3.3 Magnetic Resonance Imaging

MRI is increasingly being used for the evaluation of breast abnormalities. The sensitivity of MRI for invasive cancer is higher than 90% , but is only 60% or less for DCIS. Ongoing studies are evaluating its role in improving the rate of successful breast conserving procedures. It is useful in the treated , conserved breast to determine whether a mammographic lesion at the site of surgery is due to scar or recurrence. It has been shown to be a valuable screening tool for high risk women between the ages of 35 and 50. MRI is the optimum method for imaging breast implants. It is also of value in assessing early response to neoadjuvant therapy in women with established breast cancer.

3.4 Biopsy

Biopsy include fine needle aspiration biopsy and core needle biopsy. FNA biopsy is a common tool used in the diagnosis of breast masses. It can differentiate between solid and cystic lesions. Core needle biopsy is the method of choice to sample nonpalpable , image−detected breast abnormalities. This technique is also preferred for the diagnosis of palpable lesions.

3.5 Wire Localized Surgical Excision

Nonpalpable breast lesions should be assessed with image−guided core biopsy , as appropriate , based on the type of abnormality. If the diagnosis is not concordant with imaging findings or there is ADH in a feld of microcalcifications that may represent DCIS , most patients should proceed to excisional biopsy for definitive diagnosis. After excision , the specimen is sent for specimen radiography to confrm that the targeted lesion has been excised. Patients who have a diagnosis of benign findings on excision should undergo a new baseline mammography 4−6 months following the surgical pocedure(Figure 18−3−1 to Figure 18−3−3).

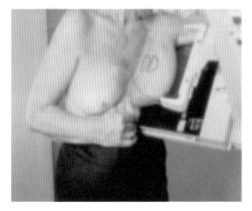

Figure 18–3–1 **Mammography**

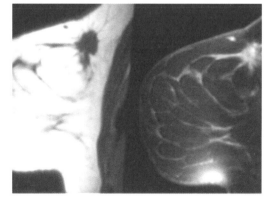

Figure 18–3–2 **MRI scan showing cancer**

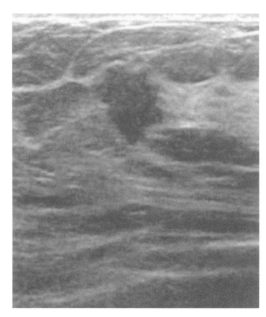

Figure 18-3-3   Ultrasound image of breast cancer

Chapter 4

Acute Mastitis

Acute mastitis is acute suppurative infection of mammary gland, much for postpartum lactation women especially in primipara for see more, often occur in the postpartum 3–4 weeks.

4.1　Etiology

(1) Postpartum galactostasis

Breast milk is the ideal medium, which is conducive to the growth and reproduction of invading bacteria.

(2) Bacterial invasion

Bacterial invasion through the broken or chapped nipple into the duct system is the main route of infection, Especially in primipara, who has no experience in lactation.

4.2　Clinical Manifestations

Breast pain, local redness and fever. With the development of inflammation, there is a rapid pulse of chills and high fever, often with enlarged lymph nodes, tenderness, and increased white blood cell count.

Local performance may vary from individual to individual. In general, the initial appearance of a cellulitis can form an abscess in a few days. An abscess can be a single or multi–room property. The abscess can broke up and the deep abscess can penetrate into the loose tissue between the breast and the pectoral muscle (which is called retromammary abscess). Severe infection can lead to septicemia.

4.3　Treatment

The principle is to eliminate the infection and empty the milk.

The early cellulitis performance is obvious when not suitable surgery, using of antibiotics can obtain good effect. The main pathogenic bacteria are staphylococcus aureus, but do not need to wait for the bacterial culture results, New penicillin Ⅱ can be used. For those allergic to penicillin, erythromycin can be used. Antibiotics can affect the health of the baby through milk, so drugs such as tetracycline aminoglycoside quinolones, sulfonamides and metronidazole should be avoided.

After the abscess formation, the main treatment is to cut the drainage in time and the pus should be tested for bacterial culture and drug sensitivity. During operation, a good anesthesia should be performed. To avoid damage to the milk tube, a milk fistula should be formed, and radiate incision should be done. The abscess of subareola of breast should be curved along the edge of the areola. Deep abscesses or after breast can make arc incision along the edge of the breast, after the cut of the gap, using finger gently separation multiple chambers of an abscess in order to drainage, if pus cavity is large, the contra-aperture drainage can be used. Contralateral breast should stop feeding, breast pump to suck milk, local heat is applied to dissipate the early inflammation. Lactation should be stopped if the infection is severe or a milk fistula is formed. Oral bromine hidden pavilion 1. 25 mg, 2 times a day, 7−14 days, or 1−2 mg diethylstilbestrol, 3 times a day, a total of 2−3 days, or intramuscular injection of estradiol benzoate, 2 mg each time, 1 time a day, to stop milk secretion.

4.4 Prevention

The key is to avoid galactostasis, prevent nipple injury, and keep it clean. Prenatal health education should be strengthened, guide the puerpera to wash the bilateral nipples with warm water and soap often, make a regular breastfeeding, etc. Every time lactation milk should be empty. It should be timely treatment if the nipple is broken or cracked. Pay attention to the oral health of baby.

Chapter 5

Mammary Dysplasia

A group of conditions marked by changes in breast tissue that are benign (not cancer). There are different types of mammary dysplasia, including some types caused by an increase in the number of cells or by the growth of abnormal cells in the breast ducts or lobes. Signs and symptoms of mammary dysplasia include irregular lumps or cysts, breast swelling or discomfort, skin redness or thickening, and nipple discharge. Most benign breast conditions do not increase the risk of breast cancer. Also called benign breast disease.

It is very important to understand this disease correctly because the clinical manifestations of this disease are sometimes confused with breast cancer.

5.1 Etiology

Endocrine disorders is the main reason.

5.2 Diagnosis

According to the clinical manifestation, the diagnosis of this disease is not difficult. But it is important to pay special attention to the breast cancer there possibly exists at the same time with the disease, should review every 3-6 months, When the localized breast hyperplasia is obvious, it should be distinguished from breast cancer. The latter is more specific, with a hard texture, which is markedly different from the surrounding mammary gland, sometimes accompanied by axillary lymph node enlargement, mammography and ultrasound will helpful for the identification of both.

5.3 Treatment

The main treatment of the disease is symptomatic treatment, which can be used in traditional Chinese medicine. Patients with severe symptoms can be treated with tamoxifen for 3 days after menstruation, twice daily, 10 mg for 15 days. The effect of this drug is better, but it has an effect on endometrium and ovary.

For the limited breast cystic hyperplasia, it should be reviewed within 7−10 days after menstruation. If the lump becomes soft, shrink or subside, it can be observed and continue to be treated with Chinese medicine. If there is no obvious subtraction of the tumor, or in the observation process, the local lesion may be malignant, and should be excised for rapid pathological examination.

Chapter 6

Tumor of Breast

The incidence of breast tumors is very high. Fibroadenoma is the most common tumor in benign breast tumors and its proportion in benign tumors is 3/4. After that, it is intraductal papilloma of the breast. In the malignant breast tumors, breast cancer (98%) is the most common tumor, and its incidence rate rises 0.2%–8% every year. Breast sarcoma(2%) is not common.

Male breast cancer is rare and its incidence is less than 1% of female breast cancer and also less than 0.1% of male cancer death.

6.1 Fibroadenoma

Exact etiology of fibroadenoma is not clear. Hormones such asestrogen may play a part in the growth and development of the tumors. A fibroadenoma is a noncancerous tumor in the breast that's commonly found in women under the age of 30. There are two types of fibroadenomas: simple fibroadenomas and complex fibroadenomas. The simple fibroadenomas' proportion is 75%. Some fibroadenomas are so small they can't be felt. The growth of the tumor is slow. When they can be felt, it's very distinct from the surrounding tissue. The edges are clearly defined and the tumors have a detectable shape. They're moveable under the skin and typically not tender. These tumors often feel like marbles, but may have a rubbery feel to them. Menstruation has no effect on the size of the lump. A physical examination is very important. The routine breast examination for fibroadenomas is breast ultrasound or mammogram imaging test. Surgical resection is the only effective method for the treatment of fibroadenoma. Pathological examination is necessary.

6.2 Intraductal Papilloma

Intraductal papillomas of the breast are benign lesions with an incidence of 2%–3% in humans. The peak age incidence was 40–50 years. These papillomas form when fibrous tissue begins to overgrow. They usually remain small in size. One of the most obvious symptoms of intraductal papilloma is nipple discharge from one milk duct. Sometimes a small lump may be felt underneath the nipple, but this is not always the case, depending on the position of the lump. One breast may enlarge slightly if the lump grows significantly, and some breast pain may be felt. Two types of intraductal papillomas are generally distinguished. The central type develops near the nipple. They are usually solitary and often arise in the period nearing menopause. On the other hand, the peripheral type are often multiple papillomas arising at the peripheral breasts, and are usually found in younger women. Surgery to remove a papilloma is usually a simple procedure. During the surgery a small incision is made near the areola, through which the papilloma and the associated milk duct are removed. Pathological examination is necessary.

The malignant transformation rate of intraductal papilloma is as high as 6% –8%. The peripheral type are associated with a higher risk of malignancy.

6.3   Phyllodes Tumors of the Breast

Phyllodes tumors, also cystosarcoma phyllodes, cystosarcoma phylloides and phylloides tumor, are typically large, fast-growing masses that form from the periductal stromal cells of the breast.

They account for less than 1% of all breast neoplasms. They are divided into benign, borderline and malignant. A large series from the M. D. Anderson Cancer Centre reported the incidence of each as benign (58%), borderline (12%), and malignant (30%). This is predominantly a tumor of adult women, with very few examples reported in adolescents. Patients typically present with a firm, palpable mass. These tumors are very fast-growing, and can increase in size in just a few weeks. Occurrence is most common between the ages of 40 and 50, prior to menopause. This is about 15 years older than the typical age of patients with fibroadenoma, a condition with which phyllodes tumors may be confused. They have been documented to occur at any age above 12 years. Malignant phyllodes tumours behave like sarcomas and can develop blood-borne metastases. Approximately 10% of patients with phyllodes tumours develop distant metastases and this can go up to 20% in patients with histologically malignant tumours. The commonest sites for distant metastases are the lung, bone, and abdominal viscera. Rare sites of metastasis like to parotid region have also been described. The common treatment for phyllodes is wide local excision. Other than surgery, there is no cure for phyllodes, as chemotherapy and radiation therapy are not effective. The risk of developing local recurrence or metastases is related to the histologic grade, according to the above-named features.

6.4   Breast Cancer

Breast cancer is the most common cancer among women in the world. One in every eight women in the United States develops breast cancer. In China, the proportion is lower, but the trend is on the rise.

6.4.1   Cause of disease

The causes of breast cancer are not clear. Estradiol and estrone have a direct relationship with breast cancer. The primary risk factors for breast cancer are being female and older age. The incidence of male breast cancer is 1% in women's breast cancer. The high incidence of breast cancer in Chinese women is 40–60 years old. Chinese patients are 10 years younger than those in western countries. Other potential risk factors include genetics, lack of childbearing or lack of breastfeeding, higher levels of certain hormones, certain dietary patterns, and obesity. Recent studies have indicated that exposure to light pollution is a risk factor for the development of breast cancer.

6.4.2   Signs and symptoms

The first noticeable symptom of breast cancer is typically a lump that feels different from the rest of the breast tissue. More than 80% of breast cancer cases are discovered when the patient feels a lump. Less frequent symptoms are nipple discharge; breast pain; erosion, retraction, enlargement, or itching of the nipple and redness, generalized hardness, enlargement, or shrinking of the breast. Rarely, lumps found in lymph nodes located in the armpits can also indicate breast cancer.

Early breast cancer is mostly a single small lump with no pain. Hard mass with unclear edge and unsmooth surface is the feature. The lump will not be propelled when the tumor invades the chest wall muscles. With the growth of the tumor volume, local eminence can be found on the breast. If the tumor invades the Cooper's ligament, we will find the dimple sign. As the tumor continues to progress, the subcutaneous lymphatics will be blocked by the tumor, orange peel skin will appears. If the tumor cells invade the skin, small nodules can occur. With the progression of the tumor, skin nodules may be fused, even ulcerated.

Lymph node metastasis of breast cancer is most common in the axillary at first. Enlarged lymph node is hard and painless and can not be propelled. Axillary nodes that are matted or fixed to skin or deep structures indicate advanced disease. Distant metastasis of breast cancer is also common. The symptoms caused bymetastatic breast cancer will depend on the location of metastasis. Common sites of metastasis include bone, liver, lung and brain. Bone or joint pains can sometimes be manifestations of metastatic breast cancer, as can jaundice or neurological symptoms.

Inflammatory breast cancer and mammary Paget's disease(MPD) are particular types of breast cancer. Inflammatory breast cancer's symptoms may resemble a breast inflammation and may include itching, pain, swelling, nipple inversion, warmth and redness throughout the breast, as well as an orange-peel texture to the skin referred to as peaud'orange. As inflammatory breast cancer does not present as a lump there can sometimes be a delay in diagnosis. The prognosis of this kind of breast cancer is poor.

The syndrome of mammary Paget's disease presents as skin changes resembling eczema, such as redness, discoloration, or mild flaking of the nipple skin. As Paget's disease of the breast advances, symptoms may include tingling, itching, increased sensitivity, burning, and pain. There may also be discharge from the nipple. Approximately half of women diagnosed with Paget's disease of the breast also have a lump in the breast. The prognosis of this kind of breast cancer is better.

6.4.3   Pathological types of breast cancer

There are many pathological types of breast cancer. The most common are the following two categories which are noninvasive epithelial cancers and invasive epithelial cancers. Noninvasive epithelial cancers include lobular carcinoma in situ (LCIS), ductal carcinoma in situ (DCIS) or intraductal carcinoma, papillary, cribriform, solid, and comedo types. Invasive epithelial cancers include invasive lobular carcinoma, invasive ductal carcinoma, tubular carcinoma, mucinous or colloid carcinoma, medullary carcinoma, invasive cribriform carcinoma, invasive papillary carcinoma, adenoid cystic carcinoma, metaplastic carcinoma. In addition to the above types, there are other rare types of cancer, such as inflammatory breast cancer and mammary Paget's disease.

6.4.4   Diagnosis

Inspection of the breast is the most important step in physical examination and should be carried out with the patient sitting, arms at sides and then overhead. Abnormal variations in breast size and contour, minimal nipple retraction, and slight edema, redness, or retraction of the skin can be identified. The most reliable diagnostic test for breast cancer is open excisional biopsy.

6.4.5   Staging of breast cancer

A perfect pathological diagnosis is the basis for the treatment of breast cancer. There are many methods of staging breast cancer. The most widely used system is that of the American Joint Committee on Cancer (AJCC2010). The contents are as follows.

(p) Primary tumor(T)

Tx: The primary tumor can not be evaluated. T0: No evidence of the primary tumor. Tis: Carcinoma in situ (lobular or ductal) and Paget's disease of the nipple without mass. T1: Tumor ≤2 cm. T1mic: Tumor ≤ 0.1cm. T1a: Tumor >0.1 cm, ≤0.5 cm. T1b: Tumor >0.5 cm, ≤1 cm. T1c: Tumor >1 cm, ≤2 cm. T2: Tumor >2 cm, ≤5 cm. T_3: Tumor >5 cm. T4: Tumor any size with extension to the chest wall or skin. T4a: Tumor extending to the chest wall (excluding the pectoralis). T4b: Tumor extending to the skin with ulceration, edema, satellite nodules. T4c: Both T4a and T4b. T4d: Inflammatory carcinoma.

(p) Nodes (N)

Nx: The status of regional lymph nodes can not be evaluated. N0: No regional node involvement, no special studies. N0 (i−): No regional node involvement, negative IHC. N0 (i+): Node(s) with isolated tumor cells spanning <0.2 mm. N0 (mol−): Negative node(s) histologically, negative PCR. N0 (mol+): Negative node(s) histologically, positive PCR. N1: Metastasis to 1−3 axillary nodes and/or int. mammary positive by biopsy. N2: Metastasis to 4−9 axillary nodes or int. mammary clinically positive, without axillary metastasis. N3: Metastasis to ≥10 axillary nodes or combination of axillary and int. mammary metastasis.

Metastasis(M)

M0: No distant metastasis. M1: Distant metastasis.

American Joint Committee on Cancer Stage Grouping

Stage 0: TisN0M0. Stage I: T1N0M0. Stage II A: T0 N1M0, T1N1M0, T2N0M0. Stage II B: T2N1M0, T3N0M0. Stage III A: T0N2M0, T1N2M0, T2N2M0, T3N1M0, T3N2M0. Stage III B: T4N0M0, T4N1M0, T4N2M0. Stage III C: Any T, N3, M0. Stage IV: Any T, any N, M1.

6.4.6   Treatment

There are many treatment methods of breast cancer. These methods include surgery, chemotherapy, radiotherapy, endocrine therapy, and targeted therapy. For patients with no distant metastasis, the operation is necessary. Patients in stage 0− II and part of patients in stage III have surgical indications. Distant metastasis and intolerance are contraindications to surgery.

6.4.6.1   Surgical treatment

Halsted's radical mastectomy has been a standard procedure for the treatment of breast cancer since 1894. It is suggested that the metastasis of breast cancer is based on the anatomical model, which is transferred from the primary lesion to the regional lymph node. However, as the scope of surgery expanded, the survival rate did not improve significantly. This fact has prompted many scholars to narrow the scope of surgery to treat breast cancer. Over the past 30 years, Fisher has done a lot of research on the biological behavior of breast cancer. He suggested that breast cancer begins with a systemic disease. Therefore, it is necessary to narrow the scope of surgery and strengthen the postoperative comprehensive adjuvant therapy.

(1) Breast−conserving surgery

It is suitable for breast cancer patients with stage I and stage II, and the breast has the proper volume, and can maintain the appearance effect after surgery. Multifocal or multi-focal lesion, no contraindication of the edge-negative to perform the operation. The cutting edge of the tumor must be negative. Radiotherapy must be given after surgery.

(2) Modified radical mastectomy

There are two types of surgery. Patey modified radical surgery is to keep the pectoralis major and remove the pectoralis minor. Auchincloss modified radical surgery is to retain the pectoralis major and pectoralis minor. There was no significant difference in survival rate between radical surgery and modified radical surgery, and the surgical style retained the pectoralis muscle, and the postoperative appearance was better, which is the commonly used surgical method.

(3) Radical mastectomy and extensive radical mastectomy

The radical mastectomy for breast cancer should include the entire breast, pectoralis major, pectoralis minor, axillary Ⅰ, Ⅱ, and Ⅲ group lymph node dissection. Extensive radical resection needs simultaneously remove the intrathoracic artery, vein and the surrounding lymph nodes (that is, the parasternal lymph nodes).

(4) Total mastectomy

The scope of surgery must be removed from the breast and pectoral fascia. This method is suitable for carcinoma in situ, small cancer and weak age. sentinel lymph node biopsy and axillary lymph node dissection. Routine axillary lymph node dissection was performed for breast cancer patients with positive axillary lymph nodes, and the range included Ⅰ, Ⅱ group of axillary lymph nodes. Sentinel lymph node is the first (station) lymph node that receives the drainage of the breast cancer lesion. According to the pathologic findings of sentinel lymph nodes, we can determine whether axillary lymph node dissection should be needed. The selection of surgical methods should be based on the patient's willingness, pathological classification, stage of disease and adjuvant treatment. Improving patient survival and improving patient quality of life is what we need.

6.4.6.2　Chemotherapy

Chemotherapy is one of the most important treatments for breast cancer. Invasive breast cancer with axillary lymph node metastasis is the indication of adjuvant chemotherapy. There are different opinions on whether the axillary lymph node negative is applied adjuvant chemotherapy. Axillary lymph node negative and, generally speaking, there are at high risk of recurrence factors, such as primary tumor diameter greater than 2 cm, histological classification is bad, hormone receptors are negative, HER2 overexpression is, appropriate application of adjuvant chemotherapy. Chemotherapy regimens are still based on anthracycline and paclitaxel. The chemotherapy should pay attention to the patient's blood routine, liver function and kidney function. Patients with anthracycline should pay attention to cardiac toxicity. Preoperative chemotherapy, also known as neoadjuvant chemotherapy, is used in locally advanced cases to reduce tumors, improve surgical chances and detect tumor sensitivity to drugs.

6.4.6.3　Endocrinotherapy

The estrogen receptor (ER) in breast cancer cells is high in hormone-dependent tumors, and these cases are effective in endocrine therapy. An important development of endocrine therapy is the application of tamoxifen. Tamoxifen is anti-estrogen drugs, its structural formula similar to estrogen. It can compete for ER with estradiol in the target organ, and tamoxifen and ER compounds can affect the transcription of DNA gene, thus inhibiting tumor cell growth. Clinical application shows that this drug can reduce the recurrence and metastasis of breast cancer after operation, and can reduce the incidence of breast cancer on the healthy side, especially for women with ER and PgR. The drug is safe and effective. Its adverse reactions include hot flashes, nausea, vomiting, venous thrombosis, eye side effects, vaginal dryness and secretion. Aromatase inhibitors can inhibit the transformation of androgen secreted by the adrenal glands into aromatization in the estrogen process, thereby reducing estradiol and achieving the goal of treating breast cancer. The newly developed aromatase inhibitors include anastrozole, letrozole, and exemestane. In postmenopausal patients, they had better efficacy than tamoxifen. But aromatase inhibitors have a higher incidence of bone related adverse reactions than tamoxifen.

6.4.6.4   Radiotherapy

Radiotherapy is one of the most common treatments for breast cancer. Axillary lymph node positive and breast-conserving surgery is the indication of radiotherapy. Radiotherapy can effectively reduce the risk of local recurrence of breast cancer.

6.4.6.5   Molecular targeted therapy

Trastuzumab is the most common targeted drug. The HER-2 gene is the main pathogenic gene of breast cancer. Trastuzumab can block the signaling pathway of the gene and thus inhibit tumor growth. There's a lot of data showing that it can improve patient survival. Targeted therapy is a new direction for future development of breast cancer treatment.

Part 19

Chest Trauma

Chapter 1

Rib Factures

Rib fractures are the most common chest injury, over 40% of patients with chest trauma has rib fractures, which are usually caused by violence. The ribs of the 1st to the 3rd are not prone to suffer from fractures since they are thick and short, and has the protection of scapula and clavicle, fractures of which usually indicate a relatively high level of violence and frequently accompanied with clavicular or scapula fracture as well as axillary vascular nerve injury. The ribs from 4th to are long and thin, leading to a high possibility of fracture. The front of the 8th to the 10th ribs is connected with the sternum by the cartilago costalis, forming the costal arch, and the front of the 11th to the 12th ribs is free and elastic. Thus, the ribs from 8th to the 12th are not easy to be fractured, and if happens, an injury in the diaphragm and abdominal viscera should be taken into consideration. Multiple fractures of multiple ribs which is known as the flail chest may cause the local chest wall out of the support of the integrity of ribs and become soft, resulting in abnormal breathing, that is, when inhaling the softened chest wall will sink in, and protrude outward when exhaling.

1.1 Clinical Manifestations

1.1.1 Symptoms

Rib fractures produce chest pain due to stimulating of the intercostal nerve, and deep breathing, cough and body position changes intensify the pain. It makes the respiratory activity of the injured side limited, breast shallowed, cough weakened, resulting in increasing the risk of airway secretions, retention, leading to atelectasis and lung infections and other complications. Displacement of the fracture ends to the inside pierces the pleura, intercostal vessels, and lung tissue to produce hemothorax, pneumothorax, subcutaneous emphysema, or hemoptysis. Displacement of fractured ends may cause delayed hemothorax and blood pneumothorax. When the pressure of the both side of the thoracic cavity is not equal, the mediastinum moves around, that is called mediastinum flutter. Chest convulsions are often accompanied by extensive pulmonary contusion. Contused pulmonary interstitial or alveolar edema might lead to disorders of oxygen diffusion, resulting in impaired lung ventilation, hypoxemia causing dyspnea, cyanosis, and even shock. Lower rib fractures might be associated with symptoms of the abdominal visceral organ (e. g. , liver, spleen, kidney).

1.1.2 Signs

The chest wall may have malformations, with obviously local tenderness and bone friction sounds. Extruding the thorax may aggravate local pain and help differentiate from soft tissue contusions.

1.2 Diagnosis

The history of thoracic trauma, local pain and tenderness in the chest wall, and thoracic compression syndrome should be clarified. The possibility of rib fracture should be considered. Chest pressure points can be touched on the chest wall. Abnormal breathing indicates multiple fractures of multiple ribs. Chest X-ray examination will observe the situation and location of the fracture, but also understand the presence of thoracic organ injury and complications. In recent years, chest CT and three-dimensional reconstruction of the ribs can be used to confirm the location and condition of the fractures, so as to be used as a guide for surgical treatment.

1.3 Treatment

The principles of treatment are effective analgesia, clearance of respiratory secretions, fixation of the thorax, and prevention of complications.

1.3.1 Closed single rib fracture

The broken ends of the fractures are supported by upper and lower full ribs and intercostal muscles. They have less dislocations, activities, and overlaps, and tend to heal spontaneously. The main purpose of fixation of the thorax is to reduce the rib end activities and pain. The chest can be fixed by using a multi-head chest strap and an elastic chest strap. This method can also be applied to multiple rib fractures in the thoracodorsal and thoracic vertebrae, where the softened range of the chest wall is small and abnormal respiratory movements are not severe.

1.3.2 Closed multiple rib fractures

Effective analgesia and respiratory management are the main treatment principles. Patients with cough weakness and retention of respiratory secretions should be performed sputum aspiration with fiberoptic bronchoscope and pulmonary physiotherapy. Patients with respiratory tract dysfunction need mechanical ventilation through tracheal intubation. Positive pressure ventilation has an "internal fixation" effect on the chest wall. Long-term chest wall floating which can not leave the ventilator can perform surgical fixation of ribs, intraoperative use of judet splint, intramedullary nail, Kirschner wire or stainless steel wire and other fixed rib stump. In recent years, there is research of floating chest being fixed by steel wire under video-assisted thoracoscope. When other indications require chest surgery, rib fixation may also be performed simultaneously.

1.3.3　Open rib fracture

Wounds on the wall of the chest require thorough debridement and use methods above to fix the broken ends. If the pleural membrane has been punctured, pleural cavity drainage is required, and antibiotics are required to prevent infection after surgery.

Chapter 2

Fractures of the Sternum

The sternal fracture is usually caused by the violence, among which the collision of the driver's chest against the steering wheel in a traffic accident is the most common situation. The majority of sternal fractures are transverse fracture, usually occurring at the junction of the manubrium sternum with the body or the body of the sternum. Multiple fractures on the side of the sternum may result in a floating sternum, leading to the flail of the chest. Sternal fracture is often associated with injury of internal thoracic viscera, such as the blunt heart injury, injury of trachea, bronchi and big vessels as well as their branches.

2.1 Clinical Manifestations

Patients with sternal fracture have obvious chest pain and cough, which is aggravated by respiratory and postural changes, accompanied with shallow breathing, weakened cough and increased respiratory secretion. The area of chest fracture is visible malformation, and local tenderness is obvious in the local part of fracture, fracture end displacement is usually the lower end moving forward, upper end backward, and sometimes the two overlap. The fracture line of the sternal fracture can be found on the lateral and oblique X-ray plates.

2.2 Diagnosis

According to the patient's history of injury, X-ray, CT three-dimensional imaging can confirm the diagnosis.

2.3 Treatment

(1) If Patients do not has a postural change of the fracture ends, major treatments are analgesia, physical therapy, and prevention of complications. Patients still can stay in bed for 2-3 weeks, elevating the shoulder area with a pillow, using a trap dressing to fix the fracture part for 2-3 weeks, and control the pain

appropriately.

(2) Displaced sternal fractures should be reset as soon as possible on the basis of a stable general condition. ①Closed reset: The angled deformity can be reset by local compression; if there is a overlapping malformations, patients should be told to get arms over-stretched, and then give a pressure to the fracture to make it reset under the local anesthesia, and then using a chest strap to fix chest for 2-3 weeks. ②Surgical reset: It is suitable for patients who need surgical treatment if the closed reduction is not successful or if there is intrathoracic organ injury.

Chapter 3

Hemothorax

Pleural hematocele is called hemothorax, and when coexisting with pneumothorax, it is called hemopneumothorax. Chest trauma and chest wall or any organ in the chest, where there is a wound communicated with pleural cavity, can lead to hemothorax or hemopneumothorax. After hemothorax occurs, the loss of blood volume not only affects the circulation function, but also compresses the lungs and reduces the respiratory area. Hemothorax pushes mediastinum forward, causing suppression on the healthy side of the lung and affecting vena cava reflux. When a large amount of blood rapidly accumulates in the thoracic cavity, exceeding the function of defiberation of lung, pericardium and diaphragmatic muscle movement. The blood accumulated in the thoracic cavity will coagulates, forming a coagulative hematocele. After the coagulation of blood clots, a fibrous plate is formed, which limits lung and thoracic activity and damages respiratory function. Besides, blood is a good medium, and bacteria entering a wound or a broken lung can grow rapidly in the accumulation of blood, causing an infectious hematocele and eventually leading to a dense hematocele. Hematocele of the pleural cavity caused by continuous massive hemorrhage is called progressive hematocele. In a few cases, delayed blooding of pleural cavity leads to the pleural hematocele, which resulted from the puncture of intercostal vessels by the movement of the fractured rib end or blood clot's falling off from the ruptured vessel.

3.1 Clinical Manifestations

3.1.1 Symptoms

Adult hematoplethorax less than 500 mL is a small amount of hematopleural thorax, which can be asymptomatic. The costal phrenic angle disappears under the X-ray examination, and the lower lung field is not clear. For further diagnosis, ultrasonic detection and localization are feasible. Between 500 mL and 1000 mL were medium-sized hemothorax, while >1000 mL was large hemothorax. In a short period of time when hemothorax is upwards of 1000 mL, patients often have a manifestation of hypovolemic shock, such as pale, thin pulse velocity, dysphoria, shortness of breath, blood pressure decrease, and symptoms of pleural effusion; moreover, X-ray examination reveales a large effusion shadow in the pleural cavity of the injured side, with mediastinum shifting to the healthy side. B-ultrasonography and CT can help diagnose hematopleural chest. Aspiration with non-coagulated blood can confirm this disease.

3.1.2　Signs

Progressive hemothorax: ① Continuously increased pulse and decreased blood pressure, or unstable blood pressure despite of blood volume supplementation. ② Volume of thoracic drainage exceeds 200 mL per hour for 3 hours. ③ The amount of hemoglobin, red blood cell count and Hematocrit are decreased continuously, and the amount of hemoglobin and red blood cell in the drainage fluid are similar to those in peripheral blood and rapidly coagulated.

Infectious hemothorax: ① with chills, fever, and other symptoms of systemic infection. ② Things of turbid or flocuculus found in thoracic drainage suggest infection. ③ Ratio of red to white blood cells reach to 100 : 1 in pleural hemocytosis. ④ General smear or bacteria cultivation is found pathogenic bacteria.

3.2　**Treatment**

A small amount of hemothorax can be absorbed without special treatment. Non-progressive hemothorax can be treated with thoracentesis or closed drainage according to the amount of blood. In principle, blood excretion should be promptly discharged to promote lung recruitment and improve lung function. What's more, using antibiotics to prevent infection is required. Since the persistence of hemothorax increases the likelihood of coagulation of coagulating hemothorax and infectious hemothorax, the indications for closed thoracic drainage should be appropriately relaxed. Progressive hemothorax should promptly perform a exploratory surgery. The coagulation hemothorax should be treated as soon as possible to remove the blood clots, and the membrane formed due to the formation of a blood clot on the pleural surface. Infectious hemothorax should ensure the drainage of pleural effusion and exclude empyema. If there is no obvious effect or poor reexpansion of the lung, surgery to remove infected hemoperitoneum should be performed as soon as possible. In recent years, video-assisted thoracoscopy has been used in the treatment of coagulation hemothorax and infectious hemothorax. It has the advantages of small surgical trauma, definite curative effect, and rapid postoperative recovery.

Chapter 4

Traumatic Pneumothorax

The incidence of traumatic pneumothorax accounts for 15% – 50% in blunt trauma. More often than not, the lungs are punctured by the broken ends of rib fractures, and the bronchial or lung tissue may be contused and wounded due to the effects of violence, or the bronchus or lung may be ruptured due to a sharp rise in airway pressure. Sharp injury or firearm injury penetrating through the chest wall and injuring the lungs, bronchus and trachea or esophagus, also cause pneumothorax. And, most of them are hemopneumothorax or pus pneumothorax. Occasionally, pyogenic pneumothorax is caused by rupture of the stomach when the closed or penetrating diaphragm ruptures. The pneumothorax can be divided into three categories: closed pneumothorax, open pneumothorax and tension pneumothorax according to the status of the pneumothorax leakage channel and the accumulation of gas in the pleural cavity and the increase in intrapleural pressure.

4.1 Closed Pneumothorax

Pleural pressure is still below the atmospheric pressure. The amount of gas accumulated in the pleural cavity determines the degree of atelectasis on the injured side. Injury of the lungs in the injured side decreases the area of lung respiration, and the ratio of ventilation blood flow is unbalanced, affecting pulmonary ventilation and the gas exchange of lung. Increased negative pressure in the injured side of the chest causes displacement of the mediastinum to the contralateral side. According to the volume and velocity of pleural cavity gas, mild patients may have no obvious symptoms, but severe cases may have dyspnea. The physical examination may reveal that the injured side of the chest is full, breathing activity is reduced, the trachea is displaced to the contralateral side, and the wounded chest smells percussion drum sound, and the breath sounds are reduced. Chest X–ray examination shows different degrees of air in pleural cavity and lung collapse, with a pleural effusion visible fluid level.

Patients with a slow pneumothorax and a small amount of pneumogas require no special treatment. Air in pleural cavity can generally be absorbed within 1–2 weeks. A large number of pneumothorax need to be pleural cavity puncture or closed thoracic drainage to rule out the accumulation of gas, prompting the lungs to expand as soon as possible.

4.2   Open Pneumothorax

The outside air enters and exits the pleural cavity as it breathes through the chest wall defect. The degree of dyspnea is closely related to the size of the pleural cavity defect. When the diameter of the chest wall defect is greater than 3 cm, the pleural cavity pressure is equal to the atmospheric pressure. Because the intrathoracic pressure in the injured side is significantly higher than that in the healthy side, the displacement of the mediastinum to the contralateral side causes significant restricted expansion of the contralateral lung. When breathing and inhalation occur, periodical inhomogeneities in the pleural pressure on both sides change. During inhalation, the mediastinum moves to the healthy side, and exhale moves back to the injured side. This pulsation and displacement of the mediastinum will affect the blood flow back to the vena cava and cause circulatory disorders.

4.2.1   Clinical manifestations

Mainly manifested as irritability, cyanosis, significant dyspnea, decreased blood pressure, and even shock. The wounded side of the chest wall gives a sucking-like sound as the gas enters and exits the chest cavity. The trachea is displaced to the contralateral side, the sound of wounded chest percussion drum and auscultation breath disappears. Chest X-ray shows a large amount of air in pleural cavity in the injured side of the chest, lung collapse, and mediastinal bias toward the healthy side.

4.2.2   Treatment

The principle of treatment is to close the chest wall defect as soon as possible and restore the pleural cavity negative pressure.

5-6 layers of vaseline gauze can be used in the size more than 4 cm above the wound edge, covering the wound, and then pressure dressing with a cotton pad. It should be as soon as possible to repair the debridement suture or chest wall defect. Thoracic closed drainage tube should be placed postoperatively.

Indications for closed thoracic drainage: ①More than moderate amount of pneumothorax, open pneumothorax or tension pneumothorax. ②After lung thoracocentesis treatment, the lungs are still unable to re-tension. ③Pneumothorax or hemopneumothorax need to use mechanical ventilation. ④Recurrence of pneumothorax or blood pneumothorax after pulling out chest tube. ⑤Thoracotomy.

4.3   Tension Pneumothorax

Tension pneumothorax is a flap formed at the trachea, bronchus or lung injury. The gas enters the pleural cavity with each inhalation and accumulates, causing the pleural cavity pressure to be higher than atmospheric pressure, also known as high pressure pneumothorax, severe collapse of the injured side of the lung, the mediastinum significantly shifted to the contralateral side, the contralateral lung compression, and vena cava backflow disorders. The intrathoracic pressure above atmospheric pressure drives the gas through the bronchus, loose tissue around the trachea or parietal pleural lacerations, or into the mediastinal or chest wall soft tissue to form mediastinal emphysema or subcutaneous emphysema of the face, neck, and chest.

4.3.1   Clinical manifestations

Patients with tension pneumothorax have extreme dyspnea, irritability, disturbance of consciousness, sweating, and cyanosis. The trachea is displaced to the contralateral side and the jugular veins are engorged with subcutaneous emphysema. The wounded side of the chest is full, the percussion is a drum sound, and auscultation of breath sound disappears. Chest X-ray examination shows a large amount of gas accumulation in the chest cavity, complete collapse of the lungs, transposition of the mediastinum, and signs of mediastinal emphysema and subcutaneous emphysema. High-pressure gas pushes the needle outwards during thoracentesis. There may be circulatory disorders.

4.3.2   Treatment

Severe pathophysiological changes caused by tension pneumothorax rapidly leads to death, so the urgent discharge of high-pressure gas in the chest is very important. In case of emergency, insert a thick needle in the second intercostal space of the midline of the collarbone, or disinfection finger sleeve at the end of the needle to block the air from entering the chest. If the patient has a penetrating wound, use a gloved finger or pliers to dilate the wound deeper to decompress it. The above measures are able to make the tension pneumothorax become an open pneumothorax. After the condition is stable, closed drainage tube is placed in the 5th to 6th intercostal midaxillary in the thoracic. Make negative pressure drainage to promote lung expansion. 24 hours after the leak stops, X-ray examination confirms that the lungs have expanded before the drainage tube could be pulled out. When continuous air leakage occurs and the lungs are difficult to expand, open chest exploration surgery or video-assisted thoracoscopic surgery should be considered.

Chapter 5

Subcutaneous and Mediastinal Emphysenia

Subcutaneous and mediastinal emphysema refers to all kinds of causes of gas through the bronchus and loose connective tissue around the trachea or parietal pleura at the crack, or into the chest wall soft tissues and mediastinal areas, forming subcutaneous emphysema and mediastinal emphysema.

5.1 Clinical manifestations

The patients with mediastinal emphysema show different severity, which is mainly related to the rate of emphysema, the amount of gas accumulation, the presence or absence of combined tension pneumothorax, and the primary diseases causing mediastinal emphysema.

Patients with a small amount of gas may be asymptomatic. When there is more gas accumulation and higher pressure, the patient may have oppression in chest, shortness of breath, pharyngeal obstruction, and poststernal pain, etc. Patients, with large gas accumulation in the mediastinum or with tension pneumothorax, often suffer from severe dyspnea, cyanosis, and even life-threatening. Physical examination often finds subcutaneous emphysema in the neck. Severe subcutaneous emphysema spreads to the face, chest, upper limbs, and even to the abdomen and lower extremities. The subcutaneous tissue is swollen. Palpation has a feeling of snow under the skin and twist pronunciation. Other patients may have characteristic signs such as clear sound after sternal bone, narrowed or disappeared heart sounds, predischarged heartbeat and bubble burst (Hamman sign) sound consistent with heartbeat. Severe patients with neck and thoracic vein backflow disorders, combined with tension pneumothorax, can still observe the corresponding signs.

5.2 Diagnosis

In addition to considering the above clinical manifestations and signs, the diagnosis of mediastinal emphysema relies mainly on chest X-ray or CT examination. Both sides of the mediastinal band-like translucent shadows could be observed on front and rear X-ray. The increase in the brightness of the posterior sternal clearance could be observed on lateral X-ray film. Chest CT shows more clearly on mediastinal emphysema, indicating that large vessels, trachea, esophagus and heart, and other important organs that are covered by gas.

5.3   Treatment

5.3.1   General treatment

In most of patients with mediastinal emphysema, after bed rest, or given antibiotics, pain, oxygen and other general treatment, gas can be gradually absorbed in $1-2$ weeks or so. A small number of patients should be fasting and given parenteral nutrition.

5.3.2   Local exhaust treatment

For patients with more gas accumulated in the mediastinum, oppression symptoms and general treatment uneffective, incision drainage decompression should be done under local anesthesia at the suprasternal notch. Those who have subcutaneous emphysema should also do skin incision on the upper chest, so as to squeezing the exhaust.

5.3.3   Primary disease treatment

For patients with primary diseases, the surgeons should repair and suture the broken trachea and air leakage esophagus, etc.

Chapter 6

Traumatic Rupture of the Trachea or Bronchi

Trachea and bronchial injuries are more common in traffic accidents and chest impact injuries, such as sharp injuries, cutting your own throat, etc. External forces act directly on the neck or trachea, causing tracheal and bronchial rupture. Intrathoracic organ damage occurs within 2.5 cm above the carina, and bronchial rupture occurs within 2.5 cm of the distal carina. Such patients are in serious condition and often die of untimely treatment. Trachea and bronchial injuries can also be seen in iatrogenic injuries, such as inappropriate tracheotomy, tracheoesophageal fistula, etc.

6.1 Main Bronchial Injury

The left principal bronchus is longer and has more chances of injury. When the principal bronchus in the mediastinum is broken and the mediastinal pleura is intact, severe mediastinal and subcutaneous emphysema appears. When the principal bronchus ruptured in the chest cavityor the mediastinal pleura is damaged, it often appears as tension pneumothorax. A completely broken principal bronchus would seal the stump with mucosal retraction, blood clots and hyperplastic granulation, resulting in complete atelectasis of the distal lung. As the bacteria can not enter the distal lung through the principal trachea, there is less secondary infection. Partially broken principal bronchial stump usually results in stenosis and incomplete lung expansion due to fibrous tissue proliferation. Bacteria enter the bronchus where drainage is impeded. They are susceptible to secondary infections, even leading to bronchiectasis and pulmonary fibrosis.

6.1.1 Clinical manifestations

It is manifested as cough, hemoptysis, dyspnea, mediastinal and subcutaneous emphysema, tension pneumothorax or tension pneumothorax. One of the following conditions should be suspected of major bronchial injury: ①Severe mediastinal and subcutaneous emphysema in chest injury. ②Tension pneumothorax. ③After the placement of closed thoracic drainage, air leakage continues and atelectasis happens. ④Chest radiographs shows atelectasis, the lung tip falls below the plane of the main bronchus, and the lateral film finds gas accumulating beneath the deep fascia of the neck. Fiberoptic bronchoscopy helps determine the diagnosis and determine the site of injury.

6.1.2 Treatment

First of all, it should maintain airway patency, correct shock and relieve tension pneumothorax. Thoracic exploration and bronchial repair should be performed as soon as possible. Early surgery helps lung recruitment maneuver and prevent bronchial stenosis, and make the operation easier. Patients with advanced surgery have atelectasis. The key to retain the ability of lungs is whether the distal lung recruitment maneuver. For lungs that can not be reexpanded, lung or total lung resection should be performed. The surgical complications include tracheal and bronchial restenosis, and bronchopleural fistulas and empyema.

6.2 Tracheal Injury

The blunt violence in the front of the neck leads to larynx trachea separation, rupture or break of the trachea, and also causes destruction of multiple tracheal cartilage rings, resulting in softening of the trachea and suffocation. The posterior displacement of the broken end of the sternal fracture would puncture the internal thoracic trachea. The most common penetrating damage is a partial or complete rupture of the trachea caused by the neck injury. Tracheal injuries are often associated with prevertebral, thyroid, esophageal, and large vessels of the neck.

6.2.1 Clinical manifestations

The clinical manifestations of blunt traumatic tracheal injury are cough, wheezing, breathing difficulty, change of pronunciation, hemoptysis, subcutaneous neck or mediastinal emphysema. Some patients have sternal fractures. Penetrating tracheal injuries could find wound in the neck and chest. Gas often escapes from the wound with breathing. Patients often have hemoptysis, neck and mediastinal emphysema.

6.2.2 Treatment

An endotracheal intubation should be performed urgently to stop the flow of blood and secretions into the distal trachea to maintain airway patency. When the trachea is transection or the larynx trachea is separated, the distal trachea may be retracted into the thoracic cavity, and a low transverse incision of the neck is needed. The paratracheal fascia is cut open. After the finger exploration, the distal end is clamped with tissue forceps and the tracheal tube is inserted. When endotracheal intubation is difficult, a fiberoptic bronchoscope can be inserted, and an endotracheal tube can be introduced. Do not use muscle relaxants when anesthesia is intubated and before thoroughly removing respiratory secretions. If there is severe contusion of the tracheal wall during repair and anastomosis, 2-4 tracheal rings may be removed and anastomosis may be performed.

Chapter 7

Pulmonary Contusion

Pulmonary contusion is a lung injury. It is mostly caused by blunt violence, causing contusion of lung and vascular tissue. In the post−injury inflammatory response, capillary permeability increases, inflammatory cell aggregates and inflammatory mediators are released, causing congestion and edema in the injured area. Large areas of pulmonary interstitial and alveolar edema cause breathlessness and lead to hypoxemia.

7.1 Clinical Manifestations

The manifestations are dyspnea, hemoptysis, bloody frothy sputum, and pulmonary rales. Hypoxemia occurs in severe cases. It is often accompanied by flail chest. X−ray appears as flaky infiltrates, which are usually more pronounced after 24−48 hours of injury. CT has higher diagnostic accuracy.

7.2 Treatment

Principles of treatment: ①Timely treatment of combined injuries. ②Maintaining airway patency. ③Oxygen inhalation. ④Limited crystal fluid input. ⑤Patients with hypoxemia and respiratory distress are actively supported by mechanical ventilation.

In patients with pulmonary contusion who have breathing difficulty, in an emergency examination of the patient, a nasal cannula or mask is used to give 100% oxygen inhalation, while analgesics are given to relieve chest pain and facilitate breathing. After the diagnosis of X−ray chest radiograph, the patient should be further treated in the hospital. In order to prevent pulmonary contusion and inflammation, antibiotic treatment is given. For example, the development of a diffuse and villous shadow on the chest radiograph suggests a possible development of acute respiratory distress syndrome.

Chapter 8

Pulmonary Laceration

Lung laceration is a lung injury. Patients with lung laceration accompanied by visceral pleural laceration may develop into hemothorax. While with complete visceral pleural membrane, it may form intrapulmonary hematoma.

8.1 Clinical Manifestations

The lung parenchyma tear ruptures the blood vessels and the bronchus. And if communicated with the pleural cavity, it might cause hemothorax, pneumothorax, or blood pneumothorax. Blood pneumothorax is the most common in penetrating injury, and the lung parenchyma tear caused by blunt trauma is mostly located in the deep with the resulting congestion and gas accumulating somewhere to form hematoma and air cavity.

8.2 Diagnosis

The diagnosis of hemopneumothorax due to laceration of the lungs is as described above. Intrapulmonary hematoma is mostly found on chest X-ray. And the lung mass, which appears round or oval with clear edges and high density, is usually absorbed by itself from 2 weeks to several months.

8.3 Treatment

Therapeutic principles: ①Timely treatment of combined injuries. ②Maintaining airway patency. ③Oxygen inhalation. ④Limited crystal fluid input. ⑤Patients with hypoxemia and respiratory distress are actively supported by mechanical ventilation.

The complications of the lung laceration (hemangiatic, pneumothorax, or pneumothorax) should be treated accordingly. Severe pneumothorax leakage or massive hemorrhage, uneffective results from the rescue of symptomatic treatment, unstable vital signs, and progressive deterioration of the disease, should be immediately opened to sew the leaking bronchus and bleeding vessels, suture the torn lung tissue, keep the lung tissue as much as possible, and do local resection of extensively torn broken lung tissue. Thoracic closed drainage should be placed postoperatively.

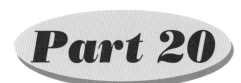

Part 20

Lungs Diseases

Chapter 1

Lung Abscess

Lung abscess is the abscess of lung tissue necrosis. The clinical features are hyperpyrexia, cough and sputum with a large number of pus and skunk. The chest X-ray image shows one or more voids containing gas and liquid. If there are multiple voids with diameter less than 2 cm, it is called necrotizing pneumonia. Pathogens may be purulent bacteria, fungi and parasites. Early pathological changes are purulent inflammation of the lung tissue, followed by necrosis and liquefaction, and finally forming abscess. Due to the widespread use of antibiotics, the incidence has decreased significantly.

Pathogens are often colonized bacteria in the upper respiratory tract and oral cavity, including aerobic anaerobic and facultative anaerobes. 90% of patients with lung abscesses are associated with infections of anaerobic bacteria with strong virulence.

Infectious substances block the bronchioles, vasculitis and small-vessel thrombosis, and pathogenic bacteria causing lung tissue purulent inflammation necrosis. The formation of lung abscess is followed by liquefaction of necrotic tissue ruptured to the bronchi. The surface of the hollow wall often has residual necrotic tissues. Lesions have a tendency to spread to the surroundings, even beyond the interlobular cleft and the adjacent lung segments. If the abscess is close to the pleura, localized fibrinous pleurisy and pleural adhesions may occur. If it is a tension abscess that ruptures into the pleural cavity, empyema or pus pneumothorax, bronchopleural fistula may form. Lung abscess could be completely absorbed, or may leave a small amount of fiber scars.

1.1 Clinical Manifestations

1.1.1 Symptoms

Patients with inhalational lung abscess often have orthodontic infection, or medical history of surgery, drunkenness, fatigue, cold and cerebrovascular disease. Acute onset, high fever (body temperature 39 – 40 ℃), with cough and sputum mucus. Inflammation involved in the parietal pleura may cause pain of the chest and is associated with breathing. When the range of lesions is large, shortness of breath may occur. There are also symptoms of systemic poisoning such as lack of energy, general malaise, and loss of appetite. If the infection is not controlled in time, it can suddenly cough up a large number of pus, phlegm and necrotic tissue in the 10–14 days after onset. In general, body temperature drops significantly after coughing up a large amount of convulsions, and the systemic toxicity symptoms decrease, and the general condition gradually returns to normal within a few weeks. If lung abscess ruptured into the pleural cavity, sudden chest pain, shortness of breath, and pus pneumothorax may appear. Blood–borne lung abscesses are more likely to have the appearance of whole–body sepsis such as chills and high fever caused by primary lesions. After a few days or weeks, coughing occurrs. The amount of sputum is small and there is little blood. Patients with chronic lung abscess often have cough, sputum, purulent sputum, recurrent fever and hemoptysis, lasting for weeks to months, accompanied with anemia, weight loss or chronic poisoning symptoms.

1.1.2　Signs

The signs are correlated to the size and location of lung abscesses. At the beginning, the lungs may have no positive signs, or may hear wet rales in the affected side. The lesions continue to develop, and bronchial breath sounds may be heard. When the abscesses of the lungs increase, an empty rale may appear. If lesions are involved in the pleura, pleural friction sound could be heard and pleural effusion liquid appears. Most of the blood–borne lung abscesses have no positive signs. Chronic lung abscesses often have clubbing fingers (toes).

1.2　Auxiliary Inspections

1.2.1　Laboratory inspections

Gram stain of sputum smear, sacral effusion and blood cultures include aerobic and anaerobic cultures, as well as antibiotic susceptibility tests are applied to identify pathogens and select effective antibiotics. Especially when pleural effusions and blood cultures are positive, the diagnostic value of pathogens is even greater.

1.2.2　X–ray examination

X–ray examination for early inflammatory shows large, dense and indistinct edges of infiltrated shadows, or thick patches of lamellae distributed in one or several segments of the lung. After the formation of necrosis and abscess, pus is excreted through the bronchus. And a round transparent area and gas–liquid plane appear in the abscess, surrounded by dense inflammatory infiltrates. The wall of the abscess is smooth or slightly irregular. After treatment with pus drainage and antibiotics, the inflammation around the lung abscess firstly absorbs, gradually shrinks to disappearance, and finally only the fibrous strand shadow remains. The wall of chronic lung abscess cavity is thicken and irregular, sometimes with multi–room.

1.2.3　CT examination

CT is more accurate to show the location and distinguishing lung abscesses with localized empyema. Smaller abscesses and pulmonary ballooning caused by staphylococcal pneumonia are also observed. And it is helpful for postural drainage and surgical treatment.

1.2.4　Fiberoptic bronchoscopy

It helps to clarify the cause and etiological diagnosis, and also could be used for treatment. If impurities are present in the airway, it could be taken out to drain the airway. If it is suspected to be tumor, pathological specimens may be taken. It also could be used to take sputum for laboratory bacteria culture. Catheter could be inserted through a fiberoptic bronchoscope, as close to or into the abscess cavity to attract pus to flush bronchus and injection of antibiotics to improve efficacy and shorten the course of the disease.

1.3　Differential Diagnosis

Patients, with a history of oral surgery, coma, vomiting, or impurities inhalation, sudden chills, high fever, cough and sputum with a large number of pus and stench, have a significant increase in the total number of leukocytes and neutrophils. And the X-ray shows thick and inflammatory shadows which have a cavity gas-liquid plane. There are cutaneous purulent lesions such as psoriasis, endocarditis in intravenous drug users, fever, cough, sputum and other symptoms. In combination with X-ray showing multiple lung abscesses in both lungs, it could be diagnosed as blood-borne lung abscesses. Blood cultures, including anaerobic cultures and antibiotic susceptibility tests, are important for determining the cause and the selection of antibiotics. Lung abscesses should be differentiated from the following diseases.

1.3.1　Bacterial pneumonia

The symptoms of early lung abscess and bacterial pneumonia are very similar in X-ray films. Streptococcus pneumoniae is commonly accompanied by cold sores, rust stains, and no large amounts of purulent sputum. X-ray shows lesions of the lobe or segments, with blurred edges. When the patients with pneumonia is treated with antibiotics, the fever does not retreat, but the cough increases with coughing up a lot of pustules, which should be diagnosed as lung abscess.

1.3.2　Secondary infection with tuberculosis

The onset of pulmonary tuberculosis is slow, long duration, long-term coughing, lack of strength, sweating, loss of appetite, or repeated bleeding. The chest X-ray shows a thicker hollow wall, no air-fluid plane, less inflammatory lesions around the hole, commonly accompanied by cords, squatting spots and nodular foci or disseminated lesions in other parts of the lungs. When it is combined with lung infections, symptoms of acute infections and coughing of purulent sputum occurs.

1.3.3　Bronchial lung cancer

Bronchial obstruction in bronchial lung cancer often causes distal pulmonary suppurative infection, but the course of lung abscess formation is relatively long. Obstructive infections treated with antibiotics are not effective because of poor bronchial drainage. Therefore, for patients over 40 years old who have recurrent infections in the same part of the lungs and poor antibiotic spasm, should consider the possibility of bronchial lung cancer which causes obstructive pneumonia. Sputum could be sent for checking cancer cells and fiberoptic bronchoscopy to confirm the diagnosis. Lung squamous cell carcinoma also occurs necrosis and liquefaction with forming a cavity, but generally with no toxicity or acute infection symptoms. And X-ray shows thicker wall cavity, residual tumor tissue making the inner wall uneven, less inflammatory infiltration area around the hole, and swollen hilar lymph nodes, hence it is not difficult to distinguish with lung abscess.

1.4　Treatment

1.4.1　Antibiotic treatment

Aspiration lung abscesses with anaerobic infections is generally sensitive to penicillium. Penicillin dosage can be determined according to the severity of the disease, and intravenously drip into the necrotic tissues. Body temperature generally falls to normal within 3-10 days, and then it can be changed to intramuscular injection. If the efficacy of penicillin is not approving, clindamycin 0. 6-1. 8 g/d, or metronidazole 0. 4 g, 3 times/day orally or intravenously. Other antibiotics such as carbapenems and beta-lactam/beta-lactamase inhibitors may also be used.

Blood-borne pulmonary abscesses are mostly infected with staphylococci and streptococci, and penicillin or cephalosporin resistant to β-lactamases may be used. MRSA infection should choose vancomycin or teicoplanin or linezolid.

The antibiotic treatment lasts for 6-8 weeks, or until the abscess and inflammation could not be observed on the X-ray, or with only a small amount of residual fibrosis.

1.4.2　Drainage of pus

It is an effective measure to improve the curative effect. For patients with uneasy to cough up viscous sputum are suggested to use expectorant or bronchodilator to facilitate fluid drainage. Those who are in better physical condition may adopt positional drainage, 2-3 times/day, 10-15 minutes each time. Bronchofiberscope is also very effective for irrigationand suction.

1.4.3　Surgical treatment

1.4.3.1　Surgical indications

(1) The abscess cavity does not shrink after 3 months of medical treatment, or the abscess cavity is too large (5 cm or more) and not easy to occlude.

(2) Major blood transfusion is ineffective or life-threatening.

(3) It is accompanied by bronchoceramic fistula, or drainage and irrigation are ineffective.

(4) Bronchial obstruction restricts airway drainage, such as lung cancer. For those who are unable to tolerate the operation, catheter may be inserted into the abscess cavity through the chest wall to drain. Patients should be evaluated before surgery for general conditions and lung function.

1.4.3.2　Pneumonectomy

Indications: ①Pulmonary tuberculosis voids. ②Tuberculous spherical lesions (tubercular tuberculosis). ③Damaged lungs. ④Tuberculous bronchial stenosis or bronchodilation scarring causing atelectasis in the lung or lobe. ⑤Repeated or persistent hemoptysis. ⑥Other indications: for instance, there are still rows of bacteria after thoracoplasty, etc.

Contraindications: ①Pulmonary tuberculosis is expanding or in the active period. ②General condition and the cardiopulmonary compensatory capacity are poor. ③Combining with tuberculosis in other extra-pulmonary organs.

Complications: ①Bronchial pleural fistula: the incidence of tuberculosis patients is high. ②Obstinate thoracic cavity with residual gas: most of the patients are asymptomatic. This cavity can maintain sterility.

③Empyema: it is caused by the residual gas after lung resection of tuberculosis, and its incidence is much higher than that of non-tuberculosis patients. ④Tuberculosis dissemination: no effective anti-tuberculosis drug treatment on preparation before surgery, active tuberculosis without effectively controlling, surgical anesthesia trauma affecting poor postoperative complications with bronchial thrombosis, etc. , and those which lead to tuberculosis spread.

1.4.3.3　Thoracectomy

Thoracic angioplasty involves the subperiosteal resection of different numbers of rib segments, which results in the subsidence of the soft tissue of the chest wall and the collapse of the underlying lungs. This is a collapse therapy. The operation can be completed in one or several stages. The bones are removed from the top to the bottom, and no more than 3-4 assistive bones are removed at a time. After compression, the chest is tied to avoid abnormal respiratory movements of the thorax.

The operation is mainly applicable to those patients whose lesions are limited, but general condition is poor and can not tolerate lobectomy, or lesions are extensive and can not tolerate one-sided pneumonectomy. The surgery has been rarely used in the past 30 years due to its limited efficacy.

Chapter 2

Spontaneous Pneumothorax

Spontaneous pneumothorax is a condition in which there is no trauma or anthropogenic factors. Pulmonary and visceral pleura are ruptured due to lung disease, and pulmonary and bronchial air escapes into the visceral pleura. The disease belongs to emergency thoracic surgery, and severe cases can be life-threatening but could be cured in time.

It is divided into primary and secondary pneumothorax. The most common cause of primary pneumothorax is the rupture of the sub-pulmonary bullae at the apex of the lung, which occurs mostly in young adults aged 25-30. The common cause of secondary pneumothorax is obstructive lung disease, such as chronic bronchitis, emphysema, tuberculosis, etc., mostly occurring in elderly patients aged 60-65 years. In addition, there are rare cases of menopausal pneumothorax and infant pneumothorax. In recent years, the incidence of spontaneous pneumothorax has increased at home and abroad, and primary pneumothorax is higher than that of secondary pneumothorax. Some researchers believe that due to the wide application of antibiotics, the cure rate of pulmonary infectious diseases is significantly increased, and the remaining pulmonary fibrosis, calcification, and proliferative pathological changes are correspondingly increased.

2.1 Pathology

It is generally believed that the disease is caused by tuberculosis. Currently, it is proposed that most cases of spontaneous pneumothorax are caused by alveolar rupture of subpleural emphysema, and are also found in subpleural lesions or hollow collapse, and tearing of pleural adhesions.

In most cases, spontaneous pneumothorax is due to rupture of subpleural anesthesia bubble, which could be congenital or acquired; the former is caused by congenital elastic fiber dysplasia, and the elasticity of alveolar wall decreases, resulting in expansion to form lung bullae. The latter is commonly formed on the basis of obstructive emphysema or fibrous lesions after inflammation. The bronchioles are half-obstructed and distorted, resulting in the formation of emphysema bubbles. The swollen emphysema bubbles degenerate due to nutrition and circulatory disturbances. The behavior of cough, sneezing, blowing, holding the air, pulling hard, laughing loudly, and strenuous exercise, increases the alveolar pressure, eventually leading to rupture of emphysema bubble, and formation of spontaneous pneumothorax.

2.2　Clinical Manifestations

It usually starts suddenly, with or without force to increase the incentive for chest pressure. 40% –60% of patients develop after severe cough, and a small number of patients may also be induced by physical activity, forced bowel movements, laxatives, and weight–bearing. Clinical manifestations of spontaneous pneumothorax is not typical, the symptoms could be light or heavy. Common manifestations include sudden chest pain, thoracic pack, shortness of breath, difficulty breathing, etc. , severe irritability, sweating, cyanosis, rapid breathing, rapid pulse, and even shock. A small number or localized pneumothorax shows no positive signs.

2.3　Auxiliary Inspections

2.3.1　Chest X–ray examination

Chest X–ray is the simplest and most reliable method for diagnosing pneumothorax. It shows the degree of lung atrophy, presence of pleural adhesions, mediastinal displacement, and pleural effusion. The typical X–ray findings of pneumothorax are that gas accumulates on the outside of the thoracic cavity or the tip of the lung, the translucency increases, there is no lung texture, and the lung collapses into a spherical shape toward the hilum. In a small amount of pneumothorax, the accumulation of gas is mostly limited to the apex of the lungs and the iliac crest. At this point, deep exhalation X–ray signs help diagnose. Some patients with spontaneous pneumothorax appear as "localized pneumothorax" due to separation of pleural adhesions.

2.3.2　Thoracic CT

It should be performed on patients with poorly repeated treatment of chest pneumothorax with chest CT and with irregular lung compression. Basically, there is a very low density of gas in the pleural cavity, accompanied by varying degrees of compression and atrophy in the lung tissue. Chest CT is more sensitive to the diagnosis of a small amount of gas in the chest. At the same time, it can be observed whether the lung edge has caused pneumothorax lesions, such as bullae, pleural adhesions.

2.3.3　Arterial blood gas examination

Due to the collapse of lung, patients forms ineffective perfusion, causing hypoxemia. In general, young and middle–aged adults are generally hypoxemic when their lungs are compressed by 20% –30% or more.

2.3.4　Pulmonary function tests

Pneumothorax may be limited to ventilatory damage when compressed more than 20%. The elderly pneumothorax often has severe pulmonary dysfunction when the compression of lung is less than 20% because of the underlying diseases. Patients with clinically suspected pneumothorax should not perform pulmonary function tests with forced respiration to avoid deterioration of the disease.

2.4   Differential Diagnosis

It is not difficult to diagnose spontaneous pneumothorax clinically. The main gist is as following: sudden chest pain, difficulty breathing, ipsilateral chest full, percussion drum sounds, auscultation breath sounds weakened or disappeared. Gas in the chest cavity could be observed by X-ray.

However, the clinical manifestations of it are often not typical, especially secondary pneumothorax is easily covered by primary disease and misdiagnosed. Therefore, the possibility of pneumothorax should be identified in the following cases: ①Sudden unexplained dyspnea, or sudden increase in shortness of breath on the basis of the original dyspnea. ②Sudden severe chest pain with dyspnea, with the exception of myocardial infarction and pulmonary infarction. ③Unexplained disease progression, short-term palpitation, sweating, pale or cyanosis, mentally handicapped. ④Sudden increase in symptoms of asthma, lungs or lungs full of wheeze, and all kinds of antispasmodic drugs and other treatment ineffective. ⑤Rapid or progressive aggravated hairpin. When those occur, chest X-rays should be quickly scheduled to confirm the diagnosis. In addition, spontaneous pneumothorax sometimes needs to be differentiated from the following diseases.

2.4.1   COPD exacerbations

Patients with spontaneous pneumothorax have prominent shortness of breath and are mostly suddenly or progressively aggravated, while cough and sputum are correspondingly milder. The exacerbation of COPD often involves climate change as a predisposing factor and respiratory infection as the leading factor. Outstanding performance is cough, aggravated cough, purulent sputum. X-ray examination helps confirm the diagnosis.

2.4.2   Lung bullae

Small or localized pneumothorax sometimes need to distinguish with lung bullae. Huge lung bullae may have chest tightness, shortness of breath and other symptoms, but these symptoms are gradually emerging. Clinical manifestations of lung bullae are relatively stable. Chest X-ray films shows that the lungs are compressed, showing increased brightness in the lesion area, sometimes occupying most of the thoracic cavity, but fine striae are still visible in areas with increased brightness.

2.4.3   Pleural effusion

Patients with pleural effusion often show chest pain and shortness of breath, but physical examination and X-ray examination for the effusion sign is different from pneumothorax.

2.4.4   Myocardial infarction and pulmonary infarction

The clinical manifestations of tension pneumothorax are sometimes similar to myocardial infarction and pulmonary infarction, manifesting as sudden severe chest pain, shortness of breath, difficult to breath, palpitation, pale or cyanotic, profuse irritability, etc., but tension pneumothorax shows significant thoracic pneumatosis sign on the affected side and contralateral tracheal displacement help to identify, and X-ray examination also helps.

2.4.5   Bronchial asthma

Some elderly patients with pneumothorax behave similarly to asthmatic attacks. Severe dyspnea may occur while the lungs is wheezy. Pleural effusion syndrome is ineffective for antispasmodic drugs, breathing difficulties after evacuation, and wheezing sounds are different from those of asthma. X-ray examinations are helpful for identification.

2.5   Treatment

The purpose for the treatment of spontaneous pneumothorax is to close the air leak with minimal trauma, surgical complications and mortality, and cost, to promote lung recruitment, and to minimize the recurrence. Therefore, different methods need to be taken according to factors such as the etiology of the patient, the course of the disease, the number of previous episodes, the occupation of the patient, and the general condition of the patient.

(1)General treatment

Including bed rest, limited activities, given oxygen, analgesic, cough, if necessary, given a small amount of sedative drugs, anti-infective treatment given when infected. If there is shock, it should be corrected as soon as possible, in addition to the general anti-shock measures. The shock, caused by tension pneumothorax, should be an emergency suction decompression; blood pneumothorax caused by hemorrhagic shock should be treated.

(2)Emergency treatment

For mild spontaneous pneumothorax (< 20%), if the patient is in good health and is asymptomatic, it can be observed non-surgically until it is absorbed. If the pneumothorax is compressed and the lung is compressed by more than 20%, it should be decompressed by suction to promote lung recruitment.

(3)Surgical treatment

Surgical treatment of spontaneous pneumothorax involves the removal of ruptured bullae and the underlying lesions that cause the lung bullae. The adhesion of the visceral wall to the visceral wall is facilitated by spraying the adhesion agent in the pleural wall or thorax. The binding of cellulose or fiberboard to the lungs promotes lung recruitment.

2.6   Complications

The diagnosis, treatment and prevention of complications are as follows.

(1)Hemostasis

It is mostly induced by pneumothorax attacks caused by vascular tear in the pleural adhesions. The condition could be light and heavy, and correlated to tearing blood vessels.

(2)Pleural effusion

The incidence of pleural effusion is 30%-40%, more than 3-5 days after the onset of pneumothorax. The effusion not only aggravates the lung collapse, but is also easy to develop into pus pneumothorax.

(3)Mediastinal emphysema

The air enters the mediastinum along the bronchial and pulmonary vascular beds to form mediastinal emphysema, usually without causing serious consequences. However, other causes of mediastinal emphysema, such as respiratory injury or esophageal perforation must be excluded.

(4)Pneumothorax

Secondary pneumothorax due to lung infection is easy to develop into pneumothorax.

Chapter 3

Benign Lung Tumors

3.1 Hamartoma

It is suggested that hamartoma is a congenital tumor-like abnormality, but not a true tumor, is possibly the abnormal mixture of normal brain tissue components. However, in recent years, most of researchers believe that hamartoma is a real tumor, derived from undifferentiated mesenchymal cells from the bronchus, and is a true benign mesenchymal tumor.

Pulmonary hamartoma is mostly solitary, with a regular and round morphology, clear at borders and sometimes lobulated, with a thin layer of fiber capsules and easily exfoliated from the lungs. The surface is yellow-white, translucent, hard and brittle, and in a few cases, it has spot-like calcification or ossification, and part of it has mucus. Most of the intraluminal tumors are polyps with a smooth surface. The pedicles with different widths are connected to the bronchial mucosa. Generally, they do not invade into the bronchial wall. The tumors are semi-occluded or completely obstructed in the lumen, resulting in secondary lesions. The components of hamartoma are extremely complicated and are mainly cartilage and fibrous tissues.

3.1.1 Clinical manifestations

Pulmonary hamartomas are mostly asymptomatic patients. The physical manifestations are pulmonary masses that are found on physical examinations, sometimes manifested as chest pains. The bronchodilators may cause obstruction of the lumen, manifested as cough with sputum and blood, repeated or persistent lung infections, atelectasis, etc. , similar to symptoms in lung cancer or tuberculosis.

3.1.2 Diagnosis and differential diagnosis

The diagnosis of pulmonary hamartoma is based on chest X-ray examination. The length of hamartoma is slowly increased, and there is no remarkable change in long-term follow-up with X-ray. The imaging features of pulmonary dysplasia are round or elliptical shadows with smooth edges and uneven density. There may be centrums, no infiltration around, and no satellite foci. "Popcorn-like" calcification and fat density are characteristic imaging manifestations of peripheral pulmonary hamartoma. Intrabronchial tumors are difficult to detect on chest X-ray films, and most of them appear lung consolidation, atelectasis, repeated or persistent infections at the distal end of the lesion, and bronchoscopy and biopsy are used to confirm the diagnosis. Peripheral pulmonary hamartoma can be diagnosed by biopsy. Pulmonary hamartoma should be identified with the following diseases.

(1) Tuberculosis

Pulmonary tuberculosis is commonly accompanied by empty ball, multiple calcifications, drainage of bronchial disease and satellite lesions.

(2) Peripheral lung cancer

X-ray findings are very similar to those of early-stage lung cancer, especially those with no hamartoma characteristics are difficult to identify before surgery. Hamartoma is often accompanied by calcification, and there are no signs of pleural depression and edge burr, voids and lymph node enlargement, hemoptysis, weight loss and other characteristics of lung cancer.

(3) Inflammatory pseudotumor

Pulmonary hamartoma is often mistaken for pneumonic pseudotumor, except for the lack of specific symptoms and signs. The imaging may be a mass of shadow, remains unchanged for a long time. However, inflammatory pseudotumors could be observed in the CT film.

3.1.3 Treatment

Pulmonary hamartoma is a benign tumor, but it is easily missed diagnosis of early peripheral lung cancer. Therefore, it is generally advocated that it is difficult to differentially diagnose for surgical treatment. The exploratory section of the chest should be explored as soon as possible so as to confirm the diagnosis. Diffuse pulmonary hamartoma is feasible for pneumonectomy. However, multiple pulmonary hamartomas tend to be treated non-surgically. In recent years, with the development of minimally invasive surgery, the use of video-assisted thoracoscopic surgery (VATS) for pulmonary wedge resection has been performed. It has the advantages of less trauma and bleeding, and rapid recovery, especially in lung function.

3.2 Fibroids

Pulmonary fibroma is a benign tumor that occurs in the fibrous tissue of the lungs and is rarely seen. Fibroids are hard, grayish, and sometimes cystic, and are located in deep lung tissues but not connected to adjacent blood vessels and bronchi.

(1) Clinical manifestations

Pulmonary fibroids generally do not have obvious symptoms, usually observed on physical examination. X-ray shows a dense shadow of the edge and with a relatively smooth border.

(2) Diagnosis

Microscopically, the edges of the tumors are neat without capsules. It is composed of irregularly arranged collagen capsules and spindle-shaped fibroblasts. The nucleus grows with unevenly distributed chromatin. The center of the tumor is glassy, showing no ossification or outward diffusion.

(3) Differential diagnosis

If physical examination reveals isolated lung shadows with neat borders, pulmonary fibroids should be diagnosed. The confirming diagnosis depends on pathological examinations. It should be distinguish with early lung cancer, pulmonary tuberculosis, and pulmonary leiomyoma.

(4) Treatment

Surgery is the primary method to excise it.

3.3 Leiomyoma

Pulmonary leiomyoma is a benign tumor that originates from the pulmonary blood vessels, bronchus, and the smooth muscle of the surrounding lung parenchyma. According to the organization of the source is generally divided into endobronchial, pulmonary vascular and lung parenchymal. Lung leiomyomas are mostly single tumors.

The pathogenesis of pulmonary leiomyoma is not yet clear. Some scholars believe that pulmonary leiomyoma occurs in the process of fiber scar formation in the lungs. In gross specimens, tumors are generally round or round-like, and gray in color. Microscopically, the tumor cells are generally spindle-shaped, parallel or cross-arranged, the cellular membrane is clear, the nucleus is generally rod-shaped. Smooth muscle cells stained with Van-Gieson are yellow and could be differentiated from fibroids and neurofibromas. Typical histological diagnosis is not difficult, electron microscopy and immunohistochemistry could be differentiated from other spindle cell tumors.

(1) Clinical manifestation

Lung leiomyomas are most common in middle and young adults, and the average age of the patient is about 35 years old. There are no obvious symptoms, and usually found by accident. A small number of patients are diagnosed with symptoms of cough and chest pain.

(2) Diagnosis

Chest X-ray examination is the preferred method of diagnosing it. Smooth muscle tumors are located in the lung parenchyma, the body is mostly round with clear border but no burr sign. In some cases, the trachea oppression and obstruction could be observed. There are no enlarged lymph nodes in hilar and mediastinum. Definitive diagnosis requires pathological confirmation after surgical resection.

(3) Treatment

Surgical resection is generally required. A small number of endobronchial lesions with no distal lung parenchymal lesions could be excised by fiberoptic bronchoscopy. A single leiomyoma should be surgical resection depending on tumor size and location. In the lung, especially for pulmonary nodules, the method of thoracoscopic lung wedge resection has obvious advantages such as less trauma and quicker recovery.

Chapter 4

Lung Cancer

Most of the lung cancers originate from the epithelium of the bronchial mucosa, and therefore also known as bronchopulmonary carcinomas. The incidence of lung cancer in the world has increased significantly. In the big cities of China, the incidence of lung cancer has occupied the first place in all kinds of tumors in men. The etiology of lung cancer is still unclear. Distribution of lung cancer in the right lung is more than the left lung, and in the upper lobe is more than that in the lower lobe.

4.1 Clinical Types

It is clinically divided into the following four types:

(1)Squamous cell carcinoma (SCC)

It is the most common type in lung cancer. The majority of the patients are male and over 50 years old. Most of them originate from larger bronchi. Although the differentiation degree of squamous cell carcinoma is different, the growth rate is still slow, the course of disease is longer, and is sensitive to radiotherapy and chemotherapy.

(2)Small cell carcinoma (undifferentiated small cell carcinoma)

The incidence of small cell carcinoma is lower than that of squamous cell carcinoma. It is often observed in men. It usually originates from large bronchi. Morphology of the cell is similar to small lymphocyte, like oatmeal, and is also called oatmeal cell carcinoma. It contains neuroendocrine granules in cytoplasm. It is highly malignant and fast growing. It has an earlier wide spread in lymphatic and blood circulation. It is sensitive to radiation and chemotherapy, but has poor prognosis.

(3)Adenocarcinoma

The patient of adenocarcinoma is relatively young, and the incidence is relatively common in women. Most of them originate from small bronchial epithelium, and a few from large bronchi. There are no obvious clinical symptoms in early stage, but in chest X-ray examination showing the appearance of round or elliptical lobular mass. Its growth is generally slower, but sometimes blood metastases occur at early stage and lymphatic metastasis occurs later.

(4)Large cell carcinoma

This type of lung cancer is rare, with about a half originating from the bronchi. The carcinoma cells are large, the cytoplasm is rich, and the nuclear is diverse and irregular. The differentiation of large cell carcinoma is low and is often detected after brain metastasis. The prognosis is poor. In addition, a few cases have different types of cancerous tissues, such as squamous cell carcinoma in adenocarcinoma, adenocarcinoma in squamous cell carcinoma or squamous cell carcinoma coexisted with small cell carcinoma.

4.2　Methods for Metastasis

There are several ways to spread and metastasize for lung cancer:

(1)Direct diffusion

After formation, the cancer grows along the bronchial wall and into the lumen of the bronchus, which can cause bronchitis. When the lumen is partially or completely blocked, it may spread directly into adjacent lung tissues through adjacent lobar lobes and pleural cavity. In addition, as the cancer continues to grow and expand, it may also invade the chest wall and other tissues in the chest and organs.

(2)Lymphatic metastasis

Lymphatic metastasis is a common way of diffusion. Small cell carcinoma may metastasize through lymph at an early stage. Squamous cell carcinoma and adenocarcinoma often spread through lymphatic metastasis.

(3)Blood metastasis

It is the manifestation of lung cancer in late stage. Hematogenous metastasis is more common in small cell carcinoma and adenocarcinoma than that in squamous cell carcinoma. Usually it directly invades the human pulmonary vein and then passes through the left heart to the organs throughout the body along with the large circulation of blood.

4.3　Clinical Manifestations

The clinical manifestations of lung cancer are closely related to the location, size, compression, invasion of adjacent organs and metastasis. Lung cancer in early stage, especially peripheral lung cancer, is usually asymptomatic and is mostly found on chest X-ray examination. Cancer in the larger bronchus after growing up, often appear irritating cough, easily mistaken for a wind cold. When the cancer continues to grow and affect drainage, secondary pulmonary infection happens with purulent sputum. Another common symptom is blood phlegm. Some patients with lung cancer may have chest tightness, wheezing, shortness of breath, fever and chest pain.

When the advanced lung cancer oppresses the adjacent organs and tissues, it may produce the following signs:①Compression or invasion of the septal nerve, causing ipsilateral muscle paralysis. ②Invasion of the laryngeal nerve, causing vocal cord paralysis and hoarseness. ③Compression of the superior vena cava, causing irritation of the facial, neck, upper limb and upper thoracic veins, edema of the subcutaneous tissue, and increased pressure of the upper limb vein. ④Sometimes the cancer invades the pleura and the chest wall, causing persistent intense chest pain. ⑤The cancer invades the mediastinum and compresses the esophagus, causing the dysphagia.

Lung cancer, also known as Pancoast's tumor, is able to invade the mediastinum and compress organs or tissues located in the upper thoracic cavity, such as the first rib, the subclavian artery and vein, the brachial plexus nerve, the cervical sympathetic nerve. Edema, brachialgia and upper limb movement disorders, ipsilateral upper eyelid drooping, pupil narrowing, enophthalmos, and other cervical sympathetic syndromes are commonly symptoms. Blood metastasis of lung cancer, depending on the invasion organs, may produce different symptoms.

4.4   Diagnosis

Early diagnosis of lung cancer is of great significance. Early treatment could get a better effect. Therefore, it should widely carry out publicity and education on cancer prevention, discourage smoking, and establish and complete the prevention and treatment network for lung cancer. Chest X-ray examination is carried out regularly for adults over 40 years old. If you do not recover from coughing for a long time or have blood sputum over the middle age, you should be vigilant and make a thorough examination. If chest X-ray finds that there is a mass shadow in the lung, the diagnosis of lung cancer should be taken into account firstly, and further detailed examination should be carried out. The opportunity of surgical treatment has been lost in definite diagnosis, so how to improve the rate of early diagnosis is a very urgent problem.

4.5   Accessory Inspections

(1)Chest X-ray and CT examination

X-ray examination is an important method for the diagnosis of lung cancer. Most of lung cancers could be radiographed via chest X-ray and CT. There are no abnormal signs on chest radiographs in early stage of central lung cancer. When the cancer blocks the bronchus, the sputum is blocked, and symptom of pneumonia occurs in the affected lung segments or lobes in the distal lung tissue. If the lumen of the bronchus is completely blocked by the cancerous tumor, atelectasis of lobe may appear. When the cancer develops to a certain size, the shadow of the hilar lung appears. As the shadow of the mass is often masked by mediastinal tissue, chest CT examination is needed. When the tumor invades adjacent lung tissue and metastasizes to hilar and mediastinal lymph nodes, there is a mass in the hilar area, or a mediastinal shadow.

(2)Sputum cytology examination

The cancer cells fell off from lung cancer is contained in sputum. In most cases, the pathological type of lung cancer can be determined. The accuracy rate of sputum examination is over 80%. Central lung cancer originating from larger bronchi, especially in cases with blood sputum, is more likely to be found in sputum.

(3) Bronchoscopy

The positive rate of bronchoscopy in the diagnosis of central lung cancer is high, and the tumor can be observed directly in the bronchial cavity.

(4) Mediastinoscopy

It directly observes the lymph nodes in the protuberance of the trachea and both sides of the bronchial region. Pathological examination is performed to determine whether lung cancer had metastasized to hilar and mediastinal lymph nodes.

(5) Positron emission tomography

Due to the abnormal glycolysis, FDG accumulates in tumor cells, showing abnormal local accumulation in PET imaging. It is used in the qualitative diagnosis of pulmonary nodules and masses. It also shows the mediastinal lymph node metastasis. At present, PET is the best and most accurate non-invasive method for the diagnosis of lung cancer.

4.6 Differential diagnosis

The differential diagnosis of lung cancer is based on the location of the tumor, the pathological type and the duration of the disease. It is easy to be confused with the following diseases.

(1)Tuberculosis

Pulmonary tuberculosis is easily confused with peripheral lung cancer. Pulmonary tuberculosis is more common in young people, the general course of the disease is longer. Lesions are often located in the posterior segment of the upper apex or the dorsal segment of the lower lobe. On the X-ray film, the mass density is not uniform, the sparse light inductive area and calcification point could be seen, and there are other scattered tuberculosis foci in the lung.

(2)Pulmonary inflammation

Obstructive pneumonia caused by early lung cancer, is easily misdiagnosed as bronchopneumonia. The symptoms of infection are obvious. The X-ray films shows blurry flaky or speckled shadows, and the density is uneven. Lung cancer is easily confused with lung abscess when central necrosis and liquefaction form cancerous cavity. Lung abscess has obvious infection symptom in acute phase, sputum amount is more and with purulent X-ray film. There are fluid plane, and pulmonary tissue or pleura around abscesses are often inflammatory. The cavity of bronchography is usually filled, and often accompanied by Trachea dilatation.

(3)Other lung tumors

Benign lung tumors, such as hamartoma, fibroma, chondroma, and sometimes need to be differentiated from peripheral lung cancer. Mediastinal lymphosarcoma is easy to be confused with central lung cancer. Mediastinal lymphosarcoma grows rapidly. Fever is common in clinic. Superficial lymph nodes in other parts are swollen. It shows bilateral trachea and hilar lymph node enlargement on the X-ray film.

4.7 Treatment

The main treatment methods of lung cancer include surgical treatment, radiotherapy, chemotherapeutic therapy, traditional chinese medicine treatment, and immunotherapy, etc. Although 80% of lung cancer patients have lost the opportunity of surgery at the time of definite diagnosis, the surgical treatment is still important and favorable.

However, none of the current treatments for lung cancer are effective. In order to improve the therapeutic effect of lung cancer, it is necessary to combine appropriate therapy with comprehensive therapy. Specific treatment options should be referred to the staging and TNM classification of lung cancer, pathological cell types, patients' cardiopulmonary function and systemic conditions, and other related factors, such as, careful and detailed comprehensive analysis before making a decision, using multidisciplinary comprehensive treatment.

4.7.1 Surgical treatment

The objective of surgical treatment is to remove, as thoroughly as possible, the primary lung cancer focus and local and mediastinal lesions lymph nodes, and as much as possible to preserve healthy lung tissue.

The extent of pneumonectomy depends on the location and size of the lesion.

4.7.2　Radiotherapy

It is a method for local elimination of lung cancer. In all types of lung cancer, small cell carcinoma is more sensitive to radiotherapy than squamous cell carcinoma, adenocarcinoma and bronchioles. Alveolar carcinoma is the lowest. According to statistics, radiotherapy alone, the 3-year survival rate is about 1000. Usually radiotherapy is combined with surgery and drug therapy in order to improve the curative rate. It is commonly used in clinic after surgery.

4.7.3　Chemotherapy

For lung cancer with low differentiation, especially small cell carcinoma, is effective. Clinically, it can be used alone in advanced lung cancer cases, to alleviate symptoms, or combining with surgery, radiotherapy and other therapy to prevent cancer metastasis and recurrence.

To improve the efficacy of chemotherapy, it is necessary to select the method of administration, determining the course of treatment, the combination of several drugs, intermittent administration, etc. It should be noted that chemical drugs are still less effective, with shorter remission period and more side effects in lung cancer.

In clinical application, the performance and dosage of drugs should be grasped, and side effects should be observed closely. In recent years, many new drugs have been designed to inhibit tumor growth based on specific targets of tumor metabolism or genes. That is, targeted therapy. At present, a variety of targeted therapeutic agents have been used in the treatment of lung cancer, but the efficacy still needs to be observed.

4.7.4　TCM treatment

According to the clinical symptoms, pulse and tongue coating of the patients, TCM treatment (traditional Chinese medicine) is applied to treat lung cancer depending on symptoms and signs.

4.7.5　Immunotherapy

In recent years, through experimental research and clinical observation, researchers find that the immune system is correlated to the growth and development of cancer, resulting in the rapid expansion of immunotherapy.

Specific measures for immunotherapy include the following:

(1)Specific immunotherapy: subcutaneously inoculated with treated autologous tumor cells or adjuvant therapy. In addition, a variety of interleukin, tumor necrosis factor, tumor ribonucleic acid and other biological products could be used.

(2)Non-specific immunotherapy: BCG, Corynebacterium brevis, transfer factor, interferon, thymus, or levamisole, etc. , are used to stimulate and enhance the immune function of human body. At present, the therapeutic effect of lung cancer is still not preferable. The long-term survival rate is low because most of the patients are in advanced stage. The prognosis is poor. Therefore, we must study and carry out new work to improve the overall effect of lung cancer treatment. To publicize and popularize the knowledge of lung cancer, to raise the vigilance of lung cancer diagnosis, to study and explore the methods of early diagnosis and to improve the early detection are urgent to implement. Moreover, further research and development of new effective drugs, improvement of comprehensive treatment methods and improved surgical techniques, are imperative as well.

Chapter 5

Metastatic Tumors of Lung

It is commonly observed that a malignant tumor originating from other parts of the body metastasizes to the lung. 20% –30% of the cases with malignant tumor (including cancer and sarcoma originating from gastrointestinal, genitourinary system, liver, bone, skin, etc.) have lung metastasis at different time points. Most of the cases metastasizes within 3 years after the onset of primary cancer, and in some cases that is 5 or 10 years after primary tumor treatment. In a few cases, lung metastases are found before primary cancer is detected.

5.1 Clinical Manifestations

Except for primary tumors, most of the clinical manifestations do not show any special clinical symptoms. It is not detected until a chest X−ray examination is performed in 10% of the patients. A few cases manifest the symptoms of cough, blood sputum, fever and dyspnea, or like that.

5.2 Diagnosis

According to the findings of chest X−ray and CT, combined with the diagnosis or disease history of primary cancer, it could be diagnosed. In most of the cases, it is multiple, varied in size, homogeneous in density, with a clear outline and round metastatic lesions. A few diseases, the X−ray findings showing only a single metastatic lesion in the lung, are similar to those of peripheral primary lung cancer. The positive rate of sputum cytology examination is very low. Bronchoscopy is not helpful for diagnosis. Sometimes, single lung metastatic tumors are difficult to distinguish with primary peripheral lung cancer.

5.3 Treatment

The treatment of pulmonary metastatic tumors is usually a manifestation of malignant tumors in advanced stage. For patients with widespread spread of metastatic tumors on both sides of the lungs, there is no surgical indication. However, surgical treatment may be performed to prolong the survival time of patients who meet the following conditions:

①The primary tumor has been thoroughly treated or controlled, and there is no local recurrence. ②Lung metastasis is not found in other parts of the body. There is only a single metastatic tumor; or, although there are several metastatic lesions, they are confined to one lobe or one side of the lung; or it is estimated that limited pneumonectomy can be performed. ③The patient is tolerated and with a preferable lung and heart function.

Surgical procedures should be based on the choice of pulmonary wedge resection, segmental resection, lobectomy, pneumonectomy; even bilateral resection through sternum median; or assisted with ultrasound scalpel for localized excision; or cryotomy. Due to the difficulty of radical resection, pneumonectomy of the whole lung is usually not performed.

Chapter 6

Primary Tumors of Mediastinum

The mediastinum is actually a space between the sternum and thoracic vertebra (including the bilateral paraspinal spine and the mediastinum on both sides). In mediastinum, there are heart, big blood vessel, esophagus, trachea, nerve, thymus, thoracic ductus, lymphoid tissues and connective adipose tissue. The mediastinum can be divided into several parts in order to identify the location of the lesion. The simple zonal method is to divide the mediastinum into the upper and lower parts by the horizontal line between the sternal angle and the lower edge of the 4th thoracic vertebra. In recent years, the mediastinal space, which contains many important organs, has been called the "visceral organ mediastinum". The mediastinal space in front of the pericardium and trachea is called anterior mediastinum, and that behind of the pericardium and trachea (including esophagus and paraspinal mediastinum) is called posterior mediastinum. Clinically, these two types of division are often combined to determine the location of the lesion.

6.1 Clinical Types

There are many tissues and organs in mediastinum, so there are many kinds of primary or metastatic tumors in mediastinal region. Benign tumors are more common in primary tumors, but some of them are malignant.

(1) Neurogenic tumors originated from sympathetic nerve and a few from peripheral nerve. Most of these tumors are located in the paraspinal spine of posterior mediastinum, and are found on one side. There is no obvious symptom. Pains may occur when the nerve trunk is compressed or malignant erosion occurs in it.

(2) Teratoma and dermoid cystoma are primarily located in the anterior mediastinum and near the front of main vessel in the heart bottom. Teratoma is primarily substantial, with different size and number of cystoma. The wall of the cystoma is often calcified and contains epidermis, dermis and sebaceous glands in addition to connective tissues. Most of the sacs are brown yellow, mixed with sebum and cholesterol nodules, and hair. In the solid parts, there are bone, cartilage, muscle, bronchus, intestinal wall and lymphoid tissue. 10% of the teratomas are malignant.

(3) Thymoma is located in the anterior superior mediastinum. It has an elliptical or a leaf-like shape, and with clear fringe. Most of it are benign with an intact envelope. But it is often identified as potential ma-

lignance clinically. It is easy to infiltrate nearby tissues and organs. About 15% of them are combined with myasthenia gravis. Some of the degenerated residual thymus contains active growth centers, often confused in the adipose tissues of anterior trachea, inferior thyroid gland, hilus of the lung, and pericardium.

6.2　Clinical Manifestations

Generally, positive signs of mediastinal tumor are rare. The symptoms are associated with tumor size, location, growth direction, speed, texture, and nature, etc. Because of its slow growth, benign tumor may grow to a considerable size in the direction of the chest cavity without symptom or with mild symptoms. On the contrary, if malignant tumors erode and progress rapidly, the symptoms emerges earlier.

6.3　Symptoms

The common symptoms include chest pain, chest tightness, irritation or compression of the respiratory system, nervous system, large vessels, and esophagus. Besides, some specific symptoms correlated to cancer also occur.

(1) Compression of the nervous system: Horner's syndrome occurs when the sympathetic trunk is compressed, and hoarseness sound appears in the compression of recurrent laryngeal nerve; compression of the brachial plexus nerve appears upper arm numbness, pain of shoulder and foot area. Sometimes compressing the spinal cord causes paraplegia.

(2) Irritation or compression of the respiratory system: It may cause severe cough, breathing difficulties, and fever, purulent sputum or even hemoptysis in broken respiratory system.

(3) Compression of the main vessels: compression of the unnamed vein leads to increased pressure in the upper limb and jugular vein. Compression of the superior vena cava may result in superior vena cava syndrome with facial upper limb swelling, superficial jugular vein irritation, and anterior thoracic vein migration.

(4) Specific symptoms: It is significant for diagnosis, such as coughing out fine hair or bean curd-like sebum is the symptom of teratoma, etc.

6.4　Auxiliary Examinations

In addition to the clinical manifestations, the following examinations are helpful for definite diagnosis.

(1) Chest imaging is an important method in the diagnosis of mediastinal tumor. X-ray fluoroscopy could be used to observe whether the mass is moving up and down with swallowing or morphological changes with respiration. The X-ray of lateral chest shows the position, density, shape, edge clarity, smoothness, calcification or bone shadow of the tumor. CT or MRI is more successful to show the relationship between the tumor and adjacent organs. Angiocardiography or bronchography, if necessary, could be further differentiated.

(2) Ultrasound scans are helpful in differentiating parenchymal, vascular, or cystic tumors.

(3) Radionuclide of iodine scan assists in the diagnosis of retrosternal goiter.

(4) Biopsy of cervical lymph node is helpful in differentiating lymphoid tumors from other malignant tumors.

(5) Tracheoscopy, esophagoscopy and mediastinoscopy are helpful for differential diagnosis, but are seldom used.

6.5 Treatment

Except for malignant lymphoid neoplasms, most of the primary mediastinal tumors are surgically treated provided there is no other contraindications. Due to that it would gradually grow up and oppress adjacent organs, or even occurs malignant changes or secondary infections, the benign tumors or cystomas without symptoms should be treated surgically. If malignant mediastinal tumors invade adjacent organs or with distant metastasis, and resection is contraindicated, should be treated with radiotherapy or chemotherapeutic agents according to pathological properties.

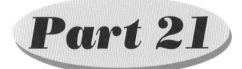

Part 21

Diseases of Esophagus

Chapter 1

Perforation

Esophageal perforation is a serious surgical emergency disease. It is extremely rare, and early symptoms are similar to those of emergency diseases in the chest and abdomen. The diagnosis and treatment are often delayed, resulting in an unfavorable outcome in some cases.

1.1 Pathogeny

Esophageal perforation and rupture could be classified according to its location and etiology. According to esophageal anatomy, it could be divided into cervical, chest and abdomen perforation. According to the etiological classification, it could be divided into the following categories: ①Spontaneous rupture. ②Iatrogenic rupture, such as esophagoscopy, dilatation therapy, intraoperative esophageal injury, etc. ③Traumatic rupture, such as bullet penetrating injury, swallowing foreign body, knife stabbing, swallowing corrosion agent, etc. ④Internal diseases of the esophagus, such as tumor, diverticulum and ulcers, etc.

Spontaneous esophageal perforation occurs due to any sudden increase in internal pressure of the esophagus that causes the internal and external pressure difference to reach a certain value in a short time. If the esophagus has basic pathological changes, it is more prone to rupture. In addition, when neurogenic diseases such as alcoholism or central nervous system are suppressed, the autonomic nervous activity is unbalanced, and the loss of esophagus and the cardia function also lead to the rupture of the esophagus.

Severe vomiting caused by various causes is the most common cause of spontaneous rupture of esophagus. It is often seen in overeating. Other causes include coughing, asthma, strong swallowing, choking, sneezing, intestinal obstruction, childbirth, pregnancy vomiting, seizures, weightlifting, and hypoglycemia. All these factors cause sudden increase in intra-abdominal pressure, forcing gastric contents to rush rapidly into the inner wall of the esophagus. There are also ruptures due to abnormal esophageal physiology or chronic wall inflammation such as chronic inflammation of the esophagus.

1.2   Diagnosis

1.2.1   Clinical manifestations

The clinical manifestations of spontaneous rupture of the esophagus is not specific, most of which are suffering from unbearable pain in the chest or upper abdomen after full meal or drunken emesis, usually severe tearing or knife cutting pain, pain aggravating with respiratory swallowing, and radiating to the back of the shoulder and after the sternum. Followingly, there is chest tightness, shortness of breath, dyspnea and pain, pleural dissection, pneumothorax, fluid pneumothorax, and so on. There are also subcutaneous emphysema in the chest and neck. The trachea is shifted to the healthy side. The upper abdomen may have signs of peritonitis. But subcutaneous emphysema does not necessarily occur rapidly after onset, and there is no subcutaneous emphysema when it is broken directly into the chest. Mediastinal burst sounds can be heard and sometimes are mistaken for pericardial fricative sounds. Most patients have liquid pneumothorax. If combined with mediastinal pleural infection, fever, septicemia and septic shock may occur. Typical clinical manifestations are vomiting, lower chest pain and subcutaneous emphysema, known as Mackler triad, which is asymptomatic in about 40% of cases.

The main clinical manifestations of esophagus perforation caused by foreign body of esophagus are as follows: subcutaneous emphysema, chest pain, high fever, swelling of the neck and tenderness, and periesophagitis, periesophagus abscess or mediastinum infection, etc.

(1) Trauma perforation injury in cervical esophagus is lighter than that in thoracic esophagus, and the prognosis is better. The early symptoms of cervical esophageal perforation include neck stiffness, local pain and vomiting. Patients often complain of neck suffocation, swallowing or head movement aggravating pain, open injury (overflow immediately from the neck wound after drinking water). The patient may have dysphonia. If the esophageal injury is not found, there will be local abscess and cervical esophageal fistula, but the signs will be obvious after 24 h. Body examination shows neck stiffness, local subcutaneous emphysema and fullness and mainly between the trachea and sternocleidomastoid muscle, and touch tenderness.

(2) Perforation and rupture of the thoracic esophagus are often found late, because their symptoms and signs are often masked by other signs of thoracic injury. The main harm of thoracic esophageal injury is the sucking effect caused by the surrounding chest negative pressure, so that the fluid in the esophagus and even the stomach is inhaled into the mediastinum and the pleural cavity. The patient is often in critical condition with symptoms of severe chest pain, extreme dyspnea, shortness of breath, and shock. Another symptom is swallowing pain, the patient will automatically spit out the saliva without swallowing. Hematemesis is also a signal worthy of attention needed emergency endoscopy check. Mediastinal emphysema may occur due to the injury of mediastinal tissue in the patient who had mediastinal inflammation in the past. More than half of the patients have subcutaneous emphysema on the neck and face in 1–12 h after injury. Perforation or rupture of the lower esophagus is usually confined to the upper abdomen and the lower part of the sternum and abdominal muscle spasm. At this time, it is most likely to be misdiagnosed as peptic ulcer perforation. In many cases, exploratory laparotomy is performed. Pain may also be misdiagnosed as myocardial infarction or acute pancreatitis.

(3) Endoscopic examination, esophageal dilatation, esophageal catheterization and even other thoracic surgery, such as mediastinal tumor removal or lobectomy, may cause iatrogenic esophageal rupture due to inadvertent operation or potential esophageal lesions. Major manifestations include esophageal endoscopy injury occuring mostly in the cervical esophagus, swallowing pain after endoscopy, and neck tenderness and subcutaneous emphysema. The damage caused by dilatation in the treatment of esophageal stricture or achalasia after the dilatation, the sternum or back pain and body temperature rise, and shock, even dyspnea, cyanosis and death may appear in severe cases. If the esophagus is injured by other thoracic operations, a large number of abnormal pleural drainage fluid may appear in the early postoperative period, or pleural effusion, high fever and other symptoms and signs may appear in the later period. Tracheoesophageal fistula after blunt chest trauma is a unique type of trauma. Coughing after swallowing is a characteristic symptom. Tracheo-esophageal fistula was found only in 0.001% of blunt chest injuries. The most common site was above the carina and the formation of fistula was related to severe blunt chest wall injuries. At the same time, the patient developed a serious and widespread infection and was quickly trapped in respiratory failure. If the patient could not be diagnosed in time or if it is not diagnosed promptly and correctly, the patient will die within 24–36 h after injury.

1.2.2　Auxiliary examination

The main manifestations of esophagus perforation or rupture in imageological examination are as follows:①mediastinal emphysema and subcutaneous emphysema. ②the widening of the mediastinum or the horizontal shadow in the mediastinum. ③pleural effusion. ④liquid pneumothorax. ⑤atelectasis and pneumonia. But the above signs are not specific. The first sign of cervical esophageal perforation is subcutaneous emphysema, which occurs on the injured side of the esophagus and expands gradually.

The free gas could be observed in the soft tissue space of the neck on the X-ray film. Thoracic esophageal rupture or perforation shows mediastinal emphysema, subcutaneous emphysema and pleural effusion. In some cases, there may be pericardial effusion, and even a "floating food sign" with diagnostic value. The chest plain film at the early stage of this disease shows "V" sign (near the paraspinal or left posterior border).

Upper gastrointestinal angiography is the most practical way to confirm diagnosis. Not only the location, size and scope of the break, but also the esophageal cancer, esophageal diverticulum and other lesions could be identified. Although esophagography is the best way to determine the esophagus perforation, it is found that the negative rate is as high as 10% with the possible reasons that the contrast medium is too thick and is not easy to overflow (such as barium); the contrast agent passes too fast (such as meglumine); The rift is in oedema, clotted or stuffed by the clots or food blocks. Therefore, negative results could not exclude the possibility of esophageal perforation.

In addition, methods for determining perforation or rupture of the esophagus include CT and fiberoptic endoscopy. The CT examination shows the manifestations of esophageal rupture: the soft tissue gas that surrounds the esophagus in the mediastinum, the adjacent esophagus with a septic cavity located in the mediastinum or thoracic cavity, and traffic between the inflatable esophagus, and the liquid and gas chamber in the mediastinum or mediastinum. The chest CT shows the density of the pleural effusion in the thoracic cavity which is obviously better than that by the chest film, and the pleural effusion with uneven density could be used as a sign that is different from other causes. The CT examination is also useful for the follow-up observation of the patients who have been treated. The post-or non-surgical treatment of patients in the thoracic cavity is also helpful.

It is controversial on the diagnosis of esophageal perforation or rupture by esophagoscopy. In some selective cases, fiberoptic endoscopy could accurately diagnose perforation and determine the location of the perforation. It is most suitable for patients with traumatic esophageal perforation. If esophagography and other examinations could not be confirmed, endoscopy is still a good method to determine esophageal rupture, but appeals to be carefully operated, or applyed in patients with hematemesis.

Other diagnostic methods include blue staining of pleural effusion could be observed with thoracic drainage tube or pleural puncture after oral administration of methylene blue diluted solution. There is another simple and effective method to confirm the diagnosis by the presence of food residue and gastric juice in the thoracic puncture and the closed drainage of the thoracic cavity, or the concentrated juice of the liquid with special odor, the increase of amylase, and the discovery of squamous epithelial cells from the salivary glands. However, some patients with esophageal rupture could not get the blue staining fluid by puncture at one time. Therefore, 1-2 times of chest puncture without blue staining fluid could not exclude the possibility of esophagus perforation or rupture.

1.2.3　Differential diagnosis

The perform of esophagus perforation is often similar to that of other cardiac and gastrointestinal diseases, and it should be identified with myocardial infarction, aortic dissecting aneurysm, peptic ulcer perforation, acute pancreatitis, acute appendicitis, pleuritis, spontaneous pneumothorax, pulmonary embolism, etc.

1.3　Treatment

There are two kinds of treatments for esophageal perforation or rupture: non-operative treatment and surgical treatment. The following factors should be taken into consideration: the causes of the injury in the esophagus, the site of the injury, the lesion of the esophagus, the time and distance of the diagnosis and treatment of the perforation or rupture, the destruction of the esophagus, the extent and scope of the intrathoracic pollution, the injury of the adjacent tissue, the age and general condition of the patients. The purpose of any treatment is to prevent further infection and necrosis of perforated tissue, to reduce pollution in adjacent areas, and to restore the integrity and continuity of the stomach and intestines and nutritional support.

1.3.1　Principles of treatment

It is difficult to control the inflammation of the mediastinum and the pleural cavity in the endoluminal secretions and gastric contents after the esophagus rupture. Therefore, infection is the main cause of the high mortality of the disease. To remove the source of infection as soon as possible, carry out effective drainage, restore the continuity of the esophagus, take early operation, simultaneously give effective antibiotics to control infection and adequate nutritional support, promote the healing of the fissure, and reduce the occurrence of complications and the mortality.

1.3.2　Non-operative treatment

1.3.2.1　Indications

It is suitable for the following: ①The injury of the apparatus, especially in the neck of the esophagus. ②The esophagus ulcerative stenosis orcardia achalasia, after the dilatation therapy, and the small perforation after the varicosis of the esophagus, fibrosis around the esophagus, and infection limited to the mediastinum. ③A few days after the perforation of the esophagus with slight symptoms. ④Critical patients with severe esophageal rupture could not tolerate major surgery because of their long onset time, serious toxic symptoms and poor general condition.

The criteria for non-operative treatment of esophagus perforation or rupture are as follows:①The perforation of the esophagus is found late, or the perforation is small. ②The perforation of the esophagus is located in the mediastinum, or between the mediastinum and the pleura of the lungs, and the contrast agent could not freely enter the adjacent body cavity. ③The limitation of the purulent cavity, the drainage fluid could drain back through the perforation, and the pleural cavity is slightly polluted. ④Without eating after the injury to the diagnosis. ⑤Non-malignant tumor of the esophagus. ⑥The symptoms and infections are mild and the physiological disorder is not obvious.

1.3.2.2　Measures

Fasting should be done immediately so as to prohibit the food continuously flowing into the mediastinum or chest cavity. At the same time, the disturbance of acid-base balance should be corrected, nutrition support should be strengthened, and effective antibiotics should be used to control infection. Broad-spectrum antibiotics should be used at least 7-14 d.

Gastrointestinal decompression tube should be indwelled with the end of the tube staying at the perforation site of esophagus, extracting the contents of the saliva and the stomach, and flushed with saline or antibiotic solution. The closed thoracic drainage tube should be retained and the tube draining the purulent cavity could be placed under the guidance of CT, and the thoracic cavity could be washed with antibiotics and liquid through the closed thoracic drainage tube. If necessary, the thoracic cavity closed drainage tube should be placed on the upper chest for pleural irrigation.

Nutrition support treatment could be used through fistulas or deep vein nutrition. The enteral nutrition after fistulas is better than intravenous nutrition. Generally, jejunostomy is used, which not only conforms to physiology, but also prevents complications caused by deep vein nutrition, and effectively prevents reflux from gastrostomy and nasal feeding. Stomal stoma could be performed at the same time to reduce pleural and mediastinal contamination through negative pressure suction. Drainage of cervical esophagus could also be performed by lavage. The use of this method must accurately record the liquid amount of enter and exit, and is only suitable for patients who is not operated.

The esophageal stents therapy have several advantages: it is not limited by the time of the onset of the disease to the implementation of treatment; due to minimally invasive operation, it reduces the patient's pain; the cost is less, and no special equipment is needed. The weakness of esophageal stent is that the esophageal stent expands the tension resulting in the enlargement of the esophagus and failure to heal; the stent has the risk of falling off and displaced, and it is difficult to maintain a longer time to ask for the function of the fistula; the long-term expansion of the esophagus may cause the esophagus ischemic necrosis, the granulation tissue proliferation, and the complications of the esophagus, and reoperation requires removal of a larger range of esophagus which is not conducive to healing.

Surgical treatment should be actively considered during conservative treatment if the patient has signs of systemic deterioration, or if there is no obvious sign of progress within 24 hours.

1.3.3　Surgical treatment

Most of the patients have a fierce attack. Therefore, once the diagnosis is confirmed or highly suspected, surgeons should actively improve the whole body condition and make an operation at the same time. Shock is not a taboo of the operation. Blood pressure of most patients increase after opening the mediastinum to remove the stuffing. No matter the time of diagnosis for the esophagus perforation, operation should be treated actively.

1.3.3.1　Principles for surgical treatment

The principles of surgical treatment for esophagus perforation or rupture are as follows:①The early post-traumatic patients should strive for surgical treatment. And the condition of the injury, especially the degree of intrathoracic contamination, should be taken into account. ②The operation scale should be small, the procedure should be simple, the operation time should be short, and the operation indications should be strictly controlled. ③Expansion of all infected and necrotic tissues, reliable closure of the wound, prevention of fistula continued to exist, drainage of infected areas should be done.

1.3.3.2　Methods

Surgical options for esophageal perforation or rupture are as follows:①Primary repair. ②The use of other tissues to strengthen the repair. ③Esophagectomy. ④Esophagus open and bypass surgery. ⑤T tube drainage. ⑥Simple thoracic drainage.

Postoperative support therapy is important, including oxygen inhalation, blood transfusion, water electrolyte and vitamin supplementation, large doses of broad-spectrum antibiotics and nutritional support. Patients who failed to repair are not repaired again. In addition to effectively draining the chest, long-term fasting should also be done and gastric stoma should be performed for tube feeding. Jejunostomy may be more suitable for preventing postoperative gastroesophageal reflux. The location of the fistula could also be determined according to the site of the wound. Jejunostomy is used for the rupture of the lower esophagus and gastrostomy is used for the rupture of the middle esophagus and thorax.

In general, the beginning, development, and prognosis of the esophagus perforation or rupture depend on the following factors:①The causes of the trauma, such as the prognosis of the injury of the apparatus is better than that of the spontaneous esophagus rupture because it can be quickly found. ②The condition of esophageal injury, such as normal esophagus, edema, infection, erosion, ulcer, fibrosis or cancer. ③The age of the wounded. ④The location of the esophagus injury. ⑤The degree of damage and the amount of pollutants. ⑥Without combined injury. In addition to iatrogenic injuries, external esophageal trauma is rarely isolated. ⑦The time from injury to hospital and surgical treatment.

Chapter 2

Hiatal Hernia and Reflux Esophagitis

2.1　Hiatal Hernia

Esophageal hiatus hernia is a disease caused by the internal organs of the abdomen (mainly the stomach) entering the chest through the hiatus of the esophagus, accounting for 90% in diaphragmatic hernia. According to anatomical defects and clinical manifestations, it is divided into four types: sliding (Type Ⅰ), single (Type Ⅱ), mixed (Type Ⅲ) and multi-organ (Type Ⅳ) esophageal hiatus hernia. Type Ⅰ is the most common, accounting for about 95%. Type Ⅱ, Ⅲ, and Ⅳ belong to the esophageal paralysis, accounting for about 5%. The incidence of esophageal hiatus is 10%–50%, which is more common in female middle-aged and older people.

2.1.1　Clinical manifestations

(1) Symptoms

Esophageal hiatal hernia lacks specific clinical manifestations, and patients often shows burning sensation, reflux or swallowing difficulty in early stage. The symptoms of sliding esophageal hiatus hernia are similar to gastroesophageal reflux disease (GERD). Dysphagia occurs when gastric tissue that penetrates the thoracic cavity compressing the distal end of the esophagus to form a mechanical obstruction, which is more common in the esophageal fistula. Further development of paraesophageal hernia occurs with obstruction, ischemia, intestinal torsion. In huge paraesophageal hernia, even critical symptoms of cardiac compression might be present. The symptoms of chest pain, upper abdominal pain, postprandial fullness, nausea, retching and other intermittent symptoms are related to local tissue ischemia and obstruction. Sliding esophageal hiatus usually causes upper gastrointestinal bleeding due to long-term cameron erosion, or even chronic hypoferric anemia.

(2) Signs

It is manifested as pain behind the sternum or under the xiphoid. The pain is mostly burning or acupuncturing, which could be radiated to the back, shoulders, neck and so on.

2.1.2　Accessory examination

(1)X-ray inspection

It is still the main method for the diagnosis of esophageal hiatal hernia. For resectable hiatal hernia (especially mild), a negative test could not rule out the disease, clinically highly suspicious cases should be repeatedly examined at a special position, such as supine head low foot high. Barium radiography displays direct and indirect signs.

(2)Endoscopy

The accurate rate for diagnosis of esophageal hiatal hernia is higher than before by endoscopic examination. And X-ray examination is complemented to assist diagnosis.

(3)Esophageal manometry

The esophageal manometry shows an abnormal picture to assist in diagnosis of esophageal hiatus hernia.

2.1.3　Differential diagnosis

Because the esophageal hiatus hernia is relatively rare, and there are no specific symptoms and signs, the definite diagnosis is more difficult. For patients with gastroesophageal reflux symptoms, older and obese, and symptoms correlated to body position should be considered in suspicious patients. The definite diagnosis needs to be checked by some instruments.

2.1.4　Treatment

For esophageal hiatal hernia with gastroesophageal reflux symptoms, medical treatment aims to control symptoms, cure esophagitis, and improve gastrointestinal motility. Surgical treatment should be considered when medical treatment is ineffective or when the risk of serious complications such as asphyxia or strangulation might occur.

Surgical methods:

(1)Transthoracic surgery: Field exposure is superior to transabdominal incision, which would fully free the esophagus and is suitable for short esophageal type, giant and mixed hernia.

(2)Transabdominal surgery: This approach avoids the chest cavity, and the impact on cardiopulmonary function is small, and is suitable for older patients, or the body and lung function of the patient is poor, or patients with chronic aspiration pneumonia and pulmonary dysfunction.

(3)Laparoscopic hiatal hernia repair and fundoplication: With the advantages of small trauma, clear image, good vision and operation in a small space, it has quickly become the first choice for the treatment of hiatal hernia.

2.1.5　Complications

Common complications in esophageal hiatus hernia include pneumothorax, subcutaneous emphysema, perforation of esophageal or gastric wall injury, intraoperative bleeding, and vagus nerve injury.

2.2　Reflux Esophagitis

Reflux esophagitis (RE) refers to the reverse flow of gastric contents (including duodenal juice) into the esophagus, causing chronic inflammation due to damage of the esophageal mucosa which leads to esophageal ulcers, stenosis and even cancerous. Reflux esophagitis is included in gastroesophageal reflux disease, and about 1/3 of patients with GERD have RE. Reflux esophagitis occurs in people of any age, and the morbidity of adults increases with age. Middle−aged and elderly people, obesity, smoking, drinking and stress are all the high−risk groups of reflux esophagitis.

2.2.1   Clinical manifestations

(1)Symptoms

Acid reflux and heartburn are the most common symptoms of reflux esophagitis and have diagnostic significance. The clinical symptoms and complications of reflux esophagitis include the following:①Pain. Temporary tingling of the chest and back is an important symptom of esophagitis, and chest tingling is a characteristic of esophagitis. ②Bleeding. The amount of bleeding is not much, especially occurs in the night or after the meal. When the lesion has deep ulcers, a large amount of bleeding occurs. ③Esophageal stenosis. 10% of severe esophagitis cause esophageal fibrosis, resulting in esophageal stricture. ④Repeated lung infections. The stomach contents goes inversely into the throat and inhaled into the lungs inducing inflammation manifested as cough, expectoration and other symptoms. ⑤Barrett's esophagus. It is a syndrome of long−term chronic gastroesophageal reflux, some of which might develop into esophageal cancer.

(2)Signs

It manifests as burning sensation (heartburn), reflux and chest pain.

2.2.2   Auxiliary inspections

(1)X−ray examination

It could be found that the lower esophageal mucosa is not smooth, visible, narrow, and creepy. When the head is at low position, it shows that the barium in the stomach is refluxing to the esophagus. Some patients have esophageal hiatus hernia.

(2)Endoscopy

Endoscopy shows the symptoms of different degrees of reflux esophagitis, clear esophageal and malignant lesions and Barrett's esophagus.

(3)Functional examination of reflux

pH measurement in the esophageal records the pH of the diurnal esophagus to determine whether there is excessive acid reflux. Common methods include the following:①Acid scavenging test, standard acid reflux test, 24h pH monitoring of esophageal or 3h pH monitoring after meal. ②Esophageal nucleus GER examination helps to find out whether there is excessive gastroesophageal reflux. ③Esophageal pressure measurement assesses the state of esophageal movement, systolic blood pressure, conduction velocity, abnormal peristaltic wave, resting pressure of upper and lower esophageal sphincter and relaxation function of esophagus.

2.2.3   Differential diagnosis

(1)Esophageal cancer. Esophagoscopy and X−ray examination could be used for identification.

(2)Peptic ulcer. It is often chronic, rhythmic, seasonal and periodic attacks. Lesions could be observed in the stomach or duodenal bulb by X−ray and gastroscopy.

(3)Esophagitis. Post−sternal pain and angina pectoris could exist alone, or sometimes at the same time, and could be alleviated with nitroglycerin, so that the identification is very difficult.

(4)Hysteria ball. It refers to the patient's complaint that the throat has a foreign body sensation, could not start swallowing, has a sense of blockage, but with no organic lesions in clinical examination. It is believed that the high reflux of the stomach causes the upper part of the esophagus to be stimulated. Sometimes it is misdiagnosed for the only symptoms in a small number of patients.

2.2.4 Treatment

Surgical treatment should be used for patients with ineffective esophageal stenosis, severe reflux symptoms, ineffective medical treatment for 3 months, incurable esophageal ulcer bleeding, moderate or above dysplasia, etc.

(1) Nissen fundoplication: It is suitable for most patients with fundus folding patients.

(2) Toupet fundoplication: It is suitable for patients with poor esophageal motility.

(3) Collis stomach angioplasty: It is suitable for esophageal shortening cases.

2.2.5 Complications

Common complications of reflux esophagitis include pneumothorax, subcutaneous emphysema, perforation of esophageal or gastric wall injury, intraoperative bleeding, and vagus nerve injury.

Chapter 3

Neoplasm

The etiology and pathogenesis of the neoplasm is still not clear. Most of the esophageal tumors are malignant, and the majority of it are cancer, followed by carcinosarcoma, leiomyosarcoma, angiosarcoma, lymphoma, etc. The benign tumor of the esophagus is rare, and most of them are derived from leiomyoma, fibroma, hemangioma, lipoma, etc., with esophageal leiomyoma accounting for about 3/4.

3.1 Liomyoma of Esophagus

3.1.1 Clinical manifestation

(1) Symptoms

In clinic, about half of the patients have no obvious symptoms, so they are often found by an X-ray or angiographic examination. The patients may have mild symptoms. The most common one is mild hypopharynx, without affecting the normal diet. Some patients may have heartburn, abdominal distension, indigestion and other symptoms of dyspepsia. A few patients may have hematemesis, black stool and other symptoms, which are mainly related to edema and bleeding on the surface of the tumor. When the tumor is very large, there would be symptoms of oppression, such as dysphagia, dyspnea. This disease has a long course and a slow development.

(2) Signs

There is no obvious sign in the patients with esophagus leiomyoma. The diagnosis are mainly determined by auxiliary examination.

3.1.2 Accessory examinations

(1) X-ray

X-ray examination is the main diagnosis method for esophagus. Combined with clinical manifestation, the patients could be definitely diagnosed by one time angiography. The main manifestation is round or oval intraluminal filling defect with smooth and sharp edge, and clear boundary to normal esophagus.

(2) Fiberesophagoscopy

Most of the esophageal leiomyomas could be diagnosed by X-ray examination. Fiberesophagoscopy is adopted to observe the swelling in the esophageal cavity. The surface of mucous membrane is smooth without folds. Occasionally, we may find obvious edge of the tumor. When swallowing, it could be observed that the mass is slightly up and down.

(3)CT and MRI

X-ray and fiberesophagoscopy are most commonly applied to make a clear diagnosis. Whereas, in a few cases, especially the middle segment leiomyoma which are easily confused with aortic aneurysm and vascular compression or malformation, CT and MRI is applied to make differential diagnosis. CT could also be used to confirm the exact location and expansion of tumor to the tube, which is conducive to the design of surgical plan and incision.

3.1.3 Differential diagnosis

(1)Malignant tumor of esophagus

Esophageal cancer is characterized by irregular filling defects and mucosal patches.

(2)Mediastinal mass

The large leiomyoma expanding to the wall of esophagus causes the soft tissue film in the mediastinum, which is easily confused with mediastinal tumor. Therefore, we should be alert to the presence of esophageal leiomyoma in the posterior inferior mediastinum and closely related to the esophagus.

3.1.4 Treatments

3.1.4.1 Expectant treatment

The patients with tumor less than 2 cm in diameter and without any symptoms, or who is not suitable for the operation due to the age, low cardiopulmonary function and other physical conditions, could be treated without operation, but need regular follow-up observation.

3.1.4.2 Surgical treatment

(1)Tumor extirpation beyond mucosa and muscular coat repair

It is preferable and suitable for patients with smaller tumors and no adhesion between tumor and mucosa.

(2)Tumor extirpation beyond mucosa under thoracoscopy

This method is suitable for patients with small tumor, non-adhesion between tumor and mucosa and non-adhesion with thoracic cavity. It has the advantages of less injury and quick recovery after operation, but it is difficult to operate.

(3)Partial esophagectomy

It is suitable for large tumors with annular growth and severe adhesion to esophageal mucosa, or with severe esophageal mucosa injury and repairing difficulty during operation. In addition, partial resection of the esophagus should also be performed for patients with malignant transformation.

3.1.5 Complications

(1)Esophageal fistula

If postoperative esophageal fistula occurs, timely thoracotomy or esophagectomy should be performed.

(2)Esophagostenosis

Esophageal stenosis may be caused by scar after operation. And esophageal dilation should be performed after operation to relieve esophageal stenosis.

(3) Canceration

It needs regular follow-up after operation.

3.2　Esophageal Cancer

3.2.1　Clinical manifestations

3.2.1.1　Symptoms

The early symptoms of esophageal cancer mainly include choking sensation when eating, and some patients have burning sensation after the sternum. Many patients have no obvious symptoms in the early stage of esophageal cancer, so they missed the best treatment time. As the disease progresses, the patient will have obvious dysphagia and there will be progressive aggravation, which is a typical symptom of esophageal cancer; the patient can also have symptoms such as vomiting, back pain and chest pain. With the disease develop to the late state, there will be symptoms such as pain, hematemesis, hoarseness, cough and others because of the infiltration or oppression to the surrounding tissue. Anemia, emaciation, and hypoproteinemia can also occur due to cachexia; if the tumor metastases distantly, the corresponding symptoms of metastasis can occur.

3.2.1.2　Classifications

(1) According to the pathological classification, it can be divided into medullary type, fungoid type, ulcerative type and constrictive type.

(2) According to the histological type, it can be divided into squamous cell carcinoma, adenocarcinoma and undifferentiated carcinoma. Squamous cell carcinoma is the most common, and the latter two are rare.

(3) The esophagus can be divided into upper, middle and lower segments in clinical. The upper segment is from the margin of the esophagus to the superior arch of the aorta, the middle segment is from the aortic arch to the lower pulmonary vein, the lower part is from the lower pulmonary vein to the cardia, the highest incidence of esophageal cancer in the middle, the lower segment is the next, and the lowest probability of esophageal cancer is in the upper esophagus.

3.2.2　Accessory examinations

3.2.2.1　X-ray

The early examination by X-ray shows that the mucous folds are limitedly thickened and fractured, the wall becomes limited stiffness, and small filling defects and niches are also found. The progressing stage is characterized by obvious stenosis of the functional mucosa, disruption of mucous membrane, larger filling defects and niches.

3.2.2.2　CT

CT examination is of great value in the diagnosis and treatment of advanced esophageal cancer. The location of the lesion and the relationship between the tumor invasion range and its adjacent structures could be identified. Moreover, it also indicates the metastasis in the mediastinal or peritoneal lymph nodes.

3.2.2.3　Endoscopic ultrasonography of esophagus

It is a combination technique of esophagus endoscopy and B-ultrasound. For esophageal cancer, especially for non-surgical esophageal cancer, it is of great value to determine the state of the disease.

3.2.3　Differential diagnosis

(1) Esophagitis: For patients with esophagitis, there is no obvious dysphagia, and the X-ray examination shows no mucosal disorder or destruction.

(2) Maga-esophagus: The patients shows dysphagia and post-sternal fullness, but X-ray shows a smooth beak-like stenosis in the lower esophagus.

(3) Leiomyoma of esophagus: The mucosa of esophageal leiomyoma is smooth and uninterrupted, and the tumor often has a clear demarcation with the mucosa of esophageal wall. The patients should be performed the pathological examination to differentiate.

3.2.4　Treatments

3.2.4.1　Surgical treatment

Surgery is the first choice for the treatment of esophageal cancer. For patients in stage 0 and stage Ⅰ, surgery should be performed actively if the general conditions is well. For patients in stage Ⅱ, the length of the lesions in the middle and lower segment less than 5 cm or the length of the lesions in upper segment less than 3 cm is suitable for surgical treatment. For patients in stage Ⅲ, the combined treatment of preoperative radiotherapy and surgery should be taken when the length of the lesion is over 5 cm and the general condition is well. For large squamous cell carcinoma, preoperative radiotherapy may be used before surgery if the possibility of resection is small and the patient is in well condition. Radical resection of esophageal cancer (gastric, jejunal and colon for esophagus) and palliative surgery (bypass, gastrostomy and intraluminal catheters) are the common modes of operation.

3.2.4.2　Radiotherapy

(1) The combined treatment of radiotherapy and surgery increases the rate of resection and improves the long-term survival rate. It is more appropriate to rest for 3-4 weeks before surgery. Metal markers are used to mark incomplete residual cancer tissues during operation, and postoperative radiotherapy is usually initiated 3-6 weeks after surgery.

(2) Simple radiotherapy is mainly used for patients with cervical and upper thoracic esophageal cancer. The operation is often difficult and accompanied with many complications, and the curative effect is not satisfactory. It also could be applied in patients with operation taboo, short lesions time, and intolerance of radiotherapy.

3.2.4.3　Chemotherapy

The combination of chemotherapy and surgery, or combination with radiotherapy or traditional Chinese medicine may improve the curative effect, relieve the symptoms and prolong the survival time of the patients with esophageal cancer. However, blood, liver and kidney functions should be checked regularly, and drug reactions should be noted meanwhile.

3.2.5　Complications

①Anastomotic fistula: It is the most severe complication after surgery of esophagus cancer. ②Stenosis of anastomotic stoma. ③Chylopleura. ④Reflux esophagitis.

Chapter 4

Esophageal Atresia

Esophageal atresia (EA) is a rare congenital anomaly characterized by discontinuity of the esophagus and a possible connection with the trachea. In 1670, Willin Durston firstly described a female infant with blind-ending upper esophageal pouch. The definition of EA with tracheoesophageal fistula (TEF) was published in the fifth edition of Thomas Gibson's The Anatomy of Human Bodies Epitomized. EA was once a lethal disease in neonate and serious chemical pneumonitis caused by aspiration and gastric reflux through abnormal connection between the trachea and esophagus is the principal cause of death from EA. Survival rate of neonate with EA has markedly improved because of advances in multidisciplinary management and innovative operational techniques.

4.1　Epidemiology

The reported incidence ranges from 1 in 2500 to 4500 live births. Some researchers reported a lower rate of EA among nonwhite population (0.55 per 10 000 births) than the white population (1.0 per 10 000 births). The male-to-female ratio is 1.26. There is increased risk for EA with the first pregnancy, increasing maternal age, and twin infants.

4.2　Etiology

The etiology of EA is unclear and its pathogenesis is controversial. There are several hypotheses as follows:

(1) Embryology

The normal development process engaged in the separation of the primitive trachea and esophagus is unclear. A wildly accepted mechanism is that the trachea and esophagus originating from the same primitive foregut, and from 5-6 weeks of embryonic life the developing trachea and esophagus are separated by lateral ingrowth of epithelial ridges. Growth speed of esophageal mesenchymal coat is faster than the cellular division in epithelial lining, causing the epithelial stretched and then interrupted.

(2)Genome

The Sonic hedgehog (Shh), a protein encoded by the SHH gene, is associated with vertebrate axial organogenesis, including foregut development and differentiation. Mice with targeted by Shh deletion develop EA-TEF. Candidate genes related to EA are HOX D group, which is involved in normal development of foreguts. The occurrence of genetic deletion, mutation, and frame-shift in HOX D will provoke potential malformation of foreguts. Recent studies found patients with deletions of FOXF gene on chromosome 16q24 and mutations in the FOXF1 gene were associated with EA-TEF.

(3)Teratogens

Successful establishment of rodent model for EA-TEF by using the adriamycin indicates the teratogenic potential of glycosidic anthracyclin antibiotics. No specific environmental risk factors leading to EA-TEF has been identified.

(4)Others

Pregnancy with Vitamin A deficiency seems to be associated with higher frequence of EA-TEF than those with sufficient supplying of vitamin.

4.3 Clinical Classification

The most useful and practical classification of EA is Gross classification, which is determined by the simple anatomic descriptions. The types of EA and incidence rates are as follows:①A:EA without TEF (7.8%).②B:EA with proximal TEF (0.8%).③C:EA with distal TEF (85.8%).④D:EA with TEF in both pouches (1.4%).⑤E:TEF without EA (4.2%).

4.4 Clinical Manifestations

4.4.1 History

Being unable to swallow in antenatal EA, the increased amniotic fluid during pregnancy is the early manifestation of EA. The first feeding of neonate is followed by vomiting, choking, and coughing.

4.4.2 Symptoms

Most newborns with EA are symptomatic in the first hours of postnatal life. The typical symptoms are as below:①Vomiting:immediate regurgitation after feeding, non-bile reflux material (feeding material) such as milk and water. ②Cyanosis:a bluish-purple discoloration of skin and mucous membranes, the presence of purple color in lip and nail with or without feeding, or worsen after feeding. ③Respiratory distress: marked by rapid shallow breathing (tachypnea) or abnormal apnea.

4.4.3 Physical signs

①Respiratory signs:rough breath sounds or bubbling rale in lung auscultation, because of gastric or feeding fluid passing through TEF into the trachea and lung, resulting in chemical pneumonitis. ②Abdominal distension:inspired air passing through TEF into the stomach, diaphragms elevating and pulmonary status worsening with the progressive abdominal distension. ③Abdominal collapse:occurring in EA without

TEF, no inspired air entering into the stomach, causing gastrointestinal collapse.

4.4.4 Associated anomalies

More than 50% neonates with EA are associated with other congenital anomalies. The common complicated malformation are as vertebral (24%), anorectal (14%), cardiac (32%), tracheoesophageal fistula (95%), renal (17%), limb or skeletal (16%), and others (11%). Compared to single anomaly, higher mortality of EA occurs in patients with multiple malformations.

4.5 Diagnosis

4.5.1 Prenatal stage

The diagnostic sensitivity of ultrasound in the prenatal stage is about 50%. With prenatal findings, including polyhydramnios and absent or a small stomach bubble, the diagnosis of EA should be considered, especially for pure EA.

4.5.2 Postnatal stage

The neonates with EA–TEF clinically present respiratory distress, feeding difficulties, and choking in the first hours of life. Related symptoms will worsen after feeding. In addition, the inability of nasogastric tube passing from the mouth or nose into the stomach strongly suggests the presence of EA.

4.5.3 Imaging study

EA or EA–TEF can be confirmed by the upper gastrointestinal contrast method. A stiff catheter is inserted into the esophagus to the point which the resistance is met. Contrast agent (diluted barium or urografin) is injected into the catheter to distend the upper esophageal pouch, then a frontal and lateral film is obtained. The presentation from films making the diagnosis of EA in details are as follows: ①EA without TEF: a small upper blind pouch of esophagus and absent of air or contrast material in stomach. ②EA with proximal TEF: a small upper blind pouch of esophagus and the presence of tracheobronchial tree. ③EA with distal TEF: a small upper blind pouch of esophagus and air in stomach or bowel. ④EA with TEF in both pouches: a small upper blind pouch of esophagus and the presence of tracheobronchial tree. ⑤TEF without EA (or H–type): difficult to determine and bronchoscopy or esophagoscopy required to confirm the diagnosis (Figure 21–4–1).

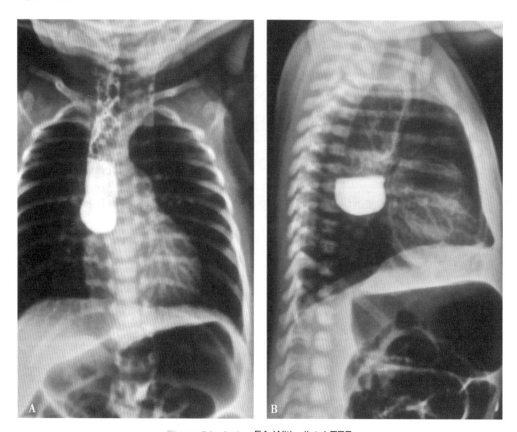

Figure 21-4-1　EA With distal TEF

Type Ⅲ EA shown the upper blind pouch of esophagusand air in gastrointestinal tract on anteroposterior (A) and lateral (B) film of upper gastrointestinal (UGI) contrast study.

4.6　Treatments

4.6.1　Preoperative managements

Chemical pneumonitis from aspiration of saliva and reflux of gastric fluid through the fistula is critical preoperative problem for the newborn with EA-TEF. The primary preoperative management is to avoid further aspiration and treat pneumonitis.

①The neonate should be kept in an upright sitting position to minimize reflux of gastric fluid up through the fistula. ②A nasogastric tube should be inserted into the upper pouch of esophagus to continuously aspirate saliva under low-pressure suction. ③Broad-spectrum antibiotics application, aerosol inhalation, and sputum aspiration are initiated to treat pneumonitis. ④Parenteral nutrition should be initiated using 5% dextrose and hypotonic saline to maintain fluid, electrolyte, and acid-base balance. ⑤Vitamin K should be administrated before operation to prevent coagulation disorder. ⑥Endotracheal intubation should be avoided to reduce risk of gastric perforation and worsen respiratory distress because of a distended abdomen from artificial ventilation through the TEF. ⑦Echocardiac evaluation should be carried out to determine whether a right sided aortic arch (about 2.5% of cases) presents which signifies a challenging repair best performed via a left thoracotomy.

4.6.2　Operative repair

（1）Operation timing

Emergency operation for EA is unnecessary. A period of 24–48 hours between diagnosis and operation can completea full assessment of neonate and treat pneumonitis. The correction of acid–base or electrolyte disorders will reduce perioperative risks and improve the outcomes of patients.

（2）Surgical method

The operation can be either open or thoracoscopic. In 1941, Gameron Haight reported the first successful open repair for EA. The first thoracoscopic repair was reported in 1999. Contrast to open repair, thoracoscopy took the longest time to complete but was associated with the shortest time for extubation, feeding, and discharge. The potential risk for brain damage due to hypoxia during thoracoscopic repair should be considered.

（3）Anesthesia

EA repair is performed under general anesthesia. Improved anesthetic techniques, such as minimal use of drugs, careful intubation of endotracheal tube providing sufficient ventilation without gas flow through TEF, and preferably artificial control of ventilation, will support successful operation repair.

（4）Operation principles

Operative interruption for neonate with EA–TEF relays greatly on the classification of anomalies. Operative principles for EA are fistula ligation and primary esophageal anastomosis created.

（5）Challenges for surgery

The most challenging types of EA are long gap type, which defined as at least 3 cm（about three vertebral bodies）between the two ends of the esophagus in pure EA. Two strategies for esophageal anastomosis are performed under tension and staged operation to stretch esophagus by placing tension on the end. The alternative methods are gastric, colonic, or jejunum replacement.

（6）Postoperative complications

The main early postoperative complications as follows: ①Leakage of esophageal anastomosis（about 20% cases）, managed conservatively with drainage and usually healing in 1–2 weeks; ②Strictures（about 40% cases）, managed with esophageal dilations; ③Vocal cord paralysis（about 5% cases）, presumably from recurrent laryngeal nerveinjury; ④Recurrent fistula（about 5% cases）, highest success rate of surgical repair.

4.7　Prognosis

4.7.1　Growth and nutrition

Poor development of uterus had been noted and nearly 50% of children had weights below 25th centile during the first 5 years of life. Aversive feeding behaviors of children caused by gastroesophageal reflux, anastomotic strictures, and esophageal disability, are major source of concern in early childhood.

4.7.2　Respiratory system

Respiratory problems, such as severe tracheomalacia and recurrent chest infection or pneumonia are common in children with EA and TEF. Respiratory morbidity decreases in frequency and severity when child reaches late adolescence.

4.7.3 Gastroesophageal morbidity

Gastroesophageal reflux is the common problem in almost 50% cases. It is expected to result in esophagitis, strictures, nutritional and respiratory problems. Esophageal disability can be seen in 75% –100% of children after operation repair. Patients have episodes of aspiration, dysphagia, food bolus obstruction and failure to thrive.

4.7.4 Musculoskeletal system

Open repair can lead to musculoskeletal morbidity, as spinal or chest deformities, "winged" scapula, . chest wall asymmetry, and ribs fusion. Modified axillary incisions or thoracoscopy techniques can reduce morbidity.

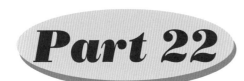

Part 22

Heart Disease

Chapter 1

The Basic Measures for Intra-cardiac Surgery

1.1 Cardiopulmonary Bypass

Cardiopulmonary bypass is a life-support technology that uses special artificial devices to extract the venous blood of cardiac out of the body for gas exchange, temperature regulation and filtration, and then sends it back to the internal arteries. Due to replacing the function of human heart and lung, the artificial device is called the heart-lung machine. The purpose of cardiopulmonary bypass is to replace cardiopulmonary function temporarily, maintain the blood supply and gas exchange of the whole body tissues and organs, and provide the operation field with or without blood for the operation of open heart surgery.

1.1.1 The structure of cardiopulmonary bypass device

It is mainly composed of artificial heart-lung machine and accessories, including blood pump (artificial heart), oxygenator (artificial lung), thermostat, variable-temperature water tank, recovery blood storage device, filter, pipeline and arteriovenous intubation, etc. The artificial heart-lung machine has the following main components.

(1) The blood pump

Blood pump is the main component that drives the unidirectional flow of oxygenated blood in vitro and sends it back to the internal arteries to replace the function of cardiac ejection. Commonly used are rotary pressure pumps and centrifugal pumps. The rotary pump uses the rotor of the pump head to turn the elastic pump pipe alternately to drive the one-way flow of blood in the pump pipe. The diameter of the pump tube determines the blood flow, and the regulated speed controls the flow. Centrifugal pump uses the drive motor and magnetic connection to drive the high speed rotation of multi-layer rotating cone or impeller in the pump to generate centrifugal force to drive one-way blood flow, which has the advantages of reducing the damage of blood components.

(2) The oxygenator

The oxygenator oxygenates venous blood, expel carbon dioxide, and replace the lungs for gas exchange. The bubble-type oxygenator mixes oxygen and venous blood into blood bubbles, which exchange gas directly in the blood bubble membrane, and then becomes oxygenated blood after defoaming and filtering. Membrane oxygenator using a breathable polymer thin film material separating oxygen and red blood cells, blood oxygenation process do not contact directly with oxygen, could significantly reduce the blood component damage and micro-air embolism.

(3) The heat exchanger

The heat exchanger, applying circulating water temperature and thermal conductive thin metal plate, reduce or increase the blood temperature of the device.

(4) The filter

The filter is a device composed of a polymer material filter mesh of 20-40 centimeter-diameter microholes, which is placed in the arterial blood supply pipeline for the effective filtration of blood components or gases.

1.1.2　Preparation for cardiopulmonary bypass

Preoperative perfusion division should learn more about the patient's condition, height, weight, surface area, hematocrit, and plasma protein concentration, etc. , fully understand the operation scheme of cardiopulmonary bypass requirements, formulate individualized cardiopulmonary bypass scheme. Select the appropriate parts, connect the cardiopulmonary bypass line, and ensure the artificial heart-lung machine is in good working condition (Figure 1). Use crystal fluid, colloidal fluid, permeable diuretics and heparin (2 mg/dL) , pre-filled artificial heart and lung machines and pipes. The electrolyte concentration of the prefilled solution should be close to that of the extracellular fluid, and the osmotic pressure is slightly higher than that of plasma, showing weak alkalinity. The prefilled liquid can eliminate the gas in the cardiopulmonary bypass device to maintain the balance of electrolyte and acid and alkali, and carries out appropriate blood dilution. Blood dilution reduces the use of blood bank to avoid blood transfusion complications; reduce blood viscosity and circulation resistance, improve microcirculation perfusion; reduce the blood component damage and coagulation mechanism disorder; prevent lung, kidney, brain and other major organ complications. At present, moderate blood dilution with a blood cell specific volume of 20% -25% or hemoglobin level of 70-80 g/L (7-8 g/dL) is mostly used.

1.1.3　Implementation of cardiopulmonary bypass

In open heart surgery, the central thoracic incision is usually used to expose the heart and free the upper and lower vena cava. In external cardiac exploration, heparin (2-3 mg/kg weight) is injected intravenously, and the total blood activation clotting time (ACT) during cardiopulmonary bypass is extended to 480-600 seconds. The ascending aorta or femoral artery is placed in the arterial intubation, and the superior and inferior vena cava are placed in the vena drainage intubation, respectively connected with the artificial cardiopulmonary bypass.

According to the needs of operation, cardiopulmonary bypass is often combined with different degree of implementation, low temperature through the blood to make the body oxygen metabolism, and reduces the expected normal temperature filling flow properly to avoid surgery left heart blood flow increased, blood component damage and myocardial damage. Heart-lung machine perfusion flow generally is 50-120 mL/(kg·min) or 2.2-2.4 L/(m² · min). The basic metabolic rate of children is high, with the perfusion flow rate of children from 10-15 kg ranging from 120-150 mL/(kg · min) , and up to 125-175 mL/(kg · min) for children with weight under 10 kg. With the support of cardiopulmonary bypass, open heart surgery often requires tightening of the lumen vein occlusion band, clamping the ascending aorta and cardiac arrest.

Open-heart surgery before and after cardiopulmonary bypass turn flow form to become systemic circulation, the aortic blood flow from the heart ejection and blood pump, venous blood respectively from the scripture, inferior vena cava intubation or not tighten vena cava, flows back into oxygenator and right atrium. During body circulation, the blood temperature is changed through the thermostat and water tank of the extracorporeal circulation device. After cardiopulmonary bypass, adequate amount of fish essence protein should be injected intravenously to stop the anticoagulant effect of heparin, and arterial intubation and superior and inferior vena cava should be removed.

1.2　Myocardial Protection

Cardiovascular surgery technology has developed greatly with the progress of cardiopulmonary bypass. The key to the implementation of cardiovascular surgery is to ensure the recovery of cardiac function on the basis of providing static and bloodless surgical vision for surgeons. Therefore, the importance of myocardial protection is self-evident. Myocardial protection is a measure and method to reduce the damage of myocardial ischemia and hypoxia during open cardiac surgery.

1.2.1　The mechanism of ischemia and ischemia-reperfusion injury

Myocardial ischemia is caused by the blocking of ascending aorta in cardiopulmonary bypass, and myocardial recovery after the opening of the ascending aorta is one of the main factors of myocardial injury.

The causes of ischemic injury during cardiac surgery include mechanical injury, drug damage, and extracorporeal circulation inflammatory injury, such as progressive disease, the operation itself as blocking the coronary circulation and causing whole heart ischemia, and the relative ischemia caused by the change of the supply and demand of blood flow and oxygen during the operation.

Ischemia-reperfusion injury is a phenomenon that tissue damage is aggravated and even irreversible injury occurs when blood flow is restored on the basis of ischemia. The mechanism of ischemia-reperfusion injury is complex. The main reasons are as follows:

1.2.1.1　Oxygen free radical hypothesis

During myocardial ischemia and reperfusion, the increase of oxygen free radicals is caused by increased xanthine oxidase, respiratory burst of neutrophils, impaired mitochondrial function, and increase of catecholamine. Oxygen free radicals damage membrane phospholipids, proteins and nucleic acids, and damage the extracellular matrix, oxygen free radicals can also induce inflammatory mediators to cause damage to cardiac muscle cells.

1.2.1.2　Calcium overload hypothesis

Intracellular Ca^{2+} concentration is positively correlated with cell damage. After ischemia-reperfusion, the recovery of Na^+-Ca^{2+} exchange, increased membrane permeability, mitochondrial dysfunction, and catecholamine increase, resulting in a large amount of intracellular Ca^{2+} flow, so that intracellular calcium overload. Calcium overload causes dysfunction of mitochondria, activates calcium dependent degrading enzymes, promotes oxygen free radical generation, causes arrhythmia, and causes myofibrils to be overcontracted, resulting in cell damage.

1.2.1.3　Leukocytes hypothesis

The possible cause of leukocytosis during perfusion is the degradation of membrane phospholipid during tissue injury, and the increase of the metabolites of arachidonate, of which leukotrienes, PGE2, platelet activating factor (PAF), and alexin and kinin have strong chemotaxis, and then attract a large number of leukocytes to enter tissue or adhere to cell endothelium. Leukocytes damage tissues by mechanical blockage and inflammatory reaction.

1.2.1.4 Myocardial energy metabolism disorder hypothesis

The physiological function of the myocardium is dependent on the sufficient supply of ATP. The level of ATP in the myocardium is closely related to the severity of myocardial ischemia and reperfusion injury.

1.2.1.5 Insulin resistance hypothesis

By virtue of prolonged cardiac ischemia–reperfusion, glucose uptake and utilization of myocardium are decreased. These effects are possibly related to insulin resistance (IR) and correlated to the decreased GLUT–4 expression and translocation to the membrane of myocytes. The depressed GLUT–4 translocation during cardiac ischemia decreases uptake of glucose, contributing to ischemic heart injury. CD36, facilitating the high–affinity uptake of fatty acids from albumin and triacylglycerol–rich lipoproteins in the heart, is also participated in the process of myocardial IR via assisting the traffic and utilization of fatty acids between the cell surface and intra–cellular compartments (specifically endosomes) during cardiopulmonary bypass. The siRNA–mediated PPAR gamma knockdown enhances the myocardial insulin resistance on myocardial ischemia reperfusion during cardiopulmonary bypass. The molecular mechanisms is due to the silence of PPAR gamma decreasing the expression of GLUT–4 and inhibiting its transportation from cytoplasm to membrane. HIF–1α, plays a regulatory role in IR, decreases the expression of insulin receptor which is a post–bypass cause of IR. Increased insulin resistance leads to excessive reliance on myocardial glycogen as an energy source and a deficit in energy substrates that contributes to cardiac dysfunction. In addition, mitogen activated protein kinase signal transduction system (MAPK), intracellular phosphatidyl inositol kinase (PI3K), endogenous NO, and growth factor (IGF–1) are also promising factors contributing to IR in myocardium.

1.2.2 Myocardial protection in cardiopulmonary bypass

Myocardial protection during cardiopulmonary bypass includes protection before cardioplegia, during cardiac arrest and after parallel phase. Myocardial protection before cardiac arrest is an important part of myocardial protection during the perioperative period of cardiovascular surgery, which is mainly to increase the energy reserve of the myocardium, improve the internal environment, keep the oxygen supply and the oxygen consumption balance. From cardiopulmonary bypass to blocking the ascending aorta, it is a pre–parallel circulation stage. This stage is mainly to ensure myocardial perfusion and full drainage of cardiac chambers.

From the beginning of the ascending aorta, the transformation of the body from the autogenous or artificial heart and lung to the artificial support of the body's respiratory cycle is completed, and the body enters the ischemic stage of the heart and lung.

The focal point of myocardial ischemia is continuously maintaining the low temperature and low metabolic state of the donor heart, providing the donor heart with the energy substrate and buffer system, maintaining the appropriate osmotic pressure, avoiding the edema and energy imbalance of the cardiac myocytes, thus providing a guarantee for the smooth recovery of the cardiac function after the surgical operation.

The key to myocardial protection is selecting the type of cardioplegia, way of perfusion and myocardial temperature. High potassium and low temperature are fundamental.

A case of crystalloid and hemophoric cardioplegia is taken as an example.

(1) The mechanism of cold crystalloid cardioplegia is to fill the myocardium with cardioplegia containing high concentration of potassium, reduce the transmembrane potential, inhibit the spread and formation

of action potential, resulting in the asystole at the diastolic stage. The hypothermia of crystalloid cardioplegia reduces the basic metabolism of myocardium and energy consumption, and ultimately increases the tolerance of myocardium to ischemia. The advantage of cold crystalloid cardioplegia is that it is effective, simple and practical. The insufficiency is as follows: ①Provide no oxygen and other rich nutrients for myocardium. ②Lack of acid-base balance and the buffer of colloid. ③The recovery of crystalloid cardioplegic solution causes excessive blood dilution. ④Discarding it may lead to the loss of blood, thus it could not meet the demand of severe myocardial injury.

（2）The hemophoric cardioplegia stops the heart in an aerobic environment, and avoid the electrical mechanical activity of consuming ATP in the short timebefore cardiac arrest. The aerobic oxidation process is carried out during cardiac arrest, but anaerobic fermentation is reduced to a lower level, which is beneficial to ATP preservation. The advantage of oxygenated cardioplegia is that it provides a better buffering capacity, higher colloid osmotic pressure and more physiological substrates and trace elements. But there are also many defects, such as agglutinin producing, red blood cell retention and platelet aggregation caused by low temperature, the increase of viscosity making the distribution more uneven, the left shift of hemoglobin tending to reduce the uptake of oxygen. The adoption of hemophoric cardioplegia must pay attention to two points, one is that the blood cooling could not be too low (15 ℃ is appropriate); two is that multiple perfusion is effective at interval of 20-30 minutes.

1.2.3　Myocardial protection in the post-parallel phase

From opening ascending aorta to the cessation of cardiopulmonary bypass, it is called post-parallel circulation stage. After opening ascending aorta, the blood flow of coronary artery restores, the spontaneous respiration recovers from artificial support. The reperfusion injury caused by cardiopulmonary ischemia injury, and the rise and fall of body temperature, would have an adverse effect on the recovery of cardiac function. In this stage, autogenous and artificial heart and lung work simultaneously, adjusting the internal environment, promoting the recovery of heart function, and smooth stopping is the key point of this stage in the management of extracorporeal circulation.

Other strategies for enhancing myocardial protection include myocardial ischemic preconditioning, cardioprotection during cardiopulmonary bypass, and the improvement of cardioplegia. Although there are many methods of myocardial protection in cardiac surgery, the primary principles are high potassium for cardiac arrest, hypothermia, metabolic reduction, heart emptied but no strain.

Chapter 2

Congenital Heart Disease

2.1 Septum Defect

2.1.1 Atrial septal defect

Atrial septal defect (ASD) is a gap, which exists alone or coexists with other cardiac malformations. The incidence of atrial septal defect is about 0.07%, which accounts for 6% –10% of congenital heart disease. Secondary ASD is a common clinical type, which accounts for 80% –90% of congenital heart diseases.

2.1.1.1 Clinical manifestations

(1) Symptoms

The clinical symptoms of simple atrial septal defect are atypical. In most of the patients, heart murmurs were found after they had physical examinations. Some patients may have palpitations and shortness of breath after activities, and most of these symptoms occur only in adulthood. Few patients shows shortness of breath, sweating, limited activity in their infancy. Some patients were treated with complicated atrial arrhythmia, mostly with supraventricular premature beat or atrial flutter and atrial fibrillation.

(2) Signs

There might be a preheart uplift in patients. When we have a auscultation on patients, a soft systolic murmur would be heard between the second and third intercostal sides of the sternum at levels of II – III. The patients who were complicated with increased pulmonary artery pressure, enhancement of second heart sounds could be heard in pulmonary valve region. The patients who were complicated with larger defects, diastolic rumbling murmur could be heard due to relative tricuspid stenosis.

2.1.1.2 Accessory examination

Patients who have the above clinical manifestations, and if they were suspected to be atrial septal defect, they should have the following examinations.

(1) Electrocardiogram

It shows right deviation of electrocardio axis and right ventricular hypertrophy.

(2) Chest X-ray

It shows increment of pulmonary blood flow, prominent of pulmonary artery segment, and enlargement of right atrium and right ventricular.

(3) Echocardiogram

This examination is used to confirm the diagnosis. Two-dimensional color Doppler ultrasound is used to estimate the size and location of the defect, and determine the location of the pulmonary vein, and the direction of the shunt.

(4) Right cardiac catheterization

It is necessary for patients who are complicated with severe pulmonary hypertension. The examination determines the direction of the shunt and the size of the flow, also calculates the pulmonary vascular resistance, so as to determine whether there is a surgical indication.

2.1.1.3　Differential diagnosis

(1) Interventricular septal defect

This disease have a more earlier and sever symptoms. Heart murmur of it is often rough in relatively lower location. Echocardiography could diagnose this disease clearly.

(2) Partial endocardial cushion defect

This disease have a more obvious and early symptoms. In the apex of heart, systolic murmurs could often be heard due to the mitral reflux. ECG often shows the left axis deviation and left anterior branch block. Echocardiography is applied to definitely diagnose this disease.

(3) Simple partial pulmonary venous malformation drainage

There are no obvious symptoms in this disease, the similar murmurs to the atrial septal defect could be find in the physical examinations. Echocardiography is appropriate to find the complete atrial septum, and determine the location of the pulmonary vein returned to the atrium.

2.1.1.4　Treatment

(1) Non-operative treatment

1) Oxygen therapy: For patients who are complicated with cardiac insufficiency or pulmonary hypertension, oxygen therapy is adopted to reduce pulmonary artery pressure and right heart afterload.

2) Drug: Cardiac stimulants is commonly used to enhance myocardial contractility, in combination with diuresis and anticoagulant therapy.

(2) Surgical treatment

Indications: The diagnosis of atrial septal defect is clear. Auxiliary examination indicates that the cardiac volume load and the pulmonary blood are both increasing, or the cardiac catheterization Q_p/Q_s is more than 1.5, which requires surgical treatment.

1) Repair of atrial septal defect under direct vision: Surgeons often use the median incision to complete the operation. But for cosmetic results, surgeons could also select right chest incision.

2) Percutaneous transcatheter closure of atrial septal defect: It is better for the patients who are central type atrial septal defect with clear defect margin.

3) Repair of superior chamber atrial septal defect: Surgeons should pay attention to preventing pulmonary venous obstruction.

2.1.1.5　Postoperative complications

(1) Aeroembolism

The aeroembolism is one of the serious complications, caused by the left heart of patients exposing to the air during the operation. If the left heart drainage tube is placed in the operation, the suction should not be too large to prevent the left heart from being too empty. In addition, when close the right atrial incision, surgeons should gently wobble left ventricle and the left atrium in order to make the bubble discharge from the perfusion needle. If the bubble spills from the perfusion needle all the time, the left heart exhaust time should be extended accordingly.

(2)Residual leakage

It is mainly caused by surgical technique defects. In addition, the adult patients with too large ASD are sometimes sutured directly because of excessive tension, which causes tear and residual leakage. Surgeons should explore the structure of the heart carefully, and use the patches reasonably in operation to reduce suture tension. Once the residual leakage occurs, if the patient are complicated with large defect, they need a second operation to repair the defect. But if the patients are complicated with small defect, surgeons could use the intervention to fill the defect.

(3)Conduction block

It is primarily caused by the injury of the atrioventricular node and conduction bundle near the coronary sinus due to suture of ASD, and the incidence is generally low.

2.1.2 Ventricular sepal defect

There is an abnormal connection between the left and right ventricles at any location of the interventricular septum. Ventricular septal defects cause blood shunting between the ventricles, and haemodynamic disturbances. Congenital ventricular septal defect (VSD)is caused by embryonic primitive ventriculoperitoneal dysplasia, including the type of simple VSD or with other cardiac malformations. Simple VSD is a very common congenital heart disease, and its incidence is about 0. 2% , accounting for 20% –40% of all congenital heart diseases. According to the anatomical position, VSD is divided into membranous, arteriosus, muscular and mixed types.

2.1.2.1 Clinical manifestations

(1)Symptoms

The symptoms of patients are related to the size of VSD, the volume of blood flow and the degree of the elevated pulmonary artery pressure. If the VSD are complicated with small fractional flow, it might be asymptomatic or mild symptoms, or be naturally closed. If the VSD is complicated with large diameter or large volume, it manifests palpitations after exercise, dyspnea, difficulty of post–birth feeding, hypoevolutism, recurrent pulmonary infection, congestive heart failure, and persistent respiratory distress. If the patients, accompanied by increased pulmonary hypertension, are not treated in time, Eisenmenger syndrome may occur, including cyanosis and right heart failure.

(2)Signs

A typical VSD murmur could be heard, it is a holosystolic murmur between the third and fourth intercostal in the left margin of the sternum. Rough murmurs are, sometimes, conducted to the whole anterior chest wall. And with the increase of pulmonary artery pressure, the murmurs become short and soft, and finally completely vanish. When the patients are complicated with pulmonary hypertension and right ventricular hypertrophy, precordial prominence might be observed.

2.1.2.2 Accessory examinations

(1)Chest X–ray

It manifests increment of pulmonary blood flow, prominent of pulmonary artery segment and enlargement of left ventricle. If the patients are complicated with severe pulmonary hypertension, enlargement of right ventricle, reduction of pulmonary blood and bilateral pulmonary arteries could be observed.

(2) Electrocardiogram

The VSD with small fraction flow may show a normal electrocardiogram, but the VSD with larger fraction flow often manifests left deviation of electric axis and the left ventricular hypertrophy. With the progression of the pulmonary hypertension, the electrocardiogram of patients would show the enlargement of right ventricular and even the right ventricular hypertrophy.

(3) Color Doppler echocardiography

It shows the location and size of the VSD. Also, it shows the relationship between the aortic valve and the three apical valve. In addition, it shows the situation of left ventricular outflow tract and the shunt.

(4) Cardiac catheterization

It is the gold standard for definite diagnosis. Patients with a relatively simple condition or complicated with less sever degree of pulmonary hypertension do not need this examination. But for patients are complicated with severe pulmonary hypertension, it is necessary to examine pulmonary artery pressure, calculate pulmonary artery resistance, and observe the results of acute pulmonary artery dilatation test before surgery.

2.1.2.3 Differential diagnosis

(1) Atrial septal defect

Primary atrial septal defect is not easily to identify with ventricular septal defect. Especially the patients who are complicated with pulmonary hypertension, it is the most reliable to use cardiac catheterization to do the examination. Echocardiography could also be used for differential diagnosis.

(2) Pulmonary stenosis

The systolic murmur of the pulmonary valve is located in the second intercostals of the left margin of the sternum, which is the systolic murmur like the ejecting hair and generally not easy to confuse with the murmurs of the ventricular septal defect.

(3) Aortic stenosis

Systolic murmurs of aortic stenosis is located in the second intercostal of right margin of the sternum, and it conducts to the carotid artery. It is generally not confused with that of the ventricular septal defect. But if the patients are complicated with the subaortic stenosis, the murmurs can be heard between the third and fourth intercostal of the left margin of the sternum. And it should also be distinguished from the murmurs of ventricular septal defects.

2.1.2.4 Treatment

(1) Non-operative treatment

1) Oxygen therapy: It is helpful for patients who are complicated with cardiac insufficiency and arterial hypertension, and reduces pulmonary artery pressure and right heart afterload.

2) Drug: Surgeons often apply cardio drugs, diuretics, vasodilators and pulmonary artery pressure drugs to treat.

(2) Surgical treatment

1) Surgical indication: ①The patients who are complicated with moderate shunt volume(VSD diameter >0.5 cm) and clinical symptoms. Also the patients' auxiliary examination shows the ventricular enlargement or load aggravation. ②The patients are combined with aortic valve prolapse and closure, right ventricular outflow tract obstruction, patent ductus arteriosus and other cardiac malformations. ③Conical septum type of VSD. ④The patients are complicated with endocarditis. ⑤If the patients who are more than 2 years old, and are complicated with small shunt volume and asymptomatic. Also it's auxiliary examination is normal, but with any of the following indicators: aortic valve prolapse, history of endocarditis or ventricular en-

largement.

2)Operative method:Usually,surgeons adopt the tracheal intubation,intravenous anesthesia,and median sternum incision to repair directly under extracorporeal circulation. The establishment of cardiopulmonary bypass is as same as the general open heart surgery. In the operation,the determination of operative heart incision depends on the type of VSD. The common way are through the right atrium,the pulmonary artery, and the right ventricle to operate.

2.1.2.5 Postoperative complications

(1)Conduction block

The incidence is high in early VSD repairing patients,which is related to the damage of anatomical structure and inadequate exposure resulting from cardiopulmonary bypass inducing arrhythmia. The incidence of complete atrioventricular block which is related to the injury of atrioventricular node and His bundle during operation,is about 1%. Conduction block is associated with different types of VSD.

(2)Residual shunt

Inadequate exposure,suture leakage,excessive suture in suture process,too small or too large patch, infection,etc. ,lead to residual shunt,with an incidence of about 5%. If the larger flow volume ($Q_p/Q_s >$ 1.5 : 1)of VSD residual shunt after operation occurs,the patients need reoperation.

(3)Aortic insufficiency

It is commonly brought about by congenital aortic valvular prolapse,or traction of aortic valve during operation. Most of them need to be repaired in time,so surgeons should explore the anatomical relationship of the aortic valve carefully.

2.2 Right Heart Valve Disease

2.2.1 Pulmonary stenosis

Pulmonary stenosis is the most common type of pulmonary outlet stenosis. The incidence of it is 8% - 10% in the congenital heart diseases,of which only 90% of the simple pulmonary stenosis. The stenosis of the funnel,the artery trunk and its branch stenosis are rare.

2.1.1.1 Clinical manifestations

(1)Symptoms

Most of the patients is 10-20 years old. The symptoms are closely related to the degree of pulmonary stenosis,there may be no symptom in the patients with mild pulmonary stenosis. But with the increase of age,the symptoms,such as poor labor endurance,fatigue and heart palpitations after becoming tired,shortness of breath,might occur gradually. Dizziness or faintness could be found in the patients with severe stenosis,and the symptoms of right heart failure such as jugular congestion,liver enlargement and lower limb edemaoccur at the late stage.

(2)Signs

The main sign is that the resonant blowing systolic ejection murmur of level Ⅲ-Ⅳ in the second intercostal of the left margin of the sternum could be heard,which conducts to the left neck or the left subclavian region. The systolic tremor in the site where the murmur is most resonant could be touched. What's more,the noise intensity varies with the degree of stenosis,the flow velocity,the blood flow and the thickness of the chest wall. In the patients with severe pulmonary stenosis,forward bulge of the left margin of the sternum could be observed because of the right ventricular hypertrophy, and heaving apex impulse in the front of the heart could be felt. If combined with atrial septal defect, the patients may have cyanosis and clubbing (toes).

2.2.1.2　Accessory examinations

(1) Chest radiography

Enlargement of the right ventricle, thickening of the pulmonary artery, conical bulge, thinning of the hilar vessels and reduction of shadows could be found.

(2) ECG

The right axis deviation, high P wave and right ventricular hypertrophy could be observed in ECG.

(3) Color Doppler echocardiography

The examination shows enlargement of the right ventricle, and the location and degree of stenosis could also be determined.

(4) Cardiac catheterization

The systolic pressure difference between the right ventricle and the pulmonary artery could be determined to be more than 1.3 kPa (10 mmHg), and the cross valve pressure gradient reflects the degree of stenosis of pulmonary artery orifice.

2.2.1.3　Differential diagnosis

(1) Atrial septal defect

The signs of mild pulmonary stenosis are similar to atrial septal defect by the electrocardiogram examination, should be paid attention to identify.

(2) Interventricular septal defect

The signs of pulmonary stenosis are similar to those of VSD by the electrocardiogram examination. But they are generally not confused due to their differences in murmurs and location.

(3) Congenital primary pulmonary artery dilatation

The clinical manifestations of it are similar to those of light pulmonary stenosis by the electrocardiogram examination, and is difficult to differentiate and diagnose the disease. If by the right ventricular catheterization, surgeons do not find the systole pressure difference or other pressure abnormalities between right ventricle and pulmonary artery, and there is no shunt at the same time. Owing to the expansion of the total arc of the pulmonary artery is found by the chest X-ray, congenital primary pulmonary artery dilatation could be definitely diagnosed.

(4) Tetralogy of Fallot

If there is a cyanosis caused by right-to-left shunt in patients of severe pulmonary stenosis with atrial septal defect, it should be differentiated from tetralogy of Fallot carefully.

2.2.1.4　Treatment

Surgery is the main treatment for pulmonary valve stenosis. There are no clinical symptoms in the patients with mild pulmonary stenosis, the patients who grow and develop normally needn't surgical treatment. Patients with moderate or severe symptoms or gradually aggravated symptoms should be treated as early as possible.

(1) Percutaneous balloon pulmonary valvuloplasty

The balloon is delivered to the pulmonary valve by interventional therapy, and the pressure on balloon causes tension in the narrow opening of valve and leads to a tear of narrow embrane, thereby relieving pulmonary valve stenosis. It is suitable for the patients with simple pulmonary stenosis. There are often complications such as arrhythmia, pulmonary valve reflux, pulmonary artery injury, etc. , after operation.

(2) Surgical treatment

1) Direct vision section of pulmonary valve at low temperature: It is only suitable for patients with simple pulmonary valve stenosis, light illness, and without secondary funnel stenosis and other associated cardiac malformations.

2) Direct visual correction under extracorporeal circulation: It is suitable for the treatment of all kinds of pulmonary artery stenosis.

2.2.1.5　Complications

Besides the common complications of open heart surgery under general cardiopulmonary bypass, there are two main points:

(1) Low cardiac output syndrome

After pulmonary artery stenosis is relieved, the blood volume of pulmonary circulation increases significantly, so we should pay attention to adequate blood volume to avoid postoperative low cardiac output syndrome. If necessary, intravenous dopamine and carisoprodol should be added to enhance myocardial contractility.

(2) Pulmonary valve insufficiency

The surgery of pulmonary valve stenosis is one of the common causes of pulmonary insufficiency.

2.2.2　Tetralogy of Fallot

It is a common congenital heart malformation, which is caused by congenital dysplasia of right ventricle. The basic pathology includes ventricular septal defect, pulmonary artery stenosis, aortic riding span, and right ventricular hypertrophy. It is the most common in children cyanotic cardiac malformation.

2.2.2.1　Clinical manifestations

(1) Symptoms

1) Cyanosis: It often occurs after exercising or crying, and would be relieved after calming. Children often appear cyanosis 3-6 months after birth, and a few might appear in adults.

2) Dyspnea and hypoxic seizures: The children often appear dyspnea and hypoxic seizures 6 months after birth. Due to the lack of tissue hypoxia and poor activity endurance, the patients often have an ecphysesis after activity. The severe cases occur anoxic seizures, loss of consciousness, and convulsions.

3) Squatting: It is a characteristic gesture of this disease. Dyspnea and cyanosis through this posture might relieve in children.

(2) Signs

Children often develop poorly, and often have different degrees of cyanosis. The clubbing finger (toe) could be found in the elder children or adult patients. In the patients, the medium-term sprayed murmurs between second and third intercostal in the left margin of sternum could be heard. The less narrow, the louder murmurs. On the contrary, the narrow is heavier, the murmurs are lighter, and even the murmurs completely disappear. Usually it is without systolic tremor.

2.2.2.2　Accessory examinations

(1) Electrocardiogram

By electrocardiogram, patients shows the right deviation of electrocardio axis, right atrial hypertrophy and right ventricular hypertrophy. Approximately 20% of the patients show the incomplete right bundle branch block.

(2) Thoracic X-ray

Via thoracic X-ray, patients shows blunt and upward heart, and prominent aortic knot. Also it shows the decrease of pulmonary blood, and enlargement of right ventricular.

(3) Laboratory examination

It shows the increasing count of erythrocytes, hemoglobin and hematocrit. Also, it shows the decrease of arterial oxygen saturation, and platelet count.

(4) Echocardiogram

Most of the patients could be definitely diagnosed by it. It determines the location and size of ventricular septal defect, the extent of aortic riding span, the stenosis or degrees of right ventricular outflow tract or pulmonary artery, the development of ventricle, and the valve condition.

(5) Cardiac catheterization and angiographic examination

Indication: ①The patients could not use the echocardiography to diagnose clearly. ②There is a large lateral branch of the body and lung, which needs to be located and plugged. ③The patients are associated with abnormal coronary artery disease. ④The lesions of the patients are complex.

2.2.2.3　Differential diagnosis

(1) Cyanotic heart disease

For example, the double outlet right ventricle. Tetralogy of Fallot often has a history of squatting. The differential diagnosis depends on careful echocardiography, if not be identified, angiography should be adopted.

(2) Eisenberg's syndrome

Both of them have different basic pathological changes and should be identified carefully.

(3) Faroe triad

Cyanosis of Faroe triad is relatively late and its squatting is rare. There is jet systolic murmurs between the second intercostal in the left margin of the sternum. The murmurs have a long duration. Chest radiograph shows enlargement of right ventricle and right atrium, and prominent of pulmonary artery segment. Echocardiography should be used to differentially diagnose.

2.2.2.4　Treatment

(1) Palliative operation

If complicated with the poor development of pulmonary vessels and small left ventricle, and the malformation of the coronary artery affecting the employ of the right ventricular outflow tract patch in the operation, should be performed the palliative operation. The second stage correction operation should be carried out later.

(2) Radical operation

This operation could relieve the stricture of the right ventricular outflow tract completely, repair the ventricular septal defect closely, restore the normal blood flow of the left ventricle to the aorta and the right ventricle to the pulmonary artery, and close the abnormal connection of the patent ductus arteriosus, the body and lung shunt. Also, it could correct the other intracardiac and extra cardiac malformations.

2.2.2.5　Postoperative complications

(1) Low cardiac output syndrome: It is the main postoperative complications after TOF radical operation, and its causes include the following: ①The children are seriously ill, especially have the dysplasia of pulmonary artery and left ventricular. ②The satisfied deformity correction, and the favorable right ventricular outflow tract dredging. ③The postoperative factors include the favorable cardiac contractile function, vol-

ume condition, and the pericardial tamponade, electrolyte disorder and arrhythmia.

(2)Arrhythmia: It is a common complication after TOF radical operation. The incidence of complete cardiac arrest after operation is 3% –5%. By controlling the body temperature and antiarrhythmic drugs, the ventricular rate could be controlled. If still do not satisfy with the heart rate and blood pressure, surgeons could use the atrial synchronous pacing to do the electrical conversion.

(3)Residual leakage of ventricular septum.

(4)Pulmonary valve reflux.

(5)Right ventricular outflow tract residual stenosis.

2.2.3　Ebstein 's malformation

The three apical valve deformity (also known as Ebstein 's malformation) means that the three apical valve leaves moving down to the right ventricle. The patients are complicated with the abnormal development, enlargement of the valvular ring, insufficiency and the formation of the atrial right ventricle, or are combined with other congenital malformations. It is a rare congenital malformation with the incidence of 0.5% –1% in the congenital heart diseases.

2.2.3.1　Clinical manifestations

(1)Symptoms

In virtue of different degrees of malformation, the patients have different manifestations. It might be asymptomatic, or with palpitations and shortness of breath. Adult patients are prone to fatigue, and are often complicated with arrhythmia or preexcitation syndrome resulting in tachycardia. Due to the right to left shunt at the atrial level, cyanosis and clubbing fingers occur. When the patients are complicated with right heart insufficiency, the venous pressure is elevated, with hepatomegaly and lower extremities edema.

(2)Signs

Left anterior chest bulges, systolic tremor could be touched, and opening sound of tricuspid anterior lobe could also be heard, with splitting of first heart sound, decrease of fourth heart sound and second heart sound of pulmonary artery.

2.2.3.2　Accessory examinations

(1)ECG

It shows the supraventricular tachycardia, atrioventricular block, complete right bundle branch block, right ventricular hypertrophy and pre–excitation syndrome.

(2)Thoracic X–ray

It shows the deficiency of pulmonary blood, the depressed pulmonary artery segment, and the oval heart or the flask heart.

(3)Echocardiogram

It is helpful for definite diagnosis, and shows the tricuspid septal valve and posterior valve descending and the anterior closure retardation. The decline of EF slope, enlargement of right atrial ventricular, and the paradoxical movement of the atrioventricular right ventricle could also be observed. Horizontal shunt and three cuspid insufficiency could be demonstrated by Color Doppler.

(4)Right cardiac catheterization and angiography

It is not commonly needed. The septal and posterior lobes going downwards could be observed. The right atrium is large, and contrast agent emptying of the right atrium and the right ventricle are delayed. We could also observe sparse pulmonary vascular shadow, and the tricuspid regurgitation. If there is an atrial septal defect or acleistocardia, the signs of right to left shunt could be seen at the atrium level.

(5)MRI and CT

It is not commonly needed.

2.2.3.3   Differential diagnosis

(1)Congenital tricuspid regurgitation:Echocardiography finds no displacement of three apical valves.

(2)Atrial septal defect with tricuspid regurgitation:There is no displacement of the tricuspid valve, and the development of valves are normal.

2.2.3.4   Treatment

The mortality is high. If the patients have operative indications,they could be surgical treated,but surgeons should avoid changing the valve in children.

(1)Tricuspid valvuloplasty

It is suitable for patients with sufficient right ventricle volume and good development of anterior lobe. There are many techniques of tricuspid valvuloplasty. The Carpentier method is widely used and its clinical effect is better.

(2)Tricuspid valve replacement

It is suitable for patients that could not undergo valvuloplasty and with severe disease.

(3)Bidirectional Green surgery

It could be helpful for the patients who have obvious right ventricular dysfunction after tricuspid valvuloplasty or replacement.

(4)Starnes operation

It is suitable for severe neonates to expand the atrial septal defect and close the tricuspid valves opening under extracorporeal circulation. Surgeons could also establish the somatic pulmonary shunt.

2.2.3.5   Postoperative complications

(1)Low cardiac output syndrome

It is the main postoperative complication,and its causes includes the following:①The children are seriously ill,especially have the dysplasia of pulmonary artery and left ventricular. ②Whether the patients satisfies deformity correction,it would determine whether this complication occurs. ③The postoperative factors include favorable cardiac contractile function,volume condition,pericardial tamponade,electrolyte disorder and arrhythmia.

(2)Arrhythmia

Such as atrioventricular block,supraventricular tachycardia,etc.

(3)Coronary artery injury

It is usually caused by tricuspid valve replacement.

2.3   Aortic Valve Stenosis

Due to congenital aortic valve dysplasia,inflammatory invasion,degenerative change,calcification and other reasons,cause the structure and morphological changes of the aortic valve leaf but with a accretive boundary. It manifests as abnormal aortic valve leaf movement during cardiac contraction,reduced open area of the valve,resulting in that the blood is obstructed in the level of aortic valve leaf and cross valve pressure occurs.

2.3.1 Clinical manifestations

2.3.1.1 Symptoms

Patients with mild stenosis always have no clinical symptoms, and some patients with moderate stenosis show symptoms of chest tightness and shortness of breath when the activity is increased. Patients with severe stenosis often have symptoms of chest pain, vertigo, syncope and heart failure. A few patients with severe stenosis have sudden death after strenuous exercises.

2.3.1.2 Signs

Systolic murmurs above level 6 in aortic valve area could be heard, is often accompanied by systolic tremor, and always transmit to the neck. Mitral valve SAM signs could be observed in patients with thickened ventricular septum, and systolic blow murmur could be heard in apical area. For young patients, upper and lower extremity blood pressure should be measured to be sure if there is a coarctation of aortic arch.

2.3.2 Accessory examinations

2.3.2.1 ECG

Left ventricular hypertrophy and strain could be found. There may be atrioventricular block, indoor block, atrial fibrillation or ventricular arrhythmia. And some patients may be normal.

2.3.2.2 Chest radiography

Left ventricle enlargement, calcification in aortic valve area can be seen, and ascending aorta often dilates after stenosis. In some elderly patients, calcification involves in the sinus of valsalva and ascending aorta wall. When coarctation of aorta coexists, intercostal vessels become thickened and incisurae costales could be found.

2.3.2.3 Echocardiography

It is used to make a definite diagnosis. It shows aortic valve thickening, deformability, calcification and limited activity well. When calcification is severe, the aortic annulus and the anterior leaflet of mitral valve could be involved. It also shows that the aortic blood flow velocity and the cross valve pressure increase. The ascending aorta is dilated after stenosis, and the ventricular septum and left ventricular wall become more thick. Some patients with severe left ventricular hypertrophy, especially the severe thickening of the upper septum, could lead to left ventricular outflow tract stenosis and SAM signs of mitral valve. The velocity of blood flow in the aortic valve and left ventricular outflow tract are found to be increased by ultrasound.

2.3.2.4 Laboratory examination

For the patients whose ultrasonic diagnosis is clear and prepared for the operation, the blood, urine routine, whole set of biochemical examinations, prothrombin time, activity, immunological examination of hepatitis B, hepatitis C, syphilis and AIDS should be carried out.

2.3.2.5 Coronary arteriongraphy

Patients with the following conditions should perform the coronary angiography: ①Older than 50 years old. ②Age between 40–50, with chest pain or other symptoms of myocardial ischemia, or high risk factors for coronary heart disease.

2.3.3   Differential diagnosis

2.3.3.1   Congenital supravalvular aortic stenosis and congenital subaortic stenosis

Patients are always young, while patients with aortic stenosis are less likely to get ill before age 20. Echocardiography is applied to definitely identify the two diseases. Occasionally, in clinical, patients of aortic stenosis combined with congenital supravalvular aortic stenosis are found and easy to be confused.

2.3.3.2   Primary hypertrophic obstructive cardiomyopathy

Echocardiography could definitely diagnose this disease. Patients often have signs of ventricular septal thickening, left ventricular outflow tract stenosis, rapid blood flow, and SAM sign of anterior mitral leaflet.

2.3.4   Treatment

2.3.4.1   Expectant treatment

Asymptomatic patients with mild and moderate aortic stenosis should undergo routine electrocardiogram, chest radiograph and echocardiography annually.

2.3.4.2   Surgical treatment

Patients with symptoms such as syncope, angina pectoris, left ventricular dysfunction, severe stenosis should be in consideration. Medical treatment is not effective and intervention or surgical treatment should be performed.

(1) Aortic valve replacement

There are two kinds of prosthetic valves: mechanical and bioprosthetic valves, including stent, stent-free and homograft valves. In general, the operative mortality is 1%−2%. The risk of operation is further increased in elderly and female patients, or with severe calcification of the ascending aorta and aortic rings, small aortic ring, and other cardiac surgery.

(2) Aortic valve borderline section

It is suitable for patients with juncture adhesion and indistinctive calcification. For children or young patients with congenital valvular aortic stenosis and two petal valve, long-term valve replacement is still needed after the incision of the junction.

(3) Percutaneous balloon catheter dilatation

It is suitable for patients with congenital aortic stenosis, and symptoms of partial aortic stenosis could be relieved by this method.

(4) Ross operation

It is suitable for children or young patients with congenital aortic stenosis. Autologous pulmonary valve is transplanted to the position of aortic valve and the pulmonary artery is rebuilt by autologous pericardium or homogenous pulmonary artery conduit.

2.3.5   Postoperative complications

(1) Prosthetic valve dysfunction. Endogenous factors causing damage of valve structure include, fracture of the mechanical valve stents or rupture and deformation of the valvular lobe, tear of the valve leaf and degeneration of the valve. Exogenous factors include choice of valve improper, and the complications, such as thrombus, excessive hyperplasia of valvular tissue, and long line knot, etc.

(2) Haemorrhage. In patients with severe aortic stenosis, the wall of ascending aorta becomes pretty thin after the post-stenotic dilatation, the incidence of bleeding in the root of the incision is very high, and

it is important to improve the suture technique to prevent it.

(3) Cardiac insufficiency, parabasilar leak and infectious endocarditis.

2.4 Malformation of Artery and Vein

2.4.1 Patent ductus arteriosus

Arterial duct is a physiological blood flow channel between the pulmonary artery and the aorta on which the fetus survives. It usually performs functional closure at 10–20 hours after birth. Most of the infants' arterial duct closes 4 weeks after birth and degenerated to the patent ductus arteriosus ligaments. For some reasons, the arterial duct could not be closed, which is called patent ductus arteriosus. It is a common congenital cardiovascular malformation, accounting for 12%–15% in congenital heart diseases. About 10% of cases coexist with other cardiovascular malformations.

2.4.1.1　Clinical manifestations

(1) Symptoms

The symptoms depend on the size of the catheter, the pulmonary vascular resistance and the associated cardiac malformations. Children with small ductus arteriosus might be asymptomatic. In patients with moderate size of the patent ductus arteriosus, the flow rate increases significantly with the decrease of pulmonary vascular resistance after birth. The children often shows developmental delay, recurrent respiratory infection and fatigue. Infants with large patent ductus arteriosus develop heart failure, scorpion, shortness of breath, tachycardia and feeding difficulties within a few weeks after birth. Premature with large ductus arteriosus is often accompanied by respiratory distress and requires intubation and ventilator support. A few of patients may be complicated by subacute endocarditis. The symptoms of pulmonary hypertension caused by patent ductus arteriosus are characterized by exertional dyspnea and no left heart failure. Pulmonary artery dilatation constracts left laryngeal recurrent nerve resulting in hoarseness. If patients often have hemoptysis, the prognosis is poor. The right to left shunt caused by terminal closure of the catheter results in differential cyanosis.

(2) Sings

Continuous mechanical murmur is the characteristic sign. The most vocal part of the murmurs is between the first and the second intercostal spaces of the left margin of the sternum, and conducts to the left subclavian. And the apical pulsation of the precardiac region is enhanced and the pulse pressure is increased.

2.4.1.2　Accessory examinations

(1) ECG

The ECG of patients with small patent ductus arteriosus can be completely normal. The change of ECG depends on the degree and time of the increase of left ventricular load and the increase of right ventricular pressure load. The increased left ventricular load shows as high left ventricular voltage or left ventricular hypertrophy. When pulmonary hypertension occurs, double ventricular hypertrophy would be found. When pulmonary hypertension is serious, right ventricular hypertrophy will be shown.

(2) Chest radiography

Ascending aorta tends to be normal in infancy, and become thicker gradually after aging. The aortic node become more enlarged, and are different from other left to right shunt malformations. The leakage of descending aorta is the characteristic change. The size of the heart is related to the fractional flow. In patients with high volume of flow or increased pulmonary arterial pressure, the pulmonary artery segment is prominent, the left and right ventricles are enlarged, and the shadow of the ductus arteriosus could be seen between the aorta and pulmonary artery.

(3) Echocardiography

Left ventricular enlargement could be found by echocardiography, which is not characteristic. The two dimensional ultrasound explores from the superior fossa of the sternum, so that the arterial catheter could be found between the descending aorta and pulmonary artery, and the thickness and length could also be measured. The shunt could be displayed by Doppler examination.

(4) Cardiac catheterization

Right heart catheterization is needed, only if the patient has severe pulmonary hypertension or whether there is a surgical indication. It defines the direction of shunting and the size of the flow, measures the pressure of the pulmonary artery and calculates the pulmonary vascular resistance.

2.4.1.3　Differential diagnosis

(1) Aortopulmonary septal defect

In the early stage of the disease with severe pulmonary hypertension, the murmurs locate between the third and fourth intercostal intercostal margin of the left margin in the sternum and are more resonant in the systolic phase. Ultrasound, CT and MRI are applied to make definite diagnosis.

(2) Ventricular septal defect combined with aortic insufficiency

The murmur is a discontinuous double phase murmur between the third and the fourth intercostals of the left margin in the sternum, and the diastolic murmur is Kazakh and conducted to the apex. The aortic valve shunts and ventricular horizontal shunt signs could be identified by ultrasound.

(3) Ruptured aneurysm of aorta

There is always a history of sudden chest pain for patients with this disease. It progresses rapidly and occurs heart failure easily. The position of murmurs is low, and the murmurs is most resonant in the diastole phase. Through the echocardiography, the high dilated aortic sinus is observed in a certain heart cavity, especially in the right ventricle.

2.4.1.4　Treatment

After the establishment of patent ductus arteriosus, surgical operation should be performed if there is no contraindication.

(1) Ligation of catheterization

This operation is suitable to infants and children with diameter below 1 cm, good elasticity of catheter wall and no moderate or serve pulmonary hypertension.

(2) Patent ductus arteriosus suture

This method is effective, and avoids the risk of recurrence or the risk of aneurysm caused by the cut wall.

(3) Closure of catheter under extracorporeal circulation

It is suitable for the patients of patent ductus arteriosus with severe pulmonary hypertension, the elder patients, patients with bacterial endocarditis, patients of ventricular septal defect or other cardiac malformation with the ductus arteriosus, patients after a first stage operation, patients with a recanalization of catheter after ligation, or patients that an accidental massive hemorrhage or acute heart failure may occur in the routine operation.

(4)Tcvsd by cardiac catherization

It is suitable for most of the patients.

2.4.1.5 Postoperative complications

The most common complications are haemorrhage, recurrent laryngeal nerve injury, pseudoaneurysm, chylothorax, and catheter recanalization.

2.4.2 Aorta coarctation

Aorta coarctation is a congenital hemodynamic stenosis in the upper segment of the aorta near the opening of the ductus arteriosus. The most serious degree of stenosis could be a lumen atresia. But unlike aortic arch interruption, the aortic wall at the both ends of the coarctation of the aorta is continuous. In some rare cases, aorta coarctation occurs in the aortic arch which is between the left common carotid artery and left subclavian artery.

2.4.2.1 Clinical manifestations

(1)Symptoms

With the decrease of pulmonary circulation resistance and the closure of ductus arteriosus, the symptoms of pale, low perfusion of the whole body, metabolic acidosis, and even the abdominal organ ischemia or necrosis might occur in the newborn with severe coarctation of the aorta. The most common symptoms of infantile patients are shortness of breath, irritability, hyperhidrosis and feeding difficulties. For the patients of older children and adults, if the lateral branch develops well, there may be only symptoms of limited movement and fatigable lower limb.

(2)Signs

It is easy to be accompanied by cardiac deformity for the patients of anterior ductal constriction. The patients always go to the hospital because of congestive heart failure during infancy. About half of the patients aggravates during the first month after birth when their ductus arteriosus is closed, and the systolic murmur could be found on the left front chest and back. The patients of postductal type is usually asymptomatic in childhood. Older children and adults often visit doctors because of upper extremity hypertension and hypertension complications. And the symptoms increase with age and the patients may suffer intermittent claudication due to lower body ischemia.

2.4.2.2 Accessory examinations

(1)Chest radiography

There may be no enlargement or just slight enlargement for the heart.

(2)ECG

There may be ventricular hypertrophy, especially the left ventricular. And if it is combined with pulmonary hypertension, there may be a combined ventricular hypertrophy. About 1/3 of the diseased children have normal electrocardiogram.

(3)Echocardiography

Transthoracic echocardiography is highly sensitive to the diagnosis of coarctation of the aorta. The two dimensional echocardiography is always used to explore from the suprasternal fossae, and shows the panorama of the long axis of the aortic arch and helps judge the location and length of aorta coarctation.

(4)CT and MRI

Through enhancement and continuous scanning of the aortic arch, it shows the location of aorta coarctation.

（5）Cardiac angiography

For the typical aortic coarctation, it is not a routine examination. But aortic angiography is still the most intuitive way for observing coarctation of the aorta, and shows the area, range, large vessels of coarctation and the collateral circulation.

2.4.2.3　Differential diagnosis

（1）Interruption of aortic arch

When the pulmonary artery resistance drops and the ductus arteriosus closes, the patients of interruption of aortic arch become critically ill and have severe abdominal organ ischemia and acidosis. Identification of severe aortic shortening and aortic arch interruption in neonates relies mainly on echocardiography.

（2）Aorto-arteritis

This disease often occurs in female adults, with the manifestations of inflammation such as fever and rapid erythrocyte sedimentation. The aorta and its primary branch are affected. The aorta stenosis is always not limited and multiple. In most of patients, it is not combined with cardiac malformation.

2.4.2.4　Treatment

（1）Medication

The antihypertensive drugs are often used to control blood pressure.

（2）Interventional therapy

It includes two methods: simple balloon angioplasty and stent implantation. Overall, interventional therapy for aorta coarctation is still in the exploratory stage.

（3）Surgical treatment

In general, once the aorta coarctation is definitely diagnosed, operation should be performed as soon as possible to relieve the difference of blood pressure between the proximal and distal ends. Excision of coarctation and end-to-end anastomosis are suitable for children with limited stenosis. The forming operation of aorta coarctation, including patch forming and artificial vascular transplantation, is suitable for the patients with long coarctation segment and is difficult to perform end-to-end anastomosis after coarctation segment excision. This operation is better for the patients over 16 years old. The main artery coarctation bypass grafting is suitable for the patients with wide constriction and the site difficult to be exposed, and that resection is difficult or with reconstruction requiring a reoperation.

2.4.2.5　Complications

The most common postoperative complications include the following:

（1）Postoperative hypertension, abdominal pain, and chylopleura.

（2）Recurrence of restenosis or coarctation of the aorta.

（3）Post-operative advanced aneurysm formation. The main reason is that the residual ductus arteriosus and artificial patch materials do not match the compliance of the natural aortic wall.

2.5　Cor Triatriatum

Cor triatriatum is a congenital cardiovascular malformation in which the left or right atrial septum is divided into two parts. It is a rare congenital heart disease that approximately accounts for 0.1% of congenital heart diseases. The right cor triatriatum is less common, only accounting for about 8% of the cor triatriatum. The proximal left atrial diaphragm which is above right rear receives the pulmonary venous blood, is called the secondary heart chamber or the third heart chamber. The distal diaphragm which is the left bottom is the intrinsic left atrium and left atrial appendage which is the real left atrium that the mitral valve communicates with the left ventricle. Both are connected by the channel of the diaphragm. This deformity can exist alone and often combined with other deformities, and the most common is atrial septal defect or complete pulmonary vein abnormal reflux. The surgical effect is better, and the pulmonary artery pressure may drop to normal after surgery. The mortality rate of infants with congestive heart failure is extremely high.

2.5.1　Histoembryology

At 3-week old embryo, the lung buds and bronchial tree emerge from the foregut and differentiate into the left main vein and right main vein via the common main vein. The left main vein later differentiates into the left sinus's left horn and further into the left superior vena cava and coronary sinus. After the right main vein is differentiated into the right sinus of the venous sinus and further into the right superior vena cava and the azygos vein, the umbilical-yolk vascular vein differentiates into inferior vena cava, venous catheter and portal vein in the future. At the 5th weeks of embryonic development, the embryo length is 9-13 mm. At this point, the left and right separation processes within the original heart chamber are nearly complete, the anterior and posterior endocardial of the atrioventricular tube are joined together, the first and second rooms have been closed, and the first and second atrial septums have been completed. The posterior wall of the original left atrium protrudes outwards from a blind tube, i. e. , the pulmonary veins. At the same time, the venules in the pulmonary veins also merge into four veins. The four veins and the pulmonary veins protruding from the posterior wall of the left atrium are connected and communicated with each other so that the blood from the pulmonary veins flows into the left atrium. The pulmonary veins continuously expand and merge with the original left atrium, forming the posterior wall of the left atrium. The four pulmonary veins are opened in the left atrium. Embryology is still not clear on the causes of the formation of cor triatriatum.

2.5.2　Clinical types

Although the pathological anatomical classification method of the cor triatriatum has its own characteristics, it does not yet have the authority of the unified classification. The common typing methods such as Loeffler, Gasnl, and Mrin are based on whether there is traffic and anatomy of traffic anatomy between the anterior chamber and the true left atrium. Van Praagh is classified according to whether there is an ectopic drainage of pulmonary veins. Some pulmonary veins are the same and are divided into complete or partial types. They are divided into simple type and complex type according to whether they are associated with other intracardiac deformities. This type of method is more practical in clinical practice.

2.5.3　Clinical manifestations

The time of symptoms is related to the size of the diaphragm hole. Severe cases of small holes occur soon after birth, with severe pulmonary congestion and shortness of breath, followed by severe pneumonia and congestive heart failure. In cases with large orifices, symptoms appear later and occur in young children or children. Cases with large openings resemble atrial septal defects and are clinically asymptomatic and living normally. They only have slight shortness of breath after the activity. In most cases, jet systolic murmurs and diastolic murmurs could be heard at the bottom of the heart. Continual noise can sometimes be heard. This is due to the high degree of obstruction. But it can also be noise-free.

2.5.4   Auxiliary examination

2.5.4.1   X-ray

The heart is mildly to moderately enlarged, with right ventricular hypertrophy predominant. There is obvious pulmonary hypertension but the left atrium is not large or only slightly increases its characteristics, the superior vena cava is expanded, the interstitial lung occurs edema, pulmonary arterial segment highlights the symptoms of pulmonary hypertension.

2.5.4.2   Electrocardiogram

Right axis deviation, right ventricular hypertrophy, increased P wave prompted right atrial hypertrophy.

2.5.4.3   Echocardiography

B-mode echocardiography shows left atrium, abnormal septal echo could be seen above the mitral valve. Pulsed Doppler ultrasound shows abnormal septum, and could observe blood flow through the septum and the size of the atrial septal defect, which is helpful for diagnosis.

2.5.4.4   Cardiac catheterization and angiography

The right heart catheter is characterized by increased pulmonary arterial wedge pressure and true left atrial pressure is low or normal. About 1/3 of the cases entering the right atrium after entering the right atrium through the atrial septal defect or oval hole into the left atrium. The left atrial angiography shows abnormal left diaphragm in the diaphragm. If showed the deputy room, no contraction could be observed in the cardiac cycle, but it would keep a constant shape. Cardiac catheter angiography is not commonly adapted in normal examination.

2.5.5   Surgical indications

The traffic holes between the secondary room with the true left atrium is actually small. Due to pulmonary vein obstruction, and pulmonary hypertension and right heart failure are gradually produced, therefore it is more appropriate for the infants and children to take the cor triatriatum operations. In severe cases, the cor triatriatum should be surgically treated once diagnosed.

2.5.6   Surgical contraindications

Older patients with severe pulmonary hypertension should consider whether their pulmonary vascular lesions are retrograde or not. People with no atria and left ventricle should pay attention to the development of their left ventricle.

2.5.7   Treatment

The primary principle of surgery is to remove the left atrium septum, so that the true and deputy rooms are fully communicated. Closing the ASD and the complex cor triatriatum requires correcting other intracardiac deformities at the same time.

Surgical procedures are performed under mild hypothermic cardiopulmonary bypass. A midline sternotomy incision is taken. The real atrial, accessory, and pulmonary venous mitral valves are exposed through the right atrial septal approach and the septum is completely removed. Patients with atrial fibrillation in the cor triatriatum can also perform maze surgery at the same time.

ASD or incision atrial septal incision can be a good exposure. If the ASD is not large enough to reveal well, the ASD can be expanded. Excision of the septum should be thorough, which is the key to correct hemodynamics once, but be careful not to over-pull the septum to prevent cutting the left atrial wall. If necessary, the septum remnants can be sutured continuously to prevent rupture of the left atrial wall. When the septum is cut, the septum is usually cut before the septum, and the left atrial appendage and the mitral valve hole can be found after the septum is pulled open. The loss of the mitral annulus should be avoided. During the operation, attention should also be paid to the exploration and correction of other complications. At the time of repairing the atrial septum, attention should be paid to the simultaneous correction of the pulmonary venous ectopic junction and the opening of the coronary sinus to the right atrium. The room was patched with polyester sheets or autologous pericardial patches. The key to the success of surgery is to completely relieve the pulmonary veins.

2.6   Double-chamber Right Ventricle

The double-chamber right ventricle is a congenital heart disease caused by one or more abnormal muscle bundles crossing the right ventricular cavity and dividing the right ventricle into a high-pressure cavity that flows into the part and a low-pressure cavity that flows out of the cavity, causing blood flow obstruction. The double-chamber right ventricle is often accompanied by other congenital heart malformations. Pathological anatomy can be divided into three types: muscle septum, muscle bundle, and hybrid, depending on the shape of the muscle bundle. Most cases with ventricular septal defect, are still combined with pulmonary valve stenosis, or aortic valve or subvalvular stenosis and other cardiac malformations.

2.6.1   Pathophysiology

Because the abnormal muscle bundle divides the right ventricle into the high pressure chamber of the proximal tricuspid valve (inflow part) and the low pressure chamber of the proximal pulmonary artery (outflow part), the right ventricle-to-pulmonary artery is obstructed. The degree of obstruction is associated with the size and number of abnormal muscle bundles, and other intracardiac deformities. If the combined ventricular septal defect is located in the high pressure chamber, the pressure of right ventricular is higher than that of left ventricular, causing different degrees of right-to-left shunt; if located below, it causes left-to-right shunt and pulmonary hypertension.

2.6.2   Clinical manifestations

It is related to the degree of bleeding and heart malformation.

2.6.2.1   Symptoms

It is easy to catch cold and fever in childhood. Palpitation, shortness of breath, fatigue, and severe stenosis cases have cyanosis.

2.6.2.2   Signs

The sternal contraction murmur of 3-4 grades could be heard between the 3rd and 4th intercostal spaces of the left sternal border. The conduction is extensive, and contraction tremors are touched. The 2nd heart sounds in pulmonary artery mostly decreases, but a few cases are normal or have hyperthyroidism.

2.6.3   Auxiliary inspections

2.6.3.1   Chest X-ray

Mild patients may have no significant changes, normal pulmonary veins texture. Severe manifestation of the right heart enlargement, the lungs and blood vessels are sparsely textured.

2.6.3.2   Electrocardiogram

Most patients have a right axis, with right ventricular hypertrophy or double-chamber hypertrophy. In a minority of patients with left ventricular hypertrophy, the R wave of lead aVR is not prominent, and the R wave is high in V_3 and V_4 leads.

2.6.3.3   Echocardiography

The funnel is normal. Anomalous myotubes protrude from the anterior wall of the right ventricle to the ventricular septum, and color Doppler ultrasound can measure the pressure gradient between the two chambers.

2.6.3.4   Catheterization and angiography

Different curves can be measured in the pulmonary artery, the funnel cavity and the right ventricular sinus. The pressure gradient between the high pressure chamber and the low pressure chamber exceeds 10 mmHg. Right ventricle angiography could determine the position and shape of abnormal muscle bundles and show a filling defect.

2.6.4   Diagnosis

The pathophysiological changes and clinical manifestations of right ventricular double-chamber heart depend on the degree of intracardiac obstruction and are affected by the presence of concomitant cardiac malformations. Severe cases may have purpura and clubbing fingers and toes. Chest X-ray and electrocardiogram lack specificity. Two-dimensional echocardiography showed no stenosis of the right ventricular infundibulum and a large third ventricle, whereas there is a stenosis caused by an abnormal muscular bundle in the ventricular body below the funnel cavity. The right heart catheterization can measure different pressure curves in the pulmonary artery, the funnel cavity and the right ventricular sinus. The pressure difference between the right and the proximal cavity of the right ventricle exceeds 1.3 kPa (10 mmHg). In severe cases, the intra-chamber pressure in the proximal part of the right ventricle exceeds the left ventricular pressure.

2.6.5   Surgical indications

(1) Pure DCRV: The pressure difference in the right ventricle which is greater than 5.3 kPa (40 mmHg), should be treated by surgery. If less than 5.3kPa (40 mmHg), it needs no immediate operation, but should take regular follow-up to observe changes. Some surgeons propose that it should be surgically treated immediately once diagnosed considering abnormal muscle bundles progressively increases.

(2) Combining with other cardiac malformations requires surgical correction and removal of abnormal muscle bundles while correcting other malformations.

2.6.6   Surgical methods

2.6.6.1   Out-of-cardiac exploration

After the pericardium is cut open, the development of the pulmonary artery is well, and its outside diameter is similar to that of the aorta. Unlike the tetralogy of Fallot, the aorta is not significantly thickened or moved to the right. The systolic tremor can be touched in the infundibulum; the right ventricular outflow tract has a transverse depression on its surface, which is the connection between the high-pressure cavity and the low-pressure cavity. A small marginal branch from the right coronary artery is obliterated. In patients diagnosed with ventricular septal defect, if the change is found during operation, it is highly suspected.

2.6.6.2　Right ventricular outflow tract path

This method is a traditional surgical method, and it is more convenient to relieve obstruction and ventricular deficiencies caused by the abnormal intraventricular muscular bundle formation. This method is more suitable for cases with higher obstruction sites and closer to the pulmonary valve. Sometimes it requires patch expansion of the right ventricular outflow tract. Because the right ventricle has more muscles that are cut off by this method, it has a certain influence on the function of the right ventricle and has been used less frequently.

2.6.6.3　Transseptal atrial approach

In most cases, tricuspid valve resection of abnormal right ventricular muscle bundles, dredging right ventricular outflow tract, can receive satisfactory results. This method requires more anatomical knowledge and clinical experience to avoid damage to the tricuspid valve chordae and coronary artery septum. For young adolescents or adult patients with severe secondary right ventricular outflow tract obstruction, if the tricuspid regurgitation abnormal muscle bundle is not thorough enough, surgeons should consider reopening the pulmonary trunk and removing the abnormally high myocolic bundles through the pulmonary valve. It is conducive to completely clearing the outflow. Compared with the right ventricular outflow tract, this method has better protection for right ventricular function and is currently used more widely.

2.7　Double Outlet Right Ventricle

The double outlet of the right ventricle originates from the right ventricle in the aorta and the pulmonary artery, or most of the aorta and the other aorta originate in the right ventricle, and the ventricular septal defect is the sole outlet of the left ventricle. Ventricular septal defect is usually larger than the diameter of the aorta, and the caliber of the ventricular septal defect is smaller than that of the aortic opening in only 10% of cases. About 60% of the ventricular septal defect is located below the aortic valve, 30% below the pulmonary valve, and a few cases have ventricular septal defect. The location of the ventricular septal defect in the middle of the aorta and pulmonary artery below the opening of the ventricular septal defect is located in the middle and lower ventricular septum and aortic opening farther. It is common for the aorta and pulmonary artery to open in the same plane and the aorta located on the right. Followed by the opening of the aorta is located right behind the opening of the pulmonary artery, and the opening of the aorta located in the right front of the opening of the pulmonary artery. The aortic opening is located in the left front of the opening of the pulmonary artery. This situation is more common in patients with inhomogenous right ventricle double outlets. 90% of the patients have the same atrioventricular relationship, the right atrium is connected to the right ventricle, the left atrium connected to the left ventricle, and the involuntary relationship accounts for only about 10%. Other pulmonary malformations include infundibular stenosis, the main aortic stenosis, the atrioventricular valve abnormalities, ventricular failure development, atrial septal defect, and coronary artery abnormalities.

2.7.1　Pathophysiology

The hemodynamic changes in the right ventricle with double outlet mainly depends on the location and size of the ventricular septal defect, and whether it is associated with pulmonary artery stenosis and its degree. When the ventricular septal defect is located under the aortic valve and no pulmonary artery stenosis, blood in the left ventricular directly flows into the aorta through the defect, and the main right ventricular blood into the pulmonary artery, pulmonary blood flow increases. It is clinically similar to simple ventricular septal defect combined with pulmonary hypertension. When the ventricular septal defect is located under the pulmonary valve and no pulmonary artery stenosis, blood of the left ventricular directly flows into the pulmonary artery through the defect, and the main right ventricular blood into the aorta. It is clinically similar to complete arterial dislocation combined with ventricular septal defect, with pulmonary congestion and severe Cyanosis. Regardless of the location and size of ventricular septal defects, if there is pulmonary artery stenosis or tetralogy of Fallot, the patients displays pulmonary ischemia and severe cyanosis.

2.7.2   Clinical manifestations

Aortic subvalvular VSD is not associated with pulmonary stenosis. Symptoms similar to large VSD, usually bruising may not be obvious, due to the presence of pulmonary congestion, manifested as shortness of breath, excessive sweating, backward development, right recurrent respiratory infections and congestive heart failure in infants, children with sternum. There are three grades of systolic murmurs and tremors in the left and right margin of the 3rd—4th intercostal space. The second tone of the pulmonary valve area is hyperactive. Sometimes the third heart sound can be heard in the apex. If left untreated, advanced pulmonary vascular disease can be progressed.

If the aortic subvalvular VSD combined with pulmonary stenosis, clinical manifestations similar to Fallot tetralogy, hair cyanosis within 1 year after birth, depending on the degree of pulmonary artery stenosis, the performance of cyanosis is different, and the child may be manifested as backward development, paralysis, or even hypoxic episodes. In the left sternal border, there are systolic murmurs and tremors in grade 3 in the intercostal space between the 3rd and 4th rib, and the second tone in the pulmonary valve area is weakened, sometimes smells the third heart sound in the apex.

Clinical manifestations of pulmonary subvalvular VSD are similar to that of complete arterial dislocation with VSD. Cyanosis, recurrent respiratory infections, and heart failure appear in infants. If accompanied by pulmonary artery stenosis, aggravate cyanosis and heart failure, the child develops backward. In the left sternal border, there are systolic murmurs and tremors in grade 3 in the intercostal space between the 3rd and 4th rib, and the second tone of the pulmonary valve area is weakened. Most children patients may die in infancy.

2.7.3   Diagnosis

Clinical manifestations are affected by the presence and location of right ventricular outflow tract and pulmonary valve stenosis and the main pulmonary artery. The patient may behave similar to VSD with pulmonary hypertension or Fallot tetralogy. Physical examination, electrocardiogram and X-ray film are not characteristically. Echocardiography can determine the relationship between VSD and large vessels, the location and size of VSD, whether there is pulmonary hypertension, and whether the atrioventricular valve is abnormal. The right heart catheter and angiography can be diagnosed and know about the development condition of the ventricular and great blood vessels and coronary arteries. Ultra-high-speed CT or MRI helps diagnose. Simple DORV can be diagnosed according to the results of the ultrasound examination and surgical treatment is performed accordingly. Complex DORV or other cardiac malformations require angiocardiography before surgery.

2.7.4 Treatments

2.7.4.1 Surgical indications

Right ventricle double outlet with VSD but without other cardiac malformations, surgical indications consistent with ventricular septal defect combined with pulmonary hypertension should be treated as soon as possible, especially the ventricular septal defect pulmonary hypertension under the pulmonary artery occurs earlier, should be operated within 2 years old. For Taussig-Bing malformation, palliative surgery is feasible. Rastelti surgery or intra-atrial ventricular septal defect repair surgery is performed 4-5 years post palliative surgery. If the condition allows, transposition of the ventricular septal defect should be repaired as much as possible before half a year old. If the right ventricle double outlet combined with pulmonary valve and right ventricular outflow tract stenosis, operation should be taken as soon as possible, and the surgical indications are consistent with Fallot tetralogy. If combined with other deformities, such as complete endocardial cushion defect, aortic valve deformity, etc., should be corrected as soon as possible. Due to different types of clinical manifestations and not timely treatment, children often die of severe complications. It is performable to select appropriate surgical options to reduce mortality according to the manifestation types.

2.7.4.2 Surgical methods

It is generally advocated that radical surgery is performed after the age of 2 years old. The purpose of the operation is as follows:

(1) An artificial tunnel is established between the ventricular septal defect and the subaortic outflow tract using a Dacron patch. Care should be taken to avoid obstruction of this connection, and it is sometimes necessary to expand the ventricular septal defect.

(2) The establishment of a pathway between the right ventricle and the pulmonary artery can be achieved by expanding the patch through the right ventricular outflow tract, incising the pulmonary valve, or connecting the right ventricle with the pulmonary artery via an artificial valved tube.

(3) Repair the concomitant malformations. It is recently reported that the mortality rate of double outlets of right ventricle in the neonatal period is as low as 4% -8%.

2.8 Double Outlet Left Ventricle

The left ventricle double(DOLV) outlet is a very rare congenital cardiovascular malformations. The two large arteries originate from the left ventricle, the two arterial openings lie in the same plane, the bilateral cones and conus muscles are not fully developed, the aortic valve, pulmonary valve, semilunar valve and mitral valve are continuous. Commonly accompanied with ventricular septal defect, pulmonary stenosis, tricuspid valve down malformation, right ventricular dysplasia, atrioventricular inconsistency, atrial and visceral anteroposterior or reversed malformations. Hemodynamic changes in the left ventricle double outlet, similar to severe tetralogy of Fallot or complete arterial dislocation combined with ventricular septal defect.

2.8.1 Pathophysiology

The hemodynamic changes of DOLV mainly depend on the location of VSD and the presence of pulmonary artery stenosis. When VSD is located under the aorta, low-oxygen-containing right ventricular blood mainly enters the aorta via VSD, and its hemodynamic changes are similar to complete transposition of the main arteries with VSD, usually accompanied with cyanosis and heart failure. Because 85% of patients with

DOLV have pulmonary stenosis, cyanosis is more pronounced. When the VSD of DOLV is located under the pulmonary artery, its hemodynamics is similar to that of a normal VSD. If accompanied with pulmonary stenosis, the hemodynamic change is similar to Fallot tetralogy, and the cyanosis is prominent but the heart failure is rare.

2.8.2   Clinical manifestations

It is associated with pathological anatomy and malformations.

2.8.2.1   Symptoms

The patients manifest different degrees of purpura, with or without pulmonary stenosis, the degree of stenosis and the location of ventricular septal defect. The cyanosis may increase with crying and activities. There may be slow growing development, and laboring breathing difficulty.

2.8.2.2   Signs

In the 3rd–4th intercostal spaces of sternal border, systolic tremors could be touched and loud systolic murmurs could be heard.

2.8.3   Diagnosis

The diagnosis of DOLV mainly depends on ultrasound and cardiac catheterization. Echocardiography shows the connection between the two main arteries and the left ventricle, VSD location, large cones and other concomitant malformations. Left and right ventricular ejections from the left and right ventricles of the two–plane film angiography are performed from the left ventricle, showing the location and number of VSD, whether there is a stenosis of the pulmonary artery, the size of the left and right ventricles, and whether it is balanced.

DOLV is a rare congenital heart malformation. Most misdiagnosed congenital heart disease as DOLV is an inhomogenous atrioventricular double outlet. The malformation morphology is located on the left side of the right ventricle. It is connected to the mitral valve and sends out two major arteries. If the degree of trabecular roughening is not noticed by cardiac angiography, the morphological right ventricle located on the left side is probably misdiagnosed as a morphological left ventricle.

2.8.4   Surgical treatments

Surgical indications should be the same as that of the double outlet right ventricle. The diagnosed case should be performed surgically. In infants with left ventricle double outlet with pulmonary congestion, early surgery or pulmonary cerclage should be preferred. If pulmonary stenosis is combined with pulmonary ischaemia, it is advisable to first perform a body–to–pulmonary shunt, and then use a valved–cardiac catheter for resection. However, if severe pulmonary vascular obstructive disease has occurred, it is a surgical contraindication.

According to the location of ventricular septal defect and whether there is pulmonary artery stenosis, combined with extracorporeal circulation at low temperature, surgery should be performed through the median sternotomy incision.

(1) The ventricular septal defect is located below the pulmonary valve without pulmonary stenosis: through a right ventricular incision, a patch is used to construct the inner tunnel and the pulmonary artery is connected to the right ventricle. If combined with pulmonary stenosis, surgeons must remove the stenosis. Outflow tract augmentation orthopedics is performed when needed.

(2) The ventricular septal defect is located below the aortic valve with or without pulmonary artery ste-

nosis: through the right ventricle incision, the patch closes the ventricular septal defect, close the pulmonary valve orifice or suture the proximal pulmonary artery, and uses a valved extracardiac catheter to connect the right ventricle with the pulmonary artery.

(3) Close the ventricular septal defect and expand the right ventricular outflow tract.

(4) Close the ventricular septal defect, suture the pulmonary valve, excise the infundibular hypertrophied muscle, employ the patch to reconstruct and expand the right ventricular outflow tract, and implant the artificial valve into the pulmonary artery.

2.9　Single Ventricle

Single ventricle is a rare congenital malformation. Its incidence in living infants is about 1 : 6500, accounting for about 1.5% of congenital heart diseases. The ventricle receives blood from both tricuspid and mitral valves or common atrioventricular valves.

2.9.1　Clinical manifestations

Most single-chamber patients have obvious congenital heart disease manifestations in the early years, such as purpura, tachycardia, or slow weight gain, which attracts attention in newborns or early in babies. Patients with more pulmonary blood are often found in early stages. Untreated single-chamber patients have a shorter natural lifespan.

2.9.2　Diagnosis

2.9.2.1　Physical examination

Achilles tendon and clubbing (toe) are seen in patients with reduced pulmonary blood flow. Increased abnormal pulmonary blood flow showed poor growth and weight loss in patients with chronic congestive heart failure. If congestive heart failure or right atrioventricular valve stenosis without atrial septal defect is happened, the jugular vein is full or engorgement. If the right side of the atrioventricular valve insufficiency is severe, the jugular vein and the liver will have systolic beats.

In the visual examination and palpation, the heart beat is shown to be diffused, and the aorta is relatively anterior in many patients, and the aortic valve is closed at the left sternal border in the percussion.

The first heart sound can be enhanced during auscultation, and the second heart sound is also strong and single. Most patients can hear loud systolic murmurs from pulmonary valve stenosis or subaortic stenosis. Patients with increased pulmonary blood flow can hear diastolic murmurs from the relative narrowing left atrioventricular valve at the apex.

2.9.2.2　Auxiliary inspections

(1) ECG examination

The results vary due to the ventricular subtypes, but most patients have ventricular hypertrophy.

(2) Chest X-ray examination

Most patients have heart shadow enlargement, pulmonary blood increase or decrease depending on whether there is pulmonary valve stenosis. Left atrial enlargement is observed in patients with increased pulmonary blood flow or atrioventricular valve insufficiency. Other aspects vary depending on the pathological anatomy of each subtype.

(3) Cardiac catheterization and angiography

It is used to confirm the diagnosis of single ventricle and its type and comorbidities. The goals and objectives of the examination include the following: ①the type of single ventricle; ②the presence and location of the chamber at the outlet; ③the spatial position of the pulmonary artery of the aorta and the room-to-chamber correlation; ④the presence and location of obstruction of the pulmonary artery or aortic blood flow; ⑤the number, position, function status of the atrioventricular valve, and its deviation and ride-over; ⑥pulmonary arterial pressure and resistance; ⑦ventricular function; ⑧pulmonary artery thickness, distribution, or twists caused by loop surgery; ⑨ malformations. Although the venous blood of the systemic circulation and pulmonary circulation is mixed in a single ventricle, the blood oxygen saturation of the pulmonary artery and the aorta can not be considered to be the same due to the different blood flow conditions in the heart chamber. Therefore, in order to accurately calculate the pulmonary circulation and the systemic circulation resistance, the blood oxygen saturation and pressure of the two arteries must be determined separately.

(4) Echocardiography examination

Two-dimensional ultrasound imaging has basically replaced invasive cardiac catheterization, and provides many aspects of observation and analysis of single ventricle patients, such as the basic anatomy of the heart, the relationship between the main arteries, cardiac malformations, pulmonary stenosis or ventricular stenosis. The new Doppler technique could quantitatively measure the extent of pulmonary artery stenosis, ventricular output obstruction, and atrioventricular valve insufficiency. Echocardiography is superior to cardiovascular imaging in understanding the morphology, deviation, and striding of the atrioventricular valve.

2.9.3　Surgical treatments

(1) Palliative surgery aims to increase (body-pulmonary artery shunt) or reduce (pulmonary artery loop) pulmonary blood flow to improve symptoms. However, palliative surgery also has its drawbacks. For instance, pulmonary artery distorting after somatic-pulmonary artery shunting often causes difficulty in reconstructive surgery. Pulmonary blood flow increasing too much contributes to heart failure due to increasing ventricular volume load; superior vena cava-pulmonary artery anastomosis (Glenn surgery) does not increase ventricular volume load, but sometimes ipsilateral pulmonary artery spasm occurs in the late stage; pulmonary artery band displaces to the distal side causing pulmonary artery distortion.

(2) Ventricular extracorporeal surgery (Fontan operation) allows the pulmonary circulation and the ventricle to directly enter the pulmonary artery from the atrium (suture the side of the atrioventricular valve and the pulmonary artery), while the remaining monoventricular special donor is used for circulation.

(3) The ventricular septum employs a large man-made fiber fabric to divided the ventricular chamber into two, and each receives the blood from one side of the atrioventricular valve and supplies the pulmonary artery and the aorta, respectively. Although the operation is complicated and difficult, the early and late mortality rates are still unsatisfactory.

Chapter 3

Acquired Heart Disease

3.1 Aortic Valve Disease

3.1.1 Aortic valve stenosis

Aortic valve stenosis is usually caused by the abnormal congenital development of aortic valve, inflammatory invasion, degenerative changes, calcification and other reasons, resulting in the changes of aortic valve structure and morphology, and the junction adhesion, manifesting abnormal systole and the decrease of open area of aortic valve. The blood flow is blocked in aortic valve, resulting in a pressure difference.

3.1.1.1 Clinical manifestations

(1) Symptoms

Patients with mild stenosis have no clinical symptoms, and patients with moderate stenosis may show chest tightness and shortness of breath when the amount of activity increases. Patients with severe stenosis often have symptoms of chest pain, dizziness, syncope, and heart failure. Severe stenosis may led to sudden death after intense exercise.

(2) Signs

The aortic valve region above level Ⅲ displays systolic murmurs, commonly accompanied by systolic tremors, and usually transmitted to the neck. In patients with significantly thickened ventricular septum, the characteristic of SAM may appear, and murmurs-like wind can be heard at the apical region in systolic motion. For young patients, blood pressures in upper and lower extremity should be measured to exclude whether its aortic arch is narrow.

3.1.1.2 Diagnosis

(1) Electrocardiograph and chest X-ray

Electrocardiograph is commonly applied to observe whether there is hypertrophy and labor loss in left ventricular. However, it could not exclude some normal patients. The chest X-ray is an effective supplementary approach to make an accurate diagnosis. X-ray appearances of the enlargement of the volume of left ventricle, the calcification in aortic valve area, and expanding of ascending aorta are often observed in stenosis. Moreover, in elder patients, calcification may invade into aorta sinus and ascending aorta wall. When it is with aortic stenosis, the intercostal blood vessels are thickened and the ribs can be seen on the chest.

(2) Echocardiography

Aortic valve stenosis could be clearly confirmed via echocardiography. Aortic valve leaves thickening, deformation, calcification, and limited activity could be obviously observed. And that, severe calcification implicate the aortic valve ring and anterior lobe of the mitral valve. Both of the velocity of aortic blood flow and the pressure difference between the valves increase. The ascending aorta dilated after stenosis, and the ventricular septum and left ventricular wall are thickened. In some cases suffering from severe hypertrophy of left ventricle, especially the severe thickening of the upper part of ventricular septum, could probably lead to a stenosis of left ventricular outflow, displaying the mitral SAM signs, and the velocity increasing of blood flow in the aortic valve and left ventricular outflow via Ultrasound test.

(3) Blood, urine and biochemical index tests

The routine blood, urine tests and biochemical index tests are indispensably required for patients who have clear echocardiography diagnosis and are scheduled to undergo surgery.

(4) Coronary angiography

In several special circumstances, as that the age of patient is over 50, or 40–50 but accompanied with other symptoms of myocardial ischemia or chest pain or coronary heart disease or else, it is extremely essential to perform coronary angiography to exclude the hazards.

3.1.1.3   Differential diagnosis

After inquiring about the patients' medical history, having an distinct understanding about the symptoms and physical examination, the surgeons can make a preliminary diagnosis. The confirming must be checked by echocardiography. Not only the ultrasonography can determine the degree of aortic valve stenosis, but also explicitly confirm the evidences of diagnosis. Whereas, it is essential to exclude several disease signs including congenital aortic stenosis and subaortic stenosis, and primary hypertrophic obstructive cardiomyopathy. The patients of congenital aortic stenosis and subaortic stenosis, who could be accurately identified by echocardiography, usually are very young and seldom perform disease symptoms before age 20. By echocardiography, hypertrophy of ventricular septal, narrow of left ventricular flow, faster blood flow, and SAM symptoms in the anterior mitral valve could be identified in the patients.

3.1.1.4   Treatment

(1) Indications for surgical treatment

The following conditions are conforming to the indications for surgical operation.

1) The patient is performing with severe aortic valve stenosis, or the transvalve length difference > 50 mmHg.

2) The patient with coronary artery disease and severe aortic valve stenosis, requires coronary artery bypass grafting.

3) The patient with ascending aorta or other heart valve lesions, accompanied by severe aortic valve stenosis, requires surgical treatment.

4) The patients with coronary heart disease, ascending aorta or heart valve disease, combined with moderate aortic valve stenosis (the average pressure difference is 30 – 50 mmHg, or the flow velocity is 3 – 4 m/s) (Graded Ⅱa), requires surgical treatment.

5) The patient with no typical symptoms, but with severe aortic valve stenosis, combined with abnormal activity, such as hypotension (graded Ⅱa), also requires operation.

（2）Methods of operation

1）Aortic valve replacement

The optional valve includes mechanical valves, biological valves with or without stent, and Homograft valves. In general, the surgical mortality rate is 1% -2%. In patients with severe calcification of aortic valvular and ascending aortic walls, or small aortic valvular rings, or combining with that who already has heart operations in the elderly and women, the risk of surgery infinitely increases.

2）Arteriotomy of aortic valve junction

It is suitable for patients with joint adhesion but without obvious calcification. Children or young patients with congenital aortic valve stenosis usually suffer from valve valvulation. After undergoing junction incision, valve replacement is still required for the long term efficacy.

3）Percutaneous balloon catheter dilation

Suitable for patients with congenital aortic valve stenosis, some aortic valve stenosis can be used to relieve symptoms.

4）ROSS surgery

It is suitable for children or young patients with congenital aortic valve stenosis. The autologous pulmonary valve is transplanted to the aortic valve position, and the pulmonary artery is reconstructed with the autologous pericardium or the same pulmonary artery duct. The autogenous pulmonary artery can still grow after transplantation to the aortic valve position. This method, in the long run, is easy to give rise to calcification and inactivation of pulmonary artery valve and artery pipeline.

3.1.1.5 Complications

There are several common complications post-operation. Incomplete closure or secondary stenosis after valvuloplasty requires reoperation.

Ruptured left ventricle, artificial valve dysfunction, bleeding peripheral leakage, thromboembolism and bleeding associated with anticoagulation, hemolysis and infectious endocarditis are also the most usual complications that are needed to pay much attentions.

3.2 Aortic Insufficiency

The blood in diastolic aorta returning to the left ventricle via aortic valve of the lesion is calledaortic insufficiency. The aortic valve is not fully closed. There are many reasons that cause the aortic valve closure to be incomplete. According to the location of the lesion, it can be divided into two types: aortic valve involvement and aortic involvement. Common causes of aortic valve involvement include congenital aortic valve abnormalities, calcified degenerative degeneration, rheumatic lesions, and infectious endocardium. The main causes of aortic involvement include non-specific dilation, equine syndrome, and dissecting aneurysms.

3.2.1 Clinical manifestations

3.2.1.1 Symptoms

Follow-up data show that the incidence of symptoms and/or left ventricular contractile dysfunction in patients with incomplete aortic valve closure has naturally progressed to an average of 4.3 %, and the average mortality rate is in about 0.2%. Patients may not display conspicuous symptoms but already has dysfunction of left ventricle.

Chronic aortic valve insufficiency may not have any obvious symptoms in the left ventricular during functionally compensatory period, but often have palpitations and breathing difficulty after fatigue. Severe cases commonly occur with night paroxysmal breathing, dyspnea and syncope. About a quarter of patients have pre-cardiac pain, and some patients can be accompanied by angina. For patients with chronic aortic valve closure symptoms, the prognosis of medical treatment in patients with dyspnea, angina or obvious heart failure is poor, similar to that of patients with symptoms of aortic valve stenosis.

3.2.1.2　Physical signs

The left ventricle expands, and the heart shifts to the left, in which it can touch the obvious pickup impulse. By stethoscope, there is diastolic water-like murmur between the 3rd and 4th rib in the left edge of the sternum, which is a high-profile, diminishing type, conducting to the apex of the heart, and happening mostly in the early and middle stage of diastole. When the patient sits with the chest leans forward and deeply inhale, the murmurs will be more apparent. Severe cases can smell Austi-Flint noise in diastolic mid-to-late at the heart apex. There are typical peripheral vascular signs: increased arterial systolic pressure, reduced diastolic pressure, and wider pulse pressure. The carotid pulse is obvious, and the mouth lips or nails have capillary pulse, and the femoral artery displaying gun sounds. In the late stage of the disease, there may be the right heart failure with rage of jugular vein, larger liver, and edema of two lower limbs.

3.2.1.3　Auxiliary inspections

(1) Electrocardiogram

With the help of electrocardiogram, it is simple to observe hypertrophy and strain in the left ventricle. In the later stage of the disease, there may be conduction blocks in indoor conduction or east branch.

(2) Chest X-ray

By means of X-ray film, the shadow of the heart expands to the bottom of the left, showing a boot-shaped appearance, the root of aorta expands, and the ratio of the heart to chest is also enlarged.

(3) Echocardiography

Echocardiography is the most sensitive and accurate non-invasive human technique for diagnosing aortic insufficiency. It is adopted to determine the reasons for the incomplete closure of the aortic valve and the shape of the valve, provide a semi-quantitative evaluation of the severity of regurgitation, and evaluate the diameter, volume, contraction function, and aortic root size of the left ventricle. Using Doppler echocardiography, the severity is semi-quantitatively evaluated based on the area and width of color regurgitation. If echocardiography is not sufficient to quantitatively evaluate left ventricular function, radionuclide imaging should be used in asymptomatic patients to assess left ventricular function at rest and to estimate the capacity of left ventricle.

3.2.1.4　Differential diagnosis

Preliminary diagnosis could be done with concerning about the medical history, the symptoms and physical examination. The confirming diagnosis must be examined by echocardiography. Ultrasonic examination can not only determine the degree of aortic valve reflux, but also primarily clarify the pathogenesis of the disease and the absence of lesions in the aortic roots. Clinically, it needs to be differentiated Gramhan-Steel with diastolic murmurs of typical aortic valve insufficiency. The latter murmur is brought about by pulmonary arterial hypertension and pulmonary arterial dilation resulting in incomplete closure of the pulmonary artery valve. It's the loudest in the pulmonary artery-sitting area. It is necessary to pay attention to the patient's systemic situation: the aortic valve closure caused by Ceseus's disease and aortic inflammation is incomplete, and the simple aortic valve replacement is prone to the occurrence of peripheral valve leakage.

3.2.1.5　Treatments

Since the closure mechanism of the aortic valve is more elaborate than that of the atrial valve, the contact surface when the valve is closed is less than that of the mitral valve and tricuspid valve, so it is difficult to take operation. The rate of residual regurgitation and reoperation is high. The surgical methods include triangular resection and suture of defoliate leaves, junction and valvular fibrous mass resection, aortic valve ring-indentation, aortic sinus folding and increased valvular ring surgery and valve folding. Also, aortic valve replacement is commonly used.

3.2.1.6　Postoperative complications

The early surgical outcome of aortic valve insufficiency depends on the etiology, the size and function of the left ventricular cavity before surgery, the presence of new coronary heart and whether there are any accidents during surgery. The total surgical mortality rate is 4.0% –8.0%. The main causes of death in the early stages of surgery are ventricular arrhythmia, left ventricular insufficiency, renal failure or multiple organ failure. The typical postoperative implications include incomplete closure or secondary stenosis, ruptured left ventricle, artificial valve dysfunction, bleeding, peripheral leakage, thromboembolism and bleeding associated with anticoagulation, hemolysis, and infectious endocarditis.

3.3　Mitral Stenosis

Mital stenosis(MS) is the adhesion and fusion of the junction when the two tips are thickened. The opening blessing or obstruction of the two-pointed valve caused by the contraction of the tendon is reduced, causing the blood flow in the left atrium to be blocked.

3.3.1　Clinical manifestations

3.3.1.1　Symptoms

The patients exhibit respiratory difficulties which could be tired or paroxysmal, and severe ones could not be flat or paroxysmal at night. Hemoptysis, phlegm with blood, pulmonary infarction, thromboembolism, hoarse voice due to the expansion of the left atrium compression laryngeal nerve, dysphagia caused by the pressure on the esophagus, are commonly observed. In addition, we can also find abdominal distension, nausea, vomiting, oliguria and edema.

3.3.1.2　Signs

With mitral appearance, the left edge of the sternum can be raised like pulse, that means the heart expands to the left, and patients with atrial fibrillation may have a short pulse. The typical stethoscopes include the first heart tone at the apex of heart, the incremental rumen noise in the middle and late diastolic stage when the patient is at the left side of the lying position accompanied by diastolic tremor. When the patient's valve is flexible, it can smell opening of the valvular, which is the main indication of taking mitral valve junction separation. In addition, there is a second tone of pulmonary artery, accompanied by mild division. When the pulmonary artery is highly dilated and functional pulmonary valve closure is incomplete, the Grahan-Steel murmur can be heard. In severe mitral stenosis, full systolic murmurs can occur in the tricuspid region, or a third heart tone(S3) from the right ventricle. In a few patients with mitral stenosis, there is no diastolic murmur at the apex of heart, known as "dumb mitral stenosis", which is due to the high stenosis of mitral valvel or the expansion of the patient's right ventricle height, occupying the heart.

3.3.2　Auxiliary inspections

3.3.2.1　Electrocardiogram

In patients with mild mitral stenosis, the electrocardiogram is normal. The characteristic electrocardiogram is changed to a P wave with an enlarged left atrium. The P wave is widened and has a bimodal type, which is called a mitral valve P wave. With the development of the disease, when the pulmonary arterial hypertension is merged, the right ventricle is increased and the electric axis is rightward. Atrial fibrillation often occurs in the late stage of the disease.

3.3.2.2　Chest X-ray

The performance is related to the degree of mitral stenosis and the stage of disease development. Cases of moderate or higher stenosis can be seen in the left atrium enlargement, pulmonary segment protrusion, and left bronchial elevation, and may have right ventricle enlargement, double pulmonary congestion, small aorta, small left ventricle, and the X-ray feature being a pear-like heart.

3.3.2.3　Echocardiography

Echocardiography is a highly specific way to make a definite diagnosis of mitral stenosis. It can be determined that the degree of stenosis, the size of the heart cavity, and the presence of thrombosis in the left atrium. Unless patients who plan to perform mitral stenosis balloon expansion, esophageal ultrasound is generally not required.

3.3.2.4　Coronary angiography

Patients over 50 years of age, except for concurrent coronary artery lesions, need to perform coronary angiography before surgery. The positive rate in routine screening is in about 10%.

3.3.3　Diagnosis and differential diagnosis

The above symptoms appear clinically. In the mitral valve stethoscope area, rumble murmu can be smelled in the middle and late stages of diastole. It can generally be further clarified as mitral valve stenosis by echocardiography examination.

The diastolic murmur should be identified with the following circumstances: Carey-Coombs murmur is the signs of active mitral valvular inflammation in acute rheumatic fever; Austin-Flint murmur is a noise that occurs in the early diastolic period when the bicuspid valve is relatively narrow; As for left atrial myxoma, there may be symptoms and signs similar to a large valve stenosis. However, the noise often appears intermittently and changes with the body position; For tricuspid stenosis, the loudest part of the sound should be between the left edge of sternum and the apex of heart. This noise is enhanced when inhaled.

3.3.4　Surgical indications

（1）Patients with severe mitral stenosis with symptoms.

（2）Patients with symptoms, moderate mitral valve stenosis, ultrasound examination confirmed left atrial thrombosis, or regular medical treatment of patients with moderate or higher cardiac enlargement.

（3）Patients with balloon dilation or mitral closure separation require: explicit mitral stenosis, smelling the sound of opening valve, ultrasound examination confirming that valve elasticity is good, without left atrial thrombosis and sinus rhythm.

（4）Mitral valve replacement: For patients with severe mitral valve stenosis, rigid valve leaves, severe calcification, severe changes in the subvalve structure, difficulty in repair, or accompanied by severe mitral valve insufficiency. Mechanical valves are suitable for young patients with atrial fibrillation and/or left atrial thrombosis and require lifelong anticoagulant therapy. Biological valves are applied to the following cases: Women of childbearing age who wish to become pregnant; It is not suitable for anticoagulant or anticoagulant treatment of patients with contraindications; Patients who are unconditionally monitored for anticoagulant therapy; Age over 60 years old, and/or combined with other disorders, secondary valve replacement patients are less likely to undergo surgery.

3.3.5 Methods of operation

(1) Mitral valve junction separation

The mitral valve junction separation has three types of percutaneous mitral valve balloon dilation, open-breasted mitral valve closure dilation, and open mitral valve opening under the extracorporeal cycle. At present, the traditional mitral valve closure dilation has been replaced by percutaneous mitral valve balloon dilation.

(2) Mitral valve replacement

There are mainly two types of mechanical valves and biological valves. According to the size of the patient's own mitral valve ring, and also according to the patient's weight, the size of the left ventricle. The size of 27 mm valve is most commonly used in adults; light weight, small left ventricular patients can choose the size of 25 mm valve.

3.3.6 Postoperative complications

Perioperative mortality rate after mitral valve stenosis replacement is between 2% to 7%, according to the foreign data. Nearly a decade, the surgical death rate in Fuwai cardiovascular hospital is between 1% to 1.5%. The typical postoperative complications include ruptured left ventricle, artificial valve dysfunction, cardiac insufficiency, bleeding, peripheral leakage, thromboembolism and bleeding associated with anticoagulant, hemolysis and infectious endocarditis.

3.4　Tricuspid Stenosis

As the structure of the tricuspid valve changes, the area of the tricuspid valve decreases, so that the blood from right atrial could not pass through the tricuspid valve successfully during the diastolic period. The most common cause of tricuspid stenosis is rheumatism, occasionally infection or congenital. Rheumatic tricuspid stenosis often coexists with tricuspid valve closure, and simple tricuspid stenosis is very rare.

3.4.1 Clinical manifestations

3.4.1.1 Symptoms

Since rheumatic fever is the most common cause of tricuspid stenosis, patients often have symptoms of rheumatic mitral valve or aortic valve disease, and the symptoms of tricuspid valve stenosis are often covered by obvious symptoms of mitral valve disease. Severe triple stenosis may have significant liver size, ascites, and lower extremities edema, but the patient has no discomfort when lying down.

3.4.1.2 Physical signs

The body is found to be enraged by the jugular vein, the left lower part of the sternum shank could be smelled and diastolic murmurs, and the first cardiechema is disrupted.

3.4.2　Auxiliary inspection

(1) Electrocardiogram: P wave with high apex, right ventricular hypertrophy in absence of atrial fibrillation.

(2) Chest X-ray flat film: right atrioventricular enlargement.

(3) Echocardiography: can be clearly diagnosed, and find the degree of valve thickening and stenosis.

(4) Right cardiac catheterization: right heart catheter examination is not usually done.

3.4.3　Surgical indications

Rheumatic mitral and/or aortic valve lesions, combined with narrow tricuspid valve, should be treated at the same time.

3.4.4　Methods of operation

(1) Tricuspid stenosis incision and valvuloplasty

Although tricuspid stenosis is small, the valve ring is often enlarged, and it is generally less common to do simple fusion junction incision, and several levels are done at the junction incision and reduction. Firstly, cut the junction between the front flap and the septum or posterior flap with a sharp knife to avoid completely cutting to the valve ring, 2-3 mm away from the valve ring. If there is a thick fusion of tendons, they must also be cut together. Then the anterior and posterior junctions were sewn separately to make tricuspid valve formation.

(2) Tricuspid valve replacement

For severe tricuspid valve lesions, tricuspid valve replacement was performed.

3.4.5　Surgical complications

Commonly observed complications contains atrioventricular block at level Ⅲ, ruptured left ventricle, artificial valve dysfunction, cardiac insufficiency, bleeding, peripheral leakage, thromboembolism and bleeding associated with anticoagulation, hemolysis and infectious endocarditis.

3.5　Tricuspid Valve Insufficiency

Any cause of abnormal tricuspid valve structure in the heart during the systolic period of the right ventricle blood flow in the right atrium is tricuspid valve closure. The insufficiency of the closure caused by abnormal tricuspid valve structure can occur in rheumatic valvusitis, infectious endocarditis, tumors, rheumatoid arthritis, radiotherapy, trauma, and equine syndrome.

3.5.1　Clinical manifestations

3.5.1.1　Symptoms

Simple tricuspid insufficiency symptoms progress slowly and can be asymptomatic for many years. Light or moderate tricuspid valve closure is not full and there are no obvious symptoms. Severe tricuspid valve closure is often accompanied by symptoms such as palpitations, shortness of breath, hepatomegaly, and edema of the lower extremities. Infectious tricuspid valve insufficiency may have a history of drug use and fever. Traumatic injuries may have a history of chest trauma, but some patients have no obvious history of trauma.

3.5.1.2   Signs

Through body examination, it observes jugular vein rage, pulsing enhancement, tricuspid hairdryer type full systolic murmurs, hepatomegaly and systolic pacemaker, may have cirrhosis, ascites, and edema of lower extremity.

3.5.2   Auxiliary inspection

(1)Electrocardiogram: P wave with high peak, hypertrophy of right ventricular.

(2)Chest X-ray flat film: enlargement of right atrioventricular.

(3)Echocardiography: It can be clearly diagnosed, and get the structure and function of the tricuspid valve, the size of the valve ring, and check for other cardiac structures that affect tricuspid valve function. Doppler ultrasound can determine the degree of tricuspid regurgitation.

(4)Right heart duct and right ventricle angiography: It is generally not required. For patients with severe pulmonary hypertension, this examination can measure pulmonary arterial pressure, pulmonary circulation resistance, and help determine right ventricular function and surgical indications.

3.5.3   Surgical indications

(1)Rheumatic mitral and/or aortic valve lesions with incomplete mitral valve closure should be treated at the same time. During mitral valve surgery, if the tricuspid valve is slightly regurgitated, even if the heart ultrasound indicates that the tricuspid valve is slightly regurgitated, the tricuspid valve ring should be intervened at the same time.

(2)Simple severe tricuspid valve closure incomplete, large amount of reflux, NYHA cardiac function in level Ⅱ-Ⅲ, should be surgical treatment.

(3)Severe tricuspid insufficiency occurs in the late stage of mitral valve replacement, irreversible pulmonary vascular lesions and incomplete right ventricular function. Patients do not improve symptoms due to tricuspid valve surgery, so the surgical indications of such patients are not clear.

3.5.4   Methods of operation

(1)Tricuspid valve plasty should be made due to the low pressure of the right heart, slow blood flow, and resulting in thrombosis. Commonly used methods include De Vega flap ring plasty and Artificial valve ring fixation. The latter method is more solid and reliable than the aforementioned method.

(2)For tricuspid valve replacement, whether functional or organic, most of the tricuspid valve changes can be performed with autologous valves. Valve replacement is considered if the valve is seriously damaged, and unable or failure to form. In addition, the blood flow in the trivalve area is slow, the incidence of artificial valve thrombosis is high, and the incidence of artificial valve dysfunction is much higher than that of left heart valve replacement. It is generally believed that biological valves have fewer opportunities for dysfunction and should be considered as an important factor in the selection of valves, such as the use of mechanical valves to recommend the selection of double-leaf valves.

3.5.5   Surgical complications

The following complications are commonly seen: atrial chamber block in level Ⅲ, ruptured left ventricle, artificial valve dysfunction, cardiac insufficiency, bleeding, peripheral leakage, thromboembolism and bleeding associated with anticoagulation, hemolysis, and infectious endocarditis.

3.6　Auricular Fibrillation

Atrial fibrillation, is a commonly rapid disorder of upper ventricular rhythm. It is usually caused by organic heart disease, heart valvular disease, and coronary heart disease, but also found in healthy people without any cause. The patient's atrial wave (F wave) is between 300 and 400 bpm. Due to the physiological "filtration" effect of the atrial node, the F wave mostly undergoes absolute interference or occult conduction in the atrial node, so the ventricular rate rarely exceeds 180 bpm when the atrial fibrillation occurs.

3.6.1　Clinical manifestations

Ventricular rate is too fast leading to hypotension or angina. If there is a longer interval after the suspension of atrial fibrillation, it may cause syncope, body circulation embolism which is common occurs in rheumatic heart disease patients. The effective contraction of the loss of the Atria and the decrease of the blood volume of the heart may cause fatigue, and anxiety caused by palpitations. The strength of the first heart tone varies, and the heart rate is absolutely irregular with short Pulse.

3.6.2　Auxiliary inspection

(1) Atrial fibrillation patients with surgical treatment of, generally have basic surgical diseases. It is mainly valvular and coronary heart disease. The auxiliary inspection is in the relevant section.

(2) The ECG of atrial fibrillation is characterized by atrial activity disorders, no independent P waves, and is characterized by baseline fluctuations or atrial waves (F waves) of varying amplitude and frequency (350–600 times per minute). The ventricular reaction is extremely irregular, the R–R interval is absolutely unequal, and the shape and amplitude of the QRS wave group are also slightly different.

(3) 24 hours of dynamic electrocardiogram monitoring has corresponding performance.

3.6.3　Surgical indications

(1) Patients whose medication is not working.

(2) An organic heart attack combined with atrial fibrillation is recommended for the same period when performing heart surgery.

3.6.4　Methods of operation

Maze surgery has undergone two improvements. Since 1993, Maze Ⅲ surgery has been applied to clinical practice. However, the operation of the maze operation is complex, time–consuming and laborious, and there are complications such as bleeding. So far, it has not been widely used, and the medical units developed are limited. In recent years, the improved maze ablation surgery with radiofrequency, microwave and freezing as the energy source for ablating atrial fibrillation has achieved good clinical efficacy. Regardless of the energy method of the field, it is used to generate penetrating damage to the atrial tissue and form scar tissue to prevent electrical activity from conducting and achieve the effect of a surgical maze operation to cut a suture. The ablation of atrial fibrillation assisted by thoracoscopy further lightens the surgical trauma and can even be applied to isolated atrial fibrillation patients. The ablation equipment also developed from unipolar ablation to bipolar ablation.

The operation is divided into left atrium bypass and right atrium bypass ablation, and the left and right heart ears are removed at the same time. Factors that affect the success rate of surgery include the following:

    (1)Preoperative left atrium diameter is greater than 60 mm.

    (2)Pre-operative sinus node is dysfunctional.

    (3)Left atrial thrombosis.

    (4)Preoperative permanent atrial fibrillation time is more than 20 years.

3.6.5　Surgical complications

Maze type Ⅲ surgery has always been the gold standard for surgical treatment of atrial fibrillation. Cox himself has reported the results of 346 maze operations, including simultaneous high-risk heart surgery. The National operative mortality rate is 2% -3% , and the total success rate of atrial fibrillation treatment is 99%. However, due to the complex operation of maze surgery and the existence of hemorrhage and other complications, it has not been widely used in clinical practice.

Postoperative implications commonly observed contains conduction block, bleeding (COX reported that 6% of patients needed to open the chest again to stop bleeding. After energy ablation, the complication decreased obviously.) , esophageal injuries(rarely happening) , recurring of the atrial fibrillation, and with that the incidence of water and sodium retention after surgery is 5% -36% , and the severe patients shows pulmonary edema, pleural effusion, and perfusion of the lungs.

3.7　Pericardial Disease

3.7.1　Chronic constrictive pericarditis

Chronic constrictive pericarditis is a chronic inflammation of the pericardium. It causes thickening, adhesion, narrowing, and even calcification, limiting the heart's diastolic function, reducing the amount of blood in the heart, and silting the venous system, resulting in malnutrition and organ failure.

3.7.1.1　Clinical manifestations

(1)Symptoms

In early stage, there could be no symptoms or only fatigue. With the aggravation of the condition, heart palpitations, shortness of breath, abdominal distension, and loss of appetite may occur. In severe cases, hepatomegaly, ascites, edema of lower extremities or systemic, and difficult to breath, are typical symptoms, especially after activities the symptoms are aggravated, and even syncope may occur.

(2)Signs

The patients are mostly chronic, with shallow veins filling, significant in jugular veins, low blood pressure, narrow pulse pressure, and increased central venous pressure, up to 1. 96 kPa(20 cmH$_2$O). There are odd veins, positive for liver and neck. The palpitation weakens or disappears, the heart boundary is normal or displaced, the heart rate is fast, the heart tone is weak and distant, and the third heart tone can be heard. When the atrial valve is not closed, it can be heard and the heart contract period murmur can be heard. When pleural effusion, the intercostal space widens, and when the pleural cavity is thick and sticky, the intercostal space narrows. The liver is swollen, the abdomen is swollen, ascites are positive, and the spleen is sometimes swollen. Lower extremities may be swollen or even edema.

3.7.1.2　Auxiliary inspection

With the above clinical manifestations, patients suspected of being the disease need to undergo the following examinations.

(1) Electrocardiogram: Common QRS wave groups have low voltage, T waves are low or inverted, P waves have traces, incomplete right bundle branch block or right ventricular hypertrophy, and some cases are accompanied by atrial arrhythmia or atrial fibrillation.

(2) Chest X-ray: The size of the heart is normal or slightly larger, the edges of the heart shadow are stiff, common pericardial calcification, and the upper vena vein shadow widens.

(3) Echocardiography: It can be seen that the pericardial thickening, calcification, atrial enlargement, ventricular cavity narrowing, and cardiac function reduction.

(4) The right heart catheter isn't usually needed.

(5) Both CT and MRI can be found to increase the thickening of the pericardium and changes in each cardiac cavity, which can help in differential diagnosis.

(6) Laboratory examinations: Hypoproteinemia with significantly reduced albumin content.

3.7.1.3　Diagnosis and differential diagnosis

Patients with palpitations and shortness of breath, with shallow veins filled, the tip of the heart carrying weakness or disappearance, weak and distant heart tone should consider the possibility of constrictive pericarditis, and echocardiography could found the thickening of the pericardium.

The disease should be distinguished with the following diseases:

(1) Myocardial disease

Cardiomyopathy patients have normal palpitations at the apex of the heart, and the vocal range of the heart is enlarged. However, with electrocardiogram, alteration is more common in the left ventricle, and the block of right bundle branch is less common. Abnormal Q waves can be mostly seen. X-ray examination of cardiomyopathy patients with the heart expanding to the sides, the upper vena cava expansion is not obvious. Ultrasonic examination of the patient can be found to expansion of the heart and hypertrophy of the myocardium. The right ventricular diastolic pressure curve in patients with cardiomyopathy is found to have no early low prolapse and late elevation signs. Identification of patients with difficulty, is viable for cardiac biopsy.

(2) Liver cirrhosis

Patients with mild constrictive pericarditis only show larger size of liver, severe and chronic patients can also be accompanied by spleen and hypersplenism, displaying the performance of cardiogenic cirrhosis. The main manifestation of cirrhosis patients is portal hypertension, and esophagealossurosis shows varicose veins. There is no elevated central venous pressure or changes in the heart in patients with cirrhosis.

(3) Heart failure due to valvular disease

Valvular disease can smell the corresponding heart murmur, edema of lower extremity is heavier, but abdominal distension is lighter. With echocardiographic examination, valvular disease can be revealed.

(4) Tricuspid stenosis

The appearance is elevated venous pressure, venous system congestion. But, with echocardiography and right heart catheter examination, the disease can be identified.

3.7.1.4　Surgical indications

(1) Chronic constrictive pericarditis with clinical symptoms should be surgically treated.

(2) If the physiological effects of narrowing are small, especially when combined with other serious diseases, surgical treatment can be postponed.

(3) Chronic constrictive pericarditis caused by tuberculosis should be operated after tuberculosis is cured; If the heart failure is aggravated, the operation should be performed as soon as possible.

3.7.1.5　Methods of operation

The thickened pericardium is removed through the middle thoracic incision and the left anterior external incision. The main advantages of the middle incision path are that the right ventricle and right ventricle can be well revealed, and it is also convenient to build a three-dimensional external circulation, but the carpel behind the left septum is not satisfactory enough to reveal. The left anterior external incision path can reveal the left ventricle, including the diaphragm, but it is not good for the adhesion near the lower vena cava. Stripping should be careful to avoid going too deep into the human myocardium or injury to the coronary arteries. The order of calcification or thickened pericardial pericardial stripping that retains the island's adhesion is left ventricular outflow-left ventricle-right ventricle-right atrium and vena cava. The stripping range is left through the front and side of the left ventricle, reaching the front of the left phrenic nerve; go right through the front wall of the right atrium to the room ditch; down to the back of the diaphragm. Stripping the right ventricle outflow to reach the pulmonary artery as much as possible, so as not to cause the right ventricle outflow obstruction, resulting in an increase in the internal pressure of the right ventricle. The stripping scope should be as far as possible beyond the atrioventricular groove, so as not to leave pressure step difference between the atrioventricular groove.

3.7.1.6　Surgical complications

(1) Heart failure: In patients with long duration of the disease, the myocardial degeneration thins and the contractile function decreases.

(2) Bleeding: Long-term hepatic congestion leads to decreased coagulation function, large surgical exfoliation, and prone to hemorrhage after surgery.

(3) Pleural effusion: It may be related to poor cardiac function, hypoproteinemia, or inflammatory reactions.

3.7.2　Pericardial tumors

Pericardial tumors are benign or malignant tumors that originate in the pericardium and do not include tumors that metastasize or infiltrate the pericardium. The incidence rate was low.

3.7.2.1　Clinical manifestations

Clinically, there are many asymptomatic patients. When the tumor presses the heart or secondary pericardial effusion, it can have symptoms such as fatigue, chest tightness, and chest pain. It is not easy to find.

3.7.2.2　Auxiliary inspections

(1) Electrocardiogram: T wave changes or arrhythmias usually occur.

(2) Chest X-ray: Enormous heart shadow or abnormal shape.

(3) Echocardiography: Visible pericardial occupied lesions, cardiac compression or pericardial effusion.

(4) CT and MRI: It could be found pericardial occupied lesions, heart pressure, and pericardial effusion, which is of diagnostic and differential diagnostic significance.

3.7.2.3　Diagnosis and differential diagnosis

Similar symptoms or pericardial effusion can occur in the following diseases, and the heart shadow increases. Heart X-ray, ultrasound, CT and magnetic resonance examination can be differentiated diagnosis.

(1) Pericardial pericardial effusion increase, but the pericardium is normal and there is no heart pressure.

(2) The cardiac tumor has increased cardiac shadow, and the occupying lesions are in the pericardi-

um.

(3) The mediastinal tumor occupying lesions are located outside the heart.

3.7.2.4   Surgical indications

Usually pericardial tumors should be treated surgically once they are diagnosed. For example, if it is a benign tumor, the operation has a good effect. If it is a malignant tumor, the operation can also be clearly diagnosed, and the tumor should be completely removed or partially removed as soon as possible to relieve the symptoms caused by the tumor.

3.7.2.5   Methods of operation

According to the location and scope of pericardial tumor, choose the chest positive and left anterior external incision, cut the envelope at the normal pericardium, completely remove the tumor, and pay attention to avoid damage to the diaphragm nerve and the heart. Benign pericardial tumors and early localized malignant pericardial tumors may be completely excised. When malignant pericardial tumors involve the myocardium or large blood vessels, surgical treatment is only palliative, including decompression and pericardial filling.

3.7.2.6   Surgical complications

Benign pericardial tumor surgical treatment effect is better, early limited and malignant pericardium after thorough resection can obtain good effect, after rest surgery effect is poor, need to combine chemotherapy or radiotherapy. However, there are several common postoperative complications, that is respiratory dysfunction caused by postoperative hemorrhage and phrenic nerve damage.

3.8   Primary Cardiac Tumors

3.8.1   Cardiac myxomas

Cardiac tumors are usually divided into two major categories: primary and secondary. Among the primary cardiac tumors, cardiac myxoma accounts for 50%, which is the most common intracardiac tumor in adults. It is generally believed that myxoma originates from the subendocardial mesenchymal tissue. When it grows up, it protrudes into the centripetal cavity. Most of it is single (90%), and the most common sites are in the left atrium (>90%). Atrial myxoma often attaches to the atrial septal fossa, or to other parts of the atrium, but may originate from the atrioventricular valve. Most of the tumors have pedicles, and move with systole. Tissues are very fragile, easily broken, resulting in peripheral arteries or cerebral vascular embolization.

Cardiac myxoma is mostly benign. If the surgical resection is not complete, the local recurrence also occurs; and the exfoliated tumor tissue continues to grow in the cerebral blood vessels and peripheral vascular epithelium, destroying the blood vessel wall to form a hemangioma.

3.8.1.1   Symptoms and signs

(1) Symptoms

1) Blockage of blood flow: Myxoma of the left atrial obstructs the mitral valve at diastolic phase and resembles rheumatic mitral stenosis, causing palpitations and shortness of breath. Dizziness or transient fainting is caused by obstruction of the mitral valve in the tumor, resulting in a lack of transient cerebral blood supply, and rest or change of position may alleviate the symptoms. Myxoma of the right atrial is similar to tri-

cuspid stenosis, which may have fatigue, anorexia, pain in the liver, abdominal distension and edema of lower extremity.

2) Systemic reactions: Because of hemorrhage, degeneration and necrosis, fever, weight loss, anemia, stomach anorexia, joint pain, urticaria, and fatigue, etc. , are considered to be caused by autoimmune reactions.

3) Arterial embolism: It shows hemiplegia, aphasia, coma, acute abdominal pain and limb pain.

4) The above three manifestations are typical symptoms, but many patients are diverse and asymptomatic when it is small.

(2) Signs

1) General nutrition, weight, spirit, blood pressure and pulse.

2) Left heart function is not omnipotent, rales of the lung, morphology of mitral valve.

3) Right heart function is not generalized. Edema of lower extremity, filling of jugular vein, and hepatomegaly.

4) Cardiac auscultation: Diastolic or systolic or dual-phase murmur could be heard in the apical region of the left atrium. The diastolic murmur in the apical region is shorter, the noise is more limited, and the first sound is hyperthyroidism. When there is pulmonary hypertension, jet sound could be heard in the pulmonary valve, the second sound is hyperactive or split. And in the right atrial myxoma, the diastolic murmur could be heard in the tricuspid region.

3.8.1.2 Auxiliary examinations

(1) Patients with cardiac myxoma, especially in severe cases of systemic reactions, has much changes in anemia, erythrocyte sedimentation rate, immunoglobulin IgM, IgG, lgA, etc. , but with no specificity.

(2) Chest X-ray: It shows signs of left atrium and right ventricular enlargement, pulmonary congestion and other similar mitral valve lesions, and signs of pulmonary hypertension.

(3) Electrocardiogram: It is similar to mitral stenosis, but atrial fibrillation is rarely seen, most of it have sinus rhythm.

(4) Echocardiography: Almost all patients can be definitely diagnosed by this test. It reveales an intensive cloud-like echo within the heart chamber. Myxoma in left atrial shows abnormal echo that could protrude into the mitral valve during diastole and re-enter the atrial cavity during systole.

(5) Magnetic resonance imaging, CT or echocardiography is sometimes difficult to differentiate right atrial myxoma with atrial thrombus. A very few myxomas located in the auricle may eventually be diagnosed by surgical procedures.

3.8.1.3 Differential diagnosis

(1) Rheumatic mitral stenosis could be identified by typical echocardiography.

(2) A small number of patients should take examinations of MRI, CT or cardiac surgery to identify atrial thrombus.

3.8.1.4 Treatment

Once diagnosed, surgery should be performed as early as possible to prevent tumor embolism, sudden death or disease. The timing of the operation depends on the condition (see below).

(1) Non-surgical treatment

Non-surgical treatment is only part of the preoperative preparation. Such as treatment of acute pulmonary edema, correction of anemia and fever; symptomatic treatment of cerebral embolism. However, if active treatment of cerebral embolism, acute pulmonary edema, cardiac arrest and other malignant events have taken, the patient is still coma, or extreme exhaustion with multiple organ dysfunction, it is not appropriate for surgery.

(2) Surgical treatment

1) Indications for surgery: As mentioned above, once diagnosed, surgery is performed as soon as possible. Unless the patient is extremely debilitated with multiple organ dysfunction, or is unconscious, it is not suitable for surgery.

2) Timing of surgery: ①Patients with simple cardiac myxoma but no systemic reactions, could select surgery, but must be arranged as soon as possible. ②The systemic responses are heavy, the disease is developing rapidly, and there are signs of danger. After excluding non-myxoma factors, emergency surgery should be taken. ③Repeated episodes of arterial embolism with death threats should be arranged for emergency surgery. ④Patients with long-term fever, ineffective treatment with large amounts of antibiotics for a period of time, could not rule out that the high heat is caused by the myxoma, should take urgent surgery and apply continue to use antibiotics. ⑤Patients have chronic heart failure, physical weakness, no supine at night, sitting breathing, hepatomegaly, ascites, edema of lower extremity, should be identified to exclude other factors, actively control heart failure, and wait until the condition is stable for surgery.

3.8.1.5　Prognosis

The treatment of myxomas has a good prognosis, and the operative mortality and recurrence rate are both low. The main factors affecting the death of surgery are preoperative cardiac function, embolization, advanced age with liver and kidney dysfunction, and combined with coronary heart disease.

3.8.2　Cardiac sarcoma

In primary cardiac tumors, nausea tumors account for 1/4, of which about 95% are cardiac sarcomas, and the rest are mainly lymphomas. Therefore, cardiac sarcoma is the most common malignant tumor in the heart, second to myxomas. Cardiac sarcoma is divided into two categories according to histology: spindle cell sarcoma, including angiosarcoma, rhabdomyosarcoma, fibrosarcoma, mucinous sarcoma and liposarcoma; round cell sarcoma. Among them, angiosarcoma is the most common, followed by rhabdomyosarcoma and fibrosarcoma. Angiosarcoma is more common in adults, and rhabdomyosarcoma and fibrosarcoma are more common in children.

Sarcomas occurs anywhere in the heart, but are common in the right heart system, especially in the right atrium. The sarcoma grows from the heart wall and may protrude into the heart chamber or the pericardial cavity. It may also protrude to the inner and outer sides at the same time. The base is generally wide and a few have pedicles. Due to the location of the tumor, the tricuspid valve, and the superior and inferior vena cava openings can be blocked, causing signs of blood flow obstruction and vena cava obstruction syndrome. The heart muscle is widely replaced by tumor tissue, which causes weakness of myocardial contraction and failure. Tumor cells invade the cardiac conduction system, may cause malignant arrhythmia. If tumors grow outside the heart and invade the epicardium, may cause bloody pericardial effusion, pericardial tamponade or chest pain. If sarcoma occurs in the left heart system, is easily be misdiagnosed as myxoma. Once a cardiac sarcoma develops symptoms, the disease progresses rapidly and the prognosis is extremely poor.

3.8.2.1　Symptoms and signs

(1) Symptoms

1) There are asymptomatic in the early stage, occasionally accompanied with non-specific symptoms such as fever and weight loss.

2) The main symptoms include local invasion of refractory heart failure, vena cava obstruction syndrome, bloody pericardial effusion or pericardial tamponade, chest pain, and various arrhythmias or conduction block.

3) The disease progresses rapidly, and distant metastasis occurs very quickly.

(2) Signs

1) General conditions: Nutrition, weight, spirit, blood pressure and pulse.

2) Right heart function is not generalized. Edema of lower extremity, filling of jugular vein, and hepatomegaly.

3) Left heart function is not omnipotent, and with double rales.

4) Whether there is arrhythmia, heart murmur, pericardial effusion or Beck triad.

3.8.2.2 Auxiliary examinations

(1) Laboratory examinations: A few patients may have non-specific changes such as anemia and increased erythrocyte sedimentation rate.

(2) Chest X-rays shows changes in pericardial effusion, or local invasion.

(3) Echocardiography is used to confirm the diagnosis.

(4) CT/MRI are a routine examination to take in the tumor invasion.

(5) Pericardial puncture and pumping its pericardial effusion to find tumor cells contributes to determine its pathological type.

(6) Malignant and benign tumors of cardiac are sometimes difficult to distinguish before surgery, but could be diagnosed in surgical exploration or autopsy.

3.8.2.3 Differential diagnosis

(1) Compared with cardiac myxoma, cardiac sarcoma progresses rapidly and has a short course of disease. Echocardiography and CT/MRI show that lesions occur in the right heart system, and the base is often wide and could be partially external invasion.

(2) Echocardiographic is used to identify various cardiomyopathy.

(3) Before diagnosing primary cardiac sarcoma, sarcoma in other parts of the body must be excluded.

3.8.2.4 Treatment

Comprehensive treatment include surgery, radiation, chemotherapy, and immunotherapy is proposed.

(1) Non-surgical treatment

It includes radiation, chemotherapy, immunotherapy, etc. However, in addition to cardiac lymphoma, the effect is not good.

(2) Surgical treatment

1) indications for surgery: definite diagnosis and local resection; undiagnosed, needing surgical exploration.

2) Once diagnosed, surgery should be taken as soon as possible.

3) Surgical method: the local lesions are removed under extracorporeal circulation, including the surrounding infiltrated tissue, and the patch with large defect should be repaired. If the sarcoma is confined to the atrioventricular valve, it should replace the prosthetic valve after removal of the tumor and valve. Due to the involvement of large pieces of cardiac tissue or metastasis, surgery is often difficult to completely cure. Although aggressive large-scale surgical resection or heart transplantation may reduce local recurrence, the risk of distant metastasis remains. Surgeons should select the scope of resection according to the condition of the lesion.

3.8.2.5   Prognosis

Cardiac sarcoma has a poor prognosis. Treatment is usually palliative. Although patients would recover quickly, they often die of distant metastasis or tumor recurrence within one year after surgery.

3.9   Hypertrophic Obstructive Cardiomyopathy

Hypertrophic obstructive cardiomyopathy is characterized by ventricular muscle hypertrophy, typically in the left ventricle, with a ventricular septum, occasionally concentric hypertrophy. The volume of the left ventricular cavity is normal or diminished. Occasionally the lesion occurs in the right ventricle. The cause of the disease is not very clear. There may be more than one person in a family, suggesting that it is related to heredity.

Patients with pheochromocytoma have more hypertrophic cardiomyopathy, and intravenous infusion of a large amount of norepinephrine would cause myocardial necrosis. In animal experiments, intravenous infusion of catecholamine causes cardiac hypertrophy. Therefore, some people think that hypertrophic cardiomyopathy is caused by endocrine disorders.

3.9.1   Symptoms and signs

3.9.1.1   Symptoms

(1) Difficulty of breathing often occurs after exertion, due to decreased left ventricular compliance, increased end–diastolic pressure, followed by elevated pulmonary venous pressure, and pulmonary congestion. Mitral regurgitation associated with ventricular septal hypertrophy aggravates pulmonary congestion.

(2) Pain in the precordial area often occurs after exertion, which is like angina pectoris, but it is not typical. It is caused by the increased oxygen supply of the hypertrophic myocardium and the relative lack of coronary blood supply.

(3) Fatigue, dizziness and fainting occur more frequently during activities. It is due to the increased heart rate, shortening the diastolic phase of the left ventricle which is poorly filled during the diastolic period, and increasing the lack of filling and reducing the amount of cardiac output. When it is active or emotional, the hypertrophic myocardial contraction is strengthened by the sympathetic action, the outflow obstruction is aggravated, and the cardiac output is suddenly reduced to induce symptoms.

(4) Palpitations is due to cardiac dysfunction or arrhythmia.

(5) Heart failure is more common in patients within advanced stage. Due to decreased myocardial compliance, ventricular end–diastolic pressure is significantly increased, followed by elevated atrial pressure, and is often combined with atrial fibrillation. In advanced patients, myocardial fibrosis is extensive, ventricular systolic function is also weakened, and heart failure and sudden death are prone to occur.

3.9.1.2   Signs

(1) The cardiac dullness expands to the left. The beats of the apex shift to the bottom left with a lifting impulse.

(2) The systolic murmur in the middle or late stage could be heard in the inner part of the apex of the lower left margin of the sternum, which is transmitted to the apex but not to the bottom of the heart. It may be accompanied by systolic tremor, which is seen in patients with ventricular outflow obstruction. Measures to increase myocardial contractility or reduce cardiac load such as digitalis, isoproterenol (2 μg/min),

isoamyl nitrite, nitroglycerin, valsalva action, physical labor or premature beat would enhance the murmurs. In contrast, any measures that weaken the contractility of the heart muscle or increase the load of the heart, such as vasoconstrictor, beta blocker, squat, and clenched fist would reduce the murmurs. About half of the patients could be heard of the murmur of mitral regurgitation at the same time.

(3)The second heart sound can be abnormally split due to the blocking of left ventricle and the delayed closure of aortic valve. The third heart sound is common in patients with mitral regurgitation.

3.9.2　Auxiliary examination

(1)Chest X-ray examination

Both of the heart shadow and the left ventricle are enlarged, but with no enlargement of ascending aorta or calcification of the leaflets. In the advanced cases, the left atrium and right ventricle may also be enlarged, and the blood vessels in the lungs are stagnation.

(2)ECG examination

It shows hypertrophy and strain of the left ventricular. Some cases showed blocking of the complete right/ left bundle branch, or left anterior branch and hypertrophy of the left atrium.

(3)Cardiac catheterization

Catheterization of the right heart shows signs of elevated pulmonary pressure or stenosis of the outflow tract in right ventricle. Catheterization of the left heart shows a significant increase in left ventricular end-diastolic pressure, and a systolic pressure difference between the left ventricular lumen and the outflow tract. The aortic or peripheral arterial pressure waveform shows a rapid rise in the ascending branch, showing a double peak and then slowly decreasing. Aortic pulse pressure decreased after ventricular systole.

(4)Selective angiography of the left atrium

The anterior lobes of mitral valvular and hypertrophy of the ventricular septum could be observed. And the left ventricular cavity is curved, and the left ventricular volume is small and the papillary muscles are thick at the end of cardiac systole.

It also could be adopted to identify the presence or absence of mitral insufficiency. Adult patients should apply coronary angiography to ascertain the presence or absence of coronary artery disease.

(5)Echocardiography

The left ventricular wall is significantly thickened, the ventricular septum is more hypertrophic than the posterior wall of the ventricle, the left ventricular cavity is small, the outflow tract is narrow and the anterior leaflets of mitral valve are displaced forward with the heart systole.

3.9.3　Treatment

3.9.3.1　General treatments

Drugs that enhance the function of cardiac systole such as digitalis, beta-receptor stimulants such as isoproterenol, or reduce cardiac load, such as nitroglycerin, aggravate obstruction of the left ventricular outflow tract. If the patient is with mitral insufficiency, infective endocarditis should be prevented.

3.9.3.2　Drug treatments

It relieves symptoms and controls arrhythmia.

(1)β-blockers reduce myocardial systole, reduce obstruction of the outflow and oxygen consumption, increase diastolic ventricular dilatation and cardiac output, and slow heart rate.

(2)Calcium antagonists have both negative inotropic effects to weaken myocardial systole, improve myocardial compliance and contribute to diastolic function. The combination of β-blocker and calcium antagonist would reduce side effects and improve efficacy.

(3) Antiarrhythmic drugs are used to control rapid ventricular arrhythmia and atrial fibrillation, and amiodarone is more commonly used. Surgeons should use electric shock if medication is not effective.

For patients have ventricular systolic dysfunction in the late stage due to congestive heart failure, the treatment is the same as heart failure. For the patients with obstructive cardiomyopathy in who drug treatment is ineffective, the interventricular phrenic mediastinum and partial incision of the hypertrophy are used to relieve the symptoms. In recent years, the dual-chamber permanent pacemaker for right ventricular and atrioventricular is used to sequentially pacing to relieve the symptoms of obstructive patients.

3.9.3.3 Surgical treatments

(1) The commonly used surgical methods include myocardiectomy through combined incision of aortic and left ventricular incision, ventricular septal and myocardial resection through transaortic incision.

(2) The operative mortality is about 10%. Common causes of death includes low cardiac output and bleeding of left ventricular incision. About 5% of cases are complicated by complete conduction block, and the incidence of conduction block in left or right bundle branch is higher.

For patients with typical clinical symptoms and ineffective medication, when the left ventricular cavity and systolic pressure difference of outflow tract exceeds 50 mmHg at rest, surgical treatment should be performed to remove the ventricular septal hypertrophy to relieve the obstruction.

Chapter 4

Ischemic Heart Disease

4.1 Ventricular Aneurysm

After extensive myocardial infarction in patients with coronary heart disease, the wall of the infarct is dilated, thinned, and full-thickness of the myocardium. The necrotic myocardium is gradually replaced by fibrous scar tissue. The thinned ventricular wall of the lesion is bulging outward, resulting in loss of mobility or abnormal movement during systole, finally forms an aneurysm. Ventricular tumors are commonly seen in the left ventricle.

4.1.1 Symptoms and signs

(1) Common symptoms: chest tightness, chest pain, expiratory dyspnea, and anhelation.

(2) Refractory and recurrent episodes of ventricular arrhythmia or congestive heart failure.

(3) Chest X-ray radiographs shows calcification, and a limited expansion of the left heart. However, when the tumor is diffusely swelled, it should be differentiated from left ventricular enlargement.

(4) Two-dimensional echocardiography or radionuclide ventriculography shows abnormal bulging in segmental systolic stage of left ventricular.

(5) In the case of cardiac palpation in patients with ventricular aneurysm, double pulsation could be felt.

4.1.2 Auxiliary examination

(1) Electrocardiogram

It shows T wave inversion, high ST-T segment, disorder of ventricular rhythm, and Q wave formation.

(2) Chest X-ray

Pulmonary congestion, enlarged heart, and sometimes tumor-like changes in the apex are observed.

(3) Echocardiography

The left atrium is enlarged with abnormal motion in the apex of the left ventricular, and the ventricular aneurysm is formed. Wall thrombus or mitral insufficiency, diastolic and systolic insufficiency could also be observed.

(4)Cardiac catheterization and angiography

Coronary and left ventricular angiography identify the major branches and locations involved in the lesion, the degree of coronary artery stenosis, the extent of ventricular aneurysm, cardiac function, and abnormalities in wall segmental motion. Pulmonary arterial pressure, left ventricular end-diastolic pressure, and ventricular ejection fraction are also measured, and the presence or absence of viable myocardium and adherent thrombosis are observed as well.

(5)Magnetic resonance imaging

The location of ventricular aneurysm and cardiac function could be detected by MRI.

4.1.3　Differential diagnosis

(1)Old myocardial infarction

In the left ventricular aneurysm, the boundary of true ventricular aneurysm is clear after pericardial incision, and the reverse movement is obvious. If the area is old myocardial infarction with unclear boundary and flowered surface, ventricular systole is significantly weakened with local myocardial thinned or not be significantly thinned.

(2)Pseudo-ventricular aneurysm

It is often caused by myocardial infarction, rupture of left ventricular free wall, pericardial encapsulation. It may also be caused by trauma or infection. Cardiac catheterization and angiography could find another tumor cavity with thin wall and connected with the ventricle cavity, thrombosis and turbulence. Generally, the opening of it is small, which is the main sign for differentiation from true ventricular aneurysm.

(3)Cardiac tumors

There is no history of coronary heart disease and myocardial infarction. MRI could detect the relationship between tumor and myocardium. Echocardiography shows the range of size and location of the tumors. Radionuclide examination is helpful for differential diagnosis.

4.1.4　Treatments

Indications for surgery:

(1)The volume of the ventricular aneurysm is small, the left ventricular end-diastolic pressure is not high without wall thrombus and abnormal heart rate, may require bypass graft surgery.

(2)The volume of the ventricular aneurysm is large and cardiac function is affected. It should be treated surgically at this case.

(3)The patient's ventricular aneurysm is huge, with EF <20% , extensive coronary artery disease and vascular lesions. If the vascular conditions are not suitable for bypass transplantation, heart transplantation should be taken.

(4)Pseudo-ventricular aneurysm is prone to rupture, bleeding and death, so that it should be actively operated.

4.1.5　Complications

(1)Low cardiac output syndrome is characterized by low blood pressure, fast heart rate, low urine output and significantly decreased cardiac output.

(2)Ventricular fibrillation in patients with cardiac arrhythmias should be maintained at K^+, Na^+ and Mg^{2+} levels, and intravenous administration of lidocaine or amiodarone should be carried out to prepare for electrical defibrillation.

(3)The renal failure：Because of poor cardiac function or having the basis of renal damage，symptoms of renal insufficiency，such as oliguria and no urine，should be handled in time and taken hemodialysis when necessary. Processing of the other complications is referring to that of coronary artery bypass grafting.

4.2   Coronary Atherosclerotic Heart Disease

Coronary atherosclerotic heart disease should be also called ischemic heart disease，referring to the stenosis of the coronary vascular cavity and the obstruction of the coronary circulation caused by coronary artery wall atheromatous lesions，and leading to insufficient blood supply，ischemia and hypoxia for the myocardia at last. The pathogenesis of coronary atherosclerosis is much complex and has not yet been fully understood. According to the a large number of epidemiological and experimental data，the main pathogenic factors are high calorie，high fat，high sugar diet，smoking，hyperlipidemia，hypertension，diabetes，obesity，excessive physical activity，tense mental labor，emotional excitement，mental tension，men over middle age，high density lipoprotein reduce a lot，dysfunction of blood coagulation and so on. A few cases may have familial genetic factors. In the past 40 years，the incidence of coronary atherosclerotic heart disease has been increasing in China.

4.2.1   Physical examination

(1)General examination：the patients' development，nutrition，weight，spirit，blood pressure and pulse.

(2)For the examination of heart，surgeons should pay attention to the following：①Whether there is uplift in the precordial area and find out the location and size of the apex. ②Whether there is a sense of lift in the apex. ③Whether the extent of the heart broaden. ④The heart rate，heart rhythm，heart sound，heart murmur.

(3)Physical examination should not be neglected：①Chest examination. ②Abdominal examination. ③Whether there are signs of circulatory system.

4.2.2   Auxiliary inspections

(1)Chest X−ray

There are always no abnormalities in the chest radiography. For the patients with hypertension，the enlargement of left ventricle，the enlargement and bending of the aorta can be observed. In patients combined with congestive heart failure，the heart is obviously enlarged and the lungs are congested.

(2)ECG

Electrocardiogram is one of the most important methods to reflect myocardial ischemia. Patients with no obvious changes in electrocardiogram could undergo the stress tests to induce electrophysiological changes of myocardial anoxia temporarily. The stress test of electrocardiogram such as double step two ladder motion test，active plate exercise test，pedaling test and glucose load test can be chosen，and we can also perform a 24 hour ECG monitor to record the dynamic electrocardiogram continuously.

(3)Other diagnostic methods

It can be chosen such as sectional echocardiography，radionuclide heart imaging，etc.

(4)Selective coronary angiography and left ventriculography

Selective coronary angiography could clearly show the left and right coronary arteries and their branches，it can not only provide evidence for the diagnosis of coronary stenosis caused by atherosclerotic lesions，but also show the exact location，scope，degree of stenosis of the vessel and the situation of the collateral vessels.

4.2.3　Clinical manifestations

(1) Symptoms

The main symptom is angina caused by transient ischemia due to imbalance between supply and demand of myocardial oxygen. They always occurs at the time of labor, emotional excitement, eating or being cold. The common sites of pain are the substernal area or the precordial area, which can radiate to the left arm, the shoulder, the interscapular region, the neck, the roar and the mandible. Sometimes it's on the upper abdomen. The property of the pain may be severe colic, squeezing pain, compression pain, tight pain, or light pain that patients feel just discomfortable. Sometimes the patients may be sweaty and have a fear of dying when there is a sharp pain. The pain usually lasts 1−10 minutes, and it will disappear after taking a rest or taking a nitroglycerin tablet.

(2) Signs

There are always no special signs, when the angina pectoris attacks, the blood pressure can be slightly increased or decreased, and the heart rate can be normal, increase or decrease. Those who with severe pain show anxious, irritable, pale, sweating, and sometimes atrial or ventricular gallop can be heard. For the patients with papillary muscle dysfunction, systolic murmurs can be heard in apical regions. And what's more, in cases of myocardial infarction, the heart rate may increase or slow down, the blood pressure may decrease, the border of cardiac dullness may increase slightly, the first heart sound in the apical area may become weak, and sometimes the third, the fourth heart sounds or diastolic galloping can be heard. There could also be the signs of various arrhythmias, shock or heart failure.

4.2.4　Clinical types

(1) Stable angina

The factors that influence the progression and prognostic of stable angina are as follows: the number of diseased coronary artery branches especially whether the left coronary artery or the anterior descending branch are involved, the function of the left ventricle, the severity of myocardial ischemia, the sex and age of the patients, whether it is combined with other diseases, and so on. For the patients that one or two coronary artery become occlusive without involvement of the left main coronary artery should be treated conservatively first and regularly reviewed. However, if the conservative treatment is ineffective and patients' work and life are seriously affected, selective coronary angiography should be performed, and the patients whose vascular cavity reduce more than 50%, especially in the left coronary artery, the left anterior descending branch and the three branches of the coronary artery, should be treated by surgical treatment.

(2) Unstable angina

For most patients of unstable angina, the degree of coronary artery occlusion is serious. Some cases have a small or scattered myocardial infarction, and may have serious arrhythmia or sudden death in short term, if the conditions of this kind of patients are not controlled for 1 weeks after active medical treatment, selective coronary angiography should be performed, and the surgical treatment should be performed as soon as possible according to the results of the examination.

(3) Acute myocardial infarction

The views of coronary artery bypass grafting are inconsistent at present, but for the patients after 2 weeks of myocardial infarction, and the patients that ST segment of the treadmill exercise test is significantly depressed, the surgical treatment should be considered to preformed.

(4) Severe ventricular arrhythmia

According to statistics, 1/3 – 1/2 occurred sudden death during 2 – 3 years follow – up in the patients that severe ventricular arrhythmias occurred in convalescent or late stage after myocardial infarction. Therefore, myocardial ischemic ventricular arrhythmias should be considered as one of the indications for coronary artery bypass grafting.

4.2.5 Differential diagnosis

(1) Cardiac neurosis

The patients often complain there is chest pain, and it is a short stinging pain or persistent pain appearing after getting tired. But patients may feel comfortable after mild activity when they are not tired. Sometimes, physical activity may not lead to chest pain or chest tightness.

(2) Angina caused by other diseases

It includes reduced coronary artery blood that caused by severe aortic stenosis or insufficiency, rheumatic fever, coronary arteritis, stenosis or occlusion of the artery orifice caused by syphilis arteritis, relative ischemia of hypertrophic myocardium, and insufficiency of partial cardiac muscle blood supply caused by congenital coronary artery malformation.

(3) Intercostal neuralgia

The pain of this disease often involves 1 – 2 intercostal, but it is not limited to the anterior chest. It often presents as a stabbing pain or burning pain, persistent pain rather than paroxysmal pain. Coughing, forced breathing and body rotation aggravate the pain and there is a pain if you press along the line of the nerve. Besides, there is a local traction pain on the arm when lifting up it.

4.2.6 Therapeutic regimen

(1) Nonoperative treatment

The prevention and medical treatment of coronary heart disease has a long history for many years. The treatment measures include adjusting diet and living habits, paying attention to mental health, applying drugs to reduce blood lipid, inhibiting platelet aggregation and controlling angina, etc. The operation of percutaneous transluminal coronary angioplasty is simple, no chest opening, and less medical costs, but the incidence of restenosis will reach 30% –40% in 6–9 months after operation. In recent years, new devices and new technique for the treatment of early coronary artery embolism and intracavitary cold laser ablation of atherosclerotic plaque and stenosis are also presented.

(2) Surgical treatment

The surgical treatment of coronary heart disease has evolved over 70 years in terms of concepts and methods. Since 1955, direct coronary artery surgery has been carried out to improve myocardial blood supply. The left anterior descending coronary artery shunt was performed by using the great saphenous vein in 1967. And then, the selective coronary angiography is widely used in clinical practice, and rapidly promotes the development of surgical treatment of coronary heart disease. In 1967, Favaloro and Effler applied the great saphenous vein for ascending aorta coronary artery bypass grafting, and introduced the operation technique in 1969. By 1971, 741 operations had been performed. In 1968, Green reported the anastomosis of the anterior descending branch of internal thoracic artery. In 1971, Flemma also reported the operation of sequential transplantation, that is, using a great saphenous vein to make multiple anastomoses with multiple branches of the coronary artery. Since then, the surgical treatment of coronary heart disease has entered a new stage. At present, there are more than 400 thousand patients that have performed coronary artery bypass grafting(CABG) in the world because of coronary heart disease,and the coronary artery bypass grafting has become the main method of surgical treatment for coronary heart disease.

4.2.7　Indications for coronary artery bypass grafting

4.2.7.1　Without symptoms or with mild angina

①The patients with significant stenosis of the left coronary artery should be treated with CABG. ②CABG should be performed for the patients whose proximal end of the left anterior descending artery and the left circumflex artery are constrictive obviously(>70%). ③For the patients with three diseased vessels, especially those with left ventricular dysfunction such as EF< 50% and/or large myocardial ischemia,this treatment is beneficial. ④CABG is recommended for patients with 1 or 2 vessel lesions include proximal stenosis of the left anterior descending artery. And CABG should be performed when the noninvasive examination confirms that there are comprehensive ischemia or left ventricular ejection fraction(LVEF) < 50%. ⑤Patients with 1 or 2 vascular lesions but the proximal of left anterior descending branch was not involved in,CABG could be in consideration,and CABG should be performed when noninvasive examination showed a large area of living myocardium and was in line with the high risk criteria.

4.2.7.2　Stable angina

①The patients with significant stenosis of the left coronary artery should be treated with CABG. ②CABG should be performed when there are significant stenosis(> 70%) in the proximal end of the left lateral branch and the left circumflex artery. ③For the patients with three diseased vessels,CABG should be performed. And LVEF<50% is more meaningful for patients' life. ④When there are 2 diseased vessel with obvious stenosis in the proximal end of the left anterior descending artery,EF<50% ,or noninvasive examination showed ischemia,CABG is recommended. ⑤When there are 1 or 2 diseased vessels without obvious stenosis in the left anterior descending branches,but the noninvasive examination shows a large area of live myocardium who were in high risk,CABG was beneficial. ⑥CABG treatment is beneficial for patients with angina who are still ineffective at the greatest degree of medicine and can accept the risk of surgery. If angina pectoris is not typical,objective ischemia evidence must be obtained. ⑦CABG should be considered for the patients with 1 diseased vessels and stenosis of the proximal left anterior descending artery. If noninvasive examination confirms that there is widespread ischemia or LVEF<50% , CABG should be applied. ⑧When there were 1 or 2 diseased vessels without stenosis in the proxima end of the left anterior descending artery,but the noninvasive examination shows moderate area of living myocardium or ischemic myocardium,CABG should be considered.

4.2.7.3　Unstable angina/non ST elevation myocardial infarction(MI)

①The patients with significant stenosis of the left main coronary artery should be treated with CABG. ②The patients whose left proximal descending branch of the left main coronary artery and the proximal end of the left circumflex artery are constrictive obviously (> 70%) are recommended to be treat by CABG. ③CABG is recommended for the patients that myocardial revascularization is not ideal or impossible,and the patients that the greatest degree of non−operative treatment is ineffective and there still exists progressive ischemia. ④If there are 1 or 2 diseased vessels with obvious stenosis in the proximal left descending bronch,CABG can be chosen. ⑤If there are 1 or 2 diseased vessels without involvement of the proximal left anterior descending artery,CABG should be considered when the percutaneous revascularization is not ideal or impossible. If the noninvasive examination shows a large area of viable myocardium and meets the high−risk criteria,CABG should be applied.

4.2.7.4 ST elevated MI

For the patients with ST elevated MI(myocardial infarction) ,emergency CABG should be performed in the following situations:①The patients that have a failed intravascular angioplasty and are associated with persistent pain or hemodynamic instability, and their coronary anatomy should be suitable for surgery. ②The patients with large area of ischemic myocardium and are not suitable for intravascular angioplasty, it is not effective to use medications, and there appears a cardiogenic shock in the patients with persistent ST elevation or left bundle branch block or posterior wall MI within 36 hours after MI, and the operation can be performed within 18 hours after shock. ③When there is a malignant ventricular arrhythmia in the patients whose left main artery stenosis is more than 50% and / or with 3 diseased vessels. ④There appears a progressive STEMI which is in the early stage(6-12 hours) in the patients who are not suitable for thrombolysis or endovascular repair, or those who are ineffective by either treatment.

4.2.7.5 Contraindication of CABG

①The patients with left ventricular dysfunction, or the patients whose left ventricular ejection fraction is less than 0.2, and the patients whose end diastolic pressure of the left ventricle is greater than 3 kPa (20 mmHg). ② The patients with irreversible chronic heart failure and severe myocardial lesion. ③The patients with systemic diseases such as severe diabetes, hypertension, renal dysfunction or pulmonary insufficiency. ④Those who are elder than 65 years old should carefully consider to accept this surgery.

4.2.8 Complications

4.2.8.1 Arhythmia

The most common arrhythmia after CABG is atrial fibrillation. It usually occurs within 1-3 days after operation, and it is often paroxysmal but can be repeated. Some can terminate voluntarily without treatment, a few may last for several weeks. It is believed to be mainly related to surgical trauma, myocardial ischemia, hypokalemia, acidosis and myocardial reperfusion. Using the β-blockers as early as possible after operation or do not stop using β-blockers before the operation is effective to prevent atrial fibrillation. The principle of treatment is to control ventricular rate and then preform cardioversion. Although β-blockers such as esmolol are effective in controlling ventricular rate, patients with left ventricular dysfunction or obstructive pulmonary disease should use it cautiously. Calcium antagonists are also effective in controlling the ventricular rate. Digitalis should be preferred when there is a left ventricular dysfunction or the systemic hemodynamics are unstable. Incidental premature ventricular contractions may occur after CABG, and it often needn't to be treated. Postoperative fatal ventricular arrhythmias, such as ventricular tachycardia and ventricular fibrillation, are not common.

4.2.8.2 Low cardiac output syndrome

The causes of low cardiac output after CABG are mainly the excessive post cardiac load and poor myocardial contractility caused by early low blood volume after operation and increased peripheral vascular resistance(SVR). Myocardial contractile dysfunction is often found in the cases of extensive and severe coronary artery disease, low left ventricular function before operation, improper protection of cardiac muscle, incomplete revascularization of myocardium, myocardial infarction and acidosis in perioperative period. There are also some other reasons of low cardiac output such as pericardial tamponade, arrhythmia and tension pneumothorax.

4.2.8.3 Perioperative myocardial infarction

There may be nonfatal myocardial infarction after CABG. The incidence of myocardial infarction in patients with unstable angina is higher than that in patients with stable angina. The causes may be related to the following factors：①Incomplete vascularization of myocardium. ②Unstable hemodynamics after operation. ③The problem of bridge vessel. In general, it can be diagnosed through new Q waves and changes of myocardial enzymes in electrocardiogram. At present, troponin is considered as the most significant diagnostic index.

4.2.8.4　Postoperative bleeding

Bleeding is one of the most common complications after CABG, and usually occurs within 24 hours after surgery. The common reasons of the bleeding include untreated small branches of vascular graft, leakage of blood from anastomotic leaks, capillary hemorrhage from the internal mammary artery, and so on. A small number of patients may blood because of the reduced coagulation function cardiopulmonary bypass.

4.2.8.5　Neurological complications

The nervous system complications are one of the fatal complications after CABG. It is mainly caused by hypoxia, embolism, bleeding and metabolic disorders. Neurological complications are independent risk factors associated with mortality after CABG.

4.2.8.6　Infections

The infection include mediastinitis, wound dehiscence, dehiscence of the sternum and the infection of the deep saphenous vein of the lower extremities. The risk factors for increased wound complications include long operation time, third chest opening after surgery, low cardiac output syndrome, respiratory insufficiency, obesity and diabetes.

4.2.8.7　Renal failure

Acute renal failure is a common complication after cardiac surgery, it is also an independent risk factor associated with mortality after CABG. The related factors of renal failure after CABG are old age, the history of moderate to severe heart failure, CABG history, type 1 diabetes mellitus and preoperative renal insufficiency(serum creatinine >1.4 mg · d).

4.2.8.8　Perioperative coronary spasm

The incidence of coronary artery spasm after CABG is higher than that of other operations in all kinds of cardiac surgery or after operation. The main reasons are the light anaesthesia, the reduced sensitivity of coronary artery to vasoconstrictor and the hyperventilation. Through Holter monitoring, about 8% of the patients' ECG after the operation supported the diagnosis of coronary artery spasm. It always occurs at the end of cardiopulmonary bypass or a little time after cardiopulmonary bypass, and a few of them occur before the transfer. The principle of treatment is to relieve spasms and prevent the development of myocardial ischemia as soon as possible, so as to relieve cardiogenic shock and arrhythmia caused by myocardial ischemia.

4.3　Coronary Heart Disease

4.3.1　Coronary heart disease with ischemic mitral inadequacy

The mitral papillary muscle inadequacy or rupture caused by coronary artery ischemic heart disease may lead to mitral insufficiency. It occurs not only in the short-term or long-term after acute myocardial infarction, but also occurs in the coronary heart disease patients without myocardial infarction, the former is called acute myocardial infarction with mitral regurgitation, and the latter is called chronic ischemic cardiomyopathy combined with mitral valve inadequacy.

4.3.1.1 Pathophysiology

The pulmonary venous pressure increases because of the mitral inadequacy, and then, the pulmonary interstitial edema or alveolar pulmonary edema happens and the oxygen of blood decreases, leading to the left ventricular dysfunction and the left ventricular dilatation. What's more, the expanded annulus of mitral valve will result in the increase of the quantity of the blood during the mitral inadequacy, and the decreased blood oxygen may further aggravate myocardial ischemia and the left ventricular dysfunction, resulting in heart failure finally.

4.3.1.2 Clinical manifestations

(1) Symptoms

The typical clinical manifestations of acute myocardial infarction complicated with mitral regurgitation: it always occurs within a few hours to 2 weeks after the acute myocardial infarction, and 2-7 days is the most. In clinical, the patients' condition always aggravate rapidly, and cardiogenic shock will occur if there is a great deal of regurgitated blood caused by ruptured papillary muscles.

(2) Signs

When there is a mild mitral regurgitation caused by the rupture of partial papillary muscles, the systolic murmurs could be heard in the apex. When the complete rupture of the papillary muscles causes massive regurgitation of the mitral valve, the left ventricular function will decrease extremely, there may be no systolic murmur in the apex, and the third cardic sound may be heard at this time.

4.3.1.3 Auxiliary examinations

If the blowing systolic murmur occurs in the apex of patients with coronary heart disease, the following examination should be performed.

(1) ECG

The myocardial ischemia or acute myocardial infarction of coronary heart disease usually combines with high voltage in the left ventricularor and arrhythmias such as atrial fibrillation and ventricular premature beat.

(2) Chest X-ray

Through the chest radiograph, the left ventricular enlargement, pulmonary congestion and pulmonary edema signs could be found. And through the examination of barium meal, the left atrium care and impression oesophagea signs could be observed.

(3) Echocardiography

The left atrium enlargement, the mitral regurgitation, the mitral annulus enlargement and the abnormal motions of the wall could be observed.

(4) Cardiac catheter and angiography

For the patients with acute myocardial infarction complicated by mitral regurgitation, a Swan-Ganz catheter should be placed at the bedside for hemodynamic monitoring. The angiography of coronary artery and left ventricular angiography identifies the degree of coronary artery disease, the status of cardiac function, and the degree of mitral regurgitation, and it also identifies that whether it combines a septal perforation or weakness of the left ventricular wall and whether there is ventricular aneurysm.

4.3.1.4 Differential diagnosis

Combing echocardiography with other auxiliary examinations, the diagnosis of this disease will be clear if it appears blowing murmur in the systole of the apex for the patients with coronary heart disease.

This disease should be identified with mitral regurgitation caused by other disease, such as the mitral valve prolapse, the traumatic mitral regurgitation, the mitral regurgitation caused by chordae or papillary muscle rupture due to infective endocarditis, and what's more, the mitral stenosis with incompetence caused by rheumatic heart disease. The etiology always could be diagnosed by combing the medical history with the coronary angiography.

4.3.1.5　Treatment

The coronary artery bypass grafting should be performed with valvoplasty or valve replacement. The operative mortality rate is about 10% , and the postoperative 5-year survival rate is 70% .

4.3.1.6　Complications

①Perioperative myocardial infarction. ②Low cardiac output syndrome. ③Complications after valve formation or replacement.

4.3.2　Coronary heart disease with valve degeneration

The old patients(age older than 60 years) have higher risk of coronary heart disease, and often suffer from degenerative changes of the aortic valve and the mitral valve at the same time. Among these diseases, the aortic valve lesions mainly manifested as calcification, stenosis, and incomplete closure of the valve. And the mitral valve lesions mainly manifested as mitral regurgitation because of the weak valve leaflets, the prolonged tendons, the slender papillary muscles, the leaflet prolapse, and the annulus expansion.

4.3.2.1　Pathophysiology

The valvular heart diseases affect the function of the ventricle by changing the preload and the postload of the ventricle, but in the patients with coronary heart disease, abnormal ventricular motions and changes of the ventricular geometric shape occurs due to the decrease of the ventricular contraction strength caused by partial ischemia or infarction of the ventricle. Those two kinds of pathophysiological changes influence each other complicatedly rather than superposing simply.

4.3.2.2　Clinical manifestations

(1)Symptoms

Patients are elderly with long medical history, and besides the symptoms of aortic valve stenosis or (and) incomplete closure and mitral regurgitation, there are still symptoms caused by coronary heart disease, such as angina, chest tightness, and precordial discomfort.

(2)Physical signs

The murmur could be heard in the precordial area of the heart. For the patients with left cardiac insufficiency, dry or wet rales at the bottom of the lungs could be heard.

4.3.2.3　Auxiliary inspection

(1)ECG

The changes of myocardial ischemia caused by coronary heart disease, and ventricular hypertrophy and heart rhythm disorders caused by valvular diseases could be observed.

(2)Chest X-ray

The signs of pulmonary congestion, pulmonary interstitial edema, cardiac enlargement and aortic vessel calcification and some others could be found.

(3)Echocardiography

The echocardiography is used to make clear the situation of the motion and function for the whole or local ventricular wall. What's more, the LVEF, valve lesions, and pulmonary arterial pressure could be identified.

(4) Cardiac catheterization and angiography

It can be used to determine the extent of coronary lesions, the ventricular function, the pulmonary artery pressure, the left ventricular end–diastolic pressure and the degree of valve stenosis or reflux.

(5) Isotope examinations

To detect the extent of hibernating myocardium due to ischemia and irreparable cardiac muscle due to infarct or scarring. And it is crucial for the determination of surgical protocols and for judging the prognosis of the operation.

4.3.2.4 Differential diagnosis

Combining the typical symptoms with the medical history, the physical examination, the echocardiography and the coronary angiography, definite diagnosis could be made. The differential diagnosis is related to coronary heart disease and valvular heart disease.

4.3.2.5 Treatment

The operative mortality rate is about 5%, slightly higher than that of simple coronary artery bypass grafting and valve surgery. The surgical complications are in consistent with coronary heart disease combined with ischemic mitral inadequacy.

(1) The valvular surgery and CABG should be operated at the same time.

(2) For the patients with senile aortic valve degeneration, the surgery of aortic valve replacement is always operated.

(3) The valvoplasty is always operated for the patients of mitral valve degeneration.

4.3.3 Chronic rheumatic heart disease

The chronic rheumatic heart disease is a common type of valvular disease in China. The incidence is gradually increasing by years due to the change of life style. Therefore, the incidence of coronary heart disease combined with rheumatic heart disease is also rising up.

4.3.3.1 Pathophysiology

The chronic rheumatic heart disease is primarily related to the lesion of the valves, and affects the cardiac and respiratory function of the patients. In the case of coronary heart disease, cardiac insufficiency and valvular hypofunction would become more serious due to myocardial ischemia, ventricular dysfunction, and ventricular morphologic changes, especially the mitral valve. If there is an acute rupture of myocardial papillary muscle or chordae tendineae at the same time, the heart failure may happen fleetly. The prognosis is very poor and the motality is definitely high.

4.3.3.2 Clinical manifestation

(1) Symptoms

Most of the patients shows symptoms of cardiac insufficiency caused by rheumatic heart disease, such as palpitation and shortness of breath after exercise, limited activity, pulmonary hypertension, and the clinical manifestations of right cardiac insufficiency and left cardiac insufficiency. Most patients have no clinical manifestations of coronary heart disease, and are only found with coronary heart disease by coronary angiography. Only a few patients show the symptoms such as angina pectoris, precordial discomfort and embolism.

(2) Signs

In the precordial area, the murmur related to valves could be heard, and for the patients with left heart dysfunction, dry or wet rales can be heard in the bottom of both lungs.

4.3.3.3　Auxiliary inspection

(1) ECG

It shows cardiac arrhythmias related to valvular lesions, such as atrial fibrillation, ventricular premature contraction, left and right ventricular muscle strain, and atrial enlargement. It is associated with or without ST-T change and old myocardial infarction caused by the ischemia of coronary heart disease.

(2) Chest X-ray

Because of the valvular disease and its secondary changes, the expanded heart image, the pulmonary hypertension and the pulmonary congestion could be observed. The patients of coronary heart disease that associate with ventricular aneurysm show the signs of enlargement of partial left ventricle.

(3) Echocardiography

It shows not only the diseased valve, the degree of disease, the condition of heart function, the size of the heart, but also the abnormal wall movement and the diastolic dysfunction of the left ventricle caused by coronary heart disease.

(4) Cardiac catheterization and angiography

Patients with valvular disease over 50 years should do the examination of coronary angiography routinely before surgery. The patients under 50 years with the signs of coronary angiography such as chest pain and showing ST-T change in the electrocardiogram or high risk factors such as hypertension, hyperlipidemia, diabetes, family history of coronary heart disease should also perform this examination before the operation.

(5) Isotope examinations

This examination can be used to know about the abnormal wall motion, the left ventricular ejection fraction, and the abnormal distribution of pulmonary blood caused by valvular disease.

4.3.3.4　Differential diagnosis

The rheumatic coronary heart disease is easy to be diagnosed clearly in terms of medical history, clinical manifestations and auxiliary examinations. But it should be differentiated from coronary heart disease combined with ischemic heart disease or degenerative valvular disease.

4.3.3.5　Treatment

Coronary heart disease combined with valvular disease should be treated by simultaneous operation. And the indication of operation is similar to that of simple rheumatic valvular heart disease and coronary heart disease. The surgical methods is the same as rheumatic valvular and coronary heart disease.

4.3.4　Coronary heart disease with carotid stenosis

Patients with coronary heart disease are often associated with carotid stenosis, and 6% -20.5% of the patients with coronary heart disease have carotid stenosis. Carotid artery stenosis is one of the important causes of ischemic stroke during the perioperative period of coronary artery bypass grafting.

4.3.4.1　Pathophysiology

The mechanism of ischemic stroke caused by coronary heart disease during the perioperative period of coronary artery bypass grafting is probably caused by embolus from atherosclerotic carotid artery, especially ulcer spots blocks can significantly increase the incidence of perioperative stroke, or insufficient distal perfusion pressure caused by carotid artery stenosis, especially in the non-pulsating blood flow state of extracorporeal circulation and low systemic arterial perfusion pressure, would result in poor brain tissue perfusion.

4.3.4.2　Clinical manifestations

（1）Symptoms

Besides the symptoms of coronary heart disease, patients may have a history of stroke or transient ischemic attack(HA), and they may also have symptoms of lightheadedness or transient blackouts. Some patients have severe peripheral vascular disease.

（2）Physical signs

Systolic murmur could be heard in the neck by examination, but the intensity of murmur don't indicate the degree of arterial stenosis, and the murmur in patients with severe stenosis may reduce or disappear.

4.3.4.3　Auxiliary inspection

（1）The carotid artery color Doppler ultrasound clearly shows the residual lumen status and plaque location. For the patients with history of neck murmurs, stroke, transient ischemic stroke and peripheral vascular lesions, this examination may be the first choice.

（2）MRI may achieve the same effect with carotid artery color Doppler ultrasound, and shows multiple lacuna cerebral infarction or brain atrophy, but the cost is higher.

（3）Pre-arteriography shows the location of carotid artery lesions and the degree of stenosis clearly, and the situation of distal vessel and collateral circulation. The disadvantage is that it may make plaque fall off and the cost is high, and surgeons should preform it with coronary angiography at the same time.

4.3.4.4　Differential diagnosis

The diagnosis mainly depends on the auxiliary examination. It should be differentiated from aortic stenosis, the latter may have symptoms such as dizziness and syncope, and the systolic murmur may transmitted to the neck, the ultrasound could confirm the diagnosis.

4.3.4.5　Treatment

For patients with-coronary heart disease combined with carotid artery stenosis, the surgery effects are discrepant due to surgical methods and patients' conditions. The surgical methods include carotid endarterectomy and carotid stent placement.

4.3.4.6　Complications

For the patients that preform coronary artery bypass grafting, thorough hemostasis is important to prevent active bleeding. Surgeons should fill the aortic incision with gauze first, and suture carefully after finishing the protamine neutralization of all the operations to prevent postoperative neck hematoma.

Chapter 5

Diseases of Great Vessels

5.1　Aortic Aneurysm

5.1.1　Thoracic aortic aneurysm

The thoracic aortic aneurysm is caused by the damage of the middle wall of the thoracic aorta, the wall of the tube becomes thinning, the ability to withstand the impact of blood flow in the blood vessel or sidewall pressure declines and to expand outward under the impact of the high pressure blood flow inside the lumen of blood vessel. The most common causes of TAA are atherosclerosis and nonspecific aortic degenerative diseases, followed by cystic necrosis of the middle layer of the aorta, syphilis, infection, injury and congenital dysplasia. With the increasingly mature technology of extracorporeal circulation and the application of polytetrafluoroethylene artificial blood vessel, the surgical treatment of this disease has reached a very high level. Once diagnosed, surgical treatment should be performed actively.

5.1.1.1　Symptoms

(1) This kind of patients are usually asymptomatic or with mild symptoms and are often found by imaging examination. When the aneurysm reaches a certain level, chest pain occurs when the adjacent mediastinal tissue is compressed. The thoracic pain of the ascending aorta is mostly located in the post sternum. The pain of the neck and jaw can occur when the arch is involved. The descending aneurysm and the thoracoabdominal aortic aneurysm can have the pain in the back, upper abdomen, and the part of the ribs.

(2) Owing to press adjacent tissue or break into the surrounding tissue, it may cause hoarseness, cough, hemoptysis, dyspnea, dysphagia, jaundice, fatal heart failure, pericardial tamponade, haememesis, pleural hematothorax, etc.

(3) Whether the patients have a history of trauma, especially the history of chest trauma; whether have a history of iatrogenic injuries such as the surgical operation of left cardiac catheter or cardiopulmonary bypass and aortic blockage; whether have a history of hypertension, hyperlipidemia, smoking history, diabetes history, and history of syphilis, endocarditis, and coarctation of the aorta.

(4) Whether there is a family history, such as Marfan syndrome, and family history of aneurysms.

5.1.1.2   Physical examinations

(1)Involvement of the aortic root leads to aortic insufficiency,when there is a arteriovenous fistula,the left ventricular failure occurs.

(2)We can touch pulsatile masses or hear vascular murmur in the lesion site.

(3)When the superior vena cava is compressed,the upper half of the body can be seen venous hyperemia and pleural effusion signs are found.

(4)If TAA breaks into the heart package,it would show signs of pericardial tamponade such as fast heart rate,weak heart sounds,engorged odd pulse and jugular vein.

(5)When haemothorax caused by TAA that breaks into chest cavity,the patients' intercostal space is full,the percussion is solid the breath sounds are weakened during the auscultation,and pleura puncture can be pumped out of the blood.

5.1.1.3   Accessory examinations

(1)Electrocardiogram

It is helpful to judge whether there is a combination of coronary heart disease or not,acute pericarditis can be found when the hematopericardium occurs.

(2)Chest X-ray films

This examination is helpful for diagnosis,it can show the shadow of the thoracic aortic aneurysm. The root aortic aneurysm and ascending aorta are showed as a significant widening of the ascending aorta shadow;the arch aortic aneurysm are showed as an obvious enlargement of the aortic knot and buckling extension;the descending aortic aneurysm are showed as a significant widening of the descending aorta shadow; the thoracic abdominal aortic aneurysm are showed as a significant widening of descending aorta and abdominal aorta shadow.

(3)Echocardiography

It can directly show the morphology of the aorta,determine whether the aortic valve and the pericardium are involved,and can show the location,size,range,pulsation and complications of the tumor;if it is pseudo aneurysm,it can show a pseudo aneurysm break,tumor cavity and lateral thrombus.

(4)Magnetic resonance imaging

①The aorta can be examined and diagnosed accurately,and the location and extent of aneurysms can be accurately distinguished. ②Learn about the situation of pericardial or pleural effusion. ③The aortic arch and its main branches can be clearly displayed,which is better than CT examination. ④Distinguishing the nature of mediastinal masses. ⑤Pseudo aneurysms show it's ruptures,lumen,and lateral thrombosis.

(5)CT examination

CT can show the extent of aortic dilatation,the diameter of the aorta and the calcification of the aortic wall. It can also show the involvement of aortic root and aortic branches,and signs of complications such as para aortic hematoma,pericardial hematoma and pleural effusion. Spiral CT can provide more information on the location,range and internal structure of TAA by three-dimensional reconstruction.

(6)Selective aortic angiography and digital subtraction angiography(DSA)

These two methods are the most classic and reliable method for diagnosing this disease,and they are the gold standard of this disease. The purpose of angiography is mainly to solve the following five points: ①Determine diagnosis. ②Determine the scope of the lesion. ③Determine the entrance and exit of the endometrium. ④Evaluate the function of aortic valve. ⑤Estimate the degree of aortic branch involvement and the circumstances of upper and lower vessels.

(7)Coronary angiography

One of the most common causes of TAA is atherosclerosis. If there are high risk factors for atherosclerosis in the middle-aged and the elderly, and other auxiliary examinations suggest atherosclerosis, coronary angiography should be performed to determine the operation plan.

5.1.1.4　Differential diagnosis

(1)Mediastinal mass

It is often confused with this disease and should be identified by DSA or selective arteriography, MRI, CT and echocardiography before operation.

(2)Central lung cancer

The atypical patients with central lung cancer are easily confused with this disease, but the sputum cells of the central lung cancer patients are positive, and the pathological specimen of the bronchoscopy can be confirmed. MRI, CT and echocardiography are helpful to identify.

(3)Esophageal cancer

The middle and lower esophageal carcinoma and descending aortic aneurysm are easily confused by X-ray plain film examination, but the esophageal cancer has a history of progressive dysphagia, and the esophagus swallowing barium and esophagoscopy can be determined.

(4)Aortic valve insufficiency caused by other causes

It should be distinguished with aortic valve insufficiency caused by other causes such as aortic valve perforation and rupture of aortic sinus aneurysm caused by endocarditis.

5.1.1.5　Treatments

Because the natural prognosis of this disease is very poor, if its diameter is greater than 5 cm, no matter whether there is any symptom, it should be operated actively once it is diagnosed. Complicated with severe heart, liver, brain, lung and kidney dysfunction, patients who are ineffective in medical treatment and patients with general cachexia are classified as contraindications.

(1)Non-operative treatment

It is suitable for the patients with serious complications such as insufficiency of heart, liver, brain, lung or kidney, and the patients with ineffective medical treatment and systemic cachexia; the patients of TAA that the diameter is less than 5 cm, asymptomatic, without progressive enlargement of the tumor, and have a shorter survival period with other diseases are all suitable for non-operative treatment too. Patients who want to choose non-operative treatment should actively use beta adrenoceptor blocker to control blood pressure and quit smoking.

(2)Surgical treatment

1)Surgical indications and surgical timing:The patients with typical symptom, whose tumor diameter is greater than 5 cm, whose tumor enlarge progressively and it is faster than 1 cm/years, and the patients without surgical contraindication should be operated at an early date.

2)Operative methods:Surgeons should choose different surgical methods according to different cause, location, size and shape of the lesion. Moderate hypothermia cardiopulmonary bypass is commonly used for aortic aneurysm resection. Benall operation and Cabrol operation are suitable for Marfan syndrome. Wheat operation is suitable for patients with non Marfan syndrome.

5.1.2　Abdominal aortic aneurysm

The abdominal aortic aneurysm(AAA)is caused by the damage of the middle wall of the abdominal aorta, the wall of the tube becomes thinner, the ability to withstand the impact of blood flow in the blood vessel or sidewall pressure declines, and then the wall expand and expand outward under the impact of the high pressure blood. It is generally considered that abdominal aortic aneurysm can be diagnosed if the diameter exceeds 3 cm. This disease is the most common aneurysm the age of patients is usually more than 50 years old, with an average age of 60 years. The most common cause of AAA is atherosclerosis, followed by Marfan syndrome(including middle layer cystic necrosis of aorta) and Takayasu arteritis. In the past 20 years, the rapid development of diagnostic methods, the treatment of before and after operation, the improvement of surgical methods, the application of new techniques and the clinical application of new high quality vascular substitutes have made thousands of patients with abdominal aortic aneurysm get the opportunity to treat them, reduce the complications and have a prolong life.

5.1.2.1　Symptoms

There may be no symptoms or mild symptoms for this kind of patients, and their diseases are always found due to physical examination, radiographic examination and abdominal surgery. When the aneurysm is large to a certain extent and there are different degrees of abdominal pain when the adjacent tissue is oppressed. The sudden severe abdominal pain is often the characteristic manifestation of the rupture of the abdominal aortic aneurysm or the acute dilatation.

5.1.2.2　Clinical manifestations

When AAA oppress the adjacent tissues, there are some manifestations such as intestinal obstruction, gastrointestinal bleeding, ureteral obstruction and hydronephrosis, obstruction of the lower extremities, and massive bleeding in the abdomen, etc.

5.1.2.3　Physical examination

(1) The pulsatile masses can be touched or the vascular murmur can be heard in the lesion site.

(2) Edema of both lower limbs can be found during the compression of the inferior vena cava.

(3) There are ischemic manifestations of arterial obstruction in lower extremities caused by atherosclerotic plaque in the aneurysm or dropping in the adherent thrombus.

(4) Abdominal aortic aneurysm ruptures into the abdominal cavity will cause hematoperitoneum, and bloody fluid will be found by abdominal puncture.

5.1.2.4　Accessory examination

(1) Abdominal X-ray film

It can show the calcification shadow of abdominal aortic aneurysm, and the obstruction of the intestine caused by AAA's compression of the intestine is a liquid plane.

(2) Abdominal ultrasound

The shape of the abdominal aorta can be observed directly, and it can show the location, size, range, pulsation and complications of the tumor. If there is a pseudoaneurysm, it can show the rupture of the pseudoaneurysm, the lumen of the aneurysm, and adherent thrombus.

(3) Magnetic resonance imaging

①The aorta can be examined and diagnosed accurately, and the location and extent of aneurysms can be accurately distinguished. ②The aortic arch and its main branches can be clearly displayed, which is better than CT examination. ③Pseudo aneurysms show it's ruptures, lumen, and lateral thrombosis.

(4) CT examination

CT shows the extent of abdominal aorta dilatation, the diameter of the aorta and the calcification of the abdominal aortic wall. CT also shows the involvement of abdominal aortic branches, and signs of complications such as periaortic hematoma, pyoperitoneum. Spiral CT can provide more information on the location, range and internal structure of AAA by three-dimensional reconstruction.

(5)Selective aortic angiography and digital subtraction angiography

DSA can be chosen when the diseases could not be diagnosed or diagnosed clearly by the methods above, and the following five points can be solved: ①Determine the diagnosis. ②Determine the scope of the lesion. ③Determine the entrance and exit of the endometrium. ④Definite the condition of the renal and renal arteries. ⑤Estimate the degree of abdominal aortic branch involvement and the circumstances of upper and lower vessels.

5.1.2.5　Differential diagnosis

It is mainly identified with middle and upper abdominal masses, such as tumor of retroperitoneal lymphatic origin, tumor of other connective tissues from retroperitoneum, pancreatic tumor, mesenteric tumor, etc. Surgeons should find out if the lumps are pulsating, and examinations of MRI, CT and echocardiography are good choices.

5.1.2.6　Treatment

Considering the evolution and prognosis of abdominal aortic aneurysm, the treatment is mainly performed by surgical treatment. Patients with serious dysfunction of heart, liver, brain, lung and kidney, who are insensitive to the medical treatment and with systemic cachexia are listed as the contraindications of the operation. Patients with infection of abdominal cavity, abdominal wall, and whole body, or with malignant or other fatal diseases whose survival time is estimated to be less than 2 years can be regarded as contraindication of operation.

(1)Non-operative treatment

It includes controlling blood pressure, regular follow-up, lowering cholesterol and symptomatic treatment. Close follow-up should be made in non-surgical treatment, especially when the size changes or lumbago and abdominal pain occur, surgical treatment should be performed as soon as possible.

(2)Surgical treatment

1)Indications and timing of operation: symptomatic patients, or patients of AAA with a diameter greater than 5-6 cm, or tumor with a progressive enlargement, or with a rupture trend, all the patients above without surgical taboos should be treated as early as possible.

2)Surgical methods: selective abdominal aortic aneurysm resection, artificial vascular transplantation, and abdominal aortic aneurysm treatment have been used in clinic as a result of minimally invasive. The method includes internal stent placement and stent graft isolation.

5.2　Aortic Dissection

Within the aortic dissection, the blood of the aorta enters the middle membrane of the aorta from the tear of the intima of the aorta, separating the middle membrane and extending along the long axis of the aorta, thus causing a pathological change that the true and false cavity of the aorta are separated. The etiology of ADA is not very clear by now, but hypertension and middle aortic diseases are considered to be the most important risk factors. The prognosis of this disease is dangerous and most of the patients die in the acute stage. The main causes of death are rupture of aortic dissection, progressive hemorrhage of septum or retroperitoneal, and acute heart failure or renal failure.

5.2.1   Clinical manifestations

(1)Main symptoms:Chest pain is the most important symptom of the disease,characterized by persistent tearing or cutting pain. The pain characteristic of dissection of the aortic dissection to the proximal end is focused on the sternum;and the dissection of the aorta dissecting to the distal end often occurs in the interscapular region of the back and can be extended to the abdomen and about 1/3 patients in the acute period show signs of shock such as pale,sweat dripping,skin and limbs cold,pulse fast and weak and shortness of breath and so on.

(2)The involvement of the aortic valve always shows the manifestation of left heart failure. It shows signs of acute myocardial ischemia or even myocardial infarction when coronary arteries are involved,which must be identified with myocardial infarction caused by coronary atherosclerotic lesions,because the emergency thrombolytic therapy for the treatment of the latter is fatal to ADA. If ADA breaks into the pericardium. It shows the manifestation of pericardial tamponade. A series of symptoms of nervous systems can be found when ADA invade in the arteries supplying the brain or spinal cord or when there is a shock caused by insufficient blood supply from the brain or spinal cord,which would cause paraplegia;When the abdominal aorta and its large branches are involved,it may cause similar manifestations to acute abdominal such as insufficiency of hepatic and renal,intestinal ischemic necrosis. If ADA compresses the esophagus and trachea,it may lead to dysphagia and dyspnea. If ADA compresses the laryngeal recurrent nerve,it will lead to hoarseness. ADA can break into the esophagus and trachea and cause hematemesis or hemoptysis,and if ADA break into the chest,it would cause coughing and dyspnea. When ADA is involved in subclavian artery and femoral artery,limb weakness,pain,paleness,cold and intermittent claudication will occur.

(3)Whether there is a history of trauma in the patients,especially chest trauma;Whether there is a history of heavy physical activity and sudden body flexion and extension;Whether there is a history of iatrogenic injury,such as left cardiac catheterization,cardiopulmonary bypass,or aortic blockage;Whether there is a history of hypertension,syphilis,endocarditis,SLE,or coarctation of the aorta;And whether there is a history of taking sweet beans or other toxic food of connective tissue.

(4)Surgeons should be clear that whether there is a history of family,such as Marfan and Ehlers-Donlas syndrome.

5.2.2   Physical examination

(1)Although there is shock in clinic,blood pressure would not drop,and it may increase in the early stage of the disease.

(2)Sudden signs of aortic insufficiency were accompanied by progressive signs of heart failure,such as galloping,lung rales,etc.

(3)We can touch the pulsatile mass or hears the murmurs in the diseased region.

(4)The beating intensity of bilateral carotid,brachial artery,radial artery or femoral artery is inconsistent,or one side disappears,or there is a significant difference between two arm blood pressure. ① If ADA breaks into the pericardium,it shows signs of pericardial tamponade,such as rapid heart rate,weak heart sound,abnormal pulse and jugular vein;②When ADA breaks into the thorax,the patient had a full intercostal space,consolidated percussion sound and weak respiratory sounds. And blood can be drawn out by thoracentesis.

5.2.3　Accessory examination

(1)ECG

It is helpful to judge whether there is a combination of coronary artery disease, acute myocardial ischemia or even myocardial infarction can be found if the coronary artery is involved. And it shows the signs of acute pericarditis when there is a pericardial blood.

(2)Chest radiography

Progressive aortic widening or irregular shape and local abnormal uplift can be found.

(3)Echocardiography

We can directly observe the shape of the aorta, determine whether the aortic valve and the pericardium are involved. And the color Doppler examination can not only determine the fracture of the interlayer and distinguish whether there is thrombus in the false cavity, but also can make clear the reflux situation of the aortic valve.

(4)Magnetic resonance imaging

There are advantages of multi position and multiplane imaging: ①The whole aorta examination can be used to identify the area of intimal tear and the range of interlayer, and to identify whether there are thrombus in the true and false cavity. If there is no blood flow in the cavity, it is closed or blocked by thrombus. ②We can clear whether the dissection affects the brachiocephalic vessels and the extent of involvement. ③Understand the condition of pericardial or pleural effusion. ④The aortic arch and its main branches can be clearly displayed, which is superior to CT examination. ⑤To identify the properties of mediastinal mass.

(5)CT

CT shows the extent of aortic dilatation, the diameter of the aorta and the calcification of the aortic wall. Enhancing CT shows intimal slices of aortic intimal tear, which is one of the specific signs of ADA diagnosis. Spiral CT provides more information on the location, range, internal structure, and location of ADA through three-dimensional reconstruction.

(6)Selective aortic angiography and digital subtraction angiography

The two methods are the most classic and reliable method to diagnose this disease, and the diagnostic rate can reach 99%.

5.2.4　Differential diagnosis

(1)Acute myocardial infarction

Most of the patients with acute myocardial infarction had a history of angina pectoris, the pain aggravates gradually and the location is limited. The two diseases all have signs of shock, but the blood pressure of acute myocardial infarction drops obviously, but that in ADA may not decrease. Through the myocardial enzyme elevation and the electrocardiogram which is shown as the figure of acute myocardial infarction, we can not exclude the ADA involved in the coronary artery combined with acute myocardial infarction.

(2)Acute abdomen

When abdominal aorta and its large branches is involved by ADA, it can lead to similar symptoms of acute abdomen, sometimes it may be misdiagnosed. It is necessary to observe the signs of vascular obstruction carefully in the corresponding parts, echocardiographic examination should be performed routinely, and the magnetic resonance examination, the selective aorta angiography and digital subtraction angiography could also be performed if it is necessary.

(3) Aortic insufficiency caused by other reasons

We should also identify ADA with the aortic insufficiency caused by other causes such as aortic valve perforation caused by endocarditis, ruptured aneurysm of the aortae sinus, and true aortic aneurysm, acute aortic interruption.

5.2.5 Treatments

The natural prognosis of ADA is dangerous, and most of the patients die in the acute period. Therefore, the patient should be sent to the intensive care unit immediately once it is suspected. No matter what type of ADA, it should start the treatment with drugs firstly. If the disease is serious, and there are the further expansion and rupture of the dissection or other complications, the emergency rescue operation should be performed. If the condition is stable, surgical indication is necessary for surgical treatment.

5.2.5.1 Non-operative treatment

Non-operative treatment is used to control pain, reduce blood pressure and ventricular contraction rate, prevent further expansion and rupture of aortic dissection. Surgeons often employ strong analgesic, sedative drugs, vasodilator and beta adrenoceptor blocker to control blood pressure and left ventricular ejection force, so as to reduce the tension of the aortic wall.

5.2.5.2 Surgical treatment

Surgical treatment is applied to remove the rupture of the inner membrane, prevent the rupture of the aortic dissection, and reconstruct the blood flow in the vascular obstruction area caused by intimal slice or false lumen.

Surgical indications:

(1) Surgical indications for acute Stanford A: ① The aortic dissection is about to peel to the proximal end and shows the following cases, we should take an operation: The aortic dissection hematoma causes aortic valve insufficiency and left heart failure. The aortic dissection involves in the coronary artery and causes acute myocardial ischemia and even myocardial infarction. The aortic dissection breaks into pericardial cavities and causes pericardial tamponade. ② When the aortic dissection is about to peel to the distal end, and cause the insufficiency of blood supply in the brain or spinal cord because of the involvement of the arteries of the brain or spinal cord, the occurrence of stroke or acute hemiplegia would not be an operative taboo. It should be operated in the emergency department. The patient could recover obviously after the operation, and it is meaningless to take an operation on the patient with brain death.

(2) Surgical indications for acute Stanford B: Surgeons often use medical treatment to treat type B patients. When the following complications occur, the surgery is considered carefully: The patients with descending aorta and abdominal aorta rupture, or severe organs and limb ischemia, need emergency surgery to restore organ and limb blood circulation. The patients with drug uncontrolled hypertension and unbearable or repeated pain need operations.

(3) Indications for chronic Stanford A: If the aortic root diameter is >5. 5 cm and/or there is moderate to severe aortic insufficiency in the patients, it needs operations.

(4) Indications for chronic Stanford B operation: The lesions is expanding like tumor, and have the risk of rupture in the dilated dissection (the inner diameter exceeds the normal value 2 folds, the internal diameter increases by >1 cm in half a year, the rapid growth to one side). Or the patients suffered from poor perfusion syndrome, which could cause ischemia of distal important organs and limb because of hematoma, need operations.

5.3　Aortitis

Multiple arteritis(also known as Takayasu arteritis)is the chronic non-specific arterial inflammation of the aorta and its main branches. Inflammation causes stenosis and occlusion of blood vessels in different parts of the aorta, and a few inflammation could cause dilatation and aneurysm formation due to the destruction of the middle layer of the artery wall. There are different clinical symptoms due to the different arteries involved. It's very common to see upper limb apnea caused by the involvement of the head and upper limb arteries. The pathogenesis of the disease has not been fully clarified. It may be an autoimmune disease, which is a category of connective tissue disease. And it mainly manifests in the large artery. But it is also suggested that it is related to endocrine disturbance and genetic factors.

5.3.1　Pathophysiology

The pathological features of this disease correspond to the clinical stage. Early(active)arterial lesions mainly show the infiltration of the middle layer of lymphocytes and the infiltration of the outer membrane of giant cell;the characteristic of chronic vascular obstruction is the obstruction of the vascular cavity caused by fibrous hyperplasia in the lesion artery. The lesions are segmental, and the arterial walls between two segments are normal. In later period, local lesions can be complicated by aneurysm formation, dilatation and calcification, which is after stenosis. The brachiocephalic artery type is often the three major branch of the aortic arch, which extends from sub-clavicle to the opening of the vertebral artery, causing ischemia of the head and upper limb;and the descending aorta and the abdominal aorta can extend to the renal and iliac arteries, causing the upper limb blood pressure was higher than the lower extremities;and the renal artery type is usually only one side or bilateral renal artery involved, combined obstinate renal hypertension and rare lower limb ischemia.

5.3.2　Diagnosis

(1)Acute stage(early stage):It mainly shows the systemic allergy symptoms:fever, fatigue, general discomfort, anorexia, sweating, emaciation, etc. It can be accompanied by arthritis and nodding red class. It also shows the Reynolds syndrome and splenomegaly.

(2)The late stage is mainly local symptoms caused by vascular stenosis and obstruction.

1)Brachiocephalic artery type

Symptoms:It mainly show the ischemia symptoms of erebral, head and face, and upper limbs. Because of the ischemia and occlusion of the carotid and vertebral arteries, patients often feel dizziness, headache, memory impairment, unilateral or bilateral visual impairment code, masticatory weakness, facial atrophy, and severe brain damage, such as hemiplegia, aphasia, syncope.

Signs:patient's unilateral or bilateral radial, axillary, and carotid artery pulse is weak or disappearing. Upper limb blood pressure could not be measured or significantly reduces, or the difference between double upper limb systolic blood pressure exceeds 20 mHg. And upper limbs blood pressure is normal or elevated. Some patients had continuous murmurs or systolic murmurs in bilateral neck, supraclavicular, and sterno-cleidomastoid muscles.

2)Thoracoabdominal aortic type

Symptoms:Ischemia causes numbness of lower limb, pain, cold sensation, fatigue and intermittent claudication. The higher blood pressure of upper limbs can cause dizziness, headache and other symptoms caused by hypertension.

Signs:bilateral or unilateral lower limb blood pressure could not be measured or significantly reduces, upper limb blood pressure is normal or elevated. Continuous or systolic murmurs can be detected near the scapula,chest,parasternal,abdomen or kidney.

3)Renal artery type

Symptoms:Lesions involve in one or both sides of the renal artery,and it may lead to persistent and severe hypertension.

Signs:The blood pressure of the extremities increased significantly. The systolic murmur could be heard in the upper abdomen or kidney.

4)Pulmonary artery type

Symptoms:It has many symptoms,such as panic and shortness of breath.

Signs:It mainly shows the signs of pulmonary hypertension and right ventricular strain. It also shows the signs of pulmonary valve systolic murmurs,and pulmonary valve second tone enhancement.

5)Mixed type

The lesions involve more than two vessels at the same time. Symptoms and signs vary according to the blood vessels involved.

5.3.3　Accessory examinations

(1)Laboratory examinations

In the acute active phase,it can be seen erythrocyte sedimentation rate increases rapidly,C reactive protein is positive,serum IgG and IgM increases.

(2)Electrocardiogram

If patients are complicated with hypertension,the electrocardiogram could be observed left ventricular hypertrophy or strain. It could observe right ventricular hypertrophy or strain in pulmonary artery type.

(3)X-ray examination

Left ventricle enlargement could be observed in thoraco-abdominal aortic and renal artery type. The reduction of lung texture,the prominent of pulmonary conus and the enlargement of right ventricle could be observed in the pulmonary artery type. Selective arteriography could be used to identify the location and extent of stenosis,but it is less useful because it is invasive.

(4)Vascular ultrasound Doppler

The degree and severity of arterial stenosis can be accurately displayed.

(5)Further examination

It includes fundus examination,radionuclide examination,TCD,lung scan,CT and MRI. They can be selected according to the specific conditions of different involved arteries.

5.3.4　Differential diagnosis

(1)Congenital coarctation of aorta:Congenital vascular malformation can be manifested as an increase in upper limbs blood pressure and reduction in the lower limbs blood pressure. But the patients suffered from congenital coarctation of the aorta from childhood,and the back along the left side of the spine could be heard systolic murmur,the rib notch can be seen on the chest X-ray,and limited stenosis of the descending aorta can be seen on the arteriography.

(2)Pulmonary artery type should be differentiated from primary pulmonary hypertension and pulmonary valves stenosis. Takayasu arteritis is very common in young women with short course and rapid progress. Irregular stenosis can be seen in the pulmonary angiography. But primary pulmonary hypertension and pulmonary valves stenosis are congenital diseases. The proximal pulmonary arteries of primary pulmonary hypertension expanded significantly, but the cavities were smooth. The stenosis of the pulmonary valve was mainly in the valve. The second tone of the pulmonary artery was often weakened.

(3) In addition, it is necessary to distinguish with thromboarteritis obliterans and atherosclerosis.

5.3.5　Treatment

The treatment of Takayasu's arteritis includes medical and surgical treatment. Medical treatment is considered in the acute period to relieve symptoms and control the progress of the disease. Surgical treatment should be performed when the arterial coarctation affects the blood supply of important organs, or have the risk of aneurysm rupture.

5.3.5.1　Surgical treatment

(1) Surgical indications

Surgical treatment is suitable for the patients in chronic period, and the state of disease is stable for more than half a year, and the lesion is limited. And it is suitable for the important organs with serious arterial stenosis, such as brain, kidney, limbs and other important organs. Also, the surgical treatment is suitable for the patients with refractory hypertension, and ineffective drug treatment.

(2) Operative methods

According to the different location of the lesion, different surgical treatment methods are as follows:

1) Brachiocephalic artery type

The brachiocephalic vascular occlusion usually causes cerebral ischemic disorder. The treatment of patients in this type is mainly used with the ascending aorta brachial vascular bypass grafting.

2) Thoracic and abdominal aorta type and renal artery type

This type of surgical treatment is suitable for upper limb hypertension and lower extremity hypotension caused by thoracic and abdominal aorta stenosis. Also, it is suitable for renal hypertension caused by renal artery stenosis. Besides, in the patients with the drug treatment ineffective, thoracic aorta abdominal aorta bypass grafting or ascending aorta abdominal aorta bypass grafting is commonly applied.

3) Generalized Takayasu arteritis

When patients are combined with three major branches of the aortic arch and extensive stenosis of the thoracic and abdominal aorta, we should combine with the above two surgical methods.

4) Pulmonary arteritis

The involved pulmonary vessels in pulmonary arteritis is often multiple, and this type frequently involves in the distal end of the lung. Therefore, surgical treatment is often difficult to carry out. The surgical treatment of this type is rarely reported.

5.3.5.2　Interventional therapy

In recent years, with the improvement of the mediator technology, percutaneous transluminal angioplasty and intravascular stent technology have also been applied to treat Takayasu arteritis, which can be used in the carotid, renal, iliac, subclavian and femoral artery limited stenosis. Recent results of patients are usually satisfactory, but the long-term effect of patients still need to be further observed.

5.3.6　Complications

After operation surgeons should pay attention to controlling blood pressure, preventing infection, increasing nutrition and rest.

(1) Artificial blood vessel compression

It is very common to see in the patients of brachiocephalic arteritis, and whose operation uses artificial vascular transplantation. This operation is from aortic arch to neck brachial vascular bypass. Because the upper mediastinum and the thoracic entrance are narrower, in addition to the local edema after the operation, both reasons would cause compression of artificial blood vessels and obstruction of venous reflux. Surgeons could select small caliber artificial blood vessels and more than two vascular anastomosis to prevent it.

(2) Occlusion of vascular bridge

During the operation, surgeons should avoid compressing and distort the artificial blood vessels.

(3) Anastomotic bleeding

Anastomotic bleeding is also one of the common complications.

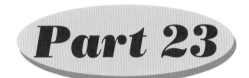

Part 23

Chest Wall Malformation

Chest wall deformities may be congenital or acquired and can be divided into three categories. The most common category is depression(pectus excavatum, PE) and protrusion deformity (pectus carinatum) of the anterior chest wall. The second category of deformities is due to failure of sternum normal development (aplasia or dysplasia) causing bifid sternum with partial or complete failure of midline fusion of the sternum resulting in ectopia cordis. In addition to the sternum, there may be aplasia of the associated structures, such as the heart, pericardium, diaphragm and anterior abdominal wall. The aplasia may also be unilateral with an absence of ribs, pectoralis muscles and breast tissue as seen in Poland's syndrome. The third category of deformities is due to trauma or pressure effects. Too early and extensive rib resection for PE repair may destroy growth centers and result in acquired asphyxiating chondrodystrophy. Abnormal pressure effects and spasticity as seen in patients with severe cerebral palsy may result in very abnormal chest configuration. Chest wall deformities are frequently familiar with several members of one family affected. The incidence of connective tissue disorders such as Marfan's syndrome and Ehlers–Danlos syndrome is markedly increased in patients with chest wall deformities. As a result, systemic weakness of the connective tissues and poor muscular development of the thorax, abdomen and spine are common and scoliosis is present in up to 19% of these patients.

Chapter 1

Pectus Excavatum

Pectus excavatum, also known as funnel chest, is the most common deformities of the anterior chest wall and characterized by a depression in the lower sternum and adjacent ribs. This result in a sunken appearance of the chest wall with the deepest at the level of xiphisternum, the deformity may be symmetric or asymmetric. For moderate to severe cases, surgical correction is necessary to alleviate symptoms and improve the quality of Patients' life.

1.1　Epidemiology

Reported prevalence has been 1/300 to 1/1000 live births. PE constitutes 90% of all chest wall deformities. There is predominance in male. The ratio of male to female is about 4 : 1. It is reported that the deformity often apparent from after birth and once the deformity is noticed, it tends to progress slowly until puberty, when rapid progression is often seen, but only 22% are noticed in the first decade of life.

1.2　Etiology

The underlying cause of PE is not well understood, many hypotheses have been suggested including the irregular growth of costal cartilage, partial fibrosis of diaphragm muscle or shortness of diaphragmatic central tendon, the obstruction of respiratory tract, musculoskeletal disorder, hereditary factor, and so on, but less of them can be confirmed or falsified.

Historically, PE is considered multifactorial in inheritance. Genetic studies support an autosomal recessive heritability, but only 40% of patients have positive family history. However, it is thought to relate to irregular growth of the cartilage that connects the sternum to the ribs especially the overgrowth of the costal cartilage but the outcome come from David VL study demonstrate that is not true.

The deformity of PE may be seen as isolated or in association with the connective tissue disorder, that is to say the PE is local repression of systematic malformation, such as Marfan syndrome and congenital scoliosis.

1.3 Pathophysiology

Patients with mild PE may not have any pathophysiological consequence which is related to the severity of the defect. Pulmonary function abnormalities range from being normal in young patients to obstructive or restrictive in older patients with marked deformity. There may be evidence of air trapping as evidenced by an increase in residual volume(RV) and the resultant increase in the ratio RV/total lung capacity(TLC). Distortion of the rib cage may result in a mechanical disadvantage for the optimum functioning of respiratory muscles and resultant air-trapping. Exercise testing may reveal cardiopulmonary limitation. The depressed sternum in severe cases may impede heart movements and affect stroke volume especially during exercise resulting in the cardiopulmonary limitation. Patient with PE may have a cardiac deviation to the left and conduction defects. Dysrhythmias such as first-degree heart block, right bundle branch block are common in PE population. A depressed sternum along with distorted cartilages and involved ribs may not only interfere with normal chest wall movements but can also cause displacement of the associated vertebrae and development of scoliosis.

1.4 Clinical Features

1.4.1 Symptoms

In addition to the characteristic indentation of the chest wall, PE may cause symptoms by compressing the underlying heart and lungs. These include shortness of breath, chest pain, palpitations, fatigue and reduced exercise tolerance. Regardless of severity, the cosmetic deformity associated with any case of PE may also result in psychological issues relating to body image and self-esteem.

The most frequent symptoms are dyspnea and chest pain on exertion, exercise intolerance. Frequent respiratory tract infections and asthma may also occur. The presence and severity of symptoms is directly related to the severity of cardiac and pulmonary compression and therefore to the severity of the deformity.

Symptoms tend to be more prevalent in older children because teenagers have a deeper deformity and a more rigid chest, whereas younger children still have a very pliable chest wall, have significant cardiac and pulmonary reserves, don't participate in competitive sports, and the deformity has not progressed to its full extent. Teenagers with PE have a poor body image and because of their exercise intolerance they stop participating in team sports which leads to isolation and feelings of worthlessness. They hate and avoid situations where they have to take their shirt off in front of other children, therefore adding to their isolation and to a downward spiral of depression and suicidal thoughts.

1.4.2 Physical examination

These patients have a classic "pectus posture" that includes thoracic kyphosis, forward sloping shoulders, and a protuberant abdomen. They tend to be very asthenic, with long limbs, delicate bone structure and poor muscular development. The pectus deformity may be localized as "cup-shaped", diffuse as "saucer-shaped", eccentric as "grand canyon" or mixed malformation with excavatum/carinatum.

1.4.3　Investigations

While PE is usually evident on examination of the chest, a number of tests may be carried out to determine the impact of the condition on the heart and lungs. These include imaging, such as a chest X-ray and CT scan, which demonstrate the extent to which the heart and lungs are compressed. An echocardiogram is helpful in characterizing how well the heart function. Other tests that may be conducted include an electrocardiogram and lung function tests.

The severity of pestus deformity should be accessed with Haller CT index since the deformity may be mild, moderate or severe and it is important to measure the severity objectively. The Haller CT index divides the internal transverse diameter of the chest by the anteroposterior diameter. The index is less than 2 in normal populations. An index greater than 3. 25 is the indication of a moderate or severe depression (Figure 23-1-1).

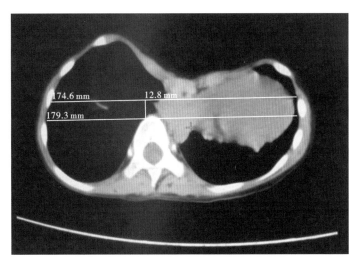

Figure 23 – 1 – 1　　Asymmetricpectus excavatum and its HI shown on chest CT scan which calculatedthrough the internal maximal transverse diameter divided by the anteroposterior diameter on the axial slice that indicates the shortest distance between the sternum and anterior surface of vertebral body

Patients with a Haller index of greater than 7 are four times more likely to have a restrictive pattern on pulmonary function testing. MRI including breath-hold MRI has been used for the morphologic assessment of thoracic deformities for the preoperative assessment of PE. A better insight of lung function in patients with PE deformity may be obtained using recently introduced techniques such as oculo-electronic plethysmography(OEP) which can show that the depressed portion of the sternum and adjacent chest wall do not move with respiration and there is a reduction in lung volume.

1.5　Management

Mild cases of PE may be managed with physiotherapy alone, which involves exercises aiming to improve posture and chest expansion. In addition, psychological counseling should be provided to those who have difficulty coping with the condition.

For moderate to severe cases, surgical correction is indicated. Surgical correction of PE reported from the beginning of 20th century, until 1949 and 1951, procedure of sternal elevation(Ravitch procedure) and "turn over" of anterior chest wall published, from then on, Ravitch procedure used widely and modified, good outcome of PE repair obtained. Since Danold Nuss introduced the minimally invasive procedure for PE repair in 1998, this procedure, known as the Nuss procedure, accepted by the pediatric surgeons and used world widely.

Surgical correction of PE most often results in significant improvements in symptoms and quality of life. These operations carry a number of risks, however, including infection, bleeding and pain postoperatively, though these risks may be lower for the Nuss procedure.

For the Ravitch procedure, the involved cartilage, xiphoid process resected completely, sternal osteotomy performed. Modification of this technique involves placement of a metallic strut behind the sternum to stabilize it. The metallic strut is removed after 6-12 months.

Nuss procedure, which is the surgical procedure of choice in most cases currently, involves placement of a titanium bar(bent to the corrected contour of the chest wall) into the pleural space through small incisions on either side of the chest, into the space between retrosternal and anterior of the heart. The bar is rotated anteriorly to press the sternal invagination from behind and sutured in place. The bar is left in place usually for 2 years, and by that time the sternum has remolded(Figure 23-1-2).

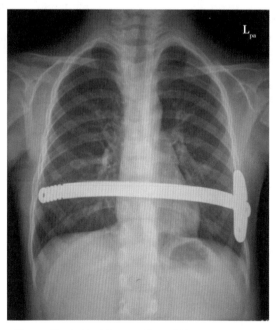

Figure 23-1-2   The position of Nuss bar shown
on anteroposterior chest X-ray
film after PE repair

Compared to Ravitch procedure, the Nuss procedure takes less time, and the patient has less blood loss. However, the postoperative recovery time is same for both procedures. Nuss procedure shows chest wall movements as normal person.

Beside the invasive procedure, vacuum bell therapy, another noninvasive technique can be selected and used in some PE patients and their deformity corrections.

Chapter 2

Pectus Carinatum

Pectus carinatum is a protrusion deformity of the chest; it may involve the upper or lower chest if the manubrium or the body of the sternum projects forward. The protrusion may be unilateral, bilateral or mixed with PE and carinatum; in some families one child may have PE and another pectus carinatum.

Pectus carinatum is much less common than PE but more common in boy. Unlike PE, pectus carinatum usually appears in late childhood and progresses rapidly during puberty, no cardiac or pulmonary compression and less influence of cardiopulmonary function. Beside the cosmetic contour of anterior chest wall, patients complain less but chest pain and less positive discovery from investigation.

Treatment is either by means of application of a pressure brace or surgical resection. Application of a pressure brace has become popular over the last 10 years however the literature on the subject is still very limited. For the invasive repair of pectus carinatum, resection of the deformed cartilages and sternal osteotomy has a long and successful history in patients with a severe deformity. Since the surgery is very invasive it should only be used in patients who have a very severe deformity, which does not respond to orthostatic pressure management, therefore, the indication of open operation for this deformity is more critical than that of PE. There is successful experience reported that repaired with Nuss procedure but more practice should be done and summarized.

Chapter 3

Sternal Defects

Sternal defects are varying, maybe partial or complete cleft with or without other malformations. Survival depends on the severity of the various abnormalities.

Partial clefts may be superior or inferior. The superior clefts are most often isolated but inferior clefts are often associated with other anomalies in the adjacent organs including the heart, pericardium, diaphragm and anterior abdominal wall. Complete sternal fissure results in ectopia cordis where the heart has no covering and sits on the chest.

Surgical repair for superior sternal clefts is easy but so difficult for inferior sternal clefts with other deformities. For the cases who suffer from completely sternal clefts with ectopia cordis, not only repairing difficult but also lower survival rate because of the chest is too small and can not accommodate the heart, therefore, closure of chest is impossible without causing heart failure.

Chapter 4

Poland's Syndrome

The condition was described by Alfred Poland and may include absence of some or all of the following: absent ribs, pectoralis major, pectoralis minor, serratus anterior, rectus abdominis and latissimus dorsi muscles. The breast may be absent (amastia) and there may be nipple deformities in male or female. There may be associated limb deformities (syndactyly, brachydactyly), absent axillary hair and limited subcutaneous fat.

The condition is usually unilateral and most common at left side. Its etiology is unknown. Surgical intervention is only required if the rib defect is large enough to cause a lung hernia or there are concerns regarding injury to the heart or lungs. Adolescent girls with amastia require breast reconstruction.

Chapter 5

Thoracic Insufficiency Syndrome Associated with Diffuse Skeletal Disorders

The thoracic insufficiency syndrome may be defined as any disorder that produces respiratory failure and prevents normal lung development. It includes both congenital and acquired disorders such as asphyxiating thoracic dystrophy(Jeune's syndrome), acquired asphyxiating osteochondrodystrophy(the result of damage to the growth centers by too early and extensive open pectus repair), spondylothoracic dysplasia(Jarcho-Levin syndrome), congenital scoliosis with multiple vertebral anomalies and fused or absent ribs(jumbled spine) and severe kyphoscoliosis as a result of severe cerebral palsy or spina bifida. These conditions are fortunately rare but repair requires complex surgical techniques if the patients exhibit respiratory insufficiency.

Part 24

External Hernia

Chapter 1

Introduction

Any organ or tissue that leave the original position, which pass through normal(or abnormal)weak(or defect)point, holes in the body and get into the other part is called hernia. An external hernia is an abnormal protrusion of intra abdominal tissue through a fascial defect in the musculoaponeurotic covering abdominal wall. About 75% of hernia occurs in the groin. Incisinal hernia comprise about 10%; umbilical about 3%; and others about 3%.

1.1 Etiology

(1)Decrease the strength of abdominal wall.

Canals where tissue pass through: inguinal canal, femoral canal, umbilical ring, etc.

Mal developed linea Alba.

Problem in healing of the abdominal incision.

(2)Increase in the intra abdominal pressure: chronic cough, constipation, enlargement of prostagland, ascites, etc.

1.2 Pathological anatomy

A hernial mass is composed of the hernia orifice, the hernia sac, covering tissues, and any contained viscera.

(1)Hernia orifice: This is composed of the layers of the abdominal wall where a hernia protruded through: The hernia is classified on the basis of the location of the orifice, for example, the inguinal hernia, the femoral hernia.

(2)Hernia sac: This covers the hernia and its size depends on the size of the hernia. Generally the covering consists of glistening peritoneum. Topographically, it may be divided into a neck, a body, and a fundus.

(3)Hernia contents: These may include any one or more of the abdominal organs. The most common ones are the omentum and the small bowel.

(4) Hernia covering: These are the layers of tissues covering the hernia sac. In an inguinal hernia the covering consists of four layers: peritoneum with properitoneal fat, transversal or cremasteric fascia, superficial perineal fascia, and skin.

1.3　Clinical Types

There is reducible hernia, nonreducible hernia, incarcerated hernia, etc.

(1) Reducible hernia: There is free mobility of the hernia contents through the hernia ring by spontaneously or with manual pressure.

(2) Nonreducible hernia: The hernia contents are fixed to the hernia ring. They may be nonreducible through incarceration, through adhesion to the hernia sac.

(3) Incarcerated hernias: The hernia contents can not be returned to the abdomen, usually because they are trapped by a narrow neck.

(4) Strangulated hernias: The contents of the sac become stuck through the hernia orifice and the blood supply is cut off so the bowel becomes ischemic. Patients have symptoms of small bowel obstruction and the hernia is tender inflammed swelling.

(5) Richter hernias: An uncommon type of hernia occurs when a part of the circumference of the bowel becomes incarcerated or strangulated in the fascial defect.

(6) Sliding hernia: A sliding hernia is a type of indirect inguinal hernia in which the wall of a viscus forms a portion of the wall of the hernia sac.

Chapter 2

Hernias of the Groin

2.1 The Inguinal Region

All hernias of the abdominal wall consists of a peritoneal sac that protrudes a weakness or defect in the muscular layers of the abdomen. The defect may be congenial or acquired.

Just outside of the peritoneum is the transversalis fascia whose weakness of defect is the major source of groin hernia. Next are found the transverses abdominis muscle, internal oblique muscle, and external oblique muscle, which are fleshy laterally and aponeurotic medially. Their aponeuroses forms investing layers of the strong rectus abdominis muscles above the semilunar line. Below this line, the aponeuroses lies entirely in front of the muscle. Between the two vertical rectus muscles, the aponeuroses meet again to form the linea alba, which is well defined only above the umbilicus. The subcutaneous layer contains Scarpa's fascia and Camper's fascia.

2.1.1 External oblique aponeurosis

The aponeurosis of external oblique muscle together with the aponeurosis of the internal oblique and transversus abdomonis, form the rectus sheath, finally, the linea alba. The aponeurosis serve as the superficial border of the inguinal canal and reflects posteriorly to form the inguinal ligament. The inguinal ligament extends from the anterior superior iliac spine to the public tubercle.

2.1.2 Internal oblique muscle

The internal oblique muscle serves as the superior(or cephalad) border of the inguinal canal. The aponeurosis of the internal oblique muscle fuses with the fibers from the aponeurosis of the transversus abdomonis near the pubic tubercle to form the conjoined tendon.

2.1.3 Transversalis fascia

The transversus abdominis muscle arises from the lateral portion of the iliopubic tract, the iliac crest, the lumbodorsal fascia, and the inner surface of the cartilage of the lower six ribs. The lower free margin of this muscle arches with the internal oblique muscle over the internal inguinal ring to form the transversus abdominis aponeurosis arch.

2.1.4   Iliopubic tract

The iliopubic tract is a fibrous condensation of endoabdominal fascia that arise from the iliopectineal arch and inserts on the anterior superior iliac spine and inner lip of the wing of ilium. The iliopubic tract is located posterior of the inguinal ligament. This structure arches over the femoral vessels, composing a portion of the femoral sheath. The iliopubic tract is located at the inferior border of the internal (deep) inguinal ring. The iliopubic insertion is along the superior border of the pubic ramus and pubic tubercle and Cooper's ligament.

2.1.5   Cooper's ligament

Cooper's ligament is a strong, fibrous band that extends laterally for about 2.5 cm along the iliopectineal pubic ramus, starting at the lateral base of the lacunar ligament.

2.2   Inguinal Canal

The adult inguinal canal is approximately 4 cm in length and is located 2−4 cm cephalad to the inguinal ligament. The inguinal canal contains either the spermatic cord or the round ligament of the uterus.

Superior wall(roof) : Medial crus of aponeurosis of external oblique, musculoaponeurotic arches of internal oblique and transverse abdominal, transversalis fascia.

Anterior wall: aponeurosis of external oblique, fleshy part of internal oblique(lateral third of canal only) , superficial inguinal ring(medial third of canal only).

Posterior wall: transversalis fascia, conjoint tendon (inguinal falx, reflected part of inguinal ligament, medial third of canal only) , deep inguinal ring(lateral third of canal only).

Inferior wall(floor) : inguinal ligament, lacunar ligament(medial third of canal only) , iliopubic tract (lateral third of canal only).

2.3   Hesselbach's Triangle

The inferior epigastric vessels serves as the superolateral border of Hesselbach's triangle. The medial border of the triangle is formed by the rectus shealth, and the inguinal ligament serves as its inferior border. A weakness of defect in the transversalis fascia, which forms the floor of this triangle, results in a direct inguinal hernia.

2.4   Femoral Canal

A femoral hernia passes beneath the inguinal ligament into the upper thigh. The predisposing anatomic feature for femoral hernias is a small empty between the lacunar ligament medially and the femoral vein laterally the femoral canal. Because its borders are distinct and unyielding, a femoral hernia has the highest risk of incarceration and strangulation.

Chapter 3

Clinical Manifestation and Diagnosis

3.1 Symptom

Most hernias produce no symptoms until the patient notice a lump or swelling in the groin, though some patients may describe a swelling, knot, or bulge in the groin appearing after physical labor or during athletics, coughing, straining, or lifting heavy weights. Frequently, hernias are detected in the course of routine physical examination. Some patients complained of a dragging sensation and, particular with indirect inguinal hernia, radiation pain into the scrotum. As a hernia enlarges, it is likely to produce a sense of discomfort or aching pain, and the patient must lie down to reduce the hernia. In most cases the swelling spontaneously regresses during rest. Persistence and simultaneous incarceration are rarely presenting symptoms. In the uncomplicated hernia spontaneous pain is rare; a feeling of a foreign body is more common. Continuing pain and tenderness in the swelling, together with nausea and vomiting, are suggestive of an incarcerated hernia. If the hernia can be reduced easily and is only minimally tender, yet with considerable pain in the area and some systemic reaction, consideration must be given to some other disease entity, such as a dissecting aortic aneurysm, a mesenteric infarction, a ruptured invertebral disc, or ureteral colic. The clinical picture, as described, may rarely represent a retrograde incarceration. For the differential diagnosis, such items as the trigger mechanism of the hernia, the temporal relationship of the symptoms, and the onset of pain are important. The appearance of a hernia is most frequently activity dependent, but other diseases, lipomas, or lymph node metastases are independent of physical activity. Direct inguinal hernias produce fewer symptoms than indirect inguinal hernias and are less likely to become incarcerated or strangulated.

Femoral hernias are notoriously asymptomatic until incarceration or strangulation occurs. Even with obstruction or strangulation, the patient may feel discomfort more in the abdomen than in the femoral area. Thus, colicky abdominal pain and signs of intestinal obstruction frequently are the presenting manifestations of a strangulated femoral hernia, without discomfort, pain, or tenderness in the femoral region.

3.2　Signs

Examination of the groin reveals a mass that may or may not be reducible. The patient should be examined in both supine and standing and also with coughing and straining, since small hernias may be difficult to demonstrate. The external ring can be identified by invaginating the scrotum and palpating with the index finger just above and lateral to the pubic tubercle. If the external ring is very small, the examiner's finger may not enter the inguinal canal, and it may be difficult to be sure that a pulsation felt on coughing is truly a hernia. At the other extreme, a widely patent external ring does not by itself constitute hernia. Tissue must be felt protruding into the inguinal canal during coughing in order for a hernia to be diagnosed.

Differentiating between direct and indirect inguinal hernia on examination is difficult and is of little importance since most groin hernias should be repaired regardless of type. Nevertheless, each type of inguinal hernia has specific features more common to it. A hernia that descends into the scrotum is almost certainly indirect. On inspection with the patient straining, a direct hernia more commonly appears as a symmetric, circular swelling at the external ring; the swelling disappears when the patient lies down. An indirect hernia appear as an elliptic swelling that may not reduce easily.

On palpation, the posterior wall of the inguinal canal is firm and resistant in an indirect hernia but relaxed or absent in a direct hernia. If the patient is asked to cough or strain while the examining finger is directed laterally and upward into the inguinal canal, a direct hernia protrudes against the side of the finger, whereas an indirect hernia is felt at the tip of the finger.

Compression over the inguinal ring when the patient strains may also help to differentiate between indirect and direct hernias. A direct hernia bulges forward through Hesselbach's triangle, but the opposite hand can maintain reduction of an indirect hernia at the internal ring.

These distinctions are obscured as a hernia enlarges and distorts the anatomic relationships of the inguinal rings and canal. In most patients the type of inguinal hernia cannot be established accurately before surgery.

A femoral hernia may present in a variety of ways. If it is small and uncomplicated, it usually appears as a small bulge in the upper medial thigh just below the level of the inguinal ligament. Because it may be detected anteriorly through the fossa ovalis femoris to present as a visible or palpable mass at above the inguinal ligament, it can be confused with an inguinal hernia.

3.3　Differential Diagnosis

Groin pain of musculoskeletal or obscure origin may be difficult to distinguish from hernia. The following local differential diagnoses are the most important ones.

(1) Lymphadenitis

Usually mistaken for an inguinal hernia. Hard lymph nodes, barely movable, without change in position and size with coughing or straining. The infectious focus can occasionally be found in the lower extremity. If there is a doubtful choice between an incarcerated femoral hernia and a lymph node, attempts at forcible reduction should be avoided and the diagnosis should be made surgically.

（2）Lipoma

Soft, does not move with coughing. Frequently of considerable size. Usually in the fossa ovalis, an important differential diagnostic consideration in femoral hernia.

（3）Varicose nodules of the saphenous vein

Common in generalized varicose disease of the lower extremity. Soft, easily movable posteriorly. No connection to the femoral canal can be demonstrated painless swelling in the inguinal area, feels like a water balloon. Superior and inferior margins are usually easily palpable. Pinkly translucent on transillumination.

（4）Tumors

Slowly progressive growth, mostly indolent, hard, nonmovable.

（5）Abscesses

Abscesses in Crohn's disease, lumbar vertebral tuberculosis, and septic urogenital diseases can enter the inguinal region along the psoas grove and appear here as a swelling.

3.4   Treatment

Inguinal hernia should be always surgically repaired following diagnosis by physical examination unless there are specific contraindications. A terminally ill, immunosuppressed, or extremely old patient may fall into the category those who should be followed without operation correction. The same advice applies to patients of all ages; the complication of incarceration, obstruction, and strangulation are greater threats than are the risk of operation. The nature history of groin hernia is one of progressive enlargement and weakening, with the potential for incarceration and obstruction of the intestine and subsequent compromise of the vascular supply to the bowel, leading to intestinal infarction. Hernia do not resolve spontaneously or improve with time.

（1）High ligation of the indirect hernia sac

A curvilinear incision approximately 2 finger breadths above the inguinal ligament. Dissection is carried through the subcutaneous tissues and the external oblique fascia is incised. Care should be taken to avoid injuring the ilioinguinal and iliohypogastric nerves. The spermatic cord is mobilized. The cremasteric muscle fibers are divided. The hernia sac is carefully dissected free from the adjacent cord structure and cleared to the level of internal inguinal ring. The hernia sac is opened and examined for visceral contents. The neck of the sac is suture ligated at the level of the internal ring, and excess sac is excised.

（2）Bassini repair

Used for indirect hernia, small direct hernia. The conjoined tendon is sutured to inguinal ligament.

（3）Halsted repair

The conjoined tendon is sutured to inguinal ligament. Transplant the spermatic cord external to the external oblique fascia.

（4）McVay repair

Used for large indirect hernia, direct hernia, recurrent hernia and femoral hernia. The conjoined tendon is sutured to Cooper's ligament from the pubic tubercle laterally to the femoral canal.

（5）Shouldice repair

A multiplayer, imbricated repair of the floor of the inguinal canal with running sutures. The transversalis fascia is incised from the internal inguinal ring to the level of the pubic tubercle. The lateral cut edge of the transversalis fascia is sutured medially to the undersurface of the internal oblique muscle. Imbrication of the tissue layers is continued by suturing the medial cut edge to the inguinal ligament. The conjoined tendon is sutured to the inguinal ligament.

(6) Lichtenstein(tension free) repair

A marlex mesh is sutured to the aponeurotic tissue overlying the pubic bone, with a continuation of this suture along the shelving edge of the inguinal ligament to a point lateral to the internal inguinal ring. The lateral edge of mesh is split to allow passage of the spermatic cord between the split limbs of the mesh. The cephalad edge of the mesh is sutured to the conjoined tendon, with the internal oblique edge overlapped by approximately 2 cm. The two tails of the lateral aspect of the mesh are sutured together, incorporating the shelving margin of the inguinal ligament just lateral to the completion knot of the lower suture.

(7) Laparoscopic hernia repair

Transabdominal properitoneal repair(TAPP).

Totally extraperitoneal approach(TEP).

Chapter 4

Other Types of Hernias

4.1　Epigastric Hernia

An epigastric hernia protrudes through the linea alba above the level of the umbilicus. The hernia may develop through one of the foramens of egress of the small paramidline nerves and vessels or through an area of congenital weakness in the linea alba.

4.1.1　Clinical findings

(1) symptoms

Most epigastric hernias are painless and are found on routine abdominal examination. If symptomatic, their presentation ranges from mild epigastric pain and tenderness to deep, burning epigastric pain with radiation to the back or the lower abdominal quadrants. The pain may be accompanied by abdominal bloating, nausea, or vomiting. The symptoms often occur after a large meal and on occasion may be relieved by reclining, probably because the supine position causes the herniated mass to drop away from the anterior abdominal wall.

(2) signs

If a mass is palpable, the diagnosis can often be confirmed by any maneuver that will increase introabdominal pressure and thereby cause the mass to bulge anteriorly. The diagnosis is difficulty to make when the patient is obese, since a mass is hard to palpate; ultrasound or computed tomography may be needed in the very obese patient.

4.1.2　Differential diagnosis

Differential diagnosis includes peptic ulcer, gallbladder disease, hiatal hernia, pancreatitis, and upper small bowel obstruction.

4.1.3　Treatment

Most epigastric hernias should be repaired. The defect can usually be closed primarily.

4.2　Incisional Hernia

About 10% of abdominal operation result in incisional hernias. The incidence of this iatrogenic type of hernia is not diminishing in spite of an awareness of the many causative factors.

(1) Etiology

The following factors are responsible for incisional hernias: poor surgical technique; postoperative wound infection; ages; general debility as in cirrhosis, carcinoma, etc; obesity; postoperative pulmonary complications; and placement of drains or stromas in the primary operative wound.

(2) Treatment

Incisional hernia should be treated by early repair. Small hernias require only a direct fascia to fascia repair for closure. Repair of large or recurrent defects is performed using nonabsorbable mesh.

Part 25

Acute Suppurative Peritonitis

Peritonitis is inflammation of the peritoneum, It can be septic or aseptic, bacterial or viral, primary or secondary, and acute or chronic. Most surgical peritonitis is secondary to bacterial contamination from the gastrointestinal tract. Usually there is an underlying pathologic process or injury to the gut and this form of peritonitis is discussed here.

Chapter 1

Anatomy and Physiology

The peritoneal cavity is a potential space containing the abdominal viscera. It develops from the primitive coelom, which is formed by a splitting of the lateral mesoderm into somatic and splanchnic layers. Originally there are two bilateral cavities separated by the developing gastronintetinal tract. The somatic mesoderm lines the body wall portion of the coelom, and the splanchnic mesoderm covers the intestine. As the embryonic body wall closes ventrally, the two coelomic cavities fuse together in the midline. In between, the developing gut is covered on both side by splanchnic mesoderm. That portion of this double layer of mesoderm from which the gut is suspended is called the mesentery. As the ventral mesentery of the intestine is resorbed, the two coelomic cavities join to become one.

The primary functions of the peritoneum have been derived by teleologic reasoning. The peritoneum does provide a frictionless surface over which the abdominal viscera can freely move, and the mesothelial lining secretes fluid that serves to lubricate the peritoneal surfaces. Normally, about 100 mL. of clear, straw colored fluid is present in the peritoneal cavity of the adult. The quality and quantity of this fluid may change with various pathologic conditions.

When required to do so, the peritoneum serves as a bi-directional dialysis membrane through which water and solutes may move. Such movement is controlled largely by the osmolar gradient. This ability of the peritoneum to absorb substances is the basis for both experimental and clinical administration of fluid, electrolytes, and blood. Isotonic saline administered intraperitoneally is absorbed at a rate of 30-35 mL. per hour after an initial equilibration phase. However, if a hypertonic fluid is used, there is a large shift of water (up to 300 to 500 mL per hour) from the intravascular space into the peritoneal cavity, which can result in hypotension and shock. Studies in humans and animals show that intraperitoneal blood is absorbed at a slower rate, but approximately 70% eventually enters the bloodstream. This absorption occurs primarily through fenestrated lymphatic channels on the undersurface of the diaphragm. Such red blood cells have a normal survival time in the circulation. Air and gases are also similarly absorbed. Air that enters the peritoneal cavity during laparotomy is present in diminishing amounts for 4-5 days.

Peritoneal dialysis is possible because of bidirectional transport across the peritoneal membrane. By adjusting that composition of the dialysate, excess water, sodium, potassium, and products of metabolism can be removed from the bloodstream. In addition, a variety of drugs can be removed with peritoneal dialysis.

Chapter 2

Diseases and Disorders of the Peritoneum

2.1 Acute Diffuse Peritonitis

Peritonitis is an inflammatory or suppurative response of the peritoneal lining to direct irritation. Peritonitis can occur after perforating, inflammatory, infectious, or ischemic injuries of the gastrointestinal or genitourinary system and without a documented source of contamination.

2.2 Cause and Pathophysiology

2.2.1 Primary peritonitis

Primary peritonitis refers to inflammation of the peritoneal cavity without a documented source of contamination. It occurs more commonly in children than in adults and in women more than in men. This latter distribution is thought to be explained by entry of organisms into the peritoneal cavity through the fallopion tubes. In children, incidence peaks in the neonatal period and again, at age 4–5 years. The patients present with an acutely tender abdomen fever, and leukocytosis. There may be a history of antecedent ear or upper respiratory tract infection. It is often difficult in this situation to differentiate between primary and secondary peritonitis, and the diagnosis ultimately may be made at laparotomy. However, children with nephrotic syndrome and, less commonly, systemic lupus erythematosus are particularly susceptible to primary peritonitis. The bacteria in these cases are usually either hemolytic streptococci or pneumococci. A diagnosis can be made by peritoneal aspiration and Gram stain after excluding pneumonia and urinary tract infection. Adults with ascites from liver disease have an increased incidence of primary peritonitis. In recent years, the bacterial flora has changed from gram positive to gram negative organisms. Thus, the distinction between primary and secondary peritonitis is more difficult to make by peritoneal aspirate alone.

2.2.2 Secondary peritonitis

Secondary peritonitis results from bacterial contamination originating from within viscera or from external sources(e. g. ,penetrating injury). It most often follows disruption of a hollow viscus. Extravasated bile and urine,although only mildly irritating when sterile,are markedly toxic if infected and provoke a vigorous peritoneal reaction. Gastric juice from a perforated duodenal ulcer remains mostly sterile for several hours, during which time it produces a chemical peritonitis with large fluid losses; but if left untreated,it evolves within 6–12 hours into bacterial peritonitis. Intraperitoneal fluid dilutes opsonic proteins and impairs phagocytosis. Furthermore,when hemoglobin is present in the peritoneal cavity,Escherichia coli growing within the cavity can elaborate leukotoxins that reduce bactericidal activity. Limited,localized infection can be eradicated by host defenses,but continued contamination invariably leads to generalized peritonitis and eventually to septicemia with multiple organ failure.

Factors that influence the severity of peritonitis include the type of bacterial contamination,the nature of the initial injury,and the host's nutritional and immune status. The grade of peritonitis varies with the cause. Clean(e. g. ,proximal gut perorations) or well localized(e. g. ,ruptured appendix) contaminations progress to fulminant peritonitis relatively slowly(e. g. ,12–24 hours). In contrast,bacteria associated with distal gut or infected biliary tract perforations quickly overwhelm host peritoneal defenses. This degree of toxicity is also characteristic of postoperative peritonitis due to anastomotic leakage or contamination. Conditions that ordinarily cause mild peritonitis may produce life threatening sepsis in a compromised host.

2.2.3　Causative organisms

Systemic sepsis due to peritonitis occurs in varying degrees depending on the virulence of the pathogens,the bacterial load,and the duration of the bacterial proliferation and synergistic interaction. Except for spontaneous bacterial peritonitis,peritonitis is almost invariably polymicrobial; cultures usually contain more than one aerobic and more than two anaerobic species. The microbial picture reflects the bacterial flora of the involved organ. As long as gastric acid secretion and gastric emptying are normal,perforations of the proximal bowel are normal,perforations of the proximal bowel(stomach or duodenum) are generally sterile or associated with relatively small numbers of gram positive organism. Perforation or ischemic injuries of the distal small bowel(e. g. ,strangulated hernia) lead to infection with aerobic bacteria in about 30% of cases and anaerobic organisms in about 10 of cases. Fecal spillage,with a bacterial load of 1012 or more organisms per gram,is extremely toxic. Positive cultures with gram negative anaerobic bacteria are characteristic of infections originating from the appendix,colon,and rectum. The predominant aerobic pathogens include the gram negative bacteria E. coli,streptococci,proteus,and the Enterobacter Klebsiella groups. Besides bacteroides fragilis,anaerobic cocci and clostridia are the prevalent anaerobic organisms. Synergism between fecal anaerobic and aerobic bacteria increases the severity of infections.

2.2.4　Clinical Manifestations

2.2.4.1　Symptoms and signs

The clinical manifestations of peritonitis reflect the severity and duration of infection of and the age and general health of the patient. Physical findings can be divided into abdominal signs arising from the initial injury and manifestations of systemic infection. Acute peritonitis frequently presents as acute abdomen. Local findings include abdominal pain,tenderness,guarding or rigidity,distention,free peritoneal air,and diminished bowel sounds signs that reflect parietal peritoneal irritation and resulting ileus. The most common symptom is pain which may be either localized or diffuse and is usually constant and of a sharp pricking character. A visceral perforation causes a severe pain of sudden onset which is usually first appreciated in the area of perforation,and upper epigastric in the case of a duodenal ulcer. Shoulder tip pain is present if the diaphragmatic peritoneum is inflamed. The pain may later become more generalized as the infection spreads. Intermittent abdominal pain may precede established peritonitis in appendicitis or strangulating obstruction. The pain often follows a period of malaise and is accompanied by anorexia, nausea and vomiting. There is usually associated constipation unless a pelvic abscess develops which can cause diarrhoea. The patient lies relatively motionless and supine with shallow respiratory excursions. The abdomen becomes increasingly rigid and board like as peritonitis develops. The knees are sometimes flexed and drawn up, reducing tension in the abdominal wall and relieving pain. Palpation of the abdomen increases the pain and should be undertaken gently when assessing abdominal guarding and rigidity which are initially voluntary and subsequently become involuntary reflexes. The site of maximum tenderness is usually related to the site of the pathology. The increasing ileus is confirmed by auscultation of the bowel sounds which diminish and finally disappear. In diffuse peritonitis the whole abdominal wall is rigid, wooden and no longer moves on respiration. The rigidity gradually resolves, if localization occurs, and a mass or abscess may become palpable through the slackening abdominal wall. If the peritonitis remains diffuse, distension and dehydration continue and end in circulatory failure, coma and death. Systemic findings include fever, chills or rigors, tachycardia, sweating, tachypnea, restlessness, dehydration, oliguria, disorientation, and, ultimately, refractory shock. Shock is due to the combined effects of hypovolemia and septicemia with multiple organ dysfunction. Recurrent unexplained shock is highly predictive of serious intraperitoneal sepsis.

The findings in abdominal sepsis are modified by the patient age and general health. Physical signs of peritonitis are subtle or difficult to interpret in either very young or very old patients or in those who are chronically debilitated, immunosuppressed, receiving corticosteroids, or recently postoperative. Diagnostic peritoneal lavage maybe employed in equivocal cases in senile or confused patients. There are virtually no false positive and only minimal false negative errors. Delayed recognition is a major cause of the high mortality rate of peritonitis.

2.2.4.2　Laboratory findings

Laboratory studies gaugethe severity of peritonitis and guide therapy. Blood studies should include a complete blood cell count. Cross matching, arterial blood gases, a blood clotting profile, and liver and renal function tests. Samples for culture of blood, urine, sputum, and peritoneal fluid should be taken before antibiotics are started. A positive blood culture is usually present in toxic patients. The demonstration of gas under the diaphragm on an erect or lateral decubitus abdominal radiograph confirms the diagnosis of perforated viscus. A serum amylase excludes acute pancreatitis as the cause of peritonitis. Peritoneal tap and lavage are occasionally useful in doubtful cases to differentiate peritonitis from other conditions. Ultrasound and computerized tomography scanning may demonstrate free peritoneal fluid, but are rarely helpful in diagnosis.

2.2.4.3　Diagnosis and differential diagnosis

The history and physical examination(leukocyte count, plain radiographs of abdomen ultrasound and computerized tomography)usually are sufficient to make the diagnosis, and no further testing is necessary.

Specific kinds of infective(e. g. , gonococcal, amebic, candidal) and noninfective peritonitis may be seen. In the elderly, systemic diseases(e. g. , pneumonia, uremia) may produce intestinal ileus so striking that it resembles bowel obstruction or peritonitis.

Familial Mediterranean fever(periodic peritonitis, familial paroxysmal polyserositis)is a rare genetically transmitted cause of acute peritonitis that primarily affects individuals southern and eastern Mediterranean genetic background. Its cause is unknown, but enzymatic defects in catecholamine metabolism and a deficiency of C5 a inhibitor in synovial fluid have been postulated. Recurring bouts of abdominal pain with direct and rebound tenderness occur along with pleuritic or joint pains. Fever and leukocytosis accompany the attacks. Renal amyloidosis is a late and serious complication.

Colchicine(1-1.5 mg daily)effective in preventing but not treating acute attacks can be used as a diagnostic test. Intravenous metaraminol infusion(10 mg)is a safe and specific provocative test that precipitates abdominal pain within 2 days in afflicted patients.

Laparotomy is often performed during the initial episodes. The peritoneal surfaces may be inflamed and there may be free fluid, but smears and cultures of peritoneal fluid are negative. Even though it may appear normal, the appendix should be removed to exclude appendicitis from the differential diagnosis in subsequent attacks. Late illness results from amyloidosis and renal failure, complications that also appear to be preventable by long term colchicines therapy.

2.2.4.4   Treatment

Fluid and electrolyte replacement, operative control of sepsis, and systemic antibioticsare the mainstays of treatment of peritonitis.

(1)Preoperative Care

1)Intravenous fluids: The massive transfer of fluid into the peritoneal cavity must be replaced by an appropriate amount of intravenous fluid. If systemic toxicity is evident or if the patient is old or in fragile health. A central venous pressure(or pulmonary artery wedge pressure)line and bladder catheter should be inserted: a fluid balance chart should be kept; and serial body weight measurements should be taken to monitor fluid requirements. Several liters of balanced salt or lactated Ringer's solution may be required to correct hypovolemia. Intravenous infusions must be given rapidly enough to restore blood pressure and urine output promptly to satisfactory level. Potassium supplements are withheld until tissue and renal perfusion are adequate. Blood is reserved for anemic patients or those with concomitant bleeding.

2)Care for advanced septicemia: Cardiovascular agents and mechanical ventilation in anintensive care unit are essential in patients with advanced septicemia.

An arterial line for continuous blood pressure recording and blood sampling is helpful. Cardiac monitoring with a Swan Ganz catheter is essential if inotropic drugs are used.

3)Antibiotics: Loading doses of intravenous antibiotics directed against the anticipated bacterial pathogens should be given after fluid samples have been obtained for culture. Initial regimens include cephalosporins or imipenem cilastatin for gram negative coliforms, ampicillin for enterococci, and metronidazole or clindamycin for anaerobic organisms. The empirically chosen antibiotic regimen should be modified after results of culture and sensitivity studies are available. Because renal impairment is often a feature of peritonitis, serum levels of potentially nephrotoxic agents(especially aminoglycosides)should be checked regularly. Antibiotics should be continued until the patient has remained afebrile with a normal white blood cell count (WBC) and a differential count of less than 3% bands.

4)Other measures: Other therapeutic measures are of secondary importance or of equivocal value. Pharmacologic doses of methylprednisolone have not been shown to be of value in controlled trials and would rarely be appropriate in light of their detrimental effects on the immune system. The experimental use of fibronectin and immune stimulating drugs(e. g. , glucan, muramyl dipeptide) or polyvalent immunoglobulins to counter sepsis related immunosuppression may soon find clinical application.

(2)Opreative management

1)Control of sepsis: The objectives of surgery for peritonitis are to remove all infected material, correct the underlying cause, and prevent late complications. Except in early, localized peritonitis, a midline incision offers the best surgical exposure. Materials for aerobic and anaerobic cultures of fluid and infected tissue are obtained immediately after the abdomen is opened. Occult pockets of infection are located by thorough exploration, and contaminated or necrotic material is removed. Routine radical debridement of all peritoneal and serosal surfaces dose not increase survival rates. The primary disease is then treated. This may require resection(e. g. , ruptured appendix or gallbladder), repair(e. g. , perforated ulcer), or drainage(e. g. , acute pancreatitis). Attempts to reanastomose resected bowel in the presence of extensive sepsis or intestinal ischemia often lead to leakage. Temporary stomas are safer, and these can be taken down several weeks later after the patient has recovered from the acute illness.

2)Peritoneal lavage: In diffuse peritonitis, lavage with copious amounts(>3 L) of warm isotonic crystalloid solution removes gross particulate matter as well as blood and fibrin clots and dilutes residual bacteria. Fears that this maneuver might spread infection to uncontaminates areas have proved to be unfounded. The addition of antiseptics or antibiotics to the irrigating solution is generally useless(e. g. , noxythiolin) or even harmful because of induced adhesions(e. g. , tetracycline, povidone induced). Antibiotics given parenterally will reath bactericidal levels in peritoneal fluid and may afford on additional benefit when given by lavage. Furthermore, lavage with aminoglycosides can produce respiratory depression and complicate anesthesia because of the neuromuscular blocking action of this group of drugs. After lavage is completed, all fluid in the peritoneal cavity must be aspirated because it may hamper local defense mechanisms by diluting opsonins and removing surfaces upon which phagocytes destroy bacteria.

Continuous peritoneal lavage for up to 3 days postoperatively with a balanced crystalloid or antibiotic containing solution is recommended by some groups. The solution is infused hourly through soft sump drains placed in the right suprahepatic and left paracolic gutters, and the effluent is collected via sump drains in the pelvic cul de sac. This method requires careful postoperative monitoring of the fluid and electrolyte status and attention to the irrigating system. Heparin may be added to reduce intraperitoneal fibrin clot formation. Postoperative lavage is unnecessary in perforated appendicitis and should be considered only in severe peritonitis associated with systemic sepsis.

3)Peritoneal drainage: Drainage of the free peritoneal cavity is ineffective and often undesirable. As foreign bodies, drains are quickly isolated from the rest of the peritoneal cavity. But they still provide a channel for exogenous contamination. Prophylactic drainage in diffuse peritonitis does not prevent abscess formation and may even predispose to abscesses or fistulas. Drainage is useful chiefly for residual focal infection or when continued contamination is present or likely to occur(e. g. , fistula). Drains are indicated for localized inflammatory masses that can not be resected or for cavities that can not be obliterated. Soft sump drains with continuous suction through multiple side perforations are effective for large volumes of fluid. Smaller volumes of fluid are best handled with closed drainage systems(e. g. , Jackson−Pratt drains). Large cavities with thick walls may be drained better by several large Penrose drains placed in a dependent position.

To achieve more effective peritoneal drainage in severe peritonitis, some surgeons have left the entire abdominal wound open to widely expose the peritoneal cavity. Besides requiring intensive nursing and medical support to cope with massive protein and fluid losses(averaging 9 L the first day), there are serious complications such as spontaneous fistulization, wound sepsis, and large incisional hernias.

An alternative method is to reexplore the abdomen every 1−3 days until all loculations have been adequately drained. The wound may be closed temporarily with a sheet of polypropylene(Marlex) mesh that contains a nylon zipper or Velcro to avoid a tight abdominal closure and to facilitate repeated opening and closing. Exploration may even be performed in the intensive care unit without general anesthesia. Available data suggest that this method should be restricted to selected patients with long standing (more than 48 hours)extensive intraperitoneal sepsis associated with multiple organ failure(high sepsis scores). The mortality rate still is about 30% in these critically septic patients.

4) Management of abdominal distention: Abdominal distention caused by ileus frequently accompanies peritonitis, and decompression of the intestine is often useful to facilitate abdominal closure and minimize postoperative respiratory problems. This is best accomplished by nasal passage of a long intestinal tube(e. g. , Baker or Dennis tube) to avoid an enterotomy and to act as a sutureless intestinal stent. A gastrostomy may be advantageous if prolonged nasogastric decompression is expected, especially in elderly patients or those with chronic respiratory disease. A feeding jejunostomy is indicated whenever prolonged nutritional support is anticipated.

(3) Postoperative care

Fluid, nutritional, and other supportive measures are continued postoperatively. Antibiotics are given for 10–14 days, depending on the severity of peritonitis. A favorable clinical response is evidenced by well sustained perfusion with good urine output, reduction in fever and leukocytosis, resolution of ileus, and a returning sense of well being. The rate of recovery varies with the duration and degree of peritonitis.

Postoperative complications can be divided into local and systemic problems. Residual abscesses and intraperitoneal sepsis. Deep wound infections, anastomotic breakdown, and fistula formation require reexploration or percutaneous drainage. Progressive or uncontrolled sepsis leads to multiple organ failure affecting the respiratory, renal, hepatic, clotting, and immune systems. Supportive measures, including mechanical ventilation, transfusion, total parenteral nutrition, and hemodialysis, are ineffectual unless primary septic foci are eliminated by combined surgical and antibiotic therapy.

2.2.5 Prognosis

The overall mortality rate of generalized peritonitis is about 40%. Factors contributing to a high mortality rate include the type of primary disease and its duration, associated multiple organ failure before treatment, and the age and general health of the patient. Mortality rates are consistently below 10% in patents with perforated ulcers or appendicitis; in young patients; in those having less extensive bacterial contamination; and in those diagnosed and operated upon early. Patients with distal small bowel or colonic perforations or postoperative sepsis tend to be older, to have concurrent medical illnesses and greater bacterial contamination, and to have a greater propensity to renal and respiratory failure; their mortality rates are about 50%.

Chapter 3

Intra−abdominal Abscesses

3.1 Pathophysiology

An intra−abdominal abscess is a collection of infection fluid within the abdominal cavity. Currently, gastrointestinal perforations, operative complications, penetrating trauma, and genitourinary infections are the most common causes. An abscess forms by one of two modes: ① adjacent to a diseased viscus(e. g. , with perforated appendix or diverticulitis) or; ② as a result of external contamination(e. g. , postoperative subphrenic abscess). In 1/3 of cases, the abscess occurs as a sequela generalized peritonitis. Interloop and pelvic abscess form if extravasated fluid gravitating into a dependent or localized area becomes secondarily infected.

Bacteria laden fibrin and blood clots and neutrophils contribute to the formation of an abscess. The pathogenic organisms arorganismse similar to those responsible fir peritonitis, but anaerobic occupy an important role. Lowering of the redox potential by E. coli is conductive to Bacteroides proliferation.

3.2 Sites of Abscesses

The areas in which abscesses commonly occur are defined by the configuration of the peritoneal cavity with its dependent lateral and pelvic basins. Together with the natural divisions created by the transverse mesocolon and the small bowel mesentery. The supracolic compartment, located above the transverse mesocolon, broadly defines the subphrenic transverse spaces. Within this area, the subdiaphragmatic(suprahepatic) and subhepatic areas of the subphrenic space may be distinguished. The subdiaphragmatic space on each side occupies the concavity between the hemidiaphragms and the domes of the hepatic lobes. The inferior limits of its posterior recess are the attachments of the coronary and triangular ligaments on the dorsal, not superior, aspect of the diaphragm. Anteriorly, the lower limits are defined on the right by the transverse colon and on the left by the anterior stomach surface. Omentum, transverse colon, spleen, and phrenocolic ligament. Although each subdiaphragmatic space is continuous over the convex liver surface, inflammatory adhesions may delimit an abscess in an anterior or posterior position. The falciform ligament separates the right and left subdiaphragmatic divisions.

The right subhepatic division of the subphrenic space is located between the undersurfaces of the liver and gallbladder superiorly and the right kidney and mesocolon inferiorly. The anterior bulge of the kidney partitions this space into an anterior(gallbladder fossa) and posterior(Morison's pouch) section.

The left subhepatic space also has an anterior and posterior part. The smaller anterior subhepatic space lies between the undersurface of the left lobe and the anterior surface of the stomach. Left subdiaphragmatic collections often extend into this anterior subhepatic area. The posterior subhepatic space is the lesser sac, which is situated behind the lesser omentum and stomach and lies anterior to the pancreas, duodenum, transverse mesocolon, and left kidney. It extends posteriorly to the attachment of the left triangular ligament to the hemidiaphragm. The lesser sac communicates with both the right subhepatic and right paracolic spaces through the narrow foramen of Winslow.

The infracolic compartment, below the transverse mesocolon, includes the pericolic and pelvic areas. The diagonally aligned root of the small bowel mesentery divides the midabdominal area between the fixed right and left colons into right and left infracolic spaces. Each lateral paracolic gutter and lower quadrant area communicates freely with the pelvic cavity. However, while right paracolic collections may track upward into the subhepatic and subdiaphragmatic space, the phrenocolic ligament hinders fluid migration along the left paracolic gutter into the left subdiaphragmatic area.

The most common abscess sites are in the lower quadrants, followed by the pelvic, subhepatic, and subdiaphragmatic spaces.

3.3　Clinical Manifestations

3.3.1　Symptoms and signs

An intra-abdominal abscess should be suspected in any patient with a predisposing condition. Fever, tachycardia and pain may be mild or absent, especially in patients receiving antibiotics. A deep seated or posteriorly situated abscess may exist in seemingly well individuals whose only symptom is persistent fever. Not infrequently, prolonged ileus sluggish recovery in a patient who has had recent abdominal surgery or peritoneal sepsis, rising leukocytosis, or nonspecific radiologic abnormality provides the initial clue. A mass is seldom felt except in patients with lower quadrant or pelvic lesions. In patients with subphrenic abscesses, irritation of contiguous structures may produce lower chest pain, dyspnea, referred shoulder pain or hiccup, or basilar atelectasis or effusion; in patients with pelvic abscesses, it may produce diarrhea or urinary urgency. The diagnosis is more difficult in postoperative, chronically ill, or diabetic patients and in those receiving immunosuppressive drugs, a group particularly susceptible to septic complications.

Sequential multiple organ failure principally respiratory, renal, or hepatic failure to stress gastrointestinal bleeding with disseminated intravascular coagulopathy is highly suggestive of intra abdominal infection.

3.3.2　Laboratory findings

Blood studies may suggest infection. A raised leukocyte count, abnormal liver or renal function test results, and abnormal arterial blood gases are nonspecific signs of infection. Persistently positive blood cultures point strongly to an intra abdominal infection is of specific value in diagnosing tubo ovarian abscess.

3.3.3　Imaging studies

3.3.3.1　X-ray studies

Plain X-ray may suggest an abscess in up 1/2 of cases. In subphrenic abscesses, the chest X-ray may show pleural effusion, a raised hemidiaphragm, basilar infiltrates, or atelectasis. Abnormalities on plain abdominal films include an ileus pattern. Soft tissue mass, air fluid levels, free or mottled gas pockets, effacement of properitoneal or psoas outlines. and displacement of viscera. Barium contrast studies interfere with and have been largely superseded by other imaging techniques. A water soluble upper gastrointestinal series may reveal soluble upper gastrointestinal series may reveal an unsuspected perforated viscus or outline perigastric and lesser sac abscesses.

3.3.3.2　Ultrasonography

Real time ultrasonography is sensitive(about 80% of cases) in diagnosing intra abdominal abscesses. The findings consist of a sonolucent area with well defined walls containing fluid or debris of variable density. Bowel gas, intervening viscera, skin incisions, and stomas interfere with ultrasound examinations, limiting their efficacy in postoperative patients. Nevertheless, the procedures readily available, portable, and inexpensive, and the findings are specific when correlated with the clinical picture. Ultrasonography is most useful when an abscess is clinically suspected, especially for lesions in the right upper quadrant and the paracolic and pelvic areas.

3.3.3.3　CT scan

CT scan of the abdomen, the best diagnostic study, is highly sensitive(over 95% of cases). Neither gas shadows nor exposed wounds interfere with CT scanning in postoperative patients, and the procedure is reliable even in areas poorly seen on ultrasonography. Abscesses appear as cystic collections with density measurements of between 0 and 15 attenuation units. Resolution is increased by contrast media(e. g. , sodium diatrizoate) injected intravenously or instilled into hollow viscera adjacent to the abscess. One drawback of CT scan is that diagnosis may be difficult in areas with multiple thick walled bowel loops or if a pleural effusion overlies a subphrenic abscess, so that occasionally a very large abscess is missed. CT or ultrasonography guided needle aspiration can distinguish between sterile and infected collections in uncertain cases.

3.3.3.4　Radionuclide scan

Radionuclide scan has a secondary but complementary role. Combined liver lung scans to delineate subphrenic pockets have been replaced by ultrasonography or CT scan. If peritoneal sepsis is clinically questionable or if the site of an abscess is uncertain, scanning with gallium 67 citrate of indium 111 labeled autologous leukocytes may sometimes disclose an abscess or another unexpected extra abdominal site of infection. These radionuclide studies are sensitive(over 80% of cases), but many false of positive errors occur as a result of nonpyogenic inflammatory conditions, bowel accumulation of labeled leukocytes, or surgical drains and other foreign bodies in postoperative patients. Leukopenia in debilitated patients can undermine the reliability of indium 111 studies. Unfortunately, leukocyte scans may not be helpful in cases where CT scans are equivocal and this fact coupled with the time consuming process has limited their clinical usefulness.

3.3.3.5　Magnetic resonance imaging

The currently long scanning time and upper respiratory motion have limited usefulness of MRI in the investigation of upper abdominal abscesses.

3.3.4　Treatment

Treatment consists of prompt and complete drainage of the abscess, control of the primary cause, and adjunctive use of effective antibiotics. Depending upon the abscess site and the condition of the patient, drainage may be achieved by operative or nonoperative methods. Percutaneous drainage is the preferred method for single, well localized, superficial bacterial abscesses that do not have fistulous communications or contain solid debris. Following CT scan or ultrasonographic delineation, a needle is guided into the abscess cavity; infected material is aspirated for culture; and a sump catheter is inserted.

Postoperative irrigation helps to remove debris and ensure catheter patency. This technique is not appropriate for multiple or deep(especially pancreatic)abscesses or for patients with ongoing contamination, fungal infections. Or thick purulent or necrotic material. Percutaneous drainage can be performed in about 75% of cases. The success rate exceeds 80% in simple abscesses but is only 25% in more complex ones; it is heavily influenced by the training and experience of the radiologist performing the drainage. Complications include septicemia, fistula formation, bleeding, and peritoneal contamination.

Open drainage is reserved for abscesses for which percutaneous drainage is inappropriate or unsuccessful. The direct extraserous route has the advantage of establishing dependent drainage without contaminating the rest of the peritoneal cavity. Only light general anesthesia or even local anesthesia is necessary, and surgical trauma is minimized. Right anterior subphrenic abscess can be drained by a subcostal incision(Clairmont incision). Posterior subdiaphragmatic and subhepatic lesions can be decompressed posteriorly through the bed of the resected twelfth rib(Nather–Ochsner incision), or by a lateral extraserous method(DeCosse incision). Most lower quadrant and flank abscesses can be drained through a lateral extraperitoneal approach. Pelvic abscesses can often be detected on pelvic or rectal examination as a fluctuant mass distorting the contour of the vagina or rectum. If needle aspiration directly through the vaginal or rectal wall returns pus, the abscess is best drained by making an incision in that area. In all cases, digital or direct exploration must ensure that all loculations are broken down. Penrose and sump drains are used to allow continued drainage postoperatively until the infection has resolved. Serial sonograms or imaging studies help document obliteration of the abscess cavity.

Transperitoneal exploration is indicated if the abscess can not be localized preoperatively, if there are several or deep lying lesions, if an enterocutaneous fistula or bowel obstruction exists, or if previous drainage attempts have been unsuccessful. This is especially likely in postoperative patients with multiple abscesses and persistent peritoneal soiling. The need to achieve complete drainage fully justifies the greater stress of laparotomy and the small possibility that infection might be spread to other uninvolved areas.

Satisfactory drainage is usually evident by improving clinical findings within 3 days of treatment. Failure to improve indicates inadequate drainage, another source of sepsis, or organ dysfunction. Additional localizing studies and repeated percutaneous or operative drainage should be undertaken urgently.

3.3.5　Prognosis

The mortality rate of serious intra abdominal abscesses is about 30%. Deaths are related to the severity of the underlying causes, delay in diagnosis, multiple organ failure, and incomplete drainage. Right lower quadrant and pelvic abscesses are usually caused by perforated ulcers and appendicitis in younger individuals. They are readily diagnosed and treated, and the mortality rates is less than 5%. Diagnosis is often delayed in older patients; this increases the likelihood of multiple organ failure. Decompensation of two major organ systems is associated with a mortality rate of over 50%. Shock is an especially ominous sign. Subphrenic, deep, and multiple abscesses frequently require operative drainage and are associated with a morality rate of over 40%. An untreated residual abscess is nearly always fatal.

Part 26

Abdominal Trauma

Because of the location and size, the abdomen is a common segment to be injured by any type of trauma. 10% of all traumatic deaths are the direct outcome of abdominal trauma, the recognition and treatment of life-threatening abdominal trauma remains a challenging task. As a surgical issue all over the world, the principles of abdominal trauma should guide all of the general surgeons to grasp the initial surgical treatment.

Chapter 1

Blunt Abdominal Trauma

1.1 Essentials

Blunt abdominal trauma is one of the commonest causes of morbidity and mortality in modern era. Usually, fall from height, traffic accidents and assaults are the frequent modes of blunt abdominal trauma. Prevalence of intra-abdominal injuries varied, efficient and rapid diagnosis was essential. Appropriate treatment was critical to ensure the survival to decrease morbidity and mortality.

The details obtained from paramedics or witnesses present at the scene of accidents are vital. Understanding of the injury mechanism is the basis of diagnostic evaluation. The medical history and any allergies should be obtained whenever possible.

1.2 Signs and Symptoms

The initial clinical assessment of patients with blunt abdominal trauma is usually complicated and notably inaccurate. The most reliable signs and symptoms are as follows: ①Pain. ②Tenderness. ③Gastrointestinal hemorrhage. ④Hypovolemia. ⑤Evidence of peritoneal irritation.

Without any significant changes in physical examination, large amounts of blood can accumulate in the peritoneal and pelvic cavities.

The following signs of physical examination would predict the potential for intra-abdominal trauma:

(1) Lap belt marks: related to small intestine rupture.

(2) Steering wheel-shaped contusions.

(3) Ecchymosis involving the flanks (Grey-Turner sign) or the umbilicus (Cullen sign): usually delayed for several hours to days.

(4) Abdominal distention.

(5) Auscultation of bowel sounds in the thorax: indicate diaphragmatic injury.

(6) Abdominal bruit: indicate underlying vascular disease or traumatic arteriovenous fistula.

(7) Local or generalized tenderness, guarding, rigidity, or rebound tenderness: peritoneal injury.

(8) Fullness and doughy consistency on palpation: indicate intra-abdominal hemorrhage.

(9) Crepitation or instability of the lower thoracic cage: indicates splenic or hepatic injuries.

1.3 Diagnosis Modalities

Diagnosis procedures should be performed after evaluation to assess abdominal injuries and determine feasibility of operative intervention.

Assessment of hemodynamic stability is the initial concern in the evaluation. Rapid evaluation for hemoperitoneum should be accomplished forthe hemodynamically unstable patient by means of diagnostic peritoneal lavage(DPL) or the focused assessment with sonography for trauma(FAST).

When the physical examination findings are inconclusive, radiographic studies of the abdomen should be adopted for the stable patients.

1.3.1 Diagnostic peritoneal lavage

Many trauma surgeons recommend DPL as the primary diagnostic technique after severe blunt abdominal trauma. The advantages of DPL are that DPL could be performed in the trauma bay and cheaper than CT.

DPL is indicated for the following patients in the setting of blunt abdominal trauma:

(1) Patients with a spinal cord injury.

(2) With multiple injuries and unexplained shock.

(3) Obtunded patients with a possible abdominal injury.

(4) Intoxicated patients in whom abdominal injury is suggested.

(5) Patients with potential intra-abdominal injury who will undergo prolonged anesthesia for another procedure.

DPL is indicated for unstable patients in whom CT scan could not be performed without delay, or for those who require emergent operative intervention for other associated trauma. DPL could be performed in the OR in order to evaluate the abdominal situation for the patients undergoing operation for an extra abdominal injury in whom an unexplained clinical deterioration occurs.

1.3.2 FAST

Bedside ultrasonography is a rapid, portable, noninvasive, and accurate examination that can be performed by emergency clinicians and trauma surgeons to detect hemoperitoneum.

The FAST protocol consists of four acoustic windows(pericardiac, perihepatic, perisplenic, pelvic) with the patient supine. An examination is interpreted as positive if free fluid is found in any of the four acoustic windows, negative if no fluid is seen, and indeterminate if any of the windows can not be adequately assessed.

1.3.3 Computed tomography

CT is the standard for detecting solid organ injuries. The advent of CT has revolutionized the care of abdominal trauma victims. CT scans provide excellent imaging of the pancreas, duodenum, and genitourinary system, allows the clinician to grade the severity of solid organ injury, identify intra abdominal fluid or air, and determine the necessity for operative intervention. Unlike DPL or FAST, CT can determine the source of hemorrhage. CT also provides information on injuries to extra abdominal sites such as the bony pelvis or mediastinum. Delayed CT is useful for accessing changes in clinical condition or for documenting healing after solid viscous injury. The inability to reliable detect hollow viscous injury is the major short coming of CT.

1.3.4   Magnetic resonance imaging

Magneticresonance imaging is another promising diagnostic tool. Owing to the acquisition time, limitations of prolonged scan and the inability to scan in the presence of ferromagnetic materials, MRI is not used to evaluate routinely. However, MRI could be a positive and valuable alternative as the technology matures.

1.3.5   Laparoscopy

As a diagnostic tool to evaluate the condition of trauma victims, the minimally invasive operation has been considered useful and popular. There are many clinical trials which have shown laparoscopy to be a good positive predictor of the need for operative intervention. As the techniques are refined and instrumentation improved, laparoscopy may acquire a more important diagnostic and therapeutic role.

1.4   Management

Treatment of blunt abdominal trauma begins at the scene of the injury and is continued upon the patient's arrival at the ED or trauma center. Management may involve nonoperative measures or operative treatment, as appropriate.

Indications for laparoscopy for patients with blunt abdominal injury include the following: ①Signs of peritonitis. ②Uncontrolled shock or hemorrhage. ③Clinical deterioration during observation. ④Hemoperitoneum findings on FAST or DPL.

Nonoperative management:

In blunt abdominal trauma, including severe solid organ injuries, selective nonoperative management has become the standard protocol. Nonoperative management strategies are based on CT scan diagnosis and the hemodynamic stability of the patient, as follows:

(1) For the most part, pediatric patients can be resuscitated and treated nonoperatively; some pediatric surgeons often transfuse up to 40 mL/kg of blood products in an effort to stabilize a pediatric patient.

(2) Hemodynamically stable adults with solid organ injuries, primarily those to the liver and spleen, may be candidates for nonoperative management.

(3) Splenic artery embolotherapy, although not standard of care, may be used for adult blunt splenic injury.

(4) Nonoperative management involves closely monitoring vital signs and frequently repeating the physical examination.

Chapter 2

Penetrating Abdominal Trauma

2.1　Surgical Treatment of Liver and Biliary Tree Trauma

2.1.1　Introduction

5% of patients suffering from trauma would face liver injury. The huge size and position under the right costal margin make the liver the most frequently injured abdominal organ. Severe liver and biliary tract injuries are still challenging trauma surgeons and lead to significant morbidity and death. Identifying those who require operative intervention, and the steps in managing liver and biliary tree injuries, is the focus of this chapter.

2.1.2　Anatomy

For the sake of planning appropriate management of injuries, it is essential to be up on hepatic and biliary anatomy. By the line of Cantlie, the liver is divided into the right and left lobes, extending from the gallbladder fossa to the left side of the inferior vena cava(IVC). The blood supply of liver is from the common hepatic artery and portal vein. The common hepatic artery branches into the gastroduodenal, right hepatic, and proper hepatic arteries. The portal vein is formed posterior to the head of the pancreas by the confluence of the superior mesenteric and splenic veins. The hepatic veins drain the liver. The right hepatic vein is formed by the superior, middle, and inferior vein branches from the right lobe. The middle hepatic vein primarily drains segments IV and V, joins the left hepatic vein just before entering the IVC. The right and left hepatic ducts join to form the common hepatic duct. The CBD is formed after receiving the cystic duct. The CBD crosses through the head of the pancreas and empties into the duodenum at the ampulla of Vater.

2.1.3　Principles of surgical treatment of liver injury

The approach to patients with abdominal trauma should focus on the patient's abdominal examination, vital signs, response to resuscitation, and imaging as indicated. Severe abdominal pain or tenderness, peritonitis, evisceration, or shock with a presumed abdominal injury warrant exploratory laparotomy(LAP). Following stab wounds, the presence of shock, evisceration, or peritonitis is a clear indication for LAP.

The initial objective of LAP is to determine whether there is exsanguinating hemorrhage and from where it emanates. Blood must be evacuated and the source identified. Primary culprits are solid organs, retroperitoneal vessels, and mesentery. The surgeon should be able to rapidly assess the liver for major lacerations, by inspecting it and palpating its surface. The approach to control of liver bleeding follows a stepwise progression. The first step in hepatic hemorrhage control is manual compression. This should be able to control the vast majority of liver bleeding. Restoration of blood volume and maintenance of tissue perfusion, correction of coagulopathy, and active warming of the patient are critical to avoid the "bloody vicious cycle" that can lead to early mortality.

Grade Ⅰ—Ⅱ lacerations(Table 26-2-1)may stop bleeding spontaneously or after a short period of packing.

Table 26-2-1 Grading of liver injuries

Grade	Types of injury	Details
Ⅰ	Hematoma	Subcapsular,<10% surface area
	Laceration	<1 cm parenchymal depth
Ⅱ	Hematoma	Subcapsular,10%-50% surface area;intraparenchymal,<10 cm diameter
	Laceration	1-3 cm parenchymal depth,<10 cm length
Ⅲ	Hematoma	Subcapsular,>50% surface area or expanding;intraparenchymal,>10 cm diameter or expanding,or ruptured
	Laceration	>3 cm parenchymal depth
	Laceration	Parenchymal disruption involving >75% of hepatic lobe or 1-3 Couinaud's segments in a single lobe
V	Laceration	Parenchymal disruption involving >75% of hepatic lobe or >3 Couinaud's segments in a single lobe
	Vascular	Juxtahepatic venous injuries
VI	Vascular	Hepatic avulsion

* Advance one grade for multiple injuries up to grade Ⅲ.

2.1.4 Principles of surgical treatment of hepatic vascular injury

Hepatic artery injuries and portal venous injuries should be repaired whenever possible. Right or left hepatic artery ligation may be necessary to control arterial hemorrhage. However, ligation of the proper hepatic artery may result in hepatic necrosis or bile duct necrosis or nonhealing of injured ducts. Portal venous ligation will generally result in liver necrosis and will obligate liver resection.

2.1.5 Principles of surgical treatment of biliary tree injury

Isolated bile duct injuries are rare, and injuries to the portal vein or hepatic artery may be lethal or result on devitalized liver. Adequate exposure and identification of all injuries is critical. Gallbladder injuries should generally be managed by cholecystectomy. It may be tempting to perform simple suture cholecystorrhaphy, but this may be associated with delayed leak or cholecystitis due to cystic duct obstruction from hematoma.

Small lacerations or cystic duct avulsions can be repaired primarily with fine absorbable monofilament suture such as polydioxanone. Transection without tissue loss may be repaired primarily, but stricture rates are reported at over 50%. Transection with tissue loss or extensive injury should be treated with Roux-en-Y choledocho or hepaticojejunostomy. Stenting of the biliary anastomosis is debated, and there are no definitive data to provide guidance.

2.2 Surgical Treatment of Spleen Trauma

2.2.1 Introduction

In the past the traditional management of splenic injury was invariably splenectomy, over the last 20 years, the importance of splenic preservation has been emphasized for preventing overwhelming postsplenectomy infection(OPSI).

2.2.2 Anatomy

The spleen is placed on left hypochondrium covered by the lower edge of the left hemithorax and rib cage. Therefore, it can easily be damaged by impact from overlying fractured ribs. The spleen shows two surfaces: The diaphragmatic surface is smooth and convex, and the visceral surface is irregular and concave and has impressions. The visceral surface of the spleen contacts the following organs: anterior surface of the left kidney, left flexure of the colon, greater curvature and fundus of the stomach, and tail of the pancreas.

Three main splenic suspensory ligaments connect the spleen with the diaphragm, left kidney, and splenic flexure of the colon. These attachments are mainly avascular except for the last which may contain small sizeable vessels.

Splenic artery provides the main blood supply to the spleen and reaches the spleen's hilum by passing through the splenorenal ligament. The artery gives rise to a superior polar artery, from where the short gastric arteries begin. The splenic artery also gives rise to superior and inferior terminal branches that enter the splenic hilum. The splenic vein provides the main venous drainage of the spleen. It runs behind the pancreas before joining the superior mesenteric vein behind the neck of the pancreas to form the portal vein.

2.2.3 Splenic injury scale

The organ injury scale of the American Association for the Surgery of Trauma(AAST)criteria for splenic injury grading are classified as follows: grade I (hematoma, subcapsular, <10% of surface area; laceration, capsular tear <1 cm in depth into the parenchyma); grade II (hematoma, subcapsular, 10%–50% of surface area; laceration, capsular tear, 1–3 cm in depth, but not involving a trabecular vessel); grade III (hematoma, subcapsular, >50% of surface area OR expanding, ruptured subcapsular or parenchymal hematoma OR intraparenchymal hematoma >5 cm or expanding; laceration, >3 cm in depth or involving a trabecular vessel); grade IV (laceration involving segmental or hilar vessels with major devascularization, i. e. , >25% of spleen); grade V (hematoma, shattered spleen; laceration, hilar vascular injury which devascularizes spleen).

2.2.4 Nonoperative management(NOM)

Isolated splenic injuries can be considered as such if the splenic laceration is the only intra-abdominal injury in absence of major associated injuries that might significantly influence outcome. After resuscitation and completion of the trauma work-up, hemodynamically stable patients with grade Ⅰ, Ⅱ, or Ⅲ splenic injuries, who have no associated intra-abdominal injuries requiring surgical intervention and without comorbidities to preclude close observation, may be candidates for NOM.

The advantages of NOM include the avoidance of nontherapeutic laparotomies (with associated cost and morbidity), fewer intra-abdominal complications, and reduced transfusion risk. Angiography with embolization is a useful adjunct to NOM. Indications to AE include CT evidence of ongoing bleeding with contrast extravasation outside or within the spleen and a concomitant drop in hemoglobin, tachycardia, and hemoperitoneum, as well as formation of pseudoaneurysm.

Indications for urgent open surgical intervention after a trial of NOM include the following:

(1) Hemodynamic instability.

(2) Evidence of continued splenic hemorrhage.

(3) Replacement of more than 50% of the patient's blood volume or need for more than 4 units of blood transfusions.

(4) Associated intra-abdominal injury requiring surgery.

Degree of hemoperitoneum itself is not an absolute contraindication to NOM. The response to fluid resuscitation should lead further treatment decision. Surgery is also indicated in the absence of major bleeding from concomitant injuries and when CT reveals splenic vascular contrast blush not amenable to angioembolization. The decision to perform splenectomy needs to be taken early in order to preempt the establishment of coagulation disorders that would be difficult to reverse.

2.2.5   Principles of surgery of spleen trauma

Splenectomy is preferably performed via a posterior approach in trauma setting. After generous packing of the abdominal quadrants and bleeding control with hilum compression, the spleen is safely and rapidly mobilized from the lateral peritoneal attachments, starting from the splenophrenic and splenorenal ligaments. This can be accomplished starting with sharp incision of the lateral attachments (with electrocautery or Metzenbaum scissors) and then continued and completed in a more easy and safe way by blunt dissection. The splenic artery and vein should be individually identified and dissected and then ligated separately with nonabsorbable sutures, keeping as close as possible to the spleen and far from the tail of the pancreas. After splenectomy, hemostasis is carefully checked in a systematic fashion by inspecting the left subphrenic area, the greater curvature of the stomach, and the short gastric vessel area, as well as the splenic hilum.

In selected cases, a minimally invasive approach can be considered, keeping in mind the limitations of laparoscopic exploration of intra-abdominal organs for blunt and penetrating abdominal trauma. The best indication for laparoscopy is for a diagnostic purpose in case of a penetrating stab wound in the left upper quadrant with suspicion of diaphragmatic tear.

2.3   Surgical Treatment of Duodenal Trauma

2.3.1   Introduction

Due to the combination of insidious and subtle onset with difficulties in diagnosis, duodenal injury remains to be a lethal injury with associated mortality up to 25%. The surgical treatment are relatively simple if the injury is promptly confirmed. Nevertheless, delayed recognition frequently occurs and is commonly associated with poor outcomes.

2.3.2　Classification

The classification system developed by the AAST is the most widely used grading system for duodenal injuries(Table 26-2-2).

Table 26-2-2　AAST grading of duodenal injury severity

Grade	Types of injury	Details
I	Hematoma	Single hematoma
	Laceration	Partial thickness
II	Hematoma	Distributed in more than one portion
	Laceration	<50% circumference
III	Lacerations	50%-75% D2
		50%-100% D1,D3,D4
IV		>75% D2
		Involves ampulla or distal CBD
V		Major disruption of duodeno-pancreatic complex,devascularization

Advance one grade for multiple injuries up to grade III. D1:first position of duodenum. D2:second portion of duodenum. D3:third portion of duodenum. D4:fourth portion of duodenum. Grade I is either intramural hematoma or partial thickness laceration. In grade II, hematomas are multiple or the laceration is full thickness but small. Grade III is a laceration that extends over 50% of the circumference. In grade IV, the laceration involves the ampulla of Vater, distal common bile duct, or extensive areas of D2. Grade V involves disruption of the whole duodeno-pancreatic complex.

2.3.3　Diagnosis

In blunt injury, patients with highly suggestive mechanisms need to be carefully considered for duodenal injury. Physical findings such as tissue contusion in the upper abdomen, lower rib fractures, or disproportionally severe epigastric pain may arouse suspicion of duodenal injury. There is no diagnostic value for blood tests(including lipase and liver function tests)in predicting duodenal injury.

Penetrating duodenal injury can be diagnosed during explorative laparotomy. Initially, hemostasis should be prioritized. When duodenal injuries are suspected based on intraoperative findings, such as hepatic flexure, stomach or liver injuries, or local signs such as bruised duodenum, saponification, or bile leak, full kocherization is performed to assess the integrity of the duodenum.

2.3.4　Nonoperative management

NOM of patients with blunt abdominal trauma and normal hemodynamics is usually successful but poses a risk of missing duodenal injuries. Usually, NOM relies on CT to exclude hollow viscus injuries. Unexplained peritoneal free fluid in CT is often described as an indicator for small bowel and duodenal injury. Nevertheless, it has not proved to be a reliable sign. Considering the poor sensitivity of CT for hollow viscus injuries, the elusive characteristic of this injury, and the deleterious consequences of delayed diagnosis, it should be emphasized that the diagnosis of duodenal injury should be based on the combination of mechanisms, clinical findings, and radiological findings. Careful inspection and interpretation by experienced radiologists and surgeons are required to detect initial duodenal injury.

Considering a lack of specific tests for excluding duodenal injuries, a diagnostic explorative laparotomy is still often required. It should be emphasized that a negative laparotomy carries minimal complication especially when compared to a delayed diagnosis of duodenal injury.

2.3.5   Principles of surgery of duodenal trauma

The key steps to successful treatment of duodenal injuries do not differ from those of the typical trauma laparotomy: identification and control of all bleeding, contamination control, and anatomical repair. These may happen as a single procedure (for isolated and limited duodenal injuries), or due to the presence of other serious injuries and physiologic derangement of the patient, the procedure may need to be truncated after bleeding and contamination control (according to the principle of damage control surgery).

The Kocher maneuver is required for duodenum exploration, it is performed at any time when injury is suspected. If an injury is detected or better visualization is required, the Kocher maneuver is extended to a complete right medial visceral rotation. This is simply achieved by dividing the peritoneum just lateral to the ascending colon in the paracolic gutter and bluntly mobilizing the colon from ileocecal valve up to hepatic flexure. The kidney is better left alone in Gerota's fascia, but if the excreting system needs to be explored, the kidney should be medialized as well.

Once hemostasis is achieved, careful evaluation of physiology, including patient temperature, lactate, and resuscitation requirements, and the severity of other injuries should be considered. In damage control settings, small bowel and colon injuries are quickly repaired or simply stapled, while the duodenum is better to be primarily repaired. If repair requires complex surgical techniques consuming time, the defect is left alone and the area needs to be drained. Further restoration of the anatomy can be performed later. It is of note that the inspection of pancreas has to be performed simultaneously as this determines definitive surgical plans.

2.4   Surgical Treatment of Pancreatic Trauma

2.4.1   Introduction

The incidence of pancreatic injuries is 1% -2% , and the detection can be difficult both preoperatively and during explorative laparotomy. The protected location in the retroperitoneum can give subtle symptoms and signs in isolated injuries leading to delayed diagnosis and management. Because the pancreas is a fixed organ in the retroperitoneum in front of a rigid vertebral column, it is prone to crush injuries following blunt trauma.

2.4.2   Classification

The American Association for the Surgery of Trauma has published the most commonly used scales for pancreatic trauma. The injuries are graded from I to V with increasing severity (Table 26-2-3).

Table 26-2-3   The American Association for the Surgery of Trauma organ injury scale for pancreas

Grade	Injury	Description
I	Hematoma	Minor contusion without duct injury
	Laceration	Superficial laceration without duct injury
II	Hematoma	Major contusion without duct injury or tissue loss
	Laceration	Major laceration without duct injury or tissue loss
III	Lacerations	Distal transection or parenchymal injury with duct injury
IV	Lacerations	Proximal transection or parenchymal injury involving ampulla
V	Lacerations	Massive disruption of pancreatic head

* Advance one grade for multiple injuries up to grade III. Proximal pancreas is to the patients' right of the superior mesenteric vein.

2.4.3 Nonoperative management

In the absence of associated injuries requiring surgical repair, pancreatic contusions and minor lacerations(grades I and II)can be treated nonoperatively. Occasionally, a minor leak or a side fistula of the pancreatic duct can be managed with an endoscopically placed stent.

2.4.4 Principles of surgery of pancreatic trauma

The key for the surgical management of pancreatic trauma is exposing the whole pancreas and assessing the state of the main pancreatic duct. Visualization of the entire pancreas can be started by transecting the-gastrocolic ligament to allow inspection of the anterior surface and inferior border of the pancrea. The Kocher maneuver mobilizing the second part of the duodenum and the pancreatic head allows the examination of the head. Additional exposure of the superior border of the head and body of the pancreas can be achieved by transection of the gastrohepatic ligament. To complete the exposure, lateral mobilization of the spleen, splenic flexure of the colon, and the dissection of the retroperitoneal attachments of the inferior border of the pancreas allow the visualization and bimanual palpation of the posterior surface of the tail and body of the gland.

The next step is the determination whether the main pancreatic duct is intact. Attempts at verifying the ductal injury with radiological means(intraoperative cannulation of the papilla through duodenotomy, intraoperative ERCP)or injecting dye are often cumbersome and unreliable. Injuries with intact main pancreatic duct(grade I – II)could be managed with peripancreatic drainage only. Injuries with ductal disruption at or to the left of the superior mesenteric vein(grade III)should be managed with distal pancreatectomy, unless the patient has severe physiological derangement. Injuries involving the main pancreatic duct at the head of the pancrea(grade IV)are challenging injuries, usually the best option is to ensure adequate peripancreatic drainage with one or two well-placed drains. In all cases, placement of peripancreatic drains should accompany any kind of pancreatic resection.

2.5 Surgical Treatment of Gastric Trauma

2.5.1 Introduction

Most of the gastric trauma(98%)are penetrating trauma, and only 2% are blunt trauma. Road traffic accidents are the most common cause of gastric rupture from blunt trauma. Other causes are falls, direct violence, cardiopulmonary resuscitation, and seat-belt injuries. Spontaneous rupture may also occur in adults after an excessive consumption of food and liquids.

2.5.2   Classification and treatment

According to the organ injury scale, gastric injuries can manifest as contusion, intramural hematoma, superficial laceration, perforation, or devascularization (Table 26-2-4).

Table 26-2-4   Grade of gastric injury and treatment

Grade *	Description of injury
I	Contusion/hematoma
	Partial thickness laceration
II	Laceration <2 cm in GE junction or pylorus
	<5 cm in proximal 1/3 stomach
	<10 cm in distal 2/3 stomach
III	Laceration >2 cm in GE junction or pylorus
	>5 cm in proximal 1/3 stomach
	>10 cm in distal 2/3 stomach
IV	Tissue loss or devascularization <2/3 stomach
V	Tissue loss or devascularization >2/3 stomach

* Advance one grade for multiple lesions up to grade III. GE: gastroesophageal.

2.5.3   Principles of surgery of gastric trauma

The operative management begins with a rapid and direct access to the entire peritoneal cavity through a midline incision. Because gastric injuries are rarely life threatening, we should follow the management of other intra-abdominal injuries that takes precedence, such as control of hemorrhage which is the first priority. After control of hemorrhage, the second issue is represented by the control of the contamination. The entire stomach should be examined carefully. Taking down of the triangular ligament of the liver and the gastrohepatic ligament or the gastrocolic omentum is necessary for particular types of gastric injuries.

In most cases, repair of the stomach with two-layer inverting closure is the treatment of choice for either blunt or penetrating injury, also to prevent bleeding from the suture line. If the injury occurs in the area of the gastroesophageal junction and it is not directly suturable, it may be necessary to perform a total gastrectomy. In case of lesions of the pylorus, in order to prevent narrow and avoid excessive pressure to the sutured line, a pyloroplasty may be considered.

At the end of the procedure, the air test is useful for assessing the integrity of the repair and searching for any untreated perforation.

2.6　Surgical Treatment of Traumatic Small Bowel and Mesentery Injuries

2.6.1　Introduction

The small bowel is the most frequently involved hollow viscus in abdominal trauma. Injuries occur more often after penetrating than blunt trauma. In the presence of free peritoneal fluid or air at radiology, an injury of the intestine must be excluded. Clinical examination and laboratory and radiological findings are useful for prompt diagnosis, but traumatic small bowel injuries remain a diagnostic challenge.

Small bowel injuries occur in 15% –26% of patients sustaining blunt or penetrating abdominal trauma, respectively. Traumatic small bowel and mesentery injuries(SBMI) can be caused by road accidents, sport accidents, falls from height, aggressions, explosions, and all causes of sudden increase of abdominal pressure. The identification of an isolated traumatic SBMI is often a challenge because of its feeble and nonspecific clinical findings, leading to an insidious delay in diagnosis and treatment, especially for blunt trauma. Laboratory tests are of little interest for identification of SBMI. DPL is the procedure of choice in detecting bowel perforations. Helical CT evaluation of the abdomen is routinely performed in all victims of abdominal trauma who are not immediately diverted to surgery. The use of abdominal CT scan has resulted in an increase in nonoperative management of solid organ injury. Concomitant simultaneous reduction of use of DPL has lessened the number of exploratory laparotomies in blunt trauma, resulting in a greater risk of delay in diagnosis of bowel perforation.

2.6.2　Classification

According to the organ injury scale, small bowel and mesentery injuries can manifest as follows (Table 26–2–5).

Table 26–2–5　Small bowel injury scale from AAST

Grade	Injury	Description
I	Hematoma	Contusion or hematoma without 2 devascularization
	Laceration	Partial thickness, no perforation
II	Laceration	Laceration <50% of circumference
III	Laceration	Laceration >50% of circumference 3 without transection
IV	Laceration	Transection of the small bowel
V	Laceration	Transection of the small bowel with segmental tissue loss
	Vascular	Devascularized segment

* Advance one grade for multiple injuries up to grade III.

2.6.3　Principles of surgery of SBMI

Timing to surgery for isolated SBMI depends on hemodynamic status of trauma victims and accuracy of diagnosis. Perforation mandates a segmental resection. Also in case of full-thickness wall injury, even without perforation, resection should be considered. Hemostasis of mesenteric hemorrhage could be enough, but sometimes, sequential ischemia of tributary tract of small bowel can force the surgeon to perform resection.

Accordingly with AAST classification of small bowel trauma, grades I and II injuries can be treated by direct reparation, while grade III resection and anastomosis must be performed if there is a vascular involvement or if reparative suture risks stenosis of intestine. In grades IV and V injuries, resection and anastomosis are mandatory.

2.7　Surgical Treatment of Colon and Rectal Trauma

2.7.1　Introduction

The management of traumatic colonic and rectal injuries is an interesting study in the evolution of trauma care in general. There are different considerations to take in to account in the management of the patient with colorectal trauma. Different considerations between blunt and penetrating injuries are important.

For hemodynamically stable patients, CT scan is used most commonly after blunt trauma. CT has the advantage over DPL as having the ability to evaluate the retroperitoneum. CT scan is also of use in patients who sustain penetrating injury to the flank to evaluate for injuries to the ascending or descending colon.

2.7.2　Classification

Colonic injuries can be described as destructive or nondestructive. Numerous classification schemes exist, and historically, the classification of injuries into these groups was important for management. Lately, however, the classification or "grading" of such injuries is less important for definitive management, but this information can be useful in the collection and analysis of data for research purposes.

2.7.3　Principles of surgery of colon and rectal trauma

Priorities in the operating room include rapid control of hemorrhage and contamination. In patients with intraperitoneal colonic or rectal injuries, the affected segment of colon should be fully mobilized by incision of the peritoneal attachments of the ascending, descending, or sigmoid portions of the colon. During the mobilization, care must be taken to visualize and preserve the ureter. The bowel must be "run" in its entirety from the ligament of Treitz to the peritoneal reflection of the proximal rectum.

An assessment of the mesentery and degree of colonic injury must be made before definitive management is undertaken. All suspicious hematomas, staining, and bruising on the colonic wall should be interrogated, as they may mask an underlying injury. Colonic injuries can be addressed with primary suture repair or with diverting ostomy. Primary repair avoids the morbidity associated with colostomy, as well as the attendant risk of the subsequent takedown operation. If the blood supply to a segment of colon is in doubt, the surgeon can perform a segmental resection. The resection does not need to include the associated mesentery, but care must be taken to ensure that the anastomosis, once created, will have an adequate blood supply.

If the diagnosis of an extraperitoneal rectal injury is made using proctoscopy, a fecal diversion can be employed as a rapid and safe manner of controlling contamination and potential pelvic soft tissue infection. The extraperitoneal rectal injury does not need to be explored and repaired and diversion is enough.

2.8　Surgical Treatment of Major Vascular Trauma

2.8.1　Introduction

Retroperitoneal vascular trauma usually presents as a retroperitoneal hematoma(RPH). The management of RPH differs based on its location, mechanism of injury, and the patient's physiological parameters, as these all imply different potentials for vascular injury. A simple and pragmatic classification is that described by Selivanov in 1982 which uses three zones of injury, central(injuries to aorta and caval vein and their main branches as well as duodenum and pancreas, zone Ⅰ), lateral(injuries to kidney and bowel vessels, zone Ⅱ), and pelvic(injuries to pelvis and iliac arteries and veins, zone Ⅲ), and this is the most commonly used in practice. This classification is valuable in facilitating decision making with regard to the management approach(Figure 26-2-1).

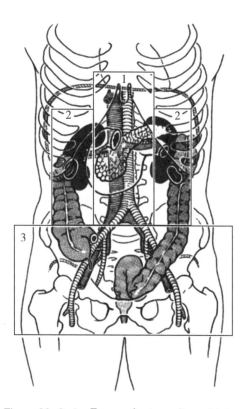

Figure 26-2-1　**Zones of retroperitoneal injury**

1 zone Ⅰ, central(injuries to aorta and caval vein and their main branches as well as duodenum and pancreas), 2 zone Ⅱ, lateral(injuries to kidney and bowel vessels), 3 zone Ⅲ, pelvic(injuries to pelvis and iliac arteries and veins).

Midline supramesocolic and inframesocolic injuries in blunt or penetrating trauma should be surgically explored as they imply an injury to the aorta, vena cava, or their major branches.

Most perirenal hematomas after blunt injuries can be managed nonoperatively, whereas perirenal hematomas after penetrating trauma should generally be explored. The exception is if the penetrating injury is minor on careful evaluation via CT. This is usually managed by observations or percutaneous drainage of the